The Mothers' and Fathers' Medical Encyclopedia

Also by Virginia E. Pomeranz, M.D.
and Dodi Schultz

The First Five Years: A Relaxed Approach to Child Care

Virginia E. Pomeranz, M.D.
and Dodi Schultz

Illustrations by Marika

The Mothers' and Fathers' Medical Encyclopedia

Little, Brown and Company
Boston Toronto

REVISED EDITION

THE FIRST EDITION OF THIS BOOK WAS PUBLISHED IN 1972
IN PAPERBACK BY NEW AMERICAN LIBRARY UNDER THE TITLE
THE MOTHERS' MEDICAL ENCYCLOPEDIA.

Library of Congress Cataloging in Publication Data

Pomeranz, Virginia E.
The mothers' and fathers' medical encyclopedia.

"The first edition of this book was published in 1972 . . . under the title The mothers' medical encyclopedia."
Bibliography: p.
1. Children — Diseases — Dictionaries. 2. Children — Care and hygiene — Dictionaries. I. Schultz, Dodi, joint author. II. Title. [DNLM: 1. Child care — Encyclopedia — Popular works. WS13 P785m]
RJ61.P68 1977 618.9'2'0003 76-48167
ISBN 0-316-71320-1

Published simultaneously in Canada
by Little, Brown & Company (Canada) Limited

PRINTED IN THE UNITED STATES OF AMERICA

To Mel and Ed, with love
and gratitude for their
faith, their encouragement,
and above all, their
enduring patience
and
to Dr. Louis Finger,
a distinguished physician and
a perceptive catalyst

Preface

Much has changed, both in the world of medicine and in our own thinking, since the writing and publication of the first edition of this book. The new title itself reflects a major and, we feel, delightful change: not only mothers, but fathers are increasingly very much involved in their children's care, in sickness and in health. This trend, we think, represents not so much "women's" liberation as *people's* liberation, a recognition that just as a woman is capable of programming a computer or driving a truck, a man is fully capable of changing a diaper, taking a temperature, or administering an antibiotic.

While the format of this new edition is much like that of the earlier one, there have been many additions and revisions. The heart of the book remains the encyclopedic listing, designed to function as a multifaceted guide: as a dictionary, defining and explaining medical terms you may hear and read about; as a first-aid manual, offering explicit instructions for coping with injuries and other emergencies major and minor; as a source of up-to-date information about all aspects of your child's health — including growth and development, preventive care, and ills both common and uncommon — from cradle through college.

There are many new entries; much material has been wholly rewritten and some has been dropped. Several antibiotics, for example, have become obsolete, while quite a few new ones have been introduced. Patterns of drug use and abuse — a topic with which parents of teenagers must, unfortunately, be familiar — have shifted, as have attitudes and legal postures on sexual activities in this age group. Tremendous strides have been made (and continue to be made) in many areas of medical research, including the development of new vaccines, heartening advances in the diagnosis and treatment of congenital disorders, and vast improvements in cancer detection and therapy. Communicable ills have assumed new worldwide patterns — some much closer to being conquered, others posing increasing problems.

The entry on poisoning — still a major threat in toddlers and preschoolers — has been handled, in this new edition, in a way we hope will prove even more useful in those crucial situations when a young life is at stake. Potentially toxic household substances have been assembled in one list rather than being scattered throughout the text. This greatly expanded list — larger, we believe, than any other published — has been included under the "Poisoning, Household Substances and Medications" entry; as an aid to fast action, emergency procedures have been repeated opposite each page of the list so that emergency-action advice is instantly available.

A vital-statistics section has again been included (Appendix E). It has been revised and updated to reflect current needs; we urge you to fill it out immediately. Additionally, four more appendices have been added: three — Appendices A, B, and C — we think will be helpful to all parents; the listing in Appendix D is, like a fire extinguisher, something every household should have and will, we hope, never need to use.

This book emphatically is not designed to substitute for the advice of your own doctor, your pediatrician or family physician, but to supplement that advice and, we hope, help you to put it to informed and intelligent use. The better you understand the various aspects of your child's health, the better the communication between physician and parent (or patient) and the more effective your physician's efforts will be.

Do bear in mind, too, that all the information in this book is necessarily of a general nature. An *average* figure — whether applying to height, weight, developmental milestones, or anything else — is just that, a statistical mean representing a mere point on the broad scale of normality. *Typical* symptoms of a particular illness or condition do not invariably occur. *Usual* or *recommended* procedures, whether therapeutic or preventive, may be judged inadvisable for an individual; if your physician's advice, based on familiarity with and examination of your youngster, conflicts with what you find here, your own doctor's judgment and guidance should be relied upon.

A number of specific products and trade names are mentioned from time to time. It should be understood that they are included for informational purposes; no endorsement or other opinion, unless specifically stated, is implied or should be inferred — and any stated opinions apply, of course, to the medications or other products as they exist at this writing.

Many people were helpful to us during the writing, and the lengthy and challenging task of revising, this book. We are grateful to them all. Our dedication singles out those to whom we are most deeply indebted. Special thanks are due to Marjorie LaRusso, R.N., whose practical experience as a pediatrics nurse and as the mother of five lively offspring provided valuable insights; to Drs. Sheldon Paul Blau, David A. Kahn, and Carl E. Pochedly, who kindly permitted us to call upon their expertise in their respective fields of rheumatology, child psychiatry, and pediatric hematology and oncology; to the American Pharmaceutical Association, the national professional pharmacists' society, for extensive information on the content of nonprescription drugs; to Little, Brown Editor in Chief Roger Donald and Executive Editors Mary Jane Walsh and Win Hodges, whose support and enthusiasm were of continuing aid and comfort; and, not least, to the hundreds of parents, grandparents, and other readers of *The Mothers' Medical Encyclopedia* whose questions, comments, and suggestions were instrumental in, and essential to, the conception and birth of *The Mothers' and Fathers' Medical Encyclopedia.*

V.E.P.
D.S.

New York City
August 1976

Contents

The Mothers' and Fathers' Medical Encyclopedia

A

Aarane: a trade name for cromolyn sodium; see ASTHMA.

abdomen: the area below the diaphragm (which is just under the ribs) — not, as is sometimes supposed, the part below the waistline; anywhere below the navel is, to a doctor, the *lower* abdomen. Within the abdomen are a great many major organs, including the stomach, liver, gallbladder, pancreas, appendix, intestines, kidneys and internal parts of the reproductive system; abdominal symptoms could signify trouble with any one of them.

Any pain in the abdomen is, of course, cause for some concern, though not necessarily alarm (see the next entry). Additionally, the doctor should be called promptly if you note any of these characteristics: swelling, bloating, rigidity, stiffness, tenderness; in an infant, the last may be evident from unusual yelping when a diaper is being fastened. "Bloating" is a somewhat relative term in a small baby; most infants normally appear a bit that way because their livers are proportionately larger, causing their little bellies to protrude, and it's a question of whether the protrusion is greater than usual.

abdominal pain: a not-to-be-ignored signal that something is wrong, and it should never be dismissed as "only" a bellyache or "just" indigestion; if something's gone wrong with a youngster's digestion, there's a reason for it. There may or may not be cause for alarm, depending partly upon the age of the child — but in any case, prompt action on your part is indicated.

Generally speaking, a serious condition may be signaled by either (a) mild but persistent pain or (b) sudden and severe pain that is not continuous but comes and goes at intervals. In either case — or even in the case of intermittent mild pain — the child should be given nothing by mouth; food, drink, a laxative or other medication, even water could make the situation worse. Unless you have discovered that your youngster has gulped down something he shouldn't have (in which case, turn to POISONING, HOUSEHOLD SUBSTANCES AND MEDICATIONS and follow the first-aid procedures outlined there), simply telephone your doctor and describe the situation, including the exact site of the pain (have the child point to it if he's old enough), the child's temperature, and any accompanying symptoms such as nausea, vomiting, or diarrhea; follow whatever instructions the doctor may give you.

In an infant, particularly under the age of one year, severe abdominal pain — especially if there is vomiting, abdominal swelling, and/or mucus-containing or bloody diarrhea — may mean a critical condition that demands emergency medical attention. (Severe abdominal pain in a small baby is usually evidenced by loud crying and by the child's either drawing his knees up or stretching his legs out stiffly.) If you cannot reach your own doctor immediately, take the baby to the nearest hospital emergency room without delay, enlisting the aid of the police if necessary.

In a young school-age child, notably between the ages of five and ten, quite the opposite situation may occur: a *non*serious Monday-through-Friday condition known to pediatricians as the "five-days-a-week bellyache." The cause is simple emotional tension, connected usually with schoolwork, and it often occurs in youngsters who are brighter than average. "My stomach hurts" is the typical complaint, and — importantly — there are *no* other symptoms: no fever, no nausea or vomiting, no loss of appetite, no diarrhea or constipation. The "hurt" is mild; it recurs each day — then vanishes during the weekend, only to appear again on Monday morning. This condition is best ignored, *once it has been diagnosed;* that initial diagnosis must be done by your doctor, not simply assumed by you.

Also see, for a discussion of typical symptoms: APPENDICITIS; COLIC; FOOD POISONING; GALLBLADDER; INTESTINAL FLU; INTESTINAL OBSTRUCTION; INTUSSUSCEPTION; MECKEL'S DIVERTICULITIS; PANCREATITIS; PEPTIC ULCER.

A-B-O incompatibility: See BLOOD GROUPS.

abortion: We refer, here, to *deliberate* abortion, which is what most people mean when they use the term. (Medically, it means *any* sudden termination of pregnancy prior to that point at which the offspring could survive independent of the mother, and what is popularly known as "miscarriage" is technically termed *spontaneous* abortion.) We don't feel it's our province to comment on moral ramifications, which will continue to be argued in the foreseeable future. We do agree with most family physicians that the termination of an accidental, unwanted pregnancy in a teenage girl — assuming that's what *she* desires — is preferable to forcing upon her the potentially traumatic alternatives of a "shotgun" marriage, single parenthood, or bearing and then giving up the child. At this writing, the permissibility of abortion has been legally established nationally, although state statutes may differ in details such as when, where, how, and by whom abortions may be performed, and whether or not minors must have parental consent. In our view, an abortion, to insure the highest degree of safety, should be performed by a qualified Doctor of Medicine.

There are presently several methods of performing an abortion, depending in part upon the duration of pregnancy.

Within the first twelve weeks of pregnancy, abortion can be effected via minor surgery performed through the vagina, a procedure called dilation and curettage, or "D and C," for short; the cervix is dilated, and the contents of the uterus removed by this route. Performed by a skilled physician within the proper period, the operation is quite safe, leaves no scars, and does not affect ability to bear children in the future. If this type of operation is attempted later in pregnancy, however, there is a high risk of infection, sterility, and other potentially critical complications. After the three-month period, abortion must be performed in some other manner. (Another early-in-pregnancy method, it should be noted, is less widely used and is considered less effective: the suction or "vacuum" method that removes the contents of the uterus by aspiration; the removal is incomplete in a significant number of cases, necessitating secondary procedures.)

One way to perform later abortion is via abdominal incision — which, like appendix removal or any other abdominal operation, is major surgery. The risks are neither greater nor smaller than those attendant upon any abdominal surgery; future births, however, may then require cesarean section. Other methods have thus been sought in order to avoid that outcome. Some have been more or less successful than others. They have all generally centered upon inducing the uterus to expel its contents via the vagina, rather than invading the uterus and forcibly removing the material.

One such, the so-called "supercoil" procedure, has proved disappointing despite early hopes. Based on the theory that the introduction of foreign matter would cause expulsion, this procedure involved the use of a mechanical device, a plastic coil — or several of them — that caused the uterus to go into contraction within 24 hours. Unfortunately, the system caused complications in a majority of cases, and a significant number of those were quite serious; they included infection, considerable blood loss and, in some cases, perforation of the uterus requiring subsequent hysterectomy.

Two methods are now favored for safety and effectiveness.

The "method of choice" — which has been in use for a number of years and has proved to have a dependably low rate of complications — is saline induction, sometimes called "salting out." In this method, fluid is removed (via a needle into the abdomen) from the amniotic sac surrounding the fetus, and is replaced by a saline solution. Uterine contractions, followed by expulsion of the uterine contents, generally occur within 48 hours.

The second, more recently introduced, is the injection of one of two drugs, PGE_2 or PGF_2-alpha (see PROSTAGLANDINS for more about this promising group of substances), with results similar to — but often a bit faster than — those obtained in saline induction. Results have not been wholly consistent, however; while dangerous complications have not usually occurred, there have sometimes been unexpected and extremely uncomfortable side effects. Further, there has been disagreement — and research continues — on which of the two drugs is preferable, how optimum dosages are to be calculated, and by what route (directly into the uterus, vaginally, or intramuscularly) the drug is best injected. Chemical variations of these prostaglandins are also under investigation.

abrasions: See SCRAPES AND

SCRATCHES. For abrasions of the *eye,* see EYE INJURIES.

abscess: a pus-filled (infected) area surrounded by inflammation. An abscess can occur anywhere in or on the body, and its seriousness depends in great part on its location. When an abscess opens — which it eventually will — its infectious contents can easily spread to cause mischief in surrounding areas; thus, the physician will usually employ special techniques to open and drain the abscess prior to that spontaneous bursting point.

For a discussion of the most common kind of abscess, see BOIL.

a.c.: See PRESCRIPTIONS.

accidents, first-aid measures: Do not panic; panic can interfere with your handling of the situation, and can be caught by the victim as well. Your first concern, whatever the nature of the accident, is respiration; if breathing has ceased or continues only with extreme difficulty, turn immediately to RESPIRATORY RESUSCITATION and follow the instructions there.

Your second concern, assuming breathing is continuing or has been restored, is extensive blood loss; if that's happening, turn to BLEEDING and follow the procedures you'll find there. Your third concern is UNCONSCIOUSNESS; your fourth, impending TRAUMATIC SHOCK. (See those entries if necessary.)

Beyond these four immediate concerns, what you should do next depends on the kind of accident and the child's specific condition. Appropriate measures are spelled out under these entries: AMPUTATION, ACCIDENTAL; BACK AND NECK INJURIES; BITES AND STINGS; BRUISES; BULLET WOUNDS; BURNS; CHOKING; CONVULSIONS; CUTS; DISLOCATION; DROWNING; EYE INJURIES; FALLS (if there is no apparent injury); FRACTURES (whether actual or suspected); HEAD INJURIES; KNEE INJURIES; NAIL INJURIES; PARALYSIS; POISONING, HOUSEHOLD SUBSTANCES AND MEDICATIONS; PUNCTURE WOUNDS (including those made by knives); SCRAPES AND SCRATCHES; SPLINTERS; SPRAINS.

accidents, prevention of: Accidents can occur anywhere — on the street, in a boat, anywhere at all. Yet each year, thousands and thousands of accidents occur in the place where a child should be safest: in his or her own home. At least six or seven thousand children under the age of fifteen *die* annually in the United States as a result of home accidents, according to the Children's Bureau of the Department of Health, Education, and Welfare. Of accidents involving youngsters, more than 50 percent occur in the home — and that leaps to 75 percent for children under the age of five.

The accidents range from falls to fires, from cuts to accidental poisoning — and most of them are preventable. The rundown that follows is not all-inclusive; it represents the *minimum* set of measures that you should take to protect your family. We believe that as a parent, you can do no less.

HOUSE RULES

Do everything you can to prevent fires. Certainly basic is the very, very careful use of matches, candles, and the like. (The first precaution is "close cover before striking.") Be sure, if you have a fireplace, that there's a protective screen in front of it. Your wiring should be adequate for your needs; be sure it's never overloaded. Buy only electrical appliances tagged with UL (Underwriters Laboratories) approval — and be sure you know how to use them safely; keep them in good repair, and replace worn cords promptly. And never leave a youngster alone in a room with a lighted stove, fire, candle, or oil lamp.

Falls are a major factor in serious injuries; many falls are fatal. Prevention of such accidents depends in part, of course, on potential victims who take the trouble to look where they're going. But conditions around the house can be contributory, too. All steps and stairways, needless to say, should be well lighted. Use only nonskid rugs, or place special antiskid mats beneath rugs. If your budget permits, replace ordinary door and window glass with safety glass. See that screens on your windows are in good repair and securely fastened; if there are no screens, put gates or bars on upper-story windows. Insist that toys be picked up, especially from stairways.

Guns should be kept unloaded and the ammunition kept under lock and key. Firearms are among the three major causes of fatal accidents in the ten-to-fourteen age group.

Be sure that knives, craft tools, and other sharp instruments are stored safely — meaning away from other implements — and that they are safely returned there after use.

When giving medicine to a child — or, for that matter, to anyone — be sure you do so in a good light. Make certain you have the right medicine, and reread the label. Allow older children to take medicine of any kind only by your permission and at your direction.

Don't use aerosol devices to chill your cocktail glasses. The stuff can kill a small child in minutes if directly inhaled.

Carbon tetrachloride — as a firefighter and as a dry-cleaning agent — has been outlawed. While it's efficient at both these jobs, it's also lethal; its fumes are toxic both inhaled and on the skin. Discard any bought-long-ago products that may contain it.

If you have a wringer-type washer, invest in an automatic safety release; it costs only a few dollars. Some two hundred thousand injuries a year are perpetrated by these machines — 60 percent of them involving people under the age of fifteen, half of those children under five — and most of them could be easily prevented.

Never permit a child to run or play with a spoon, fork, lollipop, ice-cream pop, or the like in his mouth.

When you bring clothes home (or have them delivered) from the dry cleaner's, destroy their plastic coverings immediately. A child can be quickly suffocated by innocent play with these clinging plastics.

Never leave a young child alone in the house, even for "just a few minutes." Many a fatal incident has taken place in just those few minutes.

Know where your youngsters are, what they are doing and playing with (and with whom), at all times, at whatever age.

OUTDOORS: STREET AND YARD

Never permit your children to play in the street, unless of course it is a special, roped-off play street where traffic is prohibited.

Establish and adhere to firm rules regarding the age at which your children are permitted to cross the street, and, of course, teach them the safety rules that must be observed: looking both ways, crossing only at corners, obeying traffic signals.

Never let an under-school-age child play unwatched — by you or some other responsible person.

If your house has a driveway, insist that your youngsters play elsewhere.

If you have a toddler, keep your yard fenced in, both to prevent the child from wandering and to prevent strange animals from wandering in.

Forbid your children to pet or touch strange animals.

Forbid your children to eat wild plants of any kind.

While your children are small, keep your garage door or barn door locked.

String clotheslines high enough so that children can't run into them.

Never permit a child under the age of twelve to operate or ride on a power lawnmower, or even to be in the vicinity when such a mower is being operated.

IN THE CAR

Insist that all members of the family use seat belts, and preferably shoulder harnesses as well. For infants and children too small for a regular seat belt, there are special harnesses, seats, and carriers available.

Lock the car doors and keep them locked while the car is in motion.

Do not permit any small heads or arms to be hanging out of the windows when the car is in motion.

Never leave a child or infant alone in a parked car.

Never permit a small child to play with a car's controls, even in your

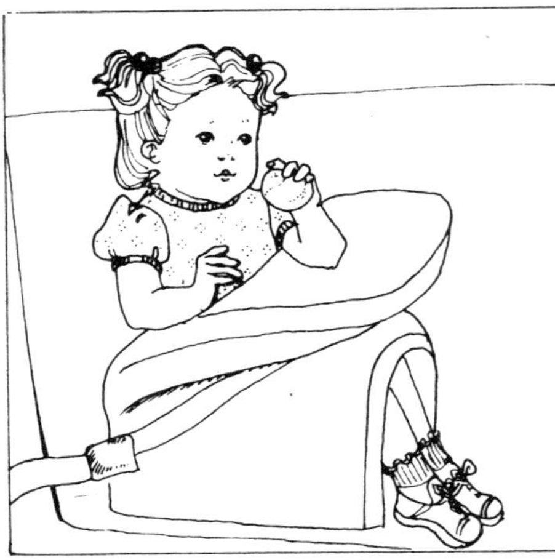

Auto Safety for Infants and Toddlers
Babies, and children weighing less than fifty pounds (22.7 kilograms), need special seats or carriers; standard seat belts are not designed for them and can in fact injure small children. Your children should always ride in the back seat, *and carrying or restraining devices you purchase for them — which should be secured by the car's built-in seat belts — should, as a minimum precaution, bear labels stating that they conform to federal standards. Even some of those are deemed inadequate by other concerned groups. Among those approved by the Committee on Accident Prevention of the American Academy of Pediatrics, at this writing, are General Motors' Infant Love Seat; Peterson model 74, for infants and toddlers from birth to fifty pounds; the Bobby-Mac 3-in-1 Baby Chair, for infants and toddlers to thirty-five pounds (16 kg); Ford's Tot-Guard* (SHOWN), *for youngsters from twenty to fifty pounds (9 to 22.7 kg); General Motors' Child Love Seat, for children from twenty to forty pounds (9 to 18 kg). Although there are harness-type devices judged acceptable by the National Highway Safety Administration, the AAP committee does not find such devices dependably secure.*

presence; this is one toy that is strictly for grown-ups.

SWIMMING AND BOATING

If you have a backyard pool, there should be a locked fence around it — even if the pool is drained.

Never let anyone dive in water of unknown depth.

Whether in pool, lake, or ocean, no one — child or adult — should ever go swimming alone; use the "buddy system": at least two persons swimming together.

In any boating or swimming situation, be sure there is an adult swimmer present for every nonswimming child — and that each adult knows for which child he or she is responsible.

Be sure you do not overload a small boat, and do not permit anyone to stand up in the boat.

On any boat of any size, from canoe to fifty-foot cruiser, every child under the age of twelve — whether or not he can swim — should wear a life jacket at all times.

Exercise extreme caution when fueling a boat. A single gallon of gasoline has the explosive power of 240 sticks of dynamite.

CHILDREN UNDER FIVE

Keep sharp instruments such as knives, scissors, and saws locked out of the reach of toddlers.

Lock up small, sharp objects that could be lethal if swallowed or aspirated: pins, needles, small pieces of jewelry. Children under the age of three or four frequently put everything into their mouths.

Fence off stairways with gates — both top and bottom — as soon as children can crawl, and keep them fenced off until the youngsters can capably negotiate stairs by themselves. Needless to say, the gates should be securely fastened in a way a child won't be able to undo.

Unused electrical outlets should be plugged with blanks (obtainable at most hardware stores) or taped over. A crawler can electrocute himself by sticking a metal object into such an outlet.

Use place mats instead of tablecloths as long as there are toddlers in your home; tablecloths are easily yanked off a table, along with the extremely hot or otherwise harmful things that may be sitting on them.

Be sure there are not dangerously wide gaps between slats of your baby's crib. Safety experts now feel the maximum gap should be no more than 2⅜ inches, and federal law so mandates (the regulation took effect early in 1974).

Keep electric cords far from crib and playpen: teething infants have been known to find them chewable — and lethal; some 40 percent of injuries associated with them are burns, primarily of small mouths.

Matches are not meant for use by this age group and should not be available to them.

Keep all household items and substances that could be swallowed, and should not be, safely locked away the minute your baby becomes mobile; crawlers and toddlers are notoriously undiscriminating about what they put into their mouths. That includes all medications, cleansers, insecticides, detergents, craft supplies, etc. Things that are used frequently, or that may

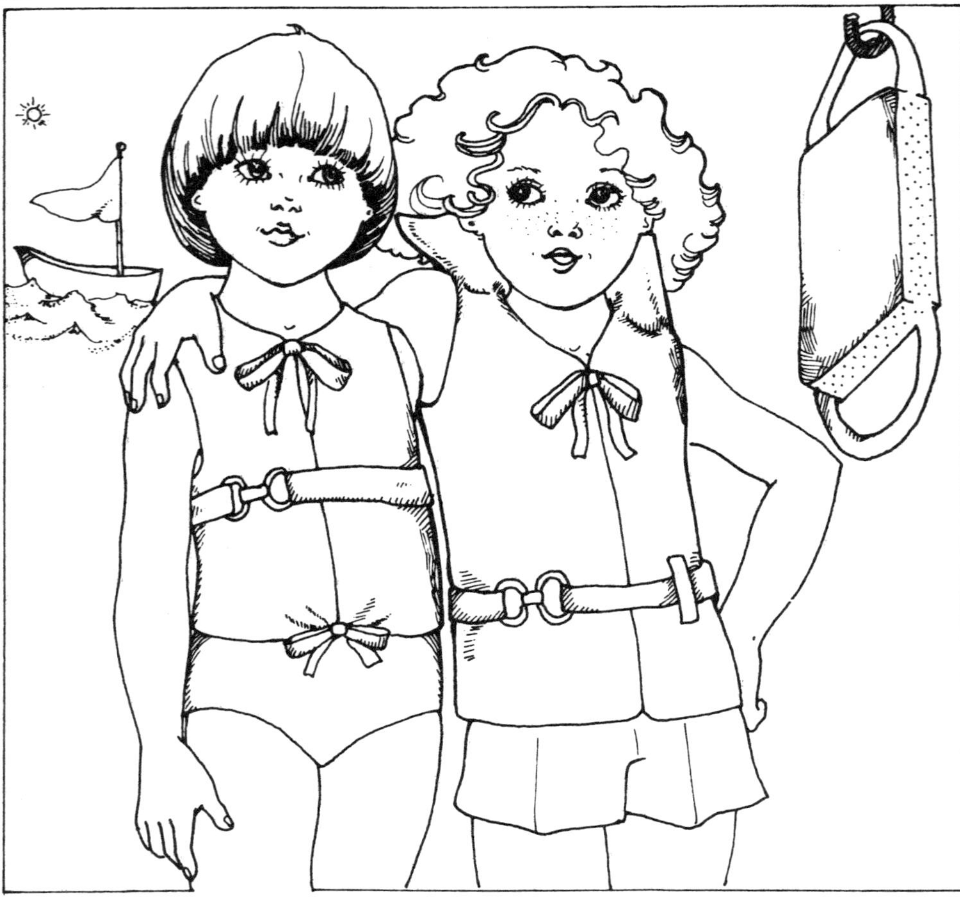

Safeguards Afloat

Buoyant flotation devices come in a number of forms; whatever types you buy, be sure they bear the official approval label of the United States Coast Guard. Approved life-preserver jackets (LEFT) *must be orange, come in two sizes for children and adults (so marked), have adjustable straps; buoyant vests* (CENTER) *may be any color, come in three sizes — adult, medium (child), and small child — and also have adjustable straps. Both of these should be adjusted beforehand for the individual who will wear them. Buoyant cushions* (RIGHT) *may be less dependable because use for seating can cause damage that destroys their buoyancy, but the straps make them handy for throwing and grasping in an emergency; if one must be slipped on in the water, it should be worn across the chest — not on the back, which can force the wearer's face downward into the water. Needless to say, all lifesaving devices should be kept readily accessible on board.*

be needed in a hurry (such as medicines) can be kept somewhere secured by a device that can be easily opened by an adult, but not by a small child; the Kindergard Child Safety Latch is a good and dependable one.

Never leave an infant of any age alone on any surface higher than the floor, for even a second. Even a week-old baby who cannot yet roll over is capable of "inching" across, and off, a bed or table.

Never leave a small child alone in a bathtub, even for an instant. A hot-water tap accidentally turned on can scald a child severely. And remember that a child can drown in a mere two inches of water. If a child is not old enough to bathe himself, he is not old enough to be in the tub unattended.

Never leave a crawler alone near the top of a stairway (which should, as previously noted, be gated in any case). Though experiments have indicated that even small tots have depth perception and an instinctive fear of falling, their muscles and coordination aren't sufficiently developed to protect them.

When you're cooking, turn the pot handles away from the front of the stove, to keep them out of the hands of curious toddlers.

Be aware that small children have limited understanding and practically unlimited curiosity, and don't underestimate their physical abilities — to climb, for example, to top shelves of bookcases or kitchen cabinets.

Never feed popcorn or nuts (or foods, such as cakes or candies, containing nuts) to a child under four; they can cause choking and block the youngster's breathing.

If your house has venetian blinds, cut open the loop of the cord with which you raise and lower the blinds; little heads can get caught in those loops.

Exclude from your small child's toy collection any toys with sharp metal parts or small things that can come loose, such as button eyes on stuffed animals or small wheels on trucks.

For additional safety guidance, see also FIRE EXTINGUISHERS; FIRE-RETARDANT CLOTHING; FOOD POISONING, PREVENTION OF; PETS; POISONING, PREVENTION OF; TOYS; TRAVEL PRECAUTIONS. Descriptions of snakes and other dangerous animals will be found under BITES AND STINGS.

acetaminophen: See PAIN RELIEVERS.

acetones: certain by-products of fat metabolism in the body. Acetones are normally present in tiny trace amounts in both the blood and the urine; excessive amounts, demonstrable by tests, tell the doctor that body fat is being rapidly consumed because ingested sugars are for some reason unavailable to completely answer the body's energy needs. Such unusual amounts are often indicative of diabetes (and someone under treatment for diabetes is tested regularly), but they may also occur, sometimes, in other conditions, including extremely high fever, severe diarrhea, and dehydration.

acetophenazine: a powerful tranquilizer; see SEDATIVES.

acetylsalicylic acid: See ASPIRIN.

Achilles tendon: See TENDONS.

achondroplasia: See DWARFISM.

Achromycin, Achrostatin: See ANTIBIOTICS; these are trade names for, respectively, tetracycline and a combination of tetracycline and nystatin.

"acid" (LSD): See PSYCHEDELICS.

acidosis: an acute (meaning, when a physician uses the word, serious) condition of overacidity in the bloodstream, usually a result of excessive fluid loss; acidosis can develop after a great deal of vomiting or diarrhea, as well as in severe and untreated diabetes. The usual symptoms of acidosis include weakness and difficulty in breathing and, typically, a distinctly "fruity" odor to the breath; coma may result if treatment is not given promptly.

acne: No one need describe acne to the distraught parent of a perhaps even more distraught afflicted teenager — and there are many of those; the agonies of acne are visited upon over 90 percent of everyone between the ages of ten and twenty-three, a span sometimes called the "acne age." The typical blackheads and pimples usually appear, unhappily, on the face, and sometimes the back, shoulders, chest, and arms as well. It's more severe, generally, in boys — but annoyingly unpredictable in girls, often blossoming several days before the start of a menstrual period, at a time of life when menstrual periods can commonly be very irregular.

Why acne? If the cause could be accurately pinpointed, the cure would be a good deal easier. There are, as it happens, a number of factors that can play a significant part. One is certainly the imbalance and change among the endocrine glands that goes on during adolescence; that, in turn, seems to encourage enlarged pores and energetic overproduction by the skin's oil glands (blackheads are simply oil glands plugged by oil and waste materials — and the black isn't dirt but oxidized oil). Another is certainly bacteria (pimples are small infections). Certain foods are probable factors. Then we come to the "maybes," which include climate, psychological factors, and hereditary predispositions.

There isn't much that can be done about that last, iffy, group of guesses — but there *are* steps that can be wisely taken by both you and your teenage son or daughter to cope with the question.

First, because infection is definitely involved, the general state of health is important. Enough rest, enough exercise, some summer sun, that sort of thing. And a generally balanced diet with emphasis on high-vitamin foods, especially vitamins B and C (see NUTRITION) — and avoidance of sweets and fats. That diet regimen can have a twofold benefit, since it will inevitably be fairly low in calories as well; one fourteen-year-old girl we know, in fact, found that her acne vanished when she went on a carefully balanced weight-watching diet.

Second, there are certain foods that don't exactly *cause* acne but seem to make it *worse.* Among the possible culprits cited by most dermatologists are: nuts; shellfish; pork; sugar-containing colas, sodas, and such; spices; fried foods; fats and oils in general; chocolate; cheeses; iodized salt; tomatoes.

Third, cleanliness does help — in removing oils, in making the skin a less fertile ground for those bacteria. That doesn't mean rough scrubbing, which can easily spread the infection. It does mean twice-a-day gentle washing — preferably with a soap containing hexachlorophene — followed by the use of an astringent, which further dries oils and tightens pores. And it means, too, keeping hair very clean (there's no such thing as too-frequent shampooing); long, oily, grimy hair can make the situation much worse.

Fourth, there are some helpful over-the-counter medications. Check the ingredients. Those containing hexachlorophene, polyoxyethylene, and/or sulfur compounds are likely to be most effective.

Finally: if none of those simple measures seem to work, and the acne persists unabated, visit a dermatologist. There are further treatments — variously involving vitamin preparations, antibiotics given internally (especially erythromycin and tetracycline) or applied topically, and other methods — that sometimes do the trick in certain individual cases; only the doctor can decide, though, whether your youngster's case may require them.

It should be added that massive doses (internally) of vitamins are *not* effective treatments for acne, despite the success of some *topical* vitamin treatments (in particular a substance called vitamin A acid, also known as retinoic acid or tretinoin). Nor are sex hormones or contraceptives.

acrodynia: a serious illness involving functional failure of the adrenal glands, evidenced typically by energy loss, muscular pain, and redness and swelling in the child's hands and feet. Happily, acrodynia is extremely rare in the United States; unhappily, it is somewhat less rare in Great Britain and continental Europe, and its usual victims are tots between the ages of four months and three years.

In the past, acrodynia was thought variously to stem from nutritional deficiencies or from infection by some unknown virus. Now, however, it has been found that the culprit is mercury poisoning — not the mercury in your thermometer (which, incidentally, is harmless even if swallowed), but the mercury used in ointments, powders, and other compounds. Such preparations are little used in the United States but are freely dispensed and still used by misguided mamas in some parts of Europe; they include Calomel (mercurous chloride, thought — wrongly — to be a cure for worms and for diarrhea), other vermifuges (antiworm preparations), ointments applied to the skin, and "teething powders."

Obviously, such preparations should be shunned. If you suspect, perhaps while traveling, that your child has this condition, see a physician quickly; treatment requires certain drugs that combine with the mercury, render it nontoxic, and eliminate it from the child's system, and the treatment is completely effective.

acromegaly: See GIANTISM; GROWTH HORMONE.

ACTH: the familiar abbreviation for adrenocorticotrophic hormone, which, translated, simply means a hormone that stimulates the adrenal glands to produce more cortisol, another hormone. ACTH is a natural secretion of the pituitary gland; it plays a role in the body's use of fats and carbohydrates, and is produced especially under conditions of stress.

This very useful substance can also be manufactured synthetically, and has been found helpful in the treatment of certain allergic conditions and various forms of arthritis. It may sometimes be administered, too, to suppress the more discomforting symptoms of pneumonia or tuberculosis. It is administered solely by injection.

Also see CORTICOSTEROIDS; ENDOCRINE GLANDS.

actinic: a technical term meaning "triggered by sunlight." Typically, the process is cumulative; probably the most heard term in common parlance is *actinic keratosis,* which is a potentially (though not actually) malignant skin growth set off by exposure to sunlight over a fairly long period of time.

acuity: accuracy or sharpness, especially of vision. See VISION for further comment.

acupuncture: As the reader must know, there has been intense interest in this ancient Oriental technique ever since 1971, when a number of Americans — including some veteran reporters, respected physicians, and government officials — returned from visits to the People's Republic of China with tales of wonders wrought by the Chinese physicians and their strange little needles. The interest sprang up, and continues, on two distinct levels. On one, there is open-minded research being carried on by both government investigators and private physicians who are anxious to learn if this method of apparently diminishing pain, or even avoiding it altogether (as in the use of acupuncture for anesthesia, which has been done even in China only since the 1950s, while acupuncture analgesia has been in use for many thousands of years), has potential for Western patients and their doctors. On quite another level, as with practically every exotic idea that captures the public imagination, unscrupulous preyers upon the chronically or acutely ill have appeared offering "miracles."

Should you be tempted to have your youngster's arthritis relieved — or any other ailment treated, or any surgical procedure accompanied — by acupuncture, there are some facts of which you should be aware.

Although acupuncture seems to play a comfortable part in the Chinese system of medicine (which, by the way, also employs the most modern medical and surgical approaches) it has not seemed, thus far, fully compatible with ours. Many physicians trained in both Eastern and Western disciplines, however, feel that acupuncture might well function as a useful adjunct to more familiar therapies, particularly for the relief of pain.

Few U.S. physicians and dentists have the necessary training to perform acupuncture correctly — i.e., according to the prescribed Oriental method. Needles of any type used without due attention to sanitary precautions can not only cause local infection, but can also transmit serious diseases.

Pending definite findings on the place of acupuncture in Western medicine, most of the states have issued regulations regarding its use; they range from extremely lax to outright banning of the practice. We think New York State's current position, which permits acupuncture under specifically limited conditions, is a sensible model and a good guideline for citizens elsewhere. Under directives issued late in 1974, acupuncture may be practiced outside an approved institution (i.e., hospital or professional school) only by licensed physicians and dentists who have also completed at least a hundred hours of special training; within approved institutions, it may also be practiced by certain others (e.g., graduates of traditional Oriental schools who have been equally well trained in acupuncture), but only under the supervision of a qualified licensed physician or dentist. In either case, the use of acupuncture is restricted to research projects designed to evaluate the technique: the state must have previously approved the project, patients must agree in writing to participate, and results and conclusions of the investigation must be made available to the state.

Acupuncture, in short, is seen by New York in the same way as the federal government views a new drug which has not yet been proved both safe and effective: as an investigational tool that should be carefully compared with — rather than replace — accepted modes of treatment, deserves to be impartially evaluated, and should be placed only in the hands of qualified individuals who will employ it with caution and discrimination. We suggest you look at it similarly, and avoid persons offering acupuncture treatment who do not meet New York's criteria.

acute: a medical term meaning appearing suddenly (as opposed to *chronic*), or quite serious, or severe (in describing a pain, for example); an acute condition generally requires prompt medical attention.

adam's apple: the popular name for the thyroid cartilage in the neck, just in front of the vocal cords; it's part of the larynx or "voice box." The adam's apple is usually more noticeable in teenage boys than in girls, and may appear especially so in a thin-necked boy; its prominence is nothing to worry about.

Adapin: a trade name for doxepin; see ANTIDEPRESSANTS.

addiction: See AMPHETAMINES; NARCOTICS; SEDATIVES. Also see DRUG ABUSE for other relevant references.

Addison's disease: an extremely serious disorder of the cortex, or outer part, of the adrenal glands, so that they don't or can't secrete the essential hormones they would normally produce; it is named for the British physician who first described the condition in the mid-nineteenth century. Many of the body's vital functions are involved. Symptoms include great fatigue; abnormally low temperature, blood pressure, and blood-sugar level; pigmentary changes in the skin; and digestive and other complications. The precise cause is unknown.

Fortunately, Addison's disease is very rare in children. It is treated, at whatever age, by speedy administration of the missing hormones, including cortisone.

Also see ENDOCRINE GLANDS.

adenitis: See LYMPH NODES.

adenoids: clumps of lymphatic tissue at roughly the point where the nasal passages descend to meet the back of the throat; their presence is perfectly normal, and they do not suddenly appear as new growths. Their name derives from the Greek *aden,* "gland," and means "glandlike."

What causes trouble is something going *wrong* with the adenoids — chiefly, if they become enlarged because of inflammation or infection. They may then interfere with proper breathing, with the result that a youngster breathes through his mouth during the day and with a great deal of snoring at night. They may block proper drainage of the middle ear, causing infection which may actually impair hearing. Their enlargement may, very commonly, be associated with infection of the tonsils.

Treatment of troublemaking adenoids depends on the extent and nature of the trouble — to be judged by your child's doctor. If the problem is mild or infrequent, the doctor may simply give antibiotics or other drugs to deal with the infection. If the problem recurs often, though, especially if hearing is seriously threatened, removal of the adenoids may be advised; the operation is simple and effective. Most ear, nose and throat specialists prefer to wait until a child is at least four years old before removing troublesome adenoids because prior to that, there is a significant possibility of regrowth; if there has been severe hearing loss, however, during those crucial years when verbal abilities are being developed, the surgery may be recommended earlier (the hearing loss is usually reversible).

adenoma: a growth in which glandlike structures are formed; it is typically circumscribed, noninvasive, and benign.

adenoviruses: See VIRUSES.

adhesion: a sticking-together of tissues that ought not to be thus connected; the trouble caused by an adhesion depends on where it's located. Tissues involved in prior surgery — especially scar tissues — are often the source of the difficulty. Adhesions in, for example, the intestines or some other part of the digestive tract can cause obstruction in the tract; since scar tissue is nonelastic, they may also cause pain if there is some kind of pull or strain at the site of the adhesion. Corrective measures may vary, and are decided by the doctor on an individual basis.

Also see LABIAL ADHESIONS, a somewhat different kind of problem.

adhesive tape: See BANDAGES.

Adiloss: a combination-of-ingredients "diet pill"; see AMPHETAMINES.

ad lib: See PRESCRIPTIONS.

adolescence: The word carries with it a number of connotations, social and otherwise, that are outside the scope of this book. Medically, adolescence is generally considered to be the period during which a boy or girl is achieving full sexual maturity (though not necessarily complete body growth). It begins with puberty — the point at which, by definition, reproduction is physically possible.

Throughout adolescence, there are continuing physical developments, accompanied by glandular and chemical changes: the growth of breasts and a broadening of the pelvis in girls; beard growth and deepening of the voice and broadening of the shoulders in boys; the appearance of pubic and axillary (underarm) hair in both sexes. There are frequently complexion problems; see ACNE. And there may be other problems as well. See DRUG ABUSE; PREGNANCY; VENEREAL DISEASES.

adrenal glands: See ENDOCRINE GLANDS.

adrenalin: a hormone produced by the adrenal glands.

Adriamycin: an anticancer agent that has proved effective against various malignancies, especially the sarcomas.

adventitious cyst: See CYST.

aerosol-sniffing: a fad recently seen among preteens and younger adolescents, in which various substances are sprayed into a paper or plastic bag, and the contents then sniffed in hope of achieving a "high." The active ingredient is the chemical fluothane. It can be extremely toxic; many deaths have been reported. Should the fad resume popularity, and you discover that your youngster is inclined to this foolish pursuit, you should do everything you can to dissuade him. It may also be wise to switch, temporarily, to nonaerosol forms of deodorant, spot remover and other household products.

For other related problems that can beset anxious parents these days, see DRUG ABUSE.

Aerosporin: a trade name for polymyxin; see ANTIBIOTICS.

afferent nerves: See NERVOUS SYSTEM.

A-Fil: See SUNSCREENS.

afterbirth: See PLACENTA.

agammaglobulinemia: a rare hereditary condition resulting in extremely low resistance to infection (often termed hypoglobulinemia), or even none at all. Its name is a combination word: *a-* meaning absence of; *gamma globulin,* that part of the blood that normally contains disease-fighting antibodies; and the suffix *-emia* referring to the blood itself. Thus someone with agammaglobulinemia lacks, or has a major deficiency in, the ability to fight invasions by disease-causing organisms. Like hemophilia, the condition is sex-linked and recessive (see HEREDITY for a full explanation of these terms); agammaglobulinemia is uncommon, and found almost exclusively in boys.

A baby with agammaglobulinemia is not in special danger within the first month or two of life; he has received a gamma globulin supply from his mother. That supply gradually declines over a period of about three months; during this period, a normal infant begins to manufacture his own gamma globulin. An afflicted child will be at the mercy of invading organisms as soon as his initial gamma globulin supply falls off, and in the past, such children invariably died in childhood. Now, however, modern medical techniques permit such a child to be given injections of gamma globulin periodically, and antibiotics have entered the picture as effective disease-fighters — so that for all practical purposes, a properly treated child with agammaglobulinemia can live a normal life.

There are sometimes slight variations in the condition from one individual to another. Some afflicted children *do* develop immunity to certain *viral* infections, such as measles or chickenpox, after having the disease. Immunizations are not usually recommended, as they can cause severe generalized reactions.

Agammaglobulinemia and the various forms of hypogammaglobulinemia are often referred to as *immune deficiency diseases.* In some of the most serious such conditions, investigators have in recent years established the lack — or possibly deficient activity — of a particular enzyme, adenosine deaminase; it is not yet clear just what role the enzyme and its activity play in resistance to infection.

ague: an old term for malaria; it was also used sometimes to denote any illness involving fever and chills.

air swallowing: See BURPING.

albino: someone lacking pigment, or color, in skin, hair, and eyes because of the rare hereditary condition called *albinism.* In classic albinism, the lack of color is complete (the pinkish tinge of skin and eyes is that of blood circulating in vessels near the surface); in other forms the lack is partial.

Genetically, the characteristic is recessive (see HEREDITY), so that both parents must be "carriers" of the trait (they need not be albinos themselves) in order to produce an albino child, and the chance of such parents producing an albino child is one in four. Albinism is found in all races and in all parts of the world, occurring about once in ten thousand births. It is more rare or less rare among certain peoples, however; among people of European descent, the incidence is only one in twenty thousand — while among certain Indian tribes of Central America it is one in 140.

Protection from sunlight is the special need of an albino child, and that protection is extremely important; it is the pigment in our skin that normally shields us from severe burning, as well as from certain skin cancers. Total sun-screening agents are available (your doctor can advise you on choosing them), and should always be applied to the child's skin when he is outdoors; even that precaution should not be relied on completely, and it is best to keep the child entirely out of the sun. An albino's eyes are photosensitive, too, and often there is some impairment of vision; an ophthalmologist should be consulted, as soon as the child reaches the age of four, about protective glasses and about corrective lenses if they are needed.

albuminuria: the presence of albumin or other proteins in the urine, a symptom (not a disease) detected by an analysis of a urine specimen. It may or may not be a matter for concern, but it *is* a signal for the doctor to investigate further; the situation is not strictly normal.

Albuminuria may signal an infection or other problem involving the urinary system or some other internal organ. Another urine specimen may be requested, both to double-check the analysis, and because albuminuria can occur temporarily — sometimes as a simple result of an unusual amount of protein in the diet, sometimes following strenuous exercise, sometimes in adolescents for no discernible reason at all. If the youngster is a boy, the doctor may ask that the specimen be taken while he is lying down; occasionally, simply standing to urinate can cause albuminuria (a phenomenon called *orthostatic* albuminuria; this is considered normal and not significant).

alcaptonuria: Don't be alarmed if your doctor tells you your child has this rare hereditary condition. In alcaptonuria, the body lacks — as the result of a minor genetic defect — a particular enzyme that normally breaks down an amino acid called alcapton; hence, that substance is excreted. Typically, the result is that the child's urine turns black upon exposure to air — which makes for very strange-looking diapers. There may also be dark-colored spots on various parts of the body. But the condition is not at all serious.

alcohol: There are three types you are likely to encounter, and if your small child has swallowed a quantity of any one of them, and that's the reason you've turned to this entry, turn immediately to POISONING, HOUSEHOLD SUBSTANCES AND MEDICATIONS.

Ethyl alcohol is liquor; you'll find it, and its effects, discussed under DRINKING.

Isopropyl alcohol is rubbing alcohol. As the label says, it's never to be used internally. Externally, it is a sometimes useful thing to have in the medicine chest, though it is not particularly good as an antiseptic for cuts, scratches, or other wounds, and it is little better than plain water as a medium for massage. It can, however, be soothing on insect bites. And it can be useful, too, in a fever-reducing sponge bath (to be given, of course, only if your doctor so recommends) — in a solution made of half rubbing alcohol, half lukewarm water.

Methyl alcohol is wood alcohol, a potent solvent used in a variety of household-craft projects. It is highly toxic, internally or externally, and should be kept under lock and key if there is a small child in the house.

aldrin: See PESTICIDES.

alexia: difficulty in achieving — or loss of — understanding of the printed word; i.e., the inability to read normally.

alimentary canal: the gastrointestinal tract (stomach and intestines) plus the pathway preceding and following it — thus, the entire tract involved in the ingestion, digestion, and absorption of food and the elimination of waste materials; the alimentary canal extends from the mouth to the anus.

alkalizers: See ANTACIDS.

alkalosis: a condition of abnormally high alkalinity in the body, upsetting its chemical balance; it has been known to result from excessive self-medication with over-the-counter antacids.

Alka-Seltzer: See ANTACIDS; PAIN RELIEVERS.

Allerest: See ANTIHISTAMINES.

allergist: See SPECIALTIES, MEDICAL.

allergy: a hypersensitivity (the "hyper" means quite a lot of) to a particular substance, manifested by specific physical reactions when that substance is encountered. The reaction is not one that everyone would clearly have (as, a burn if the skin is touched by flame), but one peculiar to an individual or group of individuals — though certain allergies do occur in many, or even most, people (an allergy to poison ivy, for one, is found in 75 percent of the U.S. population).

A substance to which someone is allergic is called — for that person — an allergen. What happens when the allergen is encountered is that the body, either instantly or within minutes or hours (rarely, days), releases substances — among them, histamine — which, in turn, trigger the outward symptoms of the reaction. Those symptoms may vary considerably, ranging from rashes and itching to sneezing and coughing, from headache to other pains to gastrointestinal flareups. Almost anything on earth is an allergen for someone, somewhere.

Encounters with the allergen can take place, generally speaking, one of four ways. They are, with some examples of each:

1) *Contact.* Poison ivy and many other plants are major culprits; the summer "Monday rash," after a weekend in the country, is often seen by doctors. Cosmetics are another example (teenage girls with this problem should switch to one of the several brands of hypoallergenic cosmetics, from which most potential troublemakers have been excluded). Among tots, an allergy to soft plastics used in nursery furniture and crib bumpers is not uncommon. And pets — dogs, cats, birds — and toys may be allergens, too.

2) *Ingestion.* That's a fancy word for taking by mouth, and almost any food can be an allergen; among the most common culprits are eggs, wheat (especially buckwheat), milk (an infant's formula can be changed to a different type, and such an allergy is usually temporary), chocolate, various fish and shellfish, nuts, pork, corn, peas, tomatoes, strawberries, oranges and other citrus fruits, synthetic flavorings in fruit-drink mixes, cheeses, and spices. Children may sometimes instinctively avoid certain foods, and the reason may be a possible allergy; it's best not to force the child to eat the food under such circumstances — just discuss the problem with your pediatrician. Ingested substances also include medication taken by mouth; allergies to a number of the antibiotics are common, and many people are allergic to such common things as aspirin.

3) *Inhalation.* Breathed-in allergens can, of course, include anything in the air — dust (including house dust), animal and bird dander, mold spores, and a broad array of pollens. Airborne allergens usually affect the respiratory tract, but may affect the mucous membranes of the eyes, as well.

4) *Injection.* As previously mentioned, there are allergies to medications, and allergy to penicillin is probably the most widespread (and one of the most serious). Materials used for immunizations can also cause trouble. The horse serum long used as the vehicle for emergency tetanus treatment has a history of causing extremely severe allergic reactions *(serum sickness)* in susceptible people; happily, a human serum is now available. And certain allergies-by-ingestion must be considered in this category as well; someone allergic to eggs, for instance, may react to certain vaccines developed in fertilized eggs (follow your own physician's advice on this subject). Allergies to insect bites and stings, in which the allergen enters directly into the bloodstream, can also be classed here.

It's hard to say just how many children have some kind of allergy. Aside from such widespread ones as allergy to poison ivy, documented figures put the estimate at a minimum 10 to 15 percent of the population, based on *reported* cases *only.* The actual figure, at least among children, is probably closer to 50 percent.

While no specific allergy is inherited (one must, in fact, encounter the allergen itself at least once prior to having the allergic reaction, in order to become *sensitized*), a *tendency* to allergy *is* inherited. If either parent has any allergies, there's a high probability of allergy in their children. If *both* parents have allergies, it is almost certain that their children will be allergic — although their allergies may be completely different from those of the parents.

There is no absolute cure for allergy. An allergy sometimes simply disappears by itself; that happens more often with allergies to particular foods than with other kinds. Most allergies persist; depending upon the allergen and the kind of reaction to it, there are a variety of controls. If possible, the ideal solution is to avoid the allergen entirely — a course that's absolutely necessary if the reaction is likely to be systemic and severe. Avoidance is the usual answer, too, to a food allergy; something else with similar nutritional benefits can be easily substituted in the diet. Antihistamines — specific drugs that act against histamine — can counter or temper allergic reactions, diminishing itching in cases of skin reactions, or permitting easier breathing when the nasal passages or sinuses are affected. And in some cases, a degree of desensitization — making the patient less likely to react, or the reaction milder — is possible, and is often the best course if the allergen is (as with certain pollens, or dust) omnipresent. Calmness may help a bit, and so may emphasis on adequate rest; both tension and fatigue seem to aggravate allergies.

Most allergic reactions are mild, or at worst temporarily uncomfortable or painful. A few, however, are quite serious, involving the entire system, and can even be fatal. Invariably, the allergen is something injected directly into the bloodstream: a serum; an injected medication such as penicillin (if there is an allergy, even penicillin by mouth is risky); the sting or bite of a particular insect. If you have discovered that your child has such an allergy, it is *vital* that you alert physicians or anyone else caring for him to that fact; that he carry a warning with him at all times; that — in the case of insect allergens — you have in the house (and carry with you when you travel) an appropriate antidote (your doctor will prescribe it).

The severe kind of allergic reaction is quite obvious. Milder allergic reactions may be much less so. If you *suspect* your child has had an allergic reaction, take the youngster to the doctor, and be able to report — preferably in writing — everything the child has encountered during the prior 72 hours: food and drink; medications of any kind; animals or birds; plants; weather conditions; insects; any new clothing, furniture, or toiletries (including ordinary items like soap and facial tissues). In that last category are the "children's cosmetics" such as bubble baths; many youngsters are allergic to them, and "bubble-bath rash" is a common post-Christmas malady.

For further discussion of various aspects of allergy, see ALLERGY TEST; ANAPHYLACTIC SHOCK; ANTIHISTAMINES; ASTHMA; BITES AND STINGS; DESENSITIZATION; HAY FEVER; HIVES; POISON IVY. If your child has one of those severe, potentially lethal allergies, also see MEDIC ALERT.

allergy test: a test undertaken by a physician, or under a physician's direction, in order to pinpoint the precise substance that has caused an allergic reaction. It's done if, in the doctor's judgment, it is important to discover the single allergen: if the symptoms are severe, unusual, or incapacitating; if a chronic, apparently allergic, condition is causing repeated infection (as, for example, continually congested nasal passages); or if generally available antihistamines and other drugs fail to relieve the reaction — so that identifying the allergen becomes crucial in order that specific measures may be instituted.

For a suspected allergy via contact, inhalation, or injection, some type of skin test will usually be used. There are several, the three most widely used being the patch test, in which a bit of the substance is put on the skin, covered, and left there usually for a 24-hour period; the scratch test, in which the skin is lightly scratched to permit instant penetration of the substance into the body, and a reaction within minutes; and an intradermal injection of a small amount of the allergen, read within minutes, and considered by many specialists the most reliable.

If the allergy involves a food, the doctor may ask you to conduct a test called an *elimination diet.* You will probably be instructed to give the child only a few foods — often foods judged to be relatively "safe" ones — for a certain period of time, then to add others, one by one, at particular intervals, and to observe the child's symptoms and reactions, until the offending food is found. It's a lengthy and sometimes tedious procedure, but it works.

allograft: See HOMOGRAFT.

alopecia: See BALDNESS.

Alpen: a trade name for ampicillin, a semisynthetic penicillin; see ANTIBIOTICS.

alphaprodine: a morphinelike synthetic drug; see NARCOTICS.

Alurate: a trade name for aprobarbital; see SEDATIVES.

Alva-Tranquil: an over-the-counter "sleep aid"; see SEDATIVES.

alveolus: one of the very smallest air cavities in the lungs; the plural is *alveoli.*

Alvodine: a trade name for piminodine, a morphinelike synthetic drug; see NARCOTICS.

Amanita mushrooms: See FOOD POISONING.

amblyopia: a relatively uncommon eye condition in which the eyes do not function in unison, or differ markedly in sight capability; vision, as a result, is dim or poor, and may even approach functional blindness. It can be caused by some types of poisoning, notably methyl (wood) alcohol. It can also result, sometimes, from a child's deliberately refraining from using one malfunctioning eye. One early clue may be a difference in the child's peripheral ("out of the corner of the eye") vision to the two sides.

If you suspect this condition, the youngster should of course be seen promptly by an ophthalmologist.

Amcill: a trade name for ampicillin, a semisynthetic penicillin; see ANTIBIOTICS.

amebiasis, amebic dysentery: See DYSENTERY.

amenorrhea: See MENSTRUATION.

amino acids: See NUTRITION.

amitriptyline: See ANTIDEPRESSANTS.

amnesia: a word used to characterize any memory loss, partial or complete (even in the latter case, skills attained before the loss — such as walking, talking, and so on — are usually retained). Amnesia can follow severe emotional shock as well as physical injury, and it may be either temporary or permanent.

amniocentesis: the withdrawal of amniotic fluid by injection through a pregnant woman's abdominal wall. First introduced in 1930, amniocentesis is now used far more widely, although it is still not a "routine" procedure. It is generally done for diagnostic purposes; it may reveal a number of things about a developing baby, including its sex, certain hereditary conditions, the degree of maturity, and so on. The risk to mother and baby, based on extensive comparative studies, is now deemed insignificant.

Amniocentesis is used when it is judged advisable in order to determine the precise status of a developing fetus, vis-à-vis treatment *in utero* (now possible in certain conditions) or consideration of a therapeutic abortion (see GENETIC COUNSELING). It is also performed (simply to withdraw a certain amount of fluid, not necessarily for analysis thereof) prior to a saline ("salting out") abortion. See ABORTION for more on the latter use.

We must add that in the majority of cases, amniocentesis performed for detection of genetic defects has resulted in parental reassurance. A survey of such procedures performed during 1974 found that in only three percent of the cases of amniocentesis performed to detect such defects were parental fears confirmed — and abortions that might otherwise have been performed on the basis of statistical probabilities were thus averted. The cases studied were all women in the fourth to sixth month of pregnancy, often called the second trimester. These results may lend support to the feeling that many malformed or genetically defective fetuses may succumb to early (first-trimester) *spontaneous* abortion or, as it is commonly known, miscarriage.

amniography: X-ray visualization of the amniotic sac.

amnion: the innermost membrane of the (amniotic) sac within which the fetus develops in the mother's uterus.

amobarbital: a barbiturate drug; see SEDATIVES.

Amoxil, amoxicillin: See ANTIBIOTICS; the first word is a trade name for the second, a semisynthetic penicillin.

AMP: See CYCLIC AMP.

amphetamines: a group of powerful and extremely dangerous drugs having virtually no desirable effects and a host of distinctly undesirable ones, sometimes including death. Amphetamines were first, and are still, promoted as appetite suppressants handy for use in weight reduction or control; they are indeed so used by some "diet doctors" (they are available by prescription only), but should not be, even for adults. Under *no* circumstances should amphetamines be given to, or taken by, a child or teenager, with two — and *only* two — exceptions to the rule: (1) Such a drug may properly be prescribed in the treatment of narcolepsy, an extremely rare condition. (2) Amphetamines, and other drugs similar to them, have been successfully used in treatment of hyperkinetic (incorrigibly overactive) children, upon whom their effect is, strangely, *opposite* to the expected one — i.e., they help to *calm* such children; such treatment is not continued beyond puberty, and does *not* cause addiction.

Amphetamines have, tragically, become an increasingly serious addiction problem among young people (even as young as thirteen or fourteen), despite the warning by some of their wiser peers that "speed kills." It therefore becomes necessary for parents to know precisely what these lethal little pills are, and what damage they are likely to do.

Included in this group of drugs, often termed "pep pills," are amphetamine sulfate, most widely known under the trade name Benzedrine ("bennies"); dextroamphetamine sulfate, marketed under the trade name Dexedrine ("dexies") as well as generically; and methamphetamine hydrochloride (Methedrine, "meth," or Desoxyn). The last soon acquired, among its devotees, the nickname "speed" — which is now generally applied to the entire group of drugs.

Additionally, and also popular with these misguided youngsters, there are combinations of amphetamines with one another or with a variety of other potent ingredients; they have been promoted (to physicians) primarily for weight reduction. They include, prominently, Dexamyl and Duodex, combinations of dextroamphetamine and amobarbital, a barbiturate; Appetrol, a blend of dextroamphetamine and meprobamate, a tranquilizer; Eskatrol, a combination of dextroamphetamine and prochlorperazine, a more powerful tranquilizer; Nobese, amphetamine plus phenobarbital, a barbiturate, and several other unpredictable ingredients; Desbutal, combining methamphetamine and pentobarbital, a barbiturate; Adiloss, methamphetamine with amobarbital; and Obetrol, a combination of four amphetamines.

Amphetamines are not, you may be told by teenage advocates of their use and abuse, narcotics — and that is correct. They *are,* however, *addictive.* As with narcotics, there is an increased tolerance level — one criterion for addictiveness — so that more and more of the drug is necessary to achieve the sought-for effect. Unlike narcotics, amphetamines do not create a *physical* dependence upon them in the body with marked withdrawal symptoms when the drug is stopped (although recent studies have suggested that severe depression, along with sleep-pattern disturbances, is not uncommon). They *do,* however, create a *psychological* dependence; this is no mere matter of "habit" but a genuine reliance nearly impossible for *anyone* to control or resist.

Just what do these drugs do? In "normal" (as in prescribed) doses, amphetamines do suppress appetite; they also, even in those small doses, have a number of side effects varying with the individual, including nervousness, insomnia, and a variety of potentially dangerous effects on the heart, circulation, central nervous system, and some of the endocrine glands. One aspirin-size amphetamine tablet carries, in addition, the stimulatory effect of approximately five cups of strong black coffee (over-the-counter caffeine tablets such as NoDoz and Comeback are each equal, by comparison, to one or two cups).

The youths who become "hooked" on amphetamines quickly exceed that dosage many times over, consuming many more of the tablets and capsules and even melting them down for injection directly into the bloodstream (thus risking serum hepatitis and tetanus in addition). What they seek is a "high" — a euphoric state of careless optimism that will blot out problems and insecurities. What they get is something quite different.

The effects — some appearing immediately, others insidiously cumulative over a period of months — are both physical and mental. Dangers of damage to the nervous and circulatory systems are, of course, multiplied. Critical disturbance of heart rhythm may occur, as may a rise in blood pressure. Extreme, life-threatening weight loss is common. Nervousness can turn to violent twitching, ultimately to convulsions. Veins are typically constricted, pupils of the eyes dilated (that is, wide open even in bright light).

There is a sense of omnipotence (e.g., traffic may be ignored in crossing streets). A minor neurosis can become a psychosis under the influence of amphetamines, and strange, bizarre behavior is commonplace; there is often paranoia, with persistent delusions and even hallucinations, and brain damage may be permanent. The "high" can become unexpectedly "low," and amphetamine addicts have been known, under such conditions, to attempt either homicide or suicide; they have sometimes succeeded.

For those who have heard it rumored that some leading athletes, particularly football players, have — despite universal rules to the contrary — used amphetamines to increase stamina and drive on the field: yes, the rumor is true. These players are extremely foolish. They have used the drugs for what is perhaps their most insidious effect: the masking of fatigue. Fatigue is the feeling that tells us to stop when we have driven our bodies too hard and too far; it is a signal that rest and renewal are needed. If that signal is ignored, or never even sent because of psychochemical interference with the nervous system, it is quite possible to simply keep going until one's heart stops. And it has happened.

These effects are not mitigated, as some suppose, by combination with barbiturates or other supposedly counteractive drugs. Nor, it should be added, are some of the nonamphetamine stimulative appetite suppressants (see DIET PILLS) any less dangerous; thrill-seekers who have turned to the latter thinking them "safer" than amphetamines should be aware that both the effects and side effects are basically the same.

Also see, for full discussion of other facets of the drug-abuse problem, AEROSOL-SNIFFING; GLUE-SNIFFING; NARCOTICS; PSYCHEDELICS; SEDATIVES.

Amphicol: a trade name for chloramphenicol; see ANTIBIOTICS.

amphotericin B: See ANTIBIOTICS.

ampicillin, Amplin: a semisynthetic penicillin and one trade name for it; see ANTIBIOTICS.

amputation, accidental: Such terrifying injuries are fortunately infrequent, but they do occur. The outcome can be directly related to how well you can control panic — both yours and the child's.

First, take measures to control hemorrhage, which may be severe; see BLEEDING.

Second, pick up the severed part and wrap it in something — preferably airtight plastic wrap followed by ice-packing, but use whatever is available. There have been successful reimplantations of fingertips, fingers, entire hands, and even arms, and further surgical restorations may be achieved in future.

Third, rush the child *and* the severed part to the nearest hospital emergency room.

Amytal: a trade name for the drug amobarbital, a barbiturate; see SEDATIVES.

Anacin: See PAIN RELIEVERS.

anaerobe: an organism that thrives in the absence of oxygen. Perhaps the best known such organism is *Clostridium tetani,* the bacillus that causes tetanus via wound infection; the deeper and narrower the wound, the less air can reach the injured tissues and the greater the danger of infection.

anal fissure: a crack in the wall of the anus, occasionally congenital but more commonly caused by irritants in the diet, by straining at an especially hard stool, by infection, or by the use of harsh laxatives (no child should ever be given *any* laxatives except by direction of a physician).

An anal fissure tends to start a vicious cycle. Because of the fissure itself, defecation is painful; thus, the child will tend to deliberately hold back, in order to avoid the severe discomfort of a bowel movement. Constipation can result, accompanied by increasing abdominal aching. When the child finally finds he can hold back no longer, the stool is unusually large — often tearing the anal wall still more, and causing bleeding (which can be seen either in the stool itself or on the toilet paper).

If your doctor discovers an anal fissure in your child, a mild laxative of the stool-softening type, such as mineral oil, may be prescribed in order to release the held-back material as rapidly and painlessly as possible; a pain reliever may also be applied locally. You may be asked to carefully regulate the child's diet in ways that will keep stools soft for a time in order to permit the fissure to heal. And because an anal fissure often occurs early in the child's toilet-training period, a certain amount of regression may occur; don't let this upset you, and don't pressure the child.

analgesia: lack, or loss, of a feeling of pain; an agent designed to effect, or aid in, achievement of that state is an *analgesic.*

analgesics: See ASPIRIN; NARCOTICS; PAIN RELIEVERS.

anaphylactic shock: a condition of shock resulting from an extreme systemic allergic reaction; it can be fatal if it is not treated promptly, usually by immediate injection of epinephrine. Substances causing anaphylactic shock are invariably allergens that get into the bloodstream, thus through the entire system, quickly — medications such as penicillin, for example, and the venom in insect stings.

Symptoms may vary but typically include extreme difficulty in breathing, coughing, extensive itching, increased pulse rate, and a bluish tinge to the skin (because of lack of oxygen); this may be followed by unconsciousness and possibly convulsions. In other instances, there may be severe nausea accompanied by vomiting.

If you suspect anaphylactic shock, lose no time; rush the child to the nearest hospital emergency room. Once the child has been treated, take appropriate precautions against future emergencies: if a medication is involved, be sure that your youngster is never again given it; if the allergy is to the sting of an insect, be sure that you keep whatever antidote is prescribed in the house at all times, and take it along whenever you travel with the child.

Also see ALLERGY; MEDIC ALERT.

Ancef: a trade name for cefazolin, one of the cephalosporins; see ANTIBIOTICS.

androgen: any one of the male sex hormones, especially testosterone or androsterone.

anemia: an abnormally low amount of hemoglobin in the blood. Hemoglobin, a substance found in red blood cells, carries oxygen to the various tissues throughout the body and also carries off waste products; thus in anemia, the tissues are being inadequately serviced. An anemic condition may be caused variously by underproduction of the red blood cells, by some malformation or malfunction of them, or by their being destroyed or lost at an abnormal rate or in extraordinary amounts.

It should at this point be evident that — whatever you may be told by tonic-peddling TV pitchmen — anemia can properly be neither diagnosed nor treated by nonmedical means. While it's perfectly true, as those commercials suggest, that weakness and fatigue are typical symptoms of anemia, they are not the only symptoms — and they themselves are symptomatic of a number of other conditions that may be more or less serious. If your doctor suspects anemia — in a child or in any member of your family — specific tests and analyses will be performed to confirm the diagnosis and to determine the underlying cause. There are many types of anemia. Some of those you are likely to hear or read about include:

Aplastic anemia — an anemia resulting from decreased formation of red blood cells by the bone marrow; it is often associated with a decrease in the number of platelets and of certain types of white cells, as well. It is frequently caused by a reaction to substances that exert a toxic effect on the bone marrow.

Hemolytic anemia — an anemia caused by too-rapid destruction of red blood cells; the cells may be broken down too fast by the spleen, and bile pigments produced by the liver as a result of that breakdown may appear in the body tissues as a yellowish cast, or jaundice. Or, some other agent may be destroying the cells. If the condition is acute, symptoms may include, among others, nausea, vomiting, and fever. Many things can cause a hemolytic anemia; among them are some types of poisoning, severe burns, certain parasitic infestations, certain infections, hereditary blood-group problems (see RH FAC-

TOR), and the venom of some snakes.

Iron-deficiency anemia — meaning, as it says, a deficiency of iron in the body. Iron is one of the factors needed for the manufacture of new red blood cells, and also plays a part in their transporting of oxygen; some is normally available from old, discarded red blood cells, but the rest must be obtained from the diet. It is possible for a child to be born with this condition if his mother suffered from a severe iron-deficiency anemia during pregnancy. Sometimes it stems from chronic infection, since persistent illness typically causes a lack of appetite which may in turn lead to malnutrition.

Pernicious anemia — an anemia related to a specific vitamin deficiency; symptoms can include gastrointestinal difficulties, as well as sensory disturbances in the limbs. It is rare in children. The manufacture of red blood cells requires Vitamin B_{12}, which in turn requires certain substances in the gastric juices for its absorption — so that a deficiency in the vitamin, or some interference with its proper absorption, may be the trouble.

Posthemorrhagic anemia — an anemia created by massive blood loss; it is the least serious of all types, since it is by definition temporary, and does not denote any failure of the body's ability to proceed with the manufacture of normal and fully functioning red blood cells. Treatment will depend upon the severity of the condition, and may or may not involve transfusion.

Sicklemia — a hereditary condition in which a chemically abnormal hemoglobin is produced; it is characterized by some or most of the red blood cells having a peculiar sickle, or crescent, shape rather than the usual rounded form. Sicklemia is found chiefly among dark-skinned peoples descended from inhabitants of tropical areas in Africa and parts of the Far East; it typically carries with it an unusually high degree of resistance to malarial infection. The anemia may be mild or serious, depending upon whether it is inherited from both parents or only from one.

Thalassemia — a condition similar to sicklemia, but somewhat rarer, and also known as Cooley's anemia or Mediterranean anemia. It occurs among Mediterranean peoples, as well as in parts of the Far East. Like sicklemia, thalassemia involves abnormal red-blood-cell structure; it sometimes includes skeletal abnormalities as well. It, too, is associated with high resistance to malaria.

Treatment of any anemia will of course depend on the cause and the physician's judgment; among the possibilities are administration of Vitamin B_{12} or iron supplements, drugs to combat infection, antitoxic agents, transfusion, and removal of the spleen.

Also see, for more details about mechanisms and conditions referred to briefly here, BLOOD CELLS; BLOOD GROUPS; FAVISM; HEREDITY; SICKLE CELL DISEASE.

anesthesiologist: See SPECIALTIES, MEDICAL.

anesthetic: an agent used to produce an absence of sensation, so that no pain will be felt, as during a surgical or other procedure. A *general* anesthetic, inhaled or injected, induces complete sleep for a specific period of time; general anesthetics include ether, thiopental (Pentothal), and others. A *local* anesthetic, usually injected, blocks certain nerves only, leaving the patient still conscious; the agent most widely used — especially in dentistry and in minor dermatological surgery — is procaine. A *topical* anesthetic is one applied, usually in ointment or liquid form, to the skin or mucous membrane in order to deaden already-existing pain, as of sunburn or a minor wound.

aneurysm: a dilation and bulging-out of the wall of an artery, with the potential danger of outright rupture of the area involved, and possibly critical hemorrhage. The degree of seriousness of an aneurysm depends upon its location; the situation is most acute if it occurs in or near the heart, brain, or other vital organ, or in a major blood vessel. An aneurysm can be caused by infection or by injury; it may also be precipitated by a congenital weakness in the artery wall. Correction of an aneurysm is surgical.

"angel dust": a street term for phencyclidine, a potent animal tranquilizer; see PSYCHEDELICS.

angina: a term originally meaning, and sometimes used as synonymous with, sore throat, although more familiar to most people as part of *angina pectoris* (chest pain). It may also refer to particular disorders involving the throat and/or mouth, such as Vincent's angina; see GUM DISORDERS.

angiography: X-ray visualization of the blood vessels.

anileridine: a morphinelike synthetic drug; see NARCOTICS.

animal bites: See BITES AND STINGS.

ankle, broken: See FRACTURES.

anorexia: a loss of, or marked decrease in, appetite; it is a typical, major symptom of appendicitis. *Anorexia nervosa* denotes such a symptom, occurring more often in teenage girls than in others and frequently resulting in severe weight loss and malnutrition, that is due not to physical illness but to emotional disturbance. An *anorexiant* is an agent that depresses the appetite; see AMPHETAMINES and DIET PILLS.

Anspor: a trade name for cephradine, one of the cephalosporins; see ANTIBIOTICS.

antacids: substances that counter a condition of hyperacidity in the stomach, a condition rare in children. Antacids should never be given to children — or taken by teenagers or adults, for that matter — without a physician's advice, and they are not designed (or effective) for other ailments of the stomach or intestinal tract, no matter how similar one's symptoms may seem to those of the jovial fellow in the commercial whose world has just been brightened by a dose of Tablet X or Liquid Y.

If your doctor *has* specifically recommended an antacid, there are quite a few available, differing chiefly in cost. One of the most effective is ordinary sodium bicarbonate, or baking soda; it's important, though, to follow the doctor's exact directions as to dosage, since too much can easily cause another problem, that of over-*alkalinity.* Similarly inexpensive are such compounds, available from your pharmacist without prescription, as magnesium carbonate U.S.P. and calcium carbonate U.S.P. (the latter, it should be noted, sometimes causes constipation).

The various brand-named antacids cost more; in some cases you are paying for additional (and probably unneeded) ingredients, in others for flavoring or ease of taking, and in many for advertising. They are of various types.

Some, the best-known of which is Alka-Seltzer, are chiefly effervescent combinations of sodium bicarbonate and aspirin. Some — such as Maalox and others — are suspensions of magnesium and aluminum hydroxides, another category of antacid chemicals. Others — usually including "gel" or "jel" in their names — are hydroxides in gel form. And still others combine two or more antacid compounds with mint flavoring for pleasant chewing; Chooz, BiSoDol mints, and Tums are familiar examples.

Generally speaking, an antacid in liquid or liquefied form, or a powder or tablet to be dissolved in water before taking it, is more dependably effective than a tablet designed to be chewed; the latter type, unless it's chewed very thoroughly, may not dissolve completely before it passes out of the stomach and into the intestine, and may thus be wasted.

antagonism: the action of a substance that opposes the action of another within the body, inhibiting it or canceling it out altogether. Such action may be desirable and deliberately encouraged (as, administering serum to combat snake venom), or undesirable and inadvertent (as an over-the-counter drug that, unknown to the patient, interferes with the beneficial effects of a medication prescribed by a physician); the word simply describes a pharmacological phenomenon.

For another, totally different type of interaction, see SYNERGISM.

antenatal: See NATAL.

antibiotics: a group of drugs, first introduced in the late 1940s, that act effectively and predictably against bacteria, and rickettsiae and some fungi as well, either killing them or severely inhibiting their growth. Some act against a few specific disease-causing organisms; others, termed "broad-spectrum" types, are effective against a great many. They may, depending on the drug and the nature of the infection, be given orally, injected, or applied topically. With a handful of exceptions, they are not effective against viruses; they are not useful for colds, flu, chickenpox, or rubella.

Rarely, antibiotics may be used — in cases where this is judged medically advisable — as preventive medication, and it is for this purpose that an antibiotic may be prescribed for, say, a youngster with flu; if the physician believes it is vital to ward off even the possibility of a secondary bacterial infection, antibiotics may be given even though they will be ineffective against the flu itself. Similarly, antibiotics may be prescribed during an epidemic for a child for whom the particular disease would pose a special danger. And antibiotics may also be given after surgery or physical injury if there is a significant danger of potential wound infection.

But these are rare and special cases. By and large, doctors try to avoid using antibiotics except when they are specifically indicated as the only effective way of dealing with organisms provably present and causing an illness. The reason is that many bacteria have turned out to be extremely resourceful, genetically speaking, and indiscriminate use of antibiotics can easily result in the creation of a new strain resistant to the antibiotic.

Some few bacteria have an apparent natural resistance. If an antibiotic is overused, the entire population (within that individual) of *non*resistant bacteria will be killed off, leaving only the resistant ones to produce future generations; and of course all such organisms spread about by that person will be the resistant kind. In carefully administered amounts, the antibiotic will deal with the disease but leave *non*-resistant bacteria to reproduce for the future.

It's for this reason that you should never buy over-the-counter antibiotic preparations — ointments, lozenges, whatever — unless your physician specifically advises you to do so; nor should you ever give to a child, or take, an antibiotic you may have in the house, without your doctor's advice.

If an antibiotic is prescribed, it's vital that you follow the exact dosage indicated. Don't ever exceed that dosage, in either amount or time period, both for the reasons we've already mentioned and because the antibiotic could destroy innocent, non-disease-causing bacteria found normally in the body, thus encouraging other problems. *Do,* on the other hand, continue the antibiotic for as long as the physician has specified, even if the symptoms of the illness seemed to have disappeared; outward symptoms can vanish well before the infection has actually been knocked out — and your doctor knows just how long the job takes.

One other important point about antibiotics is the possibility of what are loosely termed "side effects." They are not uncommon, although some of the drugs are more likely than others to give rise to untoward effects, and the effects may vary considerably from one individual to another. Some are distinctly minor in comparison with the usefulness of the treatment; others are extremely serious, even potentially lethal.

If an antibiotic has been prescribed for your child, you should keep your eyes open. Watch for any of these: a rash; unusual drowsiness; headache or dizziness; unexpected pain of any kind, anywhere; any gastrointestinal discomfort or change in frequency or consistency of bowel movements; any respiratory difficulties. Report any such symptom to your child's doctor promptly. Let the doctor judge whether it is a symptom of the illness or a possible reaction to the medication; let the doctor decide, too, if a reaction is a serious one, if the drug should be discontinued, if anything should be given to counteract the reaction. And, of course, follow your doctor's instructions, whatever they may be. (One "side effect" that may sometimes occur in older girls is discussed separately; see MONILIASIS.)

Should you discover that your child has an allergy to an antibiotic, it's vital that this information be given to anyone who might subsequently treat him; though the first reaction may be a mild rash, a second reaction — especially to an *injected* antibiotic — could be extremely serious, even fatal. Such information should be promptly recorded in the back of this book (APPENDIX E). We urge, too, that the youngster carry the warning with him at all times, if he is old enough to go to school or even play away from home; see MEDIC ALERT.

Following is a list of some of the more widely used antibiotics. It is intended — except in the cases of chloramphenicol and clindamycin, where specific warnings are needed — simply as general information about the various drugs your doctor may prescribe and/or use, and it is not presented as a comprehensive listing.

amphotericin B (Fungizone) — the leading antifungal drug, considered the drug of choice in most severe systemic fungal infections. Notable exceptions include tinea (ringworm) and localized *Candida* infections. (See candicidin, miconazole, and nystatin, three other medications on this list.)

bacitracin (Baciguent) — a drug that, as you may surmise from the trade name mentioned, is used only in topical (on-the-skin) form. It acts effectively against *Staphylococcus* and *Streptococcus,* which are responsible for the vast majority of skin and mucous-membrane infections.

Bacitracin is also combined with other antibiotics in a number of topical medications: with neomycin in Bacimycin; with polymyxin in Polysporin; with both of them in Biotres, Mycitracin, Neo-Polycin, and Neosporin.

candicidin (Candeptin, Vanobid) — a fungicidal agent, particularly effective against vulvovaginal infection, i.e., moniliasis; it comes both in ointment form and in tablets for vaginal insertion. It's important to keep using the medication for the full prescribed course (usually two weeks), in order to really get rid of the infection, even though symptoms may be relieved within two or three days.

cephalosporins — a group of semisynthetic agents developed over the past decade that act against Gram-positive coccal infections — they are particularly effective against strep — and also some bacilli; they are given to combat a number of skin, respiratory, and urinary-tract conditions. They are chemically related to the penicillins, and there is some crossover sensitivity, although many people allergic to penicillin can be successfully treated with one of this group; the physician may turn to the cephalosporins if penicillin is for some reason contraindicated, or if the bacteria involved have proved resistant to penicillin.

There are a number of cephalosporins available, and others are currently being developed; some are designed for oral use in liquid or tablet form, others strictly for injection. Among the latter are cefazolin (Ancef, Kefzol), cephaloridine (Loridine), cephalothin (Keflin), and cephapirin (Cefadyl). The oral cephalosporins include cephalexin (Keflex), which has proved useful in a broad range of skin, ear, and systemic infections and is somewhat less likely to cause gastrointestinal upsets than some other antibiotics; cephaloglycin (Kafocin), a specific against certain urinary-tract infections (but not in babies under a year of age, since its safety for this group has not been established); and cephradine (Anspor, Velosef), which was introduced in late 1974 and is, like cephalexin, available in liquid form for infants and small children.

chloramphenicol (Amphicol, Chloromax, Chloromycetin, Mychel) — a powerful broad-spectrum antibiotic with a range of effectiveness similar to that of the tetracyclines. It should not be used internally — that is, injected or given by mouth — *except* possibly for typhoid fever or other life-threatening conditions that have failed to respond to other, more desirable antibiotics, since there are a number of potentially hazardous side effects. In some, there are severe allergic reactions. Others develop serious gastrointestinal problems.

The main danger posed by chloramphenicol, however, is that the drug may possibly cause a critical anemia by attacking the bone marrow and interfering with the production of red blood cells; this condition can sometimes develop months after the drug has been administered. There have also been occasional cases of leukemia in which chloramphenicol has been implicated. Most physicians in this country are well aware of these risks and avoid the drug as much as possible. Travelers should be warned, though, that in some other countries, chloramphenicol and products containing it are actually sold over the counter as freely as aspirin.

To preclude the necessity of chloramphenicol's ever being used internally, it's wise to see that all members of your family are vaccinated against typhoid before visiting any area where that disease is endemic; the question of treatment then need never arise.

Chloramphenicol *is* safely used *topically*, notably in certain ear infections; the foregoing warnings do not apply in such use.

clindamycin (Cleocin) — a limited-use antibiotic that's effective against Gram-positive cocci, staph and strep infections in particular. It's a useful alternative in situations where there is hypersensitivity to penicillin and erythromycin, and it is now felt that clindamycin should be employed *only* in such situations. The reason is not the possibility of allergic reactions, which is fairly small (it does exist, and there is also cross-sensitivity with lincomycin, from which clindamycin was derived), but the significant number of serious intestinal reactions that have been encountered since this drug was introduced in 1971. Some investigators have reported a 20 percent incidence of severe, debilitating diarrhea; in a possible 10 percent, acute colitis — leading to megacolon and subsequently the necessity for major surgery — has occurred, and at least four dozen deaths have been attributed to such conditions. If your child has been given clindamycin and any degree of diarrhea whatever is noted by the child or by you, *stop the drug immediately* and call your physician; do *not* give the youngster an antidiarrheal medication.

clotrimazole (Lotrimin) — an antifungal agent approved in 1975 for topical use. It is chemically similar to miconazole and active against the same sort of organisms, possibly against some bacteria as well. (An oral form has been under study but is contemplated for use only in life-threatening systemic infections, since the adverse effects are frequent and serious.)

erythromycin (Bristamycin, E-Mycin, Erypar, Erythrocin, Ethril, Ilosone, Ilotycin, Pediamycin) — one of the safest of all the antibiotics, with gastrointestinal reactions uncommon and allergic ones rare. Erythromycin (the brand names listed actually include some slight chemical variations) is the top alternative for a host of conditions in which penicillin is the drug of choice but is deemed inadvisable for a particular patient, including strep infections, syphilis, diphtheria, pneumococcal pneumonia, and rat-bite fever — and is *the* drug of choice for whooping cough. It is typically injected or taken orally, but is also available for topical application (in certain eye infections).

gentamicin (Garamycin) — a powerful antibiotic given (by injection; it is not administered orally) only to combat extremely serious systemic infections, including staph and various septicemias. Like the older drug neomycin, it has been known to cause both ear and kidney damage, and is even more potent than neomycin; it is thus avoided unless the critical nature of the infection makes the risk worthwhile. It is also available in topical-application form, and the warnings do not apply with such use; physicians generally try to avoid it, however, because of the better-than-average possibility of development of resistant organisms, which also tend to be resistant to some other, chemically related, drugs (kanamycin, neomycin, streptomycin).

gramicidin — an antibiotic of limited usefulness that is not employed by itself at all; it is, however, combined with some other antibiotics for topical use, notably with neomycin in Spectrocin.

griseofulvin (Fulvicin, Grifulvin, Grisactin) — a major antifungal drug, especially active against the organisms that cause tinea (ringworm) of the skin, scalp, and nails (it is not effective against moniliasis or thrush). It is given orally.

kanamycin (Kantrex) — another potent antibiotic with specific uses, kanamycin is given by injection only in cases of severe systemic infection caused by particular strains of bacteria, since large injected doses can cause both ear and kidney damage. Orally (that risk does not apply) kanamycin is the number two drug (after ampicillin) in the treatment of shigellosis, or bacillary dysentery.

lincomycin (Lincocin) — an antibiotic very closely related to clindamycin (which was derived from lincomycin) and having similar uses and side effects.

miconazole (MicaTin, Monistat) — a recently introduced fungicidal agent that in two topical (cream) forms appears to be quite effective against certain fungal infections, in particular athlete's foot (MicaTin) and moniliasis (Monistat), the latter including both the vulvo-vaginal type and the occasional diaper rash involving such organisms. It is not used in thrush or — simply because its safety has not yet been verified — for moniliasis during pregnancy.

neomycin (Mycifradin, Myciguent, Neobiotic) — another limited-use antibiotic, neomycin was formerly given by injection to combat a number of infectious organisms, but has been superseded by safer agents, since administration of neomycin by this route carries quite a high risk of toxic effects on ears and kidneys. It is now given orally for some intestinal infections, and used topically especially in infections of the eyes.

Neomycin is also combined with other antibiotics in a number of useful topical medications; see the comments under bacitracin and gramicidin.

nystatin (Mycostatin, Nilstat) — an antifungal agent effective against localized Candida infections, i.e., of the skin or mucous membranes (including both thrush and moniliasis); it may be prescribed in either oral or topical-application form. There also exist some combination products (Achrostatin V, Comycin, Declostatin, Terrastatin, Tetrastatin, Tetrex-F) that pair nystatin with one or another of the tetracyclines, on the theory that such a formulation will prevent the fungal overgrowth that is a not-uncommon nuisance resulting from therapy with those broad-spectrum antibiotics. Most medical authorities find these fixed combinations somewhat irrational, since they provide only a bare minimum of nystatin (pointless if it's not needed, too little if it is), and feel that it's better to take the nystatin separately if it's needed, whether for curative or prophylactic purposes.

penicillins — not a single drug but now a group including both natural and semisynthetic substances, the penicillins remain the drug of choice in treating the vast majority of bacterial infections. The naturally occurring penicillins may be injected or given orally; some of the semisynthetics may also be given either way, but most are designed to be taken solely by mouth.

The natural penicillins are the most likely of the antibiotics to spark severe allergic reactions, and must be avoided if an allergy has become evident (see the general comments earlier in this entry). It should be added that, contrary to prior belief, a rash reaction is not necessarily predictive of severe hypersensitivity: one limited study on this question found (via actual allergy testing) that among a group of people who believed themselves allergic to penicillin, only 15 percent actually were, while allergy was demonstrated in about eight percent of a group with no prior intimation of it.

The semisynthetics are possibly safer so far as allergic reactions are concerned. Although occasional rashes and gastrointestinal upsets do occur, they may or may not suggest allergy. Physicians' views on this subject do vary, however, and some feel that if there has been any suspicious reaction to any of the penicillins, all of them should be avoided except as a very last resort. Obviously, your own doctor's judgment, based on your child's past experiences, should be relied upon.

The trade names of the penicillins can usually be recognized; almost invariably, they include at least a syllable or two of the original word.

Natural penicillins include "the" penicillin, benzyl penicillin, usually called penicillin G, in several slight chemical variations and combinations (Bicillin, Crysticillin, Crystifor, Dramcillin, Duracillin, G-Recillin, Hyasorb, Kesso-Pen, Palocillin, Pedacillin, Pentids, Permapen, Pfizerpen, Sugracillin, and others); and penicillin V or phenoxymethyl penicillin (Compocillin, Ledercillin, Robicillin, Penapar, Pen-Vee, Uticillin, V-Cillin, Veetids, and others), which is given only orally and is more resistant to destruction by gastric acid than the penicillin G preparations.

The semisynthetics have multiplied in recent years to a point of perplexing confusion to physicians and patients alike. We shall not even attempt to mention them all. The leading one is ampicillin (Alpen, Amcill, Amplin, Omnipen, Penbritin, Pensyn, Polycillin, Principen, Totacillin), which has proved extremely useful and even more effective than penicillin G against certain infectious organisms, and is in fact now the first-choice drug for shigellosis (bacillary dysentery), respiratory infections and meningitis caused by a little-known but widespread bacterium called *Hemophilus influenzae* (there's no connection with flu, which is caused by a virus), one type of rat-bite fever, and possibly typhoid fever.

Other semisynthetic penicillins include amoxicillin (Amoxil, Larotid), carbenicillin (Geocillin, Geopen, Pyopen), cloxacillin (Tegopen), dicloxacillin (Dynapen, Pathocil, Veracillin), floxacillin (Floxapen), hetacillin (Versapen), methicillin (Staphcillin), nafcillin (Unipen), oxacillin (Bactocill, Prostaphlin), phenethicillin (Darcil, Maxipen, Syncillin), and propicillin (Cetacillin, Oricillin).

Why the proliferation of what are frequently only minor variations? In many cases, we can only echo the question. In some, however, there are special advantages (aside from the continuing effort to decrease the risk of allergic reactions). Several have been demonstrated to zero in on certain disease-causing organisms extraordinarily effectively: carbenicillin, for example, is now the first-choice weapon against a bacillus called *Pseudomonas aeruginosa,* which is among the more common causes of conjunctivitis and some ear and urinary-tract infections. Others are more effective against certain bacteria that seem to resist attack by penicillin G; some staphylococci are among the latter, and several of the semisynthetics can take over in such instances. And the chemical variations have resulted, in some instances, in drugs that are especially useful in particular parts of the body due to their rates of excretion, times of absorption, and the like.

polymyxin (Aerosporin) — a fairly limited antibiotic so far as internal administration goes, but the second-choice drug (after carbenicillin) in combating *P. aeruginosa* infections; it acts against a variety of other bacteria — but less effectively than most other antibiotics — and poses the risk of dangerous kidney reactions. Topically, polymyxin is more useful, and there are also products that combine it with other agents for such use, giving a wider spectrum of action when the bacteria causing the problem (and there may be more than one) cannot be precisely identified; it's relatively safe, since topical application is the least risky route. Typically, such products combine polymyxin with bacitracin (Polysporin) or with bacitracin and neomycin (Biotres, Mycitracin, Neo-Polycin, Neosporin).

rifampin (Rifadin, Rimactane) — an antibiotic developed in Europe and introduced in this country in 1971, specifically for the treatment of tuberculosis. Taken orally — usually in combination with one or more other medications, notably a drug called isoniazid — it has been found to effect earlier control over the infection, as compared with streptomycin. Rifampin has a special eccentricity which is understandably scary if one is not forewarned (but is harmless): it may turn all body excretions — urine, stools, saliva, sweat, tears — a bright red-orange.

spectinomycin (Trobicin) — a recently introduced specific agent against gonorrhea, now the preferred medication for that venereal disease in cases where both penicillin and ampicillin are contraindicated because of allergy or bacterial resistance. It is administered only by injection, and has not been proved safe for children.

streptomycin — the first antibiotic marketed (1947), which has now taken a back seat to drugs that pose less risk of possible adverse effects and are also more effective. It remains, however, the first-choice drug (the tetracyclines rank second) against plague and tularemia, although most physicians try to avoid it even in these instances. Streptomycin is given only by injection.

tetracyclines — the leading group of broad-spectrum antibiotics, effective (although not generally the first-choice drugs) against a wide range of infections, with the notable exceptions of strep and staph. They *are* the first-choice drugs against brucellosis, cholera, rickettsial infections, psittacosis (parrot fever), trachoma, relapsing fever, and a couple of the minor venereal diseases; they are also the leading alternatives — in cases of allergy to the penicillins or other first-choice drugs — in meningitis, tetanus, whooping cough, and syphilis, and tend to be preferred to streptomycin for tularemia and plague.

This group includes both natural and semisynthetic substances, among them tetracycline and its salts (Achromycin, Bristacycline, Cyclopar, Panmycin, Robitet, Steclin, Sumycin, Tetracyn, Tetrex), chlortetracycline (Aureomycin), demeclocycline (Declomycin), doxycycline (Doxy-II, Doxychel, Vibramycin), methacycline (Rondomycin), minocycline (Minocin, Vectrin), oxytetracycline (Terramycin), and nolitetracycline (Syntetrin). Some are available in multiple forms; others are intended for use only by injection, or only by mouth.

As with the proliferating penicillins, doubt has been expressed in some quarters that this extensive array of variations is necessary. Organisms resistant to one tend to be resistant to others as well. Rates of absorption do vary somewhat, however, as do serum levels, so a physician may choose to prescribe one rather than another for those reasons; side effects — which tend, by and large, to be noncritical in nature — may also vary somewhat from one to another.

There are three main types of possible side effects of which parents should be aware, with the tetracyclines.

First, there are often mild but uncomfortable intestinal reactions (tetracycline itself tends to be less likely to cause such reactions than other members of the group). These occur because the drugs' sweeping antibacterial action can temporarily upset the normal balance of harmless organisms in the intestines. (For the same reason, there is a higher than usual possibility of the development of moniliasis in women and teenage girls.)

Second, the tetracyclines may cause photosensitivity in some people — an increased susceptibility to sunburn, even from fairly brief exposure; at this writing, demeclocycline appears most likely to pose this risk, minocycline least so. It is best to avoid exposure to the sun when any of these drugs is being taken.

Third, the tetracyclines can affect developing teeth (not teeth that have already formed, even though they may not have erupted), so that the teeth, when they appear, are stained yellow — a condition otherwise harmless, but certainly undesirable. For this reason, physicians generally avoid prescribing tetracyclines, unless absolutely necessary, for youngsters under the age of seven or eight, the age at which the permanent teeth at the front of the mouth are usually fully developed.

tobramycin (Nebcin) — a new, injectable antibiotic introduced in 1975 for the treatment of serious, potentially life-threatening infections of the bloodstream, central nervous system, lower respiratory tract, and urinary tract involving Gram-negative strains of bacteria. Like gentamicin and other useful but potent antibiotics to which it is chemically related, tobramycin can have toxic effects on the ears and kidneys. Hence, it is employed only in severe infections in which less hazardous agents have proved ineffective or are contraindicated; in carefully controlled dosages, for only a limited period of time; and with the patient under continuous observation in the hospital.

antibodies: substances produced by the body in response to, and as a counterattack against, the entrance of specific infectious organisms or of foreign bodies (including transplanted tissue). They may be produced naturally; or, their production may be stimulated by injecting a small quantity of an antigen in order to provoke the defense (which is the usual method of immunization). Or, if antibodies are needed in a great hurry — faster than the patient's own body can build up an effective supply — antibodies previously produced by someone else can be provided by injecting gamma globulin.

Also see GAMMA GLOBULIN; IMMUNITY; IMMUNIZATION; TRANSPLANTS.

antidepressants: powerful, and potentially toxic, drugs designed to combat emotional depression. They include two distinct chemical groups — the monamine oxidase (MAO) inhibitors, so-called because of the nature of their action on the nervous system, and the tricyclics, a term referring to their chemical structure. The former include isocarboxazid (Marplan), phenelzine (Nardil), and tranylcypromine (Parnate). Prominent tricyclic antidepressants include amitriptyline (Elavil, and also combined with perphenazine in Estrafon and Triavil), desipramine (Norpramin, Pertofrane), doxepin (Adapin, Sinequan), imipramine (Imavate, Presamine, Tofranil), nortriptyline (Aventyl), and protriptyline (Vivactil). None of these drugs are used in children under teen age, with one exception.

That exception is imipramine, which — alone among the tricyclics — has been found useful in dealing with persistent enuresis (nighttime bedwetting) in children age six and up. If this medication has been prescribed for your youngster, administer it very carefully, and be aware of the potential danger; overdoses can be, and have been, lethal. The usual dosage for this purpose is 25 or 50 milligrams, sometimes 75 or 100 mg in older children. Imipramine normally comes in 10-, 25- and 50-mg tablets. There is a chemically slightly different substance, trade-named Tofranil-PM, in which the single dosage is 150 mg; it is not intended for this purpose, and *should not be so used.*

antigens: any substances — bacteria, for example — that stimulate the body to manufacture special substances — antibodies, for example — in response. An *allergen,* which provokes an allergic reaction, is a special kind of antigen.

antihistamines: drugs designed to counteract or suppress a histaminic (allergic) reaction. Most have a slight sedative (drowsy-making) effect as well, although that varies considerably among the various antihistamines and with individual reactions. Antihistamines are *not* effective treatments for common colds or for other respiratory problems in which an infection, rather than an allergic reaction, is involved.

It's not a good idea to buy over-the-counter antihistamine preparations, for a number of reasons. One is that they may be a great waste of money, far more expensive (and far less effective, because most contain too little antihistamine) than a physician would prescribe. Another is that they usually are not merely antihistamines, but contain other ingredients, such as sympathomimetic decongestants, as well (the widely advertised product Allerest is one such, as are Novahistine and virtually all "sinus" medicines). And third and most important, the condition in question may not be an allergic one at all, and may require an entirely different type of treatment; only your physician can make that judgment.

If your doctor does prescribe antihistamine pills for your youngster (for a very small child, a liquid form may be specified instead), it's worthwhile to discuss the possibility of having the prescription written for the generic drug rather than a brand name if the pills are to be taken over a long period; the price difference may be considerable. There are many antihistamines; among the most widely used are chlorpheniramine maleate (available generically as well as by the trade names Chlor-Trimeton, Histaspan, Teldrin, and others, and among those least likely to cause drowsiness), diphenhydramine hydrochloride (best known by the trade name Benadryl, but also available generically and especially effective against allergy-related itching), and pyrilamine maleate. Cyproheptadine (Periactin; it is not available generically) is a prescription antihistamine given orally — in syrup or tablet form — to combat extensive itching such as that associated with hives, chickenpox, poison ivy, or multiple insect bites.

Sometimes, if the allergy is a persistent, chronic condition, the physician — often an ear, nose, and throat specialist — may prescribe small quantities of a number of different antihistamines, asking that each be used for a period of days and that the child then switch to another; this is done, because the effects *are* often so very individual, in order to find the one that is most effective and has the least number of undesirable side effects for the particular patient.

Antihistamines, alone or in combination with other medications, are also used — sometimes effectively and properly, sometimes not — in non-allergy situations. For comments on those, see COLD PILLS; DECONGESTANTS, NASAL; MOTION SICKNESS; SEDATIVES.

anti-inflammatories: There are a number of medications that act effectively against inflammation in various sites. The most broadly used, and an extremely effective one, is aspirin. The corticosteroids also reduce inflammation, as well as other kinds of symptoms (see that entry for a full discussion). Both of these are used for a variety of conditions — aspirin of course quite often, the corticosteroids in situations where the physician deems them necessary and desirable — in both children and adults.

Additionally, there are more powerful drugs designed specifically for use during acute flareups in chronic arthritic disorders, prominently indomethacin (Indocin) and two closely related drugs called butazones — oxyphenbutazone (Oxalid, Tandearil) and phenylbutazone (Azolid, Butazolidin). All three are extremely potent medications and are used only for brief periods; with all three, there are potentially critical side effects, including allergies and a great many toxicities (there is also potential cross-sensitivity between indomethacin and aspirin, even though they are not related chemically; that is, someone allergic to one may also have an allergic reaction to the other), and any untoward reactions must be reported to the prescribing physician promptly.

None of these three powerful drugs is considered safe for children under the age of fourteen.

antipyretic: a medication that acts to reduce fever (for which the medical term is pyrexia); the best-known example is aspirin.

antiseptic: a substance, designed for external or topical use on the skin or mucous membrane, inhibiting the growth of bacteria. A generation ago, it was thought desirable to keep antiseptics such as merbromin solution (Mercurochrome) and tincture of iodine in the family medicine chest. The thinking has changed. These substances are highly toxic if accidentally swallowed; further, they do no special good for the average wound, and may in fact interfere with the body's natural defenses against infection.

A small wound, after being thoroughly cleansed with soap and water, is best left open to the air to heal; in the case of a more serious injury, it should be left to the physician treating the wound to decide if the application of an antiseptic or other medication is desirable.

antitoxin: a substance developed in blood serum to fight *(anti)* the effects of a specific poison *(toxin)* resulting from a disease, bite, injury, etc. Antitoxins are chiefly produced from animal serum (especially that of horses), which is then purified for injection into humans; since some persons have serious allergic reactions to horse serum, antitoxins are increasingly being produced in human serum (tetanus antitoxin is now available in human-serum form).

Emergency antitoxin treatment is at this writing available for, among other things, botulism, diphtheria, scorpion stings, snakebite, some spider bites, and, as previously noted, tetanus.

antitussive: a cough remedy.

antivenin: antitoxin given to counter the effects of a venom, as in snakebite.

Antivert: a trade name for meclizine; see MOTION SICKNESS.

antrum: one of the antral sinuses; see SINUSES.

anus: the opening at the end of the rectum, through which fecal matter is discharged; its opening and closing is regulated by a circular muscle called the anal sphincter.

Itching around the anus, especially if it happens at night, may indicate that a child has pinworms, a condition much more common than most people think; see WORMS.

Also see, for comments on other special anal problems, ANAL FISSURE; HEMORRHOIDS; STENOSIS OF THE ANUS.

aorta: See BLOOD VESSELS.

APC tablets: pain relievers combining aspirin, phenacetin, and caffeine. They are potentially dangerous, and should not be given to a child or taken by anyone; phenacetin has been implicated in kidney disorders, and the federal government now requires a warning to be stated on products containing it. The ingredient has simply been removed from some such products; among these are Anacin (now containing only aspirin and caffeine) and Excedrin (now consisting of aspirin, two other related analgesics, and caffeine). Other preparations, notably Empirin Compound and Bromo-Seltzer, still include it.

For full discussion of these and other products promoted for the treatment of minor discomforts, see PAIN RELIEVERS.

Apgar score: a method, devised by the late anesthesiologist Virginia Apgar, of quickly evaluating the status of a newborn infant by using a sort of "checklist" on which numerical values are assigned — at one minute, and again at five minutes, after birth — to such items as heart rate, reflexes, and the like; the top "score" is ten. It may be repeated a specific number of hours later if it is considered desirable to double-check for either deterioration or improvement in the baby's condition.

aphasia: loss of the power of speech, usually due to an injury or illness involving the central nervous system; the word describes a condition, not the cause or prognosis (it may or may not be permanent).

aplastic anemia: See ANEMIA.

apnea: absence of, or marked deficiency in, respiration.

apophysis: the growing part of a long bone.

appendicitis: an inflammation of the appendix (see the next entry); it is unusual in a child under the age of five.

Symptoms of appendicitis may vary, and it does *not* usually begin with an intense pain in the lower right part of the abdomen. The first symptom is, very consistently, a general abdominal discomfort accompanied by loss of appetite. (If a child asks for food and eats eagerly, appendicitis can be ruled out.) Gradually, the pain will usually settle in that lower right area, which becomes rigid and tender to the touch. There may also be nausea or vomiting, and sometimes a low fever develops.

If your youngster exhibits *any* of these symptoms, appendicitis should be suspected. Give the child absolutely nothing to eat or drink — no food, no water, no laxatives or aspirin or any other medication. Have the child lie down and rest, and phone your doctor immediately. A sudden cessation of the pain is *not* a signal for you to relax; it could mean that the appendix has ruptured, and the child is in even greater danger (see PERITONITIS). If that happens, and you cannot reach your own doctor right away, rush the child to the nearest hospital emergency room.

Acute appendicitis is dealt with by surgery and possibly the administration of antibiotics.

appendix: a vermiform (worm-shaped) projection from a section of the large intestine, in the lower right part of the abdomen. The appendix is a vestigial organ, one that may have played some useful role at a prior time in human evolution, but has absolutely no function now. If it becomes inflamed, however, it can stir up a great deal of trouble (see the preceding entry); frequently, it is removed in the course of other abdominal surgery in order to eliminate the possibility of such trouble.

appetite: A child's appetite can vary even as an adult's can, and for many of the same reasons. Like grown-ups, youngsters tend to want less to eat in hot weather, and a somewhat smaller appetite on sticky summer days is nothing to be concerned about. A child's appetite is apt to be small, too, when he is sick, whether or not the illness has any direct connection with gastrointestinal problems (if it does, of course, you'll follow the doctor's specific instructions on diet); don't force him to eat, but simply offer small amounts of foods or liquids you know he likes and are easy to digest.

Infants, too, have variable appetites, although if you're nursing you're not especially aware of that fact. If you're bottle-feeding your baby, you'll be able to see that the amount consumed from feeding to feeding can vary a good deal. Remember that despite the fact that you measure out formula with scientific precision, your youngster's not a machine, and will be more or less hungry at some times than at others.

All these comments notwithstanding, you *should* discuss with your doctor any sudden and unexplained changes in your child's appetite. Either an abrupt loss of appetite *or* an unusual increase could be a symptom of something requiring medical consultation and is properly a cause for concern.

Also see BOTTLE FEEDING; BREAST FEEDING; FOOD, SOLID; OVERWEIGHT; UNDERWEIGHT; WEANING.

appetite suppressants: See AMPHETAMINES; DIET PILLS.

Appetrol: the trade name for an appetite suppressant; see AMPHETAMINES.

aprobarbital: See SEDATIVES.

arachidonic acid: a precursor of one of the prostaglandins believed involved in the inflammatory process (see PROSTAGLANDINS); its production is inhibited by aspirin and certain other anti-inflammatory drugs.

arbovirus: See VIRUSES.

Aristocort: See CORTICOSTEROIDS.

arm, broken: See FRACTURES.

Arrestin: See COUGHS.

arteries: See BLOOD VESSELS.

arthralgia: pain in a joint or joints, from whatever cause.

arthritis: inflammation and painful swelling in a joint or joints; the word is a descriptive one, and does not denote any particular type of arthritis or the reason for it. A number of things may cause arthritis, in addition to the conditions collectively known as the arthritic disorders (see the next paragraph, and also DERMATOMYOSITIS, LUPUS, and SCLERODERMA). It can result from injury to a joint. It is a typical accompaniment of certain systemic infections, notably rheumatic fever and — in adults and teens, less often in small children — rubella. It may also go along with such diverse infectious conditions as hepatitis (of which it is sometimes the first symptom), gonorrhea, tuberculosis, meningitis, and colitis, as well as with psoriasis (which is not an infectious disease) and with a few malignancies. It may on occasion signal a hypersensitive reaction to a medication. All of these are nonchronic, and treatment involves dealing with the cause rather than the symptom.

Rheumatoid arthritis (RA) is uncommon in children, but it does occur; children account for about one in twenty RA patients. It may take one of two forms.

One is essentially the same as RA in adults, develops gradually, and is likely to follow the same chronic flare-and-remission pattern as adult RA; persistent arthritis that continues into (or first appears in) the teens is likely to be this type.

The second, J(for juvenile)RA (although any nonspecific arthritis in a child is frequently referred to as JRA), also known as Still's Disease, typically comes on fairly suddenly, is often accompanied by fever and rash, sometimes includes enlargement of the spleen and lymph nodes, and may be self-limited — disappearing within weeks, months, or years with or without specific treatment. This second type does seem to have many characteristics of infection, although no infectious agent has been found, and no known anti-infection drugs are effective.

Either type is treated more or less symptomatically on an individual basis. Among the medications that have proved useful are analgesics such as aspirin; more potent painkillers if necessary; corticosteroids; and gold salts (a specific for RA), the use of which is called *chrysotherapy* or, less commonly, *aurotherapy*. The child's general health should also be safeguarded with adequate rest, a balanced diet, and protection from infection.

There are two other points of which parents should be aware. One is the question of rubella vaccination. In some children with RA, vaccination can aggravate the condition. That vaccination should properly have taken place at the age of one year. But if you have a child with RA who has for some reason not been vaccinated, you should know that many leading rheumatologists feel that the vaccination should be postponed until the arthritis has been in remission for quite a while, and it is a good idea to discuss the question with your pediatrician or family physician.

The other is that a serious eye condition called iridocyclitis, an inflammation of both the iris and certain other structures in the eyeball, occurs in a small but significant percentage of children with JRA, and prompt treatment is necessary to prevent scarring that could lead to visual loss. There are certain blood tests that can be helpful in predicting potential risk, including one that pinpoints something called rheumatoid factor, which is found in some 75 percent of (adult) RA patients; iridocyclitis appears highly unlikely to occur in children who manifest this factor, and may be related strictly to the typical juvenile type of RA. In any case, we would urge parents of an RA patient to have the child's eyes examined by an ophthalmologist at regular intervals (the condition can be detected only with the use of special instruments).

arthrocentesis: the withdrawal of fluid from a joint, usually to analyze it for the presence of infectious organisms.

artificial respiration: See RESPIRATORY RESUSCITATION.

ascaris: the technical term for the most prominent kind of roundworms; see WORMS.

ascites: a medical term meaning an accumulation of fluid in the abdomen. Ascites usually signals a kidney problem such as nephrosis, but may occasionally be symptomatic of other conditions including cardiac diseases, tumors, and liver problems.

ascorbic acid: another term for vitamin C; see NUTRITION.

aseptic: an adjective denoting the absence of bacteria. It might be used to describe, for example, a wound — and would then mean that the injury is free of infection. The word might also be used to characterize a particular condition, as in the phrase *aseptic necrosis* — meaning a necrosis (degeneration of tissue) not caused by infectious organisms.

aspartame: See SWEETENERS.

asphyxiation: If the problem is a foreign object the child has swallowed, see CHOKING; if smoke inhalation or carbon monoxide inhalation is involved, see GAS POISONING.

aspiration: medically, a word having two different meanings. One, the accidental drawing of a foreign body or substance into the airways; the other, the withdrawal of air or fluid from the body by suction.

aspirin: a mild antipain drug (analgesic), chemically termed acetylsalicylic acid (its name comes from *a*cetyl and *spir*aeic acid, the former name for salicylic acid), that also reduces fever, soothes inflammation, and acts as a mild "tranquilizer." Properly used, it is probably the most dependable and effective of all nonprescription drugs; *im*properly used, it is undoubtedly one of the most dangerous.

Aspirin is perfectly safe (with some

precautions and exceptions we'll come to) in normal dosage. For teenagers and adults, that is two five-grain tablets (the regular adult size), repeated in no fewer than four hours. For children, it is whatever dosage your physician specifies of the children's size (1¼-grain) tablets; if your child takes aspirin with difficulty, discuss with your doctor the advisability of using such variations as flavored tablets, aspirin in chewing-gum form, or rectal suppositories. (In a pinch, a tablet or capsule can be given rectally, although the former can be irritating and requires a lot of lubricant.)

There are a number of special precautions you should take in keeping and giving aspirin — but first, a brief comment on the product itself. It has not been demonstrated that any additives, extra ingredients, or "buffering" make aspirin either more effective, faster acting, or less likely to upset the stomach. Further, your doctor's specification of aspirin does not mean aspirin plus caffeine (the "combination of ingredients" you hear so much about) or plus anything else. It's most economical to buy the lowest priced U.S.P. aspirin you can find; if you prefer a brand name, fine — but make it plain aspirin. Any slight digestive sensitivity, which some people do have, can be tempered by giving the aspirin when there is food in the stomach, or by taking the aspirin with a *full* glass of water.

Now, for those important rules.

Don't store a large quantity of aspirin under conditions of high temperature or humidity, since these conditions cause the aspirin to decompose. Discard aspirin that is crumbly rather than firm, or that has a vinegary odor.

Don't keep aspirin — children's or adult size, flavored or plain — where any small child has access to it. Aspirin in large quantities can be highly toxic — in inverse proportion to the size of the person taking the overdose. In the past, aspirin has *headed the list* of substances responsible for accidental poisoning. Federal law now requires safety caps on aspirin and products containing it, but the safety factor is operative only if *you* follow directions carefully and close the bottle securely in the first place.

Don't ever give aspirin to a child under ten unless a physician has specifically directed that you do so — and then be sure to follow the dosage specified (which may not be the same as that suggested on the label).

Don't give aspirin for a severe pain (even a headache) or fever of unknown origin until the problem has been professionally diagnosed; aspirin can easily mask significant symptoms vital to the diagnosis. It is especially important not to give aspirin (or any other substance by mouth) if there is abdominal pain, since it could make the situation worse.

Don't continue giving a child aspirin, even if the doctor has suggested it, if the child has any unexpected or unusual reaction to it — a rash, for example, severe intestinal discomfort, or bleeding from any site. Such reactions may mean allergy. Call your doctor promptly if they appear.

Also see, for comment on other over-the-counter analgesics, PAIN RELIEVERS. Stronger antipain medications are discussed under NARCOTICS.

asthma: a chronic allergic condition

affecting the bronchial tubes; it afflicts some 6.5 million Americans and is the leading chronic problem in children. When a reaction or "attack" occurs, the muscle tissue of the tubes constricts spasmodically, squeezing the air passages; their inner lining swells, further narrowing the conduits; and secretions are produced that block the airways still more.

In an attack, the result of the various reactive events is a lack of air reaching the lungs, coupled with a feeling of choking. Typically, exhalation is particularly strained and there is a wheezing or whistling sound as the air is forced out. Attacks may last minutes or hours and can occur at any time, but are frequently worse at night. In an extremely severe attack, there may be cyanosis (a bluish tinge to the lips and skin) due to lack of oxygen.

Immediate treatment in an asthma attack may require the injection of epinephrine (adrenalin) and/or another drug that will have the effect of relaxing the bronchial tubes; if the condition has been previously pinpointed, you will have on hand medication, oral or by inhalation, prescribed by your doctor. (*Don't* depend on products you may see advertised on television or elsewhere.) If your child has asthma, your own doctor has doubtless instructed you on the appropriate steps to take, possibly including alerting the physician in case professional help is needed; those steps should be taken quickly and calmly.

There are also a number of steps parents can take *between* attacks to make them less frequent and less severe, and possibly avert them altogether.

One is medication taken on a regular basis, generally by inhalation; it typically works to reduce the severity of attacks and can even help prevent them by raising resistance to attack-triggering allergens. The most promising one, at present, is cromolyn sodium, first introduced in England in 1967 and approved for U.S. use in 1973; marketed here as Aarane and Intal, it has been found especially effective in children, though it has not yet been declared safe for those under the age of five.

Another major step parents can take is to track down, and help your child avoid, the elements that trigger attacks. Most asthmatic children, if they were extensively tested, would probably display multiple allergies; usually, however, some detective work on the part of parents can finger the chief culprit or culprits. They are almost always airborne — things breathed in by the child; the way to pinpoint them is to relate attacks to exposure to likely candidates. Among the latter are animal danders (dogs, cats, birds, etc.); certain pollens (to be suspected if the attacks are seasonal); bacteria normally present in the respiratory tract (there is a special vaccine available to combat this); animal fibers in fabrics; feathers in furnishings; and — by far the most common — ordinary house dust. For perhaps a quarter of asthmatic children, aspirin is also a trigger.

It is probably wise to see that the child's room contains no rugs, draperies, feather-filled pillows, or stuffed animals; to enclose wool blankets in synthetic covers, mattresses in plastic; to forbid pets in the room; and to wet-mop and -dust frequently (when the child is out of the room). If the nemesis narrows down to house dust, talk to your doctor about the possibility of desensitization treatments.

Emotional upset can occasionally trigger asthma attacks. As can, even more commonly, airborne but otherwise nonallergenic irritants. Among the latter are common air pollutants, chalk dust (a child with asthma is not a good candidate for blackboard monitor), and simple inhalation of cold air (in very brisk weather, the child should wear earmuffs or an ear-covering cap, perhaps a ski mask or a scarf wrapped over nose and mouth as well). You should also guard your child — so far as it's possible — from colds and flu; talk to your doctor about vaccination for the latter.

Finally, four major questions that often bother parents.

One: Will a move to another part of the country help? Usually, no, but if the allergens (or suspected allergens) involve pollens or airborne molds peculiar to your locale, the answer may possibly be yes; the question should be thoroughly discussed with your doctor, and if a move seems advisable, a waste of money can be avoided by first trying a few weeks' or months' "trial" stay in the new location.

Another: Do foods play a role? Again, usually, no — but there are exceptions. When foods are asthma triggers, they are commonly among those most often involved in hives: nuts, chocolate, wheat foods (especially buckwheat), milk, eggs, oranges, shellfish, synthetic flavorings in children's fruit-drink mixes. Your doctor can pinpoint any of these possibilities by elimination tests.

A third: How about removal of tonsils and adenoids? The answer is the same as that for any other child. If they are overgrown and are frequent sources of infection, yes; otherwise, no.

The fourth: Can a child outgrow asthma? Many do (how many adults do you know who have asthma?); the odds seem statistically best if the condition starts after the age of three. In general, attacks — even if they don't disappear altogether — usually become less severe over the years, partly because the bronchial tubes grow as the child does and are thus less easily blocked. By the time a boy or girl who previously needed desensitization treatments reaches college age, a prescribed regimen of antihistamines may provide sufficient control.

astigmatism: a visual defect involving a distortion in the shape of the lens of the eye so that it is unable to focus properly; its cause is unknown, although it is possible there are hereditary factors. The lens is flexible, and the tiny muscles that hold it in place will automatically try to correct the problem. If they succeed, vision will be accurate, but there will be symptoms such as a feeling of fatigue in the eyes, and possibly accompanying headache; if they don't succeed, vision will be distorted.

Astigmatism is corrected by glasses that compensate for the defective lens shape and, if necessary, for the nearsightedness or farsightedness that sometimes accompanies the condition. If the astigmatism is slight, the glasses may be prescribed only for reading; in a more serious astigmatism, the glasses are usually worn continuously. In occasional cases, the condition will disappear by itself after corrective glasses have been worn for a time.

If you suspect astigmatism in your child, a prompt visit to an ophthalmologist is in order; periodic vision examinations should in any case begin as soon as the youngster starts to read and take place as often thereafter as the doctor may recommend.

asymptomatic: without symptoms. The term may be used to describe a condition (the lack of reaction to the detectable presence of infectious organisms, for example, or a particular stage of an illness) or an individual.

Atarax: a trade name for hydroxyzine. See MOTION SICKNESS; SEDATIVES.

ataxia: loss of, or decrease in, muscular coordination, for whatever cause. Several types, all rare, are known to be hereditary; they include, prominently, Friedrich's ataxia, a recessive disorder which involves the spine basically and generally also affects the legs and, later, the arms.

atelectasis: a medical term describing the condition of a lung that is wholly or partly collapsed, whether at birth, because the lungs have failed to expand properly, or later as a result of a disease, a foreign body in the bronchial tubes, or injury to the chest.

athlete's foot: a highly contagious fungus infection of the feet, medically termed *tinea pedis,* and also known as ringworm (from the way the infection typically spreads out in a widening ring, not because there is any worm involved).

Athlete's foot can be effectively prevented by keeping children's feet dry inside their shoes and socks; the fungus likes warm, moist, enclosed space in which to operate. Teach children to dry their feet very thoroughly after bathing. Avoid shoes made of nonporous plastics that allow no ventilation. Sprinkle a little talcum inside the socks if feet tend to perspire a lot; in warm weather, let the youngsters go barefoot in the house and yard. The disinfectant footbaths often found in gymnasiums and at public swimming pools do help, but the solutions rapidly become diluted and so must be changed frequently if they are to do any good.

Typical symptoms of athlete's foot are familiar to anyone who has seen the condition; there is extensive cracking, peeling, and eventually blistering — especially on, between, and around the toes — often accompanied by itching. The problem can usually be dealt with successfully by a number of commercially available preparations. Soaking in a footbath of four tablespoons of Burow's solution (aluminum acetate) to each quart of hot water can be helpful. For ambulatory treatment, special antifungal powders and ointments (Desenex and Tinactin are two effective brands) can be obtained at your drugstore.

If there's no improvement after a few days, or if the situation worsens, do take the child to the doctor; there are more powerful fungicides, often needed in truly stubborn cases, that are available only by prescription. It's possible, too, for certain other conditions, including some allergic reactions, to manifest symptoms that are, to the untrained eye, quite similar; your doctor will know the difference.

atopic eczema: See ECZEMA.

atresia: the congenital absence of a normal, essential opening; anal atresia, for example, means that the normal channel through which the rectum empties is absent or is obscured by overgrown membrane. *Biliary* atresia — the absence of a normal bile duct, which results in backup of bile into the liver — affects about one in every twenty thousand babies born in this country. Atresia anywhere requires surgical correction.

Atromid-S: a trade name for clofibrate; see LIPIDS.

atrophy: a wasting-away or shrinking of tissue with time and lack of use — as of a muscle in a leg that has been in a cast for a lengthy period; such atrophy in children is usually quickly reversible, far more quickly than in adults.

atropine: a drug derived from the belladonna plant, and also manufactured synthetically; it is a smooth-muscle relaxant and dilator and works by paralyzing certain nerve endings when that effect is judged medically necessary. It is used in ophthalmology to dilate the pupils for examination of the interior of the eyes; in severe bronchitis, and sometimes prior to surgery, to relax spasms and to dry up secretions; to quicken the heartbeat in certain cases; and occasionally, usually in small amounts or in combination with other drugs, to calm intestinal spasms (but see the warning under DIARRHEA).

Atropine is highly toxic in large amounts; immediately apparent symptoms are dilated pupils, flushing, and extremely high fever (for first-aid treatment, see POISONING, HOUSEHOLD SUBSTANCES AND MEDICATIONS).

audiologist: See HEALTH PROFESSIONALS.

aura: a warning sensation felt prior to the onset of an episode involving the nervous system, as in epilepsy and migraine; in the latter, the sensation is longer lasting and generally referred to as a *prodrome.*

Aureomycin: a trade name for chlortetracycline, one of the tetracyclines; see ANTIBIOTICS.

auricle: See HEART.

aurotherapy: treatment with gold salts; see ARTHRITIS.

autism: an uncommon but by no means rare emotional problem that can afflict small children; it is also known as autistic syndrome. Generally evident before the age of three, it is typified by a group of symptoms which include a lack of normal emotional response (especially to people), a preference for the company of inanimate objects rather than parents or playmates, difficulty in communicating, and compulsive insistence on sameness and consistency.

The autistic child usually is disinclined to snuggle or be hugged. He is content to be alone in his crib or playpen, perhaps with a few special toys. He often follows a rigid pattern in moving about, and may insist that furniture and other objects be arranged in rigid patterns as well, shrieking shrilly and angrily if changes are made.

The causes of autism are not known, but more and more research into the problem has indicated that it may be congenital and there may be some biochemical aberration, possibly involving enzymes (it is not known to be hereditary, nor is handling by the parents at fault). Autistic children are not generally of below-average intelligence, and may in fact possess unusually good memories; a perhaps significant number of such children have been found to have musical talent.

Some cases of autism are more serious than others, but generally, if the diagnosis is made and treatment started early, the prognosis is good. It *is* necessary for the child to have continuing therapy over a period of time in a school or other institution specializing in the treatment of such children.

autoimmune: describing a condition, generally of unknown cause, in which the body's normal infection-fighting apparatus seems to be directed against the body's own tissues; the collagen diseases and rheumatoid arthritis are often referred to as autoimmune disorders.

autonomic: See NERVOUS SYSTEM.

Aventyl: a trade name for the drug nortriptyline; see ANTIDEPRESSANTS.

axilla: the armpit; the adjective is *axillary*. You are likely to hear the term most often in connection with temperature taking or with the enlargement of lymph nodes, some of which are located there.

azathioprine: See IMMUNOSUPPRESSANTS.

Azolid: a trade name for phenylbutazone; see ANTI-INFLAMMATORIES.

Azulfidine: a trade name for salicylazosulfapyridine; see SULFA DRUGS.

B

baby lotion: The commercial preparations are both safe and effective, and are usually pleasantly scented (which is a plus for you rather than for baby). But just as effective, and considerably less expensive, for use in the diaper area are zinc oxide and ordinary petroleum jelly; the former works best for some infants, the latter for others.

baby oil: It's of no particular use for babies — and should never be used as a sun-tanning preparation, as some teen-aimed advertising has urged; it offers no protection, can cause severe burning.

baby powder: Be sure that your baby powder does not contain zinc stearate; this substance can be extremely harmful to the baby's lungs if it is inhaled. The most economical baby powder is probably ordinary cornstarch; it's perfectly workable, and considerably cheaper.

Baciguent: a trade name for bacitracin; see ANTIBIOTICS.

bacillary dysentery: See DYSENTERY.

bacillus: See BACTERIA.

Bacimycin, bacitracin: See ANTIBIOTICS; the first word is a trade name for a medication combining bacitracin and neomycin.

backache: a malady traceable to a great variety of causes, including too-soft mattresses, ailments involving internal organs (as, the kidneys), diseases of the spine, pulled muscles or ligaments; the cause might even lie elsewhere, since a leg or foot problem, for example, can throw the body — thus, the back — out of alignment. If your youngster complains of backache, a check with your physician is in order; don't attempt to diagnose it yourself.

back and neck injuries: In any fall or similar accident involving the back or neck, treat the injury as a suspected spinal fracture; it will not hurt to do so, and it could be quite harmful *not* to do so. If the child is unable to move either arms or legs, or if sensation is lacking in either hands or feet, possible fracture should be even more strongly suspected.

Whether or not the latter situation prevails, the first rule is: *do not move the child* unless there is imminent danger of even worse injury, as in a fire. The wrong move, if there is indeed a fracture, could cause paralysis or even death. If the accident has occurred outdoors, and the weather is cold, simply cover the child with whatever is handy, and send for medical help immediately. *Don't* give anything to eat or drink (even water), or any kind of medication.

If the child *must* be moved out of a dangerous situation, the movement

Carry with Care

If a child who has a possible skull, neck, or spinal fracture must *be moved before professional care arrives — because of an immediate threat to life, such as fire — the movement must be done with extreme care in order to prevent further injury (in the case of a neck or spine fracture, the spinal cord is in imminent peril). A flat, rigid support, such as a wide board or door, should be used; once the child is correctly positioned on the makeshift "stretcher," ties should be used to prevent moving or shifting during transport.*

If the injury is a possible spinal fracture, *the child should be carried face down, arms bent with hands above the head.* ***If the skull or neck may be fractured*** *carry the child in a supine position, arms at sides, and don't let the child's head turn or roll to one side or the other.*

If the child is found lying in the proper position for transport, two people — or three, if needed and available — should lift him gently, very slightly, just enough to let others slide the "stretcher" beneath.

If the child is found in the opposite position — here a child whose spine may be fractured has been found on his back — he must be turned, but with continuing support. Two people should hold the stretcher over the child, as close as possible to him, with arms crisscrossed as in the illustration.

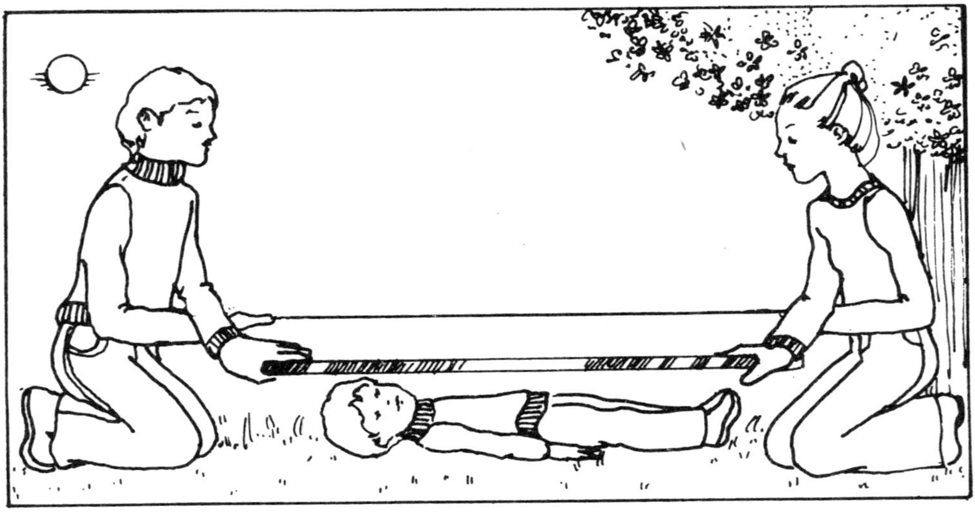

must be accomplished with as little disturbance to the neck and back as possible. (See the accompanying illustrations.) Have two or three other persons help, if possible. Get the child onto something flat — a door or a firm board — on the back, and keep the head and back carefully aligned while shifting the child onto the board; don't place a pillow or anything else under the head. And be sure the head does not roll to either side while he is being transported. Once you have the child out of the dangerous situation, get medical help as fast as possible.

Other types of back injuries are less serious, usually of the twist or pull variety; typically there is sudden pain at the time of the twist, followed by gradual stiffening, and the injury is a probable muscle strain. Apply heat — as, a

Two or three others — depending on the size of the child and how many people are available — should slip their hands beneath the child and press his body firmly against the "stretcher." The firm support continues as the board is turned through 180 degrees, until it is again horizontal and the child is in the correct position on it.

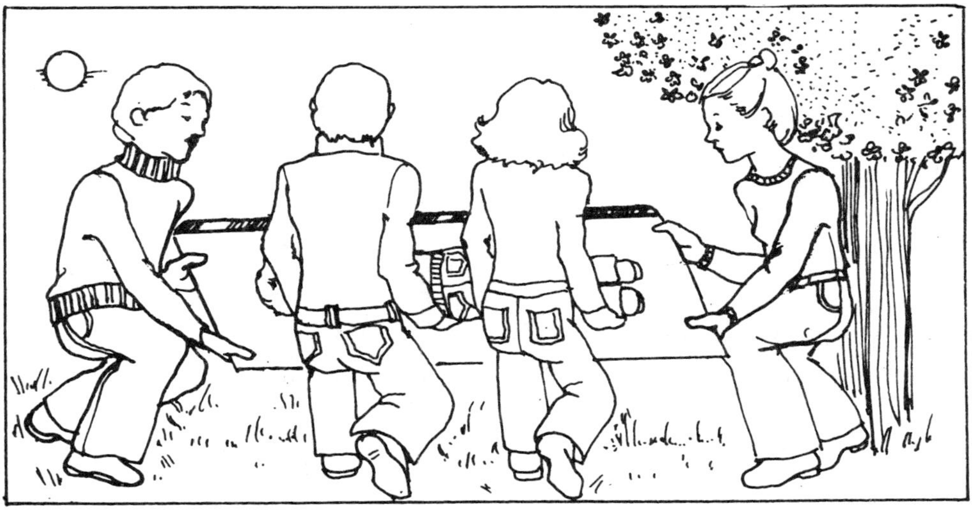

Here, the child is being carried correctly in the case of suspected spinal fracture, with ties to keep both legs and trunk from shifting about.

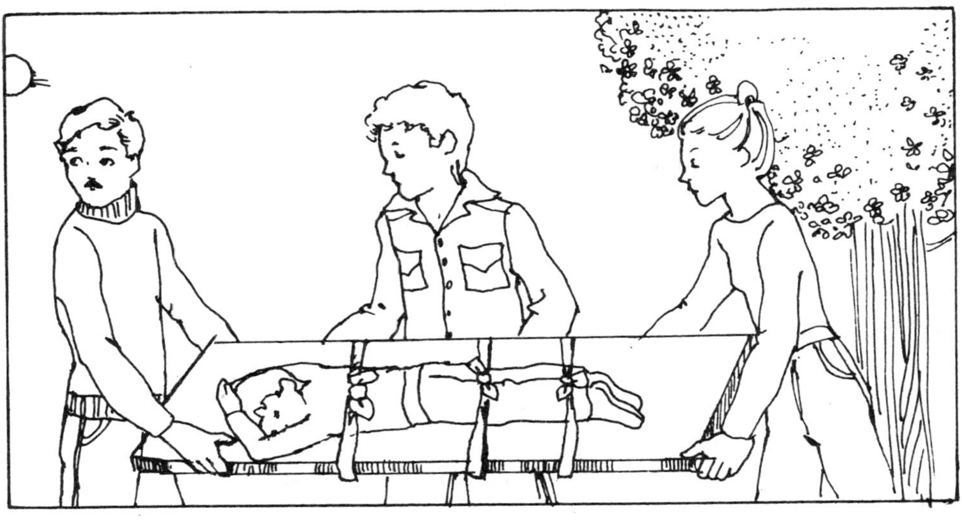

In case of a possible skull or neck fracture, the child should be transported on his back. An additional tie around the head, plus objects at each side — use blocks of wood, rolled towels or clothing, or whatever is available — help to prevent accidental head movement.

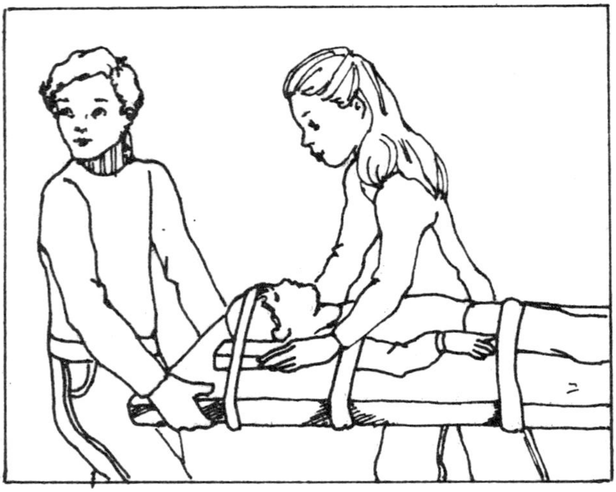

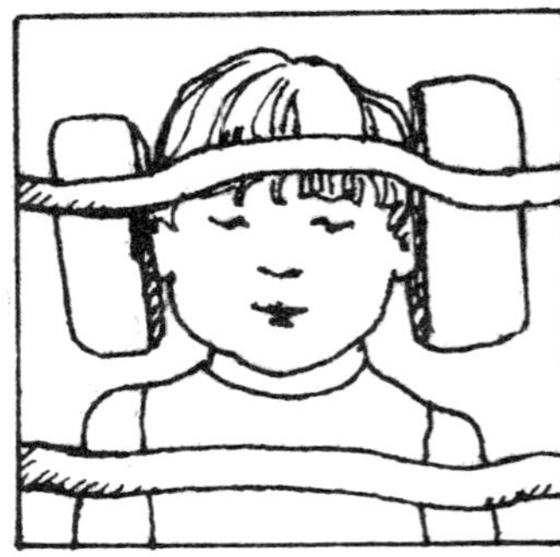

hot bath or a heating pad — and have the youngster rest in whatever position is most comfortable. Rarely does such an injury require medical attention (rest and time are the only cures), but it's a good idea to give your doctor a call and describe the problem, in case special advice or an examination of the child is indicated.

bacteria: a group of small, single-celled organisms, popularly called "germs," that cause a variety of diseases (although it should be noted that there are some harmless bacteria normally in the body as well). There are three classes of bacteria: the rod-shaped *bacillus* (diphtheria and tuberculosis are among the ills caused by bacilli); the more or less round *coccus* (diseases caused by cocci include pneumonia and the staph and strep infections); and the screw-shaped *spirochete* (spirochetes are responsible for cholera and syphilis, among others).

For a discussion of other major kinds of disease-causing organisms, see FUNGUS; RICKETTSIA; VIRUSES.

Bactocill: a trade name for oxacillin, a semisynthetic penicillin; see ANTIBIOTICS.

baking soda: another term for sodium bicarbonate; see ANTACIDS. Baking soda is also useful, in a tub-full of water, as an anti-itch bath.

balanitis: an inflammation of the penis or the clitoris.

baldness: hair loss, or absence, beyond the norm, medically called *alopecia.* Hair is normally shed and replaced continually; in adolescents and adults, this goes on at a rate of 25 to 100 hairs per day (the average head has a complement of 80,000 to 140,000; the number is usually lowest in redheads, highest in blondes, with brunettes falling somewhere in between). Medically, there are four main classifications of baldness; only three of these occur in youngsters.

Alopecia totalis is extremely rare and means, as its name implies, a complete loss or absence of hair — on the head and everywhere else (the other kinds of baldness pertain specifically to the hair on the head). It has been reported both congenitally (at birth) and as making a sudden appearance later. The cause is unknown, and no effective treatment has been found as yet.

Alopecia areata is the medical term for patchy baldness occurring in small-to-large areas on the head; it is not uncommon. Mechanical stress of some kind is often the culprit —rough yanking with a comb, too-tight ponytails, too tightly wound rollers, a child's habit of pulling at his or her hair, for example. Infections, toxic substances, and allergies can cause this problem, too, and sometimes patchy baldness (especially at the back of the head) is the first visible sign of ringworm of the scalp. Take your youngster to the doctor if the cause isn't immediately apparent. Once the cause of the condition has been determined and dealt with, the prognosis for regrowth is usually good.

Postinfectious alopecia is uncommon. It is, as you might guess, baldness that occurs after an infectious illness (it may be several months after); the illnesses most often involved are meningitis, pneumonia, and typhoid fever. This type of baldness can also occur following surgery or serious injury. It is usually temporary, with complete regrowth within six months or so.

The fourth kind of baldness is, of course, the familiar *male-pattern type* that is unlikely to concern you as a parent; it may begin as early as the twenties or as late as the seventies, or not at all. Male-pattern baldness is hereditary, and the gene involved is dominant but sex-limited; that is, it may be inherited from only one parent, but it will result in baldness in the later years only in the presence of male hormones. If a girl inherits the gene from one parent, there will be no effect, and if from both parents there may be a slight thinning of the hair in her later years; in either case, she can pass the gene on to her own children, thus affecting the future hirsuteness of her sons and grandsons. The baldness pattern itself — at what rate the hair recedes, whether or not the baldness eventually becomes total, and so on — varies from one family to another.

The incidence of male-pattern baldness also differs among races; it is most common among Mediterranean peoples, less so among other Caucasians, still less among Blacks, and least common among Orientals and American Indians.

bandages: Wounds requiring really extensive bandaging also require medical attention; there are a few bandages, however, that it's wise to have on hand for emergencies and for coping with smaller wounds and minor injuries, and some are referred to from time to time throughout this book. These are:

two-inch roller bandage for holding gauze or a splint in place (you'll find the subject of splinting covered under FRACTURES);

sterile gauze squares, individually

packaged in sealed envelopes, in two- and three-inch sizes, preferably the nonstick type;

adhesive tape — there's a hypoallergenic kind available, and it's the best type to have, since many youngsters are allergic to the ordinary kind;

adhesive strip bandages — Band-Aids and Curads are two widely sold brands — for protection of minor cuts and scratches;

a two-inch Ace elastic bandage for emergency use in case of a fractured rib and for use (but only on your doctor's instructions) on sprains and strains;

tubular gauze (Surgitube) for use on injured fingers and toes (try drugstores specializing in surgical supplies);

butterfly adhesives, which can be made

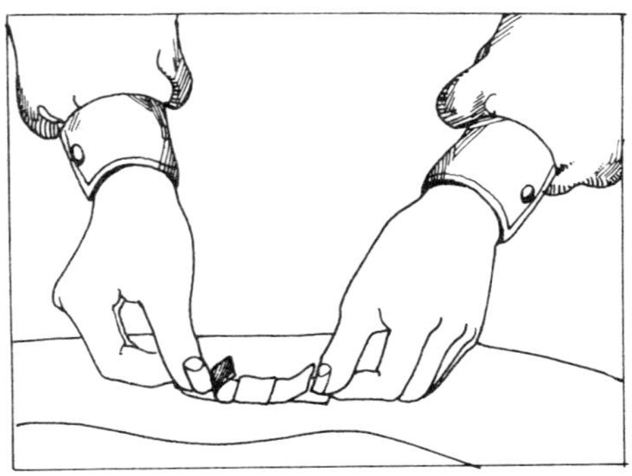

Keep It Clean
Adhesive strip bandages are packaged individually to assure that the gauze pad applied directly to a wound remains sterile; your fingering the gauze negates that precaution. Instead, apply the bandage as shown: grasp the flaps covering the gauze, turn the bandage over and apply the gauze directly to the wound without touching it yourself; continue pulling toward the ends until the flaps come away, then press the adhesive firmly.

Butterfly Bandage

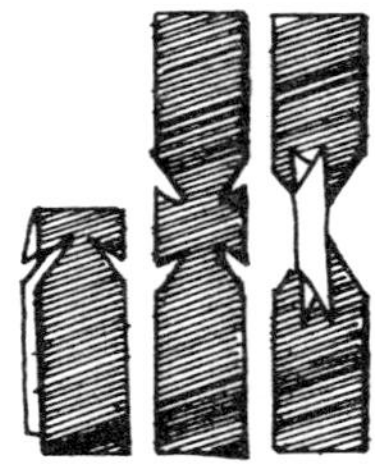

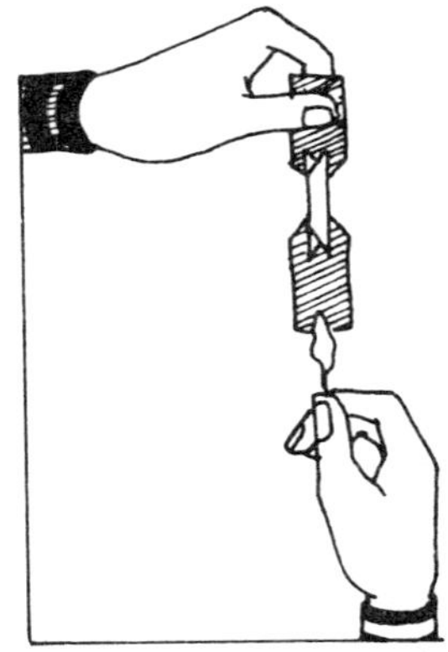

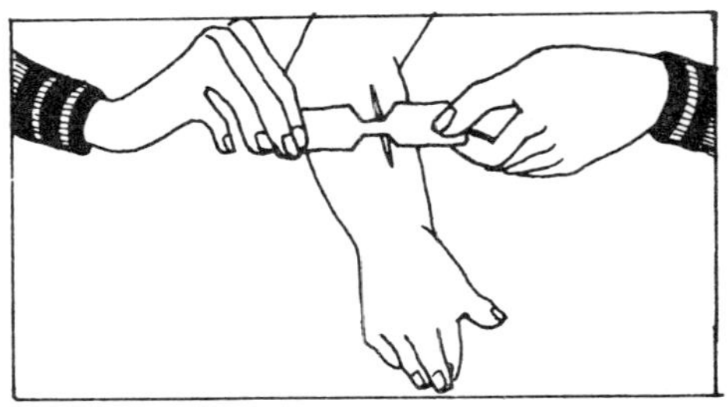

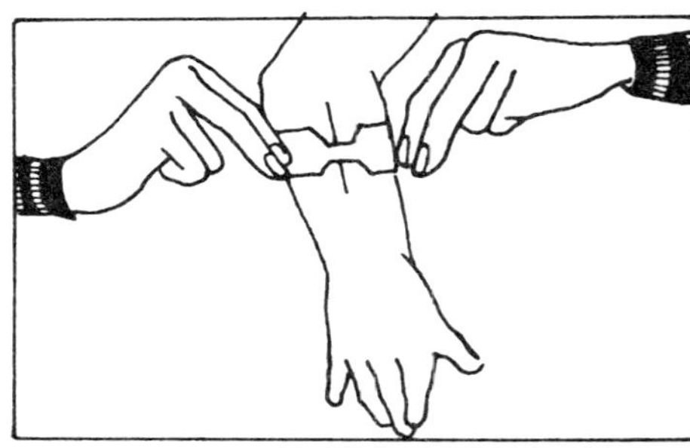

Butterflies are handy for small but slightly gaping cuts. Start with a piece of adhesive tape about an inch (2.5 cm) in width, three to four inches (7.5 to 10 cm) long. Fold in half, sticky side (indicated by shading in illustration) out; cut a notch at each side as shown. Unfold, then bend the two small flaps in to the sticky side, forming a nonsticky "bridge." Flame the adhesive ends briefly; that will make them adhere more securely. Holding that "bridge" slightly off-center, press down one end firmly; then pull the edges of the cut together and press down the other end. A gauze dressing can be applied over the butterfly, and should be if you think the area is likely to get dirty. For a longer cut, use two or three butterflies in a row.

by scissoring from adhesive tape or can be bought in ready-to-use form (buy the medium and large sizes only, since the smallest ones are too small to be really useful). Butterflies are especially useful for small but tricky cuts and have in general replaced stitching for many of the arm and leg wounds youngsters are prone to (facial cuts are, however, something else again, and should always be seen by a doctor). Their successful application may take a little practice, which it's best to do before a mishap occurs. See the illustration for how-to specifics.

Bang's disease: See BRUCELLOSIS.

barbiturates: See SEDATIVES.

barefoot walking: Walking shoeless is fine for your toddler's feet, and there's no real need to put shoes on him at all until he's ready to go out on the street. Indoors, or outdoors on sand or grass, going barefoot provides excellent foot-muscle development and exercise for any youngster; naturally, this doesn't apply if there's something potentially injurious around — such as hookworms in some parts of the southeastern United States, or sharp shell fragments littering a beach, or a great many splinters in a wood floor.

barium enema: a special diagnostic procedure in which the physician gives an enema with a fluid mixture of barium sulfate (a completely harmless compound) in order to make the large intestine opaque so that it will be visible on an X ray. The procedure is uncomfortable, but not painful. There may be a slight temporary constipation — or less commonly, diarrhea — afterward, and stools will be temporarily light in color.

Bartholin's cyst: really not a cyst in the usual sense, but actually an abscess — similar to a boil — occurring at the juncture of the vulva and vagina and involving lubricatory glands known as Bartholin's glands.

basal metabolism: See METABOLISM.

BCG vaccine: an antituberculosis vaccine widely used in Europe; the letters stand for Bacillus Calmette-Guerin. It is also an effective leprosy preventive in susceptible children, and is used for that purpose in parts of the world where the disease is endemic. In the United States, where widespread tuberculosis is a rarity and leprosy does not pose a serious threat, BCG vaccine is used only in dealing with special public-health problems involving those diseases and is not available to private physicians.

There has also been suggested the possibility — based on animal tests — that BCG vaccine may prevent certain types of cancer; such use of it is, at this time, purely experimental.

bedbug bites: See BITES AND STINGS.

bedsores: ulcerations in the skin resulting from constant pressure when a patient has spent a very long time in bed in a single position; they are quite uncommon in children. Occasional moving of the patient (assuming the condition permits it), periodic sponging, and frequent changing of bed linen usually prevent the problem. If bedsores do occur, they must be promptly treated by a physician in order to prevent extensive tissue damage.

bed-wetting: This problem generally decreases after the age of two, although it sometimes continues for several years, gradually growing less and less frequent; nighttime control is achieved after daytime control, so of course when bed-wetting ceases depends in part on when the youngster manages to stay dry during waking hours. Full control is generally achieved at an earlier age by girls, because they have a relatively greater bladder capacity than boys do.

Some children sleep unusually soundly and simply aren't conscious of the having-to-go sensation. Try to avoid giving fluids just before the child goes to sleep — and hustle him into the bathroom as soon as he awakens (a good deal of wetting occurs in that first few minutes).

Consistent or frequent bed-wetting after the age of about five is a medical problem, termed *enuresis*. The cause could be some emotional factor, or there could be a physical difficulty in the bladder or another part of the urinary tract. Sudden bed-wetting after a youngster has apparently achieved complete control could signal diabetes, or possibly an infection. Don't attempt to diagnose it yourself. Take the youngster to the doctor, who will analyze the child's urine and conduct a thorough examination to get at the precise cause. If no organic cause is found, you might discuss the possibility of a prescription drug that has sometimes proved helpful; see ANTIDEPRESSANTS.

For a discussion of the whole subject of achieving bladder and bowel control, see TOILET TRAINING.

bee stings: See BITES AND STINGS.

belladonna: See ATROPINE.

Bellergal: See MIGRAINE.

Bell's palsy: See FACIAL PALSY.

bellyache: See ABDOMINAL PAIN.

Benadryl: a trade name for diphenhydramine. See ANTIHISTAMINES; MOTION SICKNESS.

benign: harmless to other tissues or parts of the body, not cancerous or spreading; the opposite of *malignant*.

"Bennies": a slang term, among drug abusers, for the drug Benzedrine.

Bentyl: a trade name for a drug containing phenobarbital, a barbiturate; see SEDATIVES.

Benzedrine: a trade name for amphetamine; see AMPHETAMINES.

benzodiazepines: a class of "minor" tranquilizers and muscle relaxants; see SEDATIVES.

benzophenones: See SUNSCREENS.

benzphetamine: an appetite-suppressant agent; see DIET PILLS.

beriberi: an illness due to a severe lack of thiamine, one of the B vitamins; see DEFICIENCY DISEASES.

Beta-Chlor: a trade name for the hypnotic chloral betaine; see SEDATIVES.

bicarbonate of soda: See ANTACIDS.

biceps: See MUSCLES.

Bicillin: a trade name for penicillin G; see ANTIBIOTICS.

bicuspids: See TEETH.

b.i.d.: See PRESCRIPTIONS.

bilateral: involving both sides of the body or, if in reference to a problem affecting paired parts of the body (ears, legs, lungs, and so on), involving both parts; the opposite of *unilateral*.

bile: a fluid secreted by the liver into the small intestine, and also stored in, and secreted from, the gallbladder. Bile performs a number of helpful functions. It aids in digestion, especially of fatty foods, and is thus an important factor in the absorption of the fat-soluble vitamins A and D. It helps to stimulate the movement of the intestine. And it serves as the vehicle for certain waste products, especially pigments from normally decomposed hemoglobin, which are eventually excreted along with digestive wastes; it is these pigments that create the characteristic color of the feces.

Various tests concerning the function of the liver make use of the last fact. The finding of the pigments where they shouldn't be, and/or their absence from the normal places, will indicate to the doctor that something has gone wrong. If, for example, there is some obstruction of the flow of bile into the intestine, there might not only be a secretion of the bile found (by special tests) in the blood, but also in the urine (which might become unusually dark) and in the skin (the condition called jaundice); at the same time, since the pigments would not be leaving by the usual route, the stools might be unusually light in color.

bilirubin: one of the pigments produced in the destruction of red blood cells; a blood test for this pigment, used especially when there is jaundice in the newborn infant, provides the physician with an indication of the seriousness of the condition and the effectiveness of treatment.

biofeedback: an experimental therapeutic technique; its name combines the root word for "life" with "feedback," essentially a term borrowed from electronics. The technique is based upon the theory that individuals can learn to control internal activities heretofore believed completely involuntary. In brief, the patient is given training during which certain diagnostic readings — e.g., blood pressure, central-nervous-system activity, heart rhythm, or temperature differentials — are taken and made continuously available to the patient, who attempts to "will" certain beneficial changes in these readings in order to avert an epileptic seizure or an arthritic flare-up, reduce blood pressure, stabilize the heartbeat, or the like. Presumably, following the course of training, the patient will be able to effect these controls anywhere, any time. It is not easy to learn, and few have mastered it, but there have been reports of success with some individuals.

biopsy: an analysis of tissue removed — surgically, or by scraping from the skin, or by withdrawal through a needle — from a living person, either to determine if the tissue is malignant, or to check for the presence of infectious organisms, or for some other purpose. A biopsy may be done during the course of an operation (typically, to determine if more extensive surgery is indicated), or the tissue may be taken especially for biopsy; postoperative examination and analysis are also routinely performed whenever surgery involves any tissue or organ removal, as a matter of standard procedure at accredited hospitals.

Biotres: a topical medication combining bacitracin, neomycin, and polymyxin; see ANTIBIOTICS.

birth control: See CONTRACEPTION.

birth injury: an injury taking place during the process of delivery, as opposed to one that might occur while the infant is still in the womb. Many kinds of mishaps can cause a birth injury, including the slip of a surgical instrument, premature separation of the placenta, a sudden twisting of the umbilical cord, and so on, and such an injury might affect any part of the body. The situation is most serious, of course, if the baby's head has been injured, since there is the possibility of the injury affecting brain or nerve tissues.

One not uncommon — and usually not serious — birth injury sometimes afflicts extra-big, broad-shouldered babies; see BRACHIAL PARALYSIS.

birthmarks: marks, of varying types, found on the skin of the newborn infant; the term may sometimes be a misnomer, since while most are present at birth, some may not appear until shortly after birth. They are of unknown cause (certainly no fault of the parents), and are not dangerous, although they are sometimes unattractive. Most birthmarks of an especially unsightly nature, though, are temporary; if they persist beyond infancy, they can usually be medically removed (the question, if it arises, should be discussed with your youngster's doctor). Among the most common kinds of birthmarks:

Capillary hemangioma is the medical term for the flat pinkish spots that usually appear on the baby's eyelids or along the midline of the face or nape of the neck. They are overgrowths of small blood vessels (capillaries) near the surface of the skin, and they always fade with time.

Mongolian spot is a bluish discoloration that occurs most often at the base of the spine but can appear on the upper back as well; it usually disappears quickly. As its name implies, it is found in many peoples of the Far East; it occurs in almost all Orientals, in fact. Mongolian spot also occurs frequently in Blacks and in the darker-skinned Caucasian peoples of India and the Middle East.

Nevus, or *mole,* is a widespread kind of birthmark, familiar to most of us; it may or may not be present at birth. A mole may or may not be raised and may or may not be hairy; its color may range from light brown to bluish-black. Moles are, of course, permanent unless they are medically removed. Hairs in a hairy mole may be cut, but shouldn't be plucked. A later change in size or color should be reported to the doctor.

Port-wine stain looks like its name — a flat, deep-red marking resulting from dilated capillaries in the upper layer of the dermis (which is, in turn, the underlayer of the skin). A port-wine stain usually does not fade as the child grows older.

Strawberry mark may be present at birth but usually appears shortly thereafter. It is a harmless tumor of the small blood vessels; its name is an accurate description of its appearance. A strawberry mark may occur anywhere on the body, but the head, face, neck, and shoulders are the most common sites. This type of birthmark usually disappears completely, although it may grow slightly larger before it begins to fade. Treatment of any kind usually results in a worse scar than leaving the mark alone to disappear spontaneously.

BiSoDol: See ANTACIDS.

bites and stings: Here we detail first-aid and other immediate steps that should be taken, depending upon the source of the bite or sting. Sometimes, there are possible delayed complications of which you should be aware; you will find references, under the various types of bites and stings, to other appropriate entries.

First, two important points.

(1) *All* bites and stings, with the exception of minor insect bites to which there is no unusual reaction, should be seen by a physician; as soon as you have taken the steps detailed here, the child should be taken to your doctor or to the nearest hospital emergency room.

(2) All bites and stings that result in fairly deep puncture wounds carry the threat of tetanus infection. (See TETANUS for a full discussion.)

BITES BY PEOPLE

Don't underestimate the seriousness of such bites; many organisms that are innocent inhabitants of the mouth can be distinctly harmful in the bloodstream. Take time, before taking the child to a physician, only to cleanse the wound and the adjacent area with soap and water and cover it with sterile gauze (or a clean handkerchief or other clean cloth, if you have no gauze). Don't put anything else on the wound.

BITES BY OTHER MAMMALS

First-aid measures are identical with those for human bites — and you should also stop to do one other thing (or see that someone else attends to it): confine the animal if at all possible. If it is a wild one and it cannot be captured, the alternative is to try to kill it; the body should be saved for examination. The reason is that there are a number of infections that can be transmitted by the bite of a mammal, wild or domestic.

For the major threat — applying to any wild mammal, and to domestic mammals unless laboratory-born and -reared (such as most gerbils, guinea pigs, and the like) — see RABIES.

If the animal was a wild one in a nontropical area, see TULAREMIA.

If a feline, see CAT-SCRATCH FEVER (it can result from either a bite or a scratch).

And if a rat, also see RAT-BITE FEVER.

BITES BY SNAKES

Any snakebite should be handled as an acute emergency. Only a few of the several thousand snakebites that occur each year in the United States are inflicted by poisonous snakes — but those few can kill. And even a nonpoisonous snake is perfectly capable of inflicting an extremely serious bite.

The two families of poisonous snakes in the United States (see illustrations) attack differently, and so do their venoms.

Coral snakes bite and hang on with a chewing motion. There is little pain or swelling at first, but the venom attacks the nervous system; among signs of poisoning are salivation, difficulty in swallowing and speaking, sweating, vomiting, abdominal pain (having nothing to do with the site of the bite), and paralysis.

Pit vipers — rattlers and moccasins — strike quickly, with their jaws open; unless the bite site is a very small one (as, a finger or toe), a puncture mark is left at each side of the bite from the extra-long fang at each side of the snake's mouth. Typical results of the bite of members of this family include severe pain, discoloration and swelling at the site of the bite, and rapid

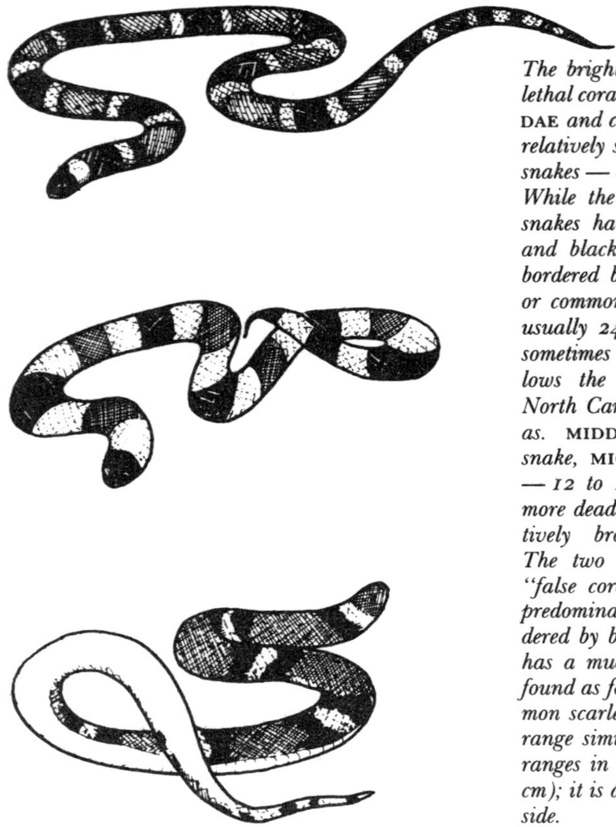

Poisonous Coral Snakes — and An Innocent Look-Alike

The bright red, black, and yellow colors of the lethal coral snakes, members of the family ELAPIDAE *and cousins of the cobras, are shared by the relatively shy and retiring, nonvenomous scarlet snakes — but in distinctively different patterns. While the corals' heads are black, the scarlet snakes have red heads; in the corals, the red and black bands never touch but are always bordered by yellow.* TOP: *the North American or common coral snake,* MICRURUS FULVIUS, *usually 24 to 30 inches (60 to 75 cm) long, sometimes more; note that a black band follows the yellow neck ring. It ranges from North Carolina south and west to central Texas.* MIDDLE: *the western or Arizona coral snake,* MICRUROIDES EURYXANTHUS, *smaller — 12 to 18 inches (30 to 45 cm)—but even more deadly; note the red band behind the relatively broader yellow "collar."* BOTTOM: *The two scarlet snakes are sometimes called "false corals," but as their name implies are predominantly red, each narrow yellow band bordered by black. The 18-inch scarlet king snake has a much broader range than the corals, is found as far north as the Great Lakes. The common scarlet snake,* shown, *has a geographical range similar to that of the common coral and ranges in size from 16 to 24 inches (40 to 60 cm); it is distinguished by its solid yellow underside.*

enlargement of nearby lymph nodes. There usually ensue weakness, sweating, nausea, and vomiting. The victim may faint. Other characteristic symptoms include a weak, rapid pulse, fever, and contracted pupils. In a very severe case, there may be internal bleeding and great difficulty in breathing. (There is one exception to the foregoing: the bite of the Mojave rattler. With this bite, there is little or no pain around the wound itself, and symptoms of poisoning are numbness at the site of the injury; numbness of the tongue, mouth, and scalp; headache; blurred vision; and respiratory distress.)

If you are sure the snake is not poisonous, first-aid measures are the same as those spelled out for bites by mammals; try to capture (or kill) the snake and save it for identification.

If you don't know, or aren't sure, if the snake is poisonous, assume the worst. Again, the snake should be saved for identification if possible. Then proceed as follows.

If the snake is definitely or probably poisonous, the first thing to do after killing or capturing the snake is — assuming you have a snakebite kit — to administer serum (antivenin), by injection. (There are two antivenins available in the United States, one for coral snakes, the other for moccasins and rattlers; hospitals in various areas stock the appropriate types.) Be sure to follow directions exactly, including any allergy test that must be done first. (If, after reading the directions, you're in doubt as to the exact amount of antivenin to inject, use a little more rather than a little less; in children particularly, proportionately more is often needed.) Then rush the child to the nearest hospital, lying down, if possible, with the wounded part a little lower than the rest of the body. The wound itself should simply be washed gently with cool water and covered with gauze or a clean handkerchief.

If you have no antivenin but can get the child to a hospital within half an hour, do so (as in preceding paragraph), at the same time taking measures to slow the circulation of the venom. If ice or extremely cold water is available, apply it to the area around the bite. If the bite is on an arm or leg, also apply a tourniquet: follow the illustrated directions under BLEEDING, be sure it's not too tight (you should be able to poke a finger under it), and loosen it, every ten minutes or so, for ninety seconds; if there is increasing swelling around the bite, move the tourniquet in advance of the swelling, i.e., toward the torso.

If you cannot reach a hospital within half an hour, you will have to make a fast attempt to remove some of the venom yourself. All the foregoing precautions — keeping the wounded part lower if possible, applying cold, using a tourniquet — should be carried out. Then take a clean knife or razor (ideally, sterile, but don't take time to do any sterilizing), bunch up the skin around the bite, and make crisscross cuts (like the letter X) over the wound; the cuts should be fairly deep, down to but not through the muscle (muscle looks like raw steak). Suck out the mixture of blood and venom through these cuts, spitting out each mouthful (venom isn't poisonous in the mouth). Continue for at least thirty minutes. Of course the child must still have professional medical care as quickly as possible.

BITES BY OTHER REPTILES

No other reptiles in the continental United States are capable of injecting a systemic poison when they bite. They can, however, inflict some extremely nasty wounds. The few that bite will not do so unless they are disturbed.

Turtles have no teeth, but a sharp, horny beak; a turtle bite can result in a serious puncture wound. There are three dangerous kinds, all found in or near fresh water: the common snapper and its larger relative the alligator snapper, which can be recognized by their long necks, powerful jaws, sharp claws, fairly long tails, and the jagged, toothlike projections at the back of the upper shell; and the "soft-shelled" turtle which has a very smooth upper shell, a very long neck, and an unusually long, sharp beak.

Turtle bites should receive the same basic first aid as mentioned ear-

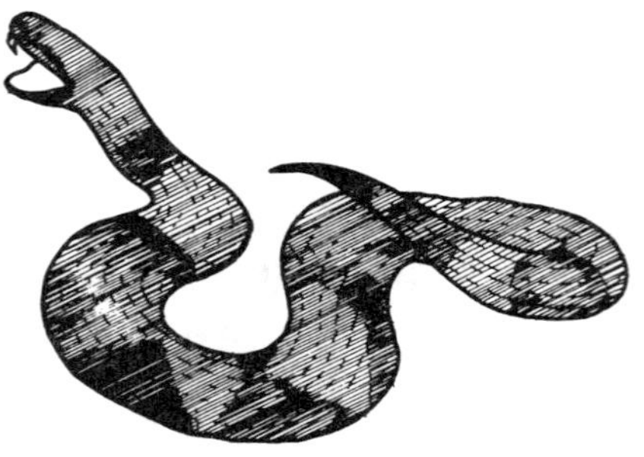

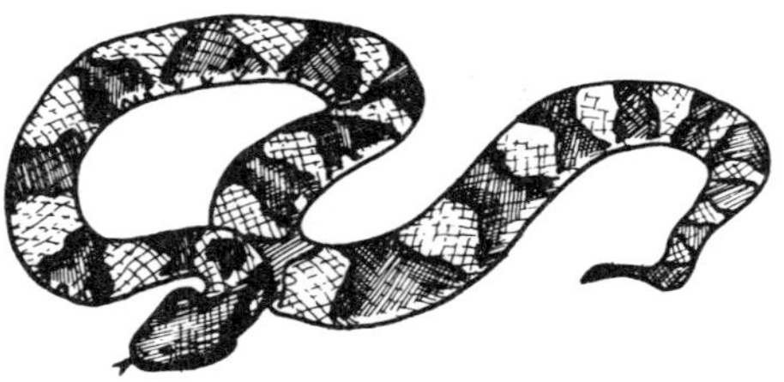

Moccasins

Like rattlers, moccasins belong to the family CROTALIDAE *or pit vipers; they are marked by tiny pits — not visible at a safe distance — at each side of the snake's head that function as heat sensors.* TOP: *The cottonmouth or water moccasin,* AGKISTRODON PISCIVORUS, *is a murky olive or brownish in hue, sometimes nearly black, with the diagonally barred pattern often indistinct except in very young snakes; it is generally three to five feet (about a meter to a meter and a half) long, but sometimes larger. The posture illustrated, in which it opens its mouth wide to reveal the white interior, is a warning display. It lurks in and about swamps and other still or slow-moving waters throughout the Southeast, westward to eastern Texas and north as far as Tennessee and Kentucky.* BOTTOM: *The highland moccasin or copperhead,* A. CONTORTRIX, *is slimmer and usually shorter than the lowland species — generally from 24 to 48 inches (60 to 120 cm) — and by and large less vicious. Its range extends from southern New England to northern Florida on the East Coast, westward to Nebraska, Kansas, Oklahoma, and Texas. Pattern and color may vary with the individual snake's age and habitat, but is usually the sort of configuration shown here, in varying shades of brown that may range from buff to rust, coffee, or taupe.*

Rattlesnakes

Rattlers are a unique group within the pit vipers, found only in the New World and mostly within the continental United States, which harbors over a dozen species; the eight most widely distributed are shown here. They are responsible for about 60 percent of poisonous bites. None are brightly colored (colors may vary from yellowish through browns and grays), and patterns may also vary, with locale and molting, from those shown here. Their distinguishing characteristic is the "rattle," an interlocking chain of hollow, horny segments that are multiplied as the snake grows; they may also break off from time to time, and a full-grown snake may have anywhere from six to — rarely — a dozen.

Few areas within the contiguous states are entirely devoid of indigenous rattlers, although they are concentrated in the West and Southwest. SHOWN, LEFT TO RIGHT AND TOP TO BOTTOM: *prairie rattler,* CROTALUS VIRIDIS, *greenish-tinged with roughly rectangular darker patches, two to five feet (60 cm to 1.5 m), with several subspecies covering the area from the Dakotas down to Texas and all points west; Massasauga rattler,* SISTRURUS CATENATUS *18 to 36 inches (45 to 90 cm), found in a diagonal sweep that extends from the Great Lakes southwestward to Arizona, New Mexico, and Texas (it lives in bogs and marshes in the East, drier country to the West); pigmy rattler,* S. MILIARIUS, *with varying spots that may appear blurry or "sooty," 15 to 30 inches (38 to 75 cm), confined to the Southeast (westward to eastern Texas, as far north as southern Missouri); eastern diamondback,* C. ADAMANTEUS, *at five (average) to nearly nine feet (1.5 to more than 2.5 m) our largest poisonous snake, distinguished by light diagonal streaks at each side of the head and tail striping, ranging near the Gulf and Atlantic coasts from Mississippi to North Carolina; sidewinder,* C. CERASTES, *with hornlike projections above its eyes and an odd, oblique gait that leaves a trail like a series of separate crochet needles, only 18 to 30 inches (45 to 75 cm), found only in sandy areas from southern Nevada southward; western diamondback,* C. ATROX, *marked much like its eastern cousin but tail stripes usually more obvious, four to seven feet (1.2 to 2.1 m), ranging from Arkansas to southeastern California*

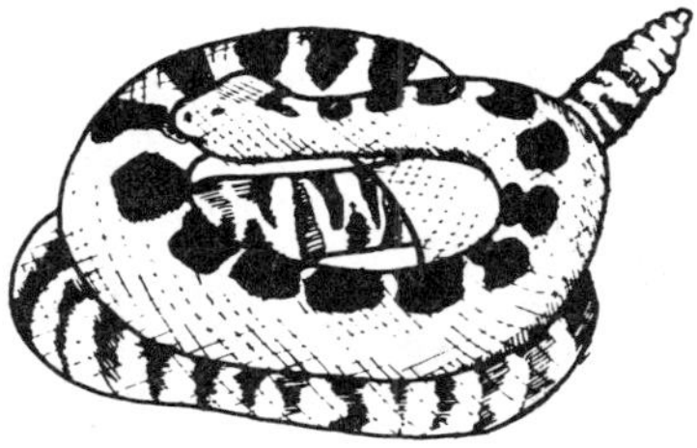

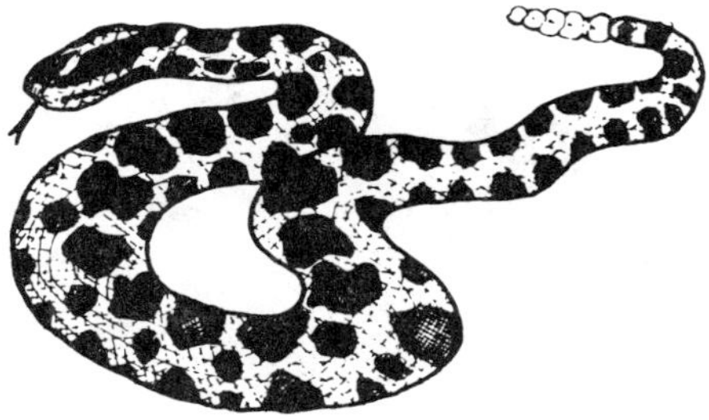

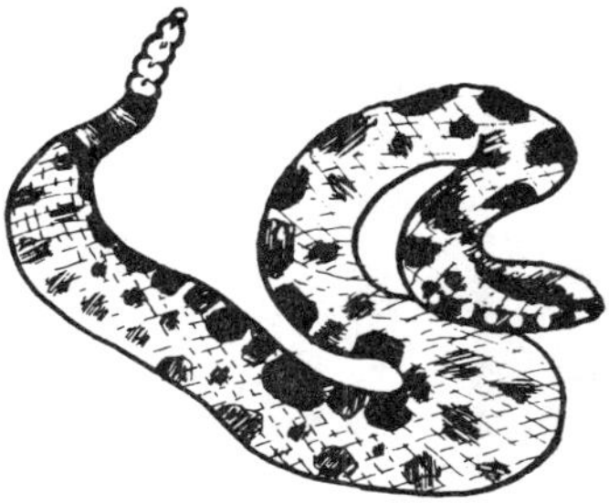

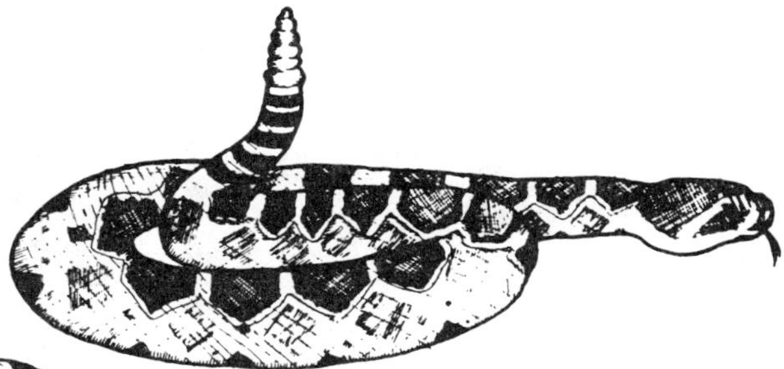

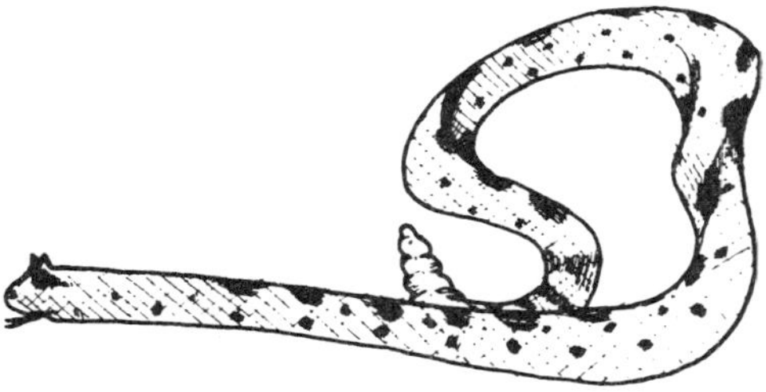

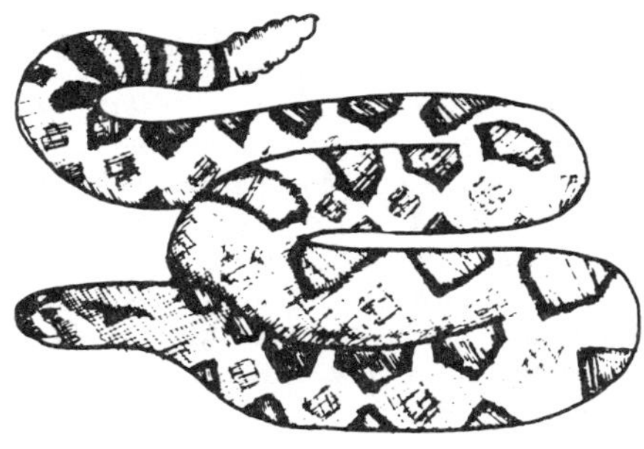

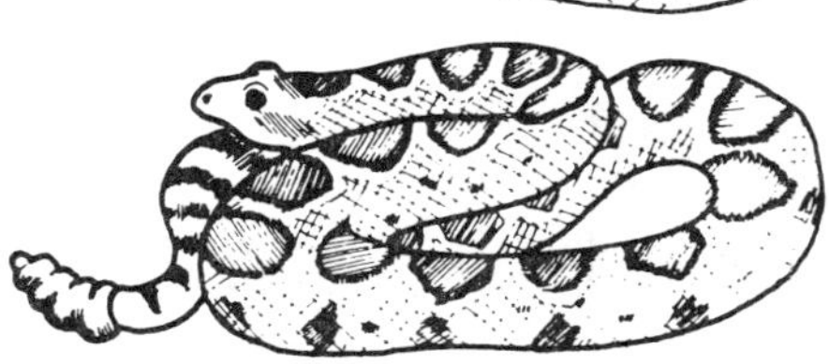

and southward; Mojave rattler, C. SCUTULATUS, *resembling the larger western diamondback but having a particularly insidious venom (see text), 30 to 40 inches (75 to 100 cm), found in the extreme Southwest from California's Mojave Desert to western Texas; timber rattler,* C. HORRIDUS, *variably patterned and sometimes appearing all black, somewhat more peaceable than other family members, about 40 inches (one meter) long but occasionally up to six feet (1.8 m), ranges from New England to northern Florida, westward as far as Texas, sometimes north to Minnesota.*

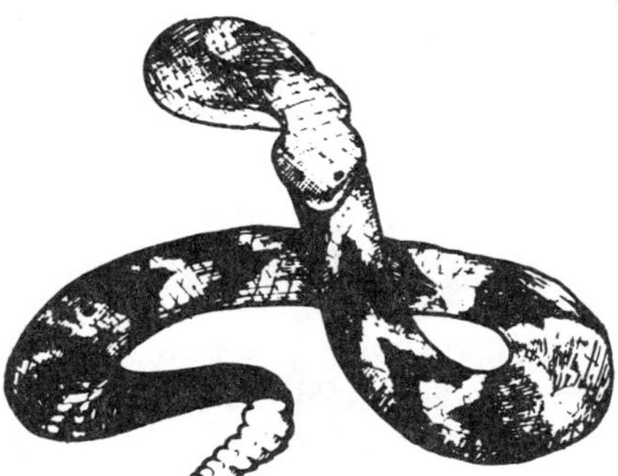

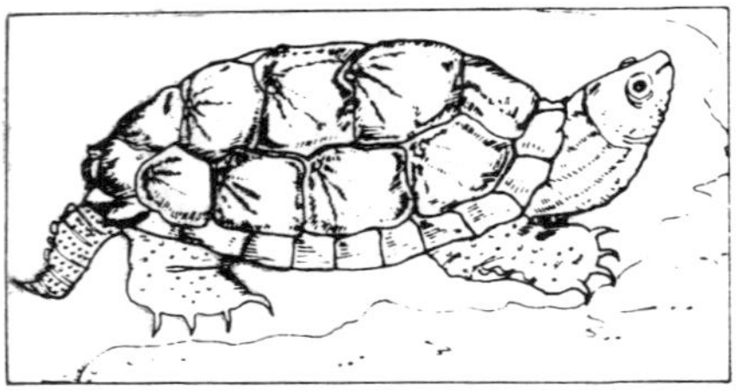

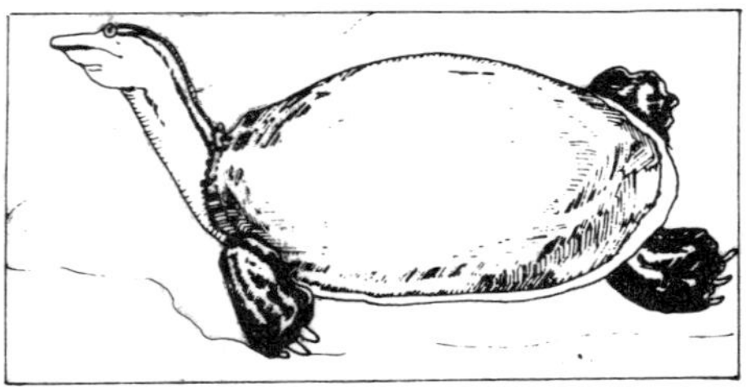

Dangerous Turtles
Turtles have no teeth and secrete no venom, but they can inflict nasty puncture wounds with their sharp beaks. TOP: *The habitat of the common snapper* (CHELYDRA SERPENTINA) *is the eastern two-thirds of the United States; it may be 18 inches (45 cm) or longer and may weigh up to 35 pounds (16 kg). Its giant relative, the alligator snapper — as large as 30 inches (75 cm), 150 pounds (68 kg) — lives chiefly along the Gulf coast, ranges northward as far as Kentucky. Note the long tail, bumpy carapace with sharp rear projections.* BOTTOM: *So-called "soft-shelled" turtles, about the size and weight of the common snapper, have smooth shells that appear nearly circular when viewed from above; there are two species, one without the tiny bumps at the front of the carapace. These turtles frequently hide by working their shells into the sand of shallow streams or ponds, only their long necks projecting.*

lier for bites in general; the strong potential for tetanus infection should be borne in mind.

Alligators and crocodiles, as is well known, are capable of inflicting critical and even lethal wounds — extensive cuts, fractures, or amputations

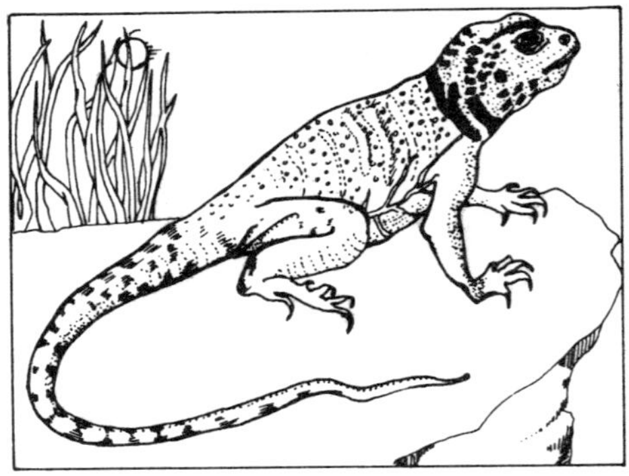

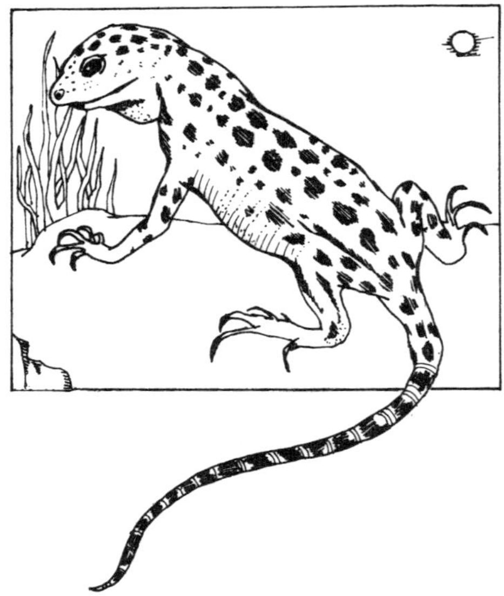

rather than mere bites. For first-aid measures, see the type of wound.

Lizards are typically placid creatures that rarely bite even if annoyed; only three types are potentially dangerous.

One of these is the collared lizard, identified by the distinctive black ring around its neck; a second is the leopard lizard, which has a leopardlike pattern on its back, along with a few bright red dots, and a horizontally striped tail. Bites by both these small

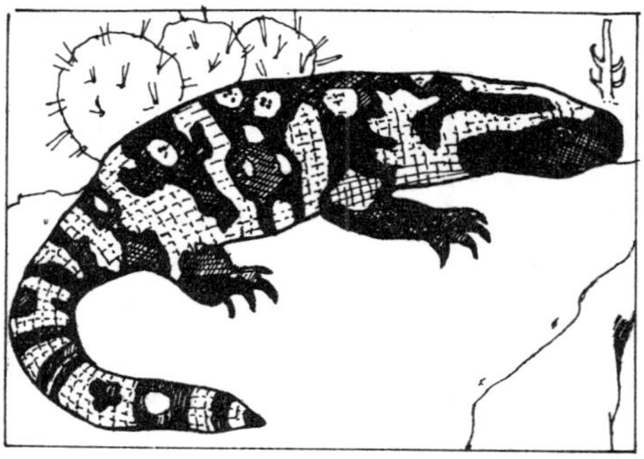

Unlovable Lizards
Most U.S. lizards have a fairly high annoyance threshold; exceptions are the three depicted here, all found in the southwest quadrant of the country. LEFT: *The collared lizard* (CROTAPHYTUS COLLARIS) *and leopard lizard* (GAMBELIA WISLIZENI) *are usually about four or five inches (10 to 12 cm) long from snout to base of tail, with the tail approximately double the body length (see text for further descriptive comment). The collared lizard is especially renowned for its speed; it has been clocked at more than sixteen miles an hour.* RIGHT: *The Gila monster,* HELODERMA SUSPECTUM, *is our only poisonous lizard and is in fact found mainly in Mexico; its range extends just slightly northward into Arizona and New Mexico. It is about two feet (a little over 60 cm) long, is of scientific interest because of its survival from ancient times, and currently enjoys protected-species status. To protect yourself, do not bother it; see text.*

lizards should be handled with the basic first-aid measures specified generally for animal bites.

The third is the large and surly Gila monster. Normally a sluggish beast, the rust-and-black Gila monster can whip about and bite with amazing speed and agility. It also secretes a venom from a gland in its lower jaw, but the poison is not injected as is a snake's, and it may or may not even seep into the wound. If it does, it will still not produce a systemic, life-threatening condition; the local reaction, however, is likely to be quite severe. A Gila monster bite, because of the possibility of that venom reaction, needs some special first-aid measures in addition to the basics, similar to some of those for snakebite: apply ice or cold compresses, if available, and, if the bite is on an arm or leg and it will take more than half an hour to reach medical care, use a tourniquet, following the prior directions for snakebite.

SCORPION STING

Scorpion venom, delivered by a stinger at the end of the tail, is both neurotoxic and hemolytic, but so far as the ones found in the United States go, fatalities are rare; the venom is not as potent as those of snakes and poisonous spiders found in this country. It is, nevertheless, a toxin, and a scorpion sting must be considered serious, especially for a small child.

The immediate result of the sting is burning pain at the site of the wound; the pain then spreads to the entire limb (arms and legs are the parts of the body stung most often). As the venom circulates, other symptoms arise — including headache, dizziness, salivation, nausea and vomiting, possibly vision and speech difficulties, respiratory problems, convulsion, and eventual shock — and a child is likely to become critically ill.

First-aid measures are minimal. Do what you can to retard circulation of the venom by applying ice, if it's available, to the site of the sting; keeping

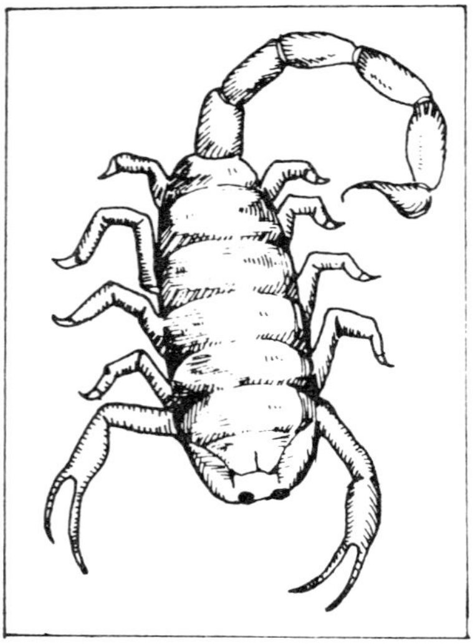

Scorpion
Scorpions cannot be mistaken for anything else; they resemble lobsters or crayfish — to which they are related. There is a curved stinger at the end of the tail. The one U.S. species that injects a venom with the sting is CENTRUROIDES SCULPTURATUS *of (chiefly) Arizona. It is smaller than some others that are not as dangerous — between 2 1/2 and 3 inches (6 to 7.5 cm) — and campers should be especially wary: stones and logs should be turned over before setting up camp, shoes and boots shaken vigorously and checked out carefully before putting them on in the morning.*

the child still, with the wounded limb lower than the rest of the body; and applying a tourniquet as for snakebite (two sections before this one). Take restorative measures if they seem necessary; see RESPIRATORY RESUSCITATION and TRAUMATIC SHOCK. Then rush the child to the hospital; there is an antivenin available, stocked by hospitals in scorpion-infested areas.

BITES BY SPIDERS, INSECTS, OTHER SMALL ARTHROPODS

By and large, with exceptions we'll specify, these bites are not serious matters. The typical localized histaminic reaction — generally itching and slight swelling — can usually be countered by applying rubbing alcohol, calamine lotion, or calamine combined with an antihistamine (Caladryl). If there are multiple bites, immersing the child in a cornstarch or baking-soda bath (put enough in to cloud the water) can relieve discomfort. Don't give the youngster antihistamines by mouth without consulting a physician.

Certainly if these measures don't work, and the itching remains unbearable, the doctor should be consulted; everything possible should be done to prevent the child from scratching (nails should, needless to say, be cut short), since scratching can very easily give rise to infection.

Any unusual symptoms beyond the localized discomfort should lead to suspicion of allergy, which requires prompt medical consultation. Such symptoms might include more extensive swelling, fever, rash, abdominal pain, and/or difficulty in breathing.

Some of those symptoms may also suggest systemic infection; a number of these creatures — in particular mosquitoes, ticks, lice, fleas, and mites — are vectors for infectious diseases. (See DENGUE; ENCEPHALITIS; MALARIA; PLAGUE; RELAPSING FEVER; TICK FEVER; TULAREMIA; TYPHOID FEVER; TYPHUS FEVER; YELLOW FEVER.) Such developments as fever, nausea or vomiting, enlarged lymph nodes,

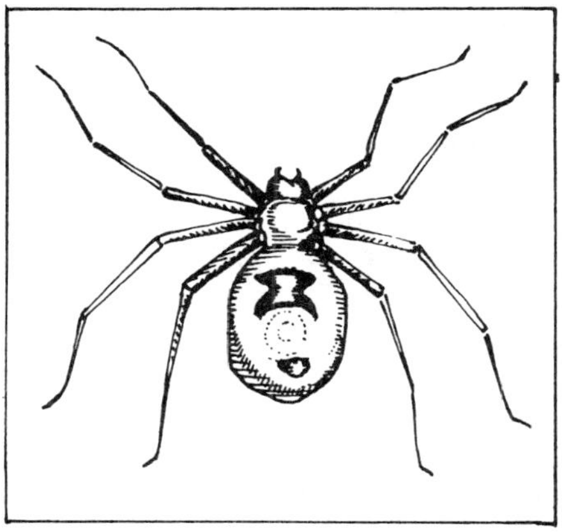

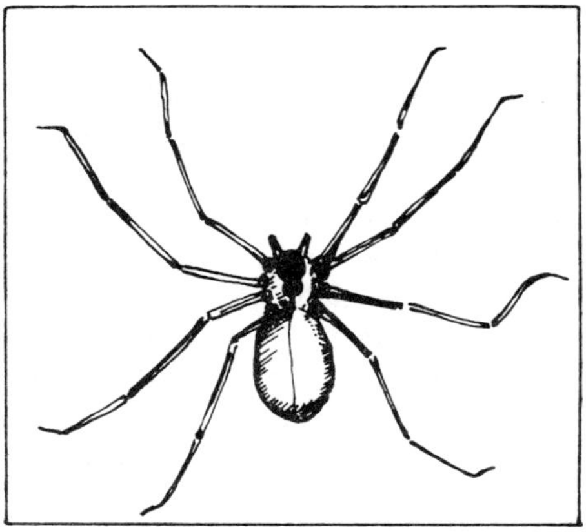

Poisonous Spiders
There are two species in our country, and both are now considered indigenous to the entire United States. See the text for the effects of their bites. LEFT: *The black widow,* LATRODECTUS MACTANS, *poses a danger, we regret to report, only via the female of the species — who, when she attacks anything else, has probably already paralyzed and consumed her mate. The spider's body is just under half an inch long (10 to 13 mm). The underside of the web-spinning female is shown here — all black, with the hourglass-shaped area and posterior spot bright red-orange: the edges of the "hourglass" can be seen from the sides. There may also be red or orange spots on the dorsal side. The area between the "hourglass" and the spot in the illustration is the spinneret from which the spider ejects her webbing material.* RIGHT: *The brown recluse or "fiddler,"* LOXOSCELES RECLUSA, *does not spin a web but lurks in dark, quiet places such as closets, behind furniture, or in unworn clothing. It is typically less than three-eighths of an inch (8 to 10 mm) long, with unusually long legs in proportion to its body. It is brown, its identifying mark a fiddle shape on the back of the head with the "neck" of the "fiddle" pointing toward the other end.*

muscle aches, marked weakness, rash, headache, abdominal pain, or breathing difficulty mean, again, that prompt medical attention is in order.

There are three possible sources of additional trouble.

The black widow spider is one of the two venomous spiders in the United States (see illustrations). Her bite first causes a sharp pain, with redness and slight swelling following quickly. The pain generally diminishes or even disappears within a few hours. But within an hour or two after the bite — if appropriate treatment is not given — symptoms of systemic poisoning will begin to appear. These typically include severe headache, muscular cramps, nausea and vomiting accompanied by abdominal cramps, sweating, salivating, and signs of impending shock; an infant or small child may go into convulsion. The possibility of death resulting is in inverse proportion to age.

There is an antivenin for the black widow bite, available only at hospitals — to one of which the child should be rushed without delay. Pause only to take basic first-aid measures, which are exactly the same (omitting the antivenin injection by you) as those for snakebite, including use of a tourniquet and sucking out the venom.

The brown recluse or "fiddler" spider, originally confined to the central and southern states, is now considered indigenous to the entire continental United States, and has been reported to have found its way to Hawaii as well. The fiddler's bite — which typically occurs at night or in a dark enclosure —at first causes only a stinging sensation, with slight to moderate discomfort. Over a period of hours — perhaps as many as eight — the pain gradually becomes intense, and a blister usually forms at the site of the bite; within 24 to 40 hours, the area will be discolored. By that time, necrosis (tissue destruction) is progressing in the deeper tissues, and if it continues, skin grafts and even extensive surgery may be needed to repair the damage.

Meanwhile, systemic effects of the poison will have become evident; they may vary somewhat from one person to another. A mild reaction usually includes nausea, abdominal cramps, chills, and some fever. In a more severe reaction, there may be a measles-like rash, a fever as high as 104° F. (40° C.), severe joint pains, and signs of impending shock.

The mere suspicion of a bite by the brown recluse means you should rush the child to the nearest hospital for emergency treatment, which generally includes the administration of cortisone (or some form thereof), antihistamines, and analgesics; care of the wound; and possibly other measures if necessary (the poison also attacks and destroys red blood cells, so transfusion may be needed). Do try to transport the child with the wounded part lower than the rest of the body, and if possible chill the area to slow the spread of the venom; *don't* apply a tourniquet, incise the wound, or take other measures.

No antivenin is yet available for the brown recluse bite, although there is hope that one may be formulated in the near future.

Ticks have a peculiar way of biting: the head of the tick actually penetrates the skin — and will remain there if the body is forcibly removed, so don't attempt such removal. Instead, cut off the tick's air supply by covering it with a thick film of petroleum jelly or butter; it will then drop off by itself.

Aside from the fact that ticks can carry tick fever and a number of other infections, they can also occasionally release a toxin. This phenomenon is not fully understood, but seems to be a largely unpredictable event involving pregnant ticks. Any sign of paralysis following a tick bite means the child should be rushed to the hospital.

INSECT STINGS

All the stinging insects are members of the order called Hymenoptera, which includes, prominently, bees, wasps, hornets, fire ants, and yellow jackets. Stings are always more painful than the wounds inflicted by biting insects, since they do contain a small amount of venom. The main problem, however, is the possibility of a severe allergic reaction; such reactions are not uncommon, and they can be lethal — so fast action is called for.

Turn to ANAPHYLACTIC SHOCK and be alert for symptoms, which, if they are going to appear, will be evident quickly.

Symptoms of a mild allergic reaction may involve only a rash and limited swelling; the reaction could be more severe on another occasion, however, and it is best to be prepared with material to counter that critical type of reaction.

If there is no reaction suggesting allergy, first — if the stinging insect is a honey bee, which leaves its stinger in the skin — remove the stinger; don't attempt to pull it out (it's very easily broken off), but remove it by scraping carefully with a clean knife or razor blade. Then apply cold compresses or, if some time has elapsed, hot compresses. For multiple stings, a warm tub filled with a full package of cornstarch can help to relieve itching. As with bites, do everything you can to prevent the child from scratching, which can trigger infection. Call your doctor if there is intractable pain or itching.

If you've learned that your child is allergic to insect stings and you think it might be very difficult to avoid the threat in future, you might discuss with your doctor the possibility of desensitization treatments, which can decrease the child's susceptibility to severe reactions. There are single extracts for the various insects, and in addition, there is a polyvalent substance for use in cases where a child — often a very small one — cannot clearly identify the insect that caused the problem; it offers protection against bees, wasps, hornets, and yellow jackets.

You can also help — whether your child is allergic or not — by the way you dress the child. These insects are attracted, for some reason, both to dark shades and to brightly colored floral patterns; light, solid colors or linear patterns are wise choices. Teens should be warned that scents (not just perfumes, but other scented cosmetics, hair sprays, etc.) also draw the insects.

CATERPILLAR STINGS

A number of caterpillars carry a minor venom in their tiny hairs or bristles — a protective device that helps safeguard this developing insect stage by discouraging natural predators. People stung by caterpillars are usually children who have poked curiously at them. The sting is quite painful, and there is usually marked swelling. The wound should be washed thoroughly, and spirits of ammonia — or rubbing alcohol, if you have no spirits of ammonia — applied to dilute the venom.

Sometimes a small child may have a severe reaction, signaled by vomiting, convulsion, or signs of impending shock (see TRAUMATIC SHOCK). If any of these occur, the child should be rushed to a hospital, and should be given no medication whatever.

If there are no such symptoms, but pain persists, the child may be given aspirin; if that doesn't do the trick, your doctor should be consulted.

STINGS OF SEA CREATURES

There are two major troublemakers lurking off U.S. continental shores — the sting ray and the Portuguese man-of-war (the tiny common jellyfish can sting, too, but with insufficient venom to cause much more than minor annoyance to anything as large as a human being).

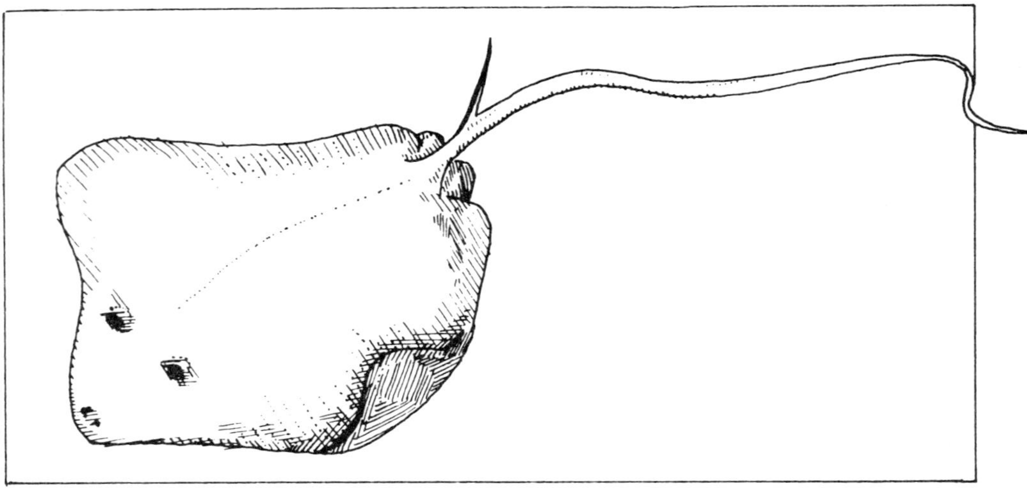

Sting Ray
In the United States, sting rays are found chiefly along the California coast; they have only occasionally been reported from the Atlantic seaboard. There are several species, ranging up to six feet (1.85 meters) across. Batlike in appearance, the rays are in fact closely related to sharks and skates: they are fish, but their skeletons are cartilaginous rather than bony; their "wings" are simply enlarged pectoral fins. The rays are bottom dwellers, feeding on plankton and other small organisms, and not vicious or prone to attack larger creatures; the barb at the base of the tail is there for defense.

The sting ray carries its venom in a defensive spike near the base of its tail (see illustration); its typical victim is an unwary wader who steps or falls on the animal. The sting of this bottom-dwelling fish is extremely painful, and the venom is also likely to trigger systemic reactions; possible symptoms of the latter include fever, vomiting, dizziness, headache, muscle spasms, and convulsions. Remove the stinger sheath if it is stuck in the wound — usually a deep puncture wound, with the potential for tetanus — and apply a tourniquet, following the tourniquet instructions for snakebite earlier in this entry. Do nothing else except rush the child to the nearest hospital.

The Portuguese man-of-war has many long tentacles, each equipped with millions of stinging cells called nematocysts; their function is the capture and paralysis of small fish and other prey — but they will cling to, and sting, anything they happen to encounter, including people. These stinging cells remain active for quite some time even if the animal has been cast up on the beach and has begun to disintegrate.

The sting produces an intense, burning pain similar to that of touching a hot iron, and the area will redden and swell fairly quickly. There are a number of potential complications, all of them critical. First-aid measures should be taken immediately, as follows.

First, remove any tentacles that may still be clinging to the victim — but *not*

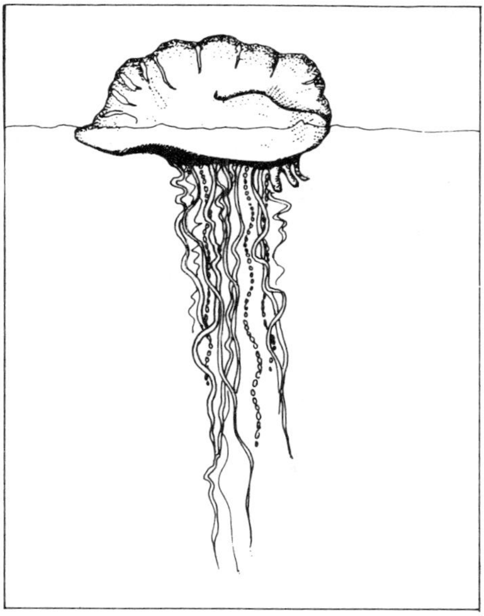

Portuguese Man-of-War
A coelenterate scientifically known as PHYSALIA PELAGICA, *this jellyfish is not actually a fish but an organism related to corals and sea anemones — not a single, sentient animal, but a colony of thousands of organisms that form its major structures: the pinkish-to-blue translucent bladder that floats on the surface, digestive organs, reproductive organs, and fishing tentacles. It is the last, ranging from 15 to 50 feet (4.6 to 15.2 meters) long or even longer, that carry the stinging cells, normally used to paralyze small fish and other prey but equally dangerous to anything they may encounter.*

Mid-ocean is the usual home of the men-of-war. Sometimes, though, they are cast up on a beach — in the United States, particularly along the Gulf coast and the Florida Atlantic shoreline. Because of the animal's primitive organization, it does not die all at once, and even apparently disintegrating tentacles may carry nematocysts — stinging cells — that are very much alive.

with your bare hands, or you may become a second victim. Cover them with alcohol or dry sand if either is available, then scrape them off, using a seashell, a piece of driftwood, or whatever is handy (or wrap something around your hands).

Next, check for signs of violent allergic reaction; see ANAPHYLACTIC SHOCK. Should such a reaction occur, it must be considered an immediate threat to life, and takes precedence over any other considerations.

Assuming you do not suspect severe allergic reaction, then check for signs of shock (see TRAUMATIC SHOCK, and follow the advice there).

When you have made sure that neither of those life-threatening conditions exists, then — and only then — turn to the wound. Apply spirits of ammonia or alcohol, whichever is readily available. It will hurt, but it will reduce the effect of the venom. Then get the child to medical aid without delay.

blackheads: pores clogged by solidified oils and waste materials; their color isn't due to dirt, but to oxidation of the oils. They're caused by a combination of excessive oiliness in the skin and a blockage of the normal avenues for release of the waste materials. Thorough regular cleansing helps, as does occasional use of one of the grainy deep-pore cleansers; it's best, too, to avoid or cut down on fats and oils in the diet. Don't try to remove blackheads at home, with mechanical devices or anything else; if extra cleansing and dietary efforts don't work, a dermatologist should be consulted.

Blackheads in teenagers are usually part of a larger problem; see ACNE.

black plague: See PLAGUE.

blackwater fever: a colloquial name for an uncommon complication of a form of malaria occurring in tropical areas; for some reason it afflicts males more frequently than females. Its characteristic symptoms include dark, bloody urine (hence, its name) and jaundice.

bladder: any saclike organ serving to store liquid (e.g., the gallbladder), but usually referring, when the word is used alone, to the urinary bladder, where urine is stored after its excretion (through the ureters) by the kidneys until it is eliminated (through the urethra). The bladder capacity of males at any age is smaller than that of females — which is why boys take longer to be toilet-trained and have more of a bed-wetting problem than girls.

For a discussion of the most common bladder ailment, see CYSTITIS.

bladder control: See TOILET TRAINING.

bleeding: Although the sight of blood can easily frighten both parent and child, it is not, *per se,* a cause for alarm; a great deal depends upon where the blood is coming from, how much, and under what circumstances. Do not panic.

Bleeding from the nose, if it is not preceded by a fall or blow, is probably not serious; see NOSEBLEED.

Bleeding from the vagina, if there has been no obvious injury, is probably not a cause for concern. In prepubertal girls, who are still investigating their bodies, there may simply be a self-inflicted scratch in the area (examine the child carefully). Menstrual periods are often very irregular in teenage girls; bleeding, even when a period is not "expected" according to the calendar, is likely to be — if there are no other symptoms — just an irregular period.

Bleeding following a blow on the head, from mouth, nose, or ears, may indicate a possible skull fracture; for emergency procedure, see HEAD INJURIES.

Bleeding from body openings following a fall or a severe blow (as being struck by a car) may indicate that there is *internal bleeding.* Symptoms might include coughed-up or vomited blood, blood from the nose, ears, or mouth, blood in the stool (or a coal-black stool); or, there may simply be symptoms of shock (typically clammy skin, nausea, shallow breathing). If internal bleeding is suspected, have the child lie down with his head lower than the rest of his body (unless a head injury is also involved, in which case his head should be elevated); loosen any tight clothing, such as collars or belts; keep him warm; and get medical care for him fast. Do *not* give him *anything,* even water, by mouth.

Any other bleeding from a body opening for which there is no apparent cause means that you should get medical attention immediately.

Bleeding from a cut or other wound is not necessarily a cause for great concern, even if there seems to be a great deal of blood; a very small cut in some areas, such as the scalp or lip, can bleed quite a lot. Apply pressure to the area with gauze or a clean handkerchief until the bleeding subsides enough so that you can investigate the exact extent of the wound.

If the injury is quite small, bleeding can be controlled by direct pressure on the wound itself. Simply hold the gauze or handkerchief firmly on the area for a few moments, until the blood starts to clot, which it will normally do fairly quickly; then either leave it to heal, or apply a butterfly or adhesive-strip bandage (see BANDAGES). If, however, bleeding continues uncontrollably from a very small injury, especially if it is a never-before-wounded infant, it may be a symptom of hemophilia, and the child must be rushed to the hospital.

A large wound, with really extensive bleeding, requires medical attention, and there are also first-aid measures you should take to prevent excessive blood loss. The condition is most critical if an artery has been cut, signaled by spurting blood, bright-red in color; extensive bleeding from a vein — darker red, flowing smoothly — is less critical, but nonetheless serious. In either case, the child must be rushed to a hospital emergency room, and in the meantime, everything possible should be done to control the bleeding.

If an arm or leg is involved, elevate it and apply pressure to the wound with gauze, a clean handkerchief, or other clean cloths (such as a torn-up sheet). Don't remove that material if the blood comes through it; simply pile additional material on top. If, despite these efforts, blood still continues to pour out of the wound, use a tourniquet; this is a last-resort measure, and must be used with care. Encircle the limb, above the injury (i.e., toward the torso), with any handy strip of cloth (necktie, roller bandage, strip torn from clothing, whatever is handy), and tie it once; then tie the ends again, around a stick (or any rod-shaped object). Twist the stick to tighten the tourniquet until the bleeding has ceased or slowed considerably. Be *sure* to release it at least every ten minutes; a continuous cut-off of blood for any longer period can cause gangrene. (See illustration on page 74.)

If another part of the body is wounded, a tourniquet cannot be used, and the pressure method described above is the only one that should be employed. And there is the possibility of another situation, which you must guard against; see TRAUMATIC SHOCK.

For comment on *blood in the urine,* see HEMATURIA.

blepharitis: a highly contagious and serious inflammation of the edges of the eyelids, caused usually by a staph or strep infection, and often following another (generalized) illness; it tends to afflict young children more often than older ones. Its appearance is unlike that of styes or other common eyelid ills: there is typically a series of tiny blisters at the roots of the lashes that may, if the condition remains untreated, eventually ulcerate and cause permanent scarring; this can, in turn, cause a distortion of the edge of the eyelid so that the lashes are twisted, turning inward against the eyeball itself. The prospects are not pleasant.

If you suspect your youngster may have blepharitis, the doctor should see him promptly; such medications as sulfa drugs and antibiotics can halt the infection quickly. Should blepharitis be diagnosed in anyone in the family, take precautions to make sure it's not spread to others — which it can be, easily — via little hands, towels, pillowcases, or slip-over-the-head clothing.

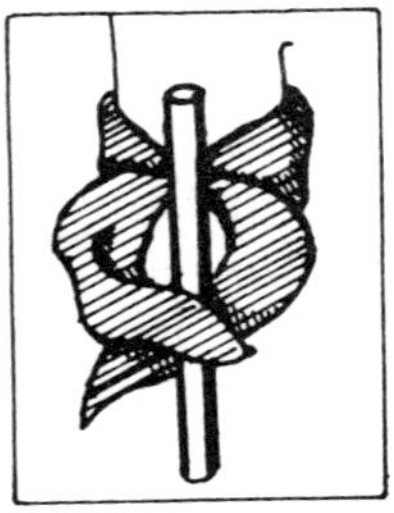

Using a Tourniquet

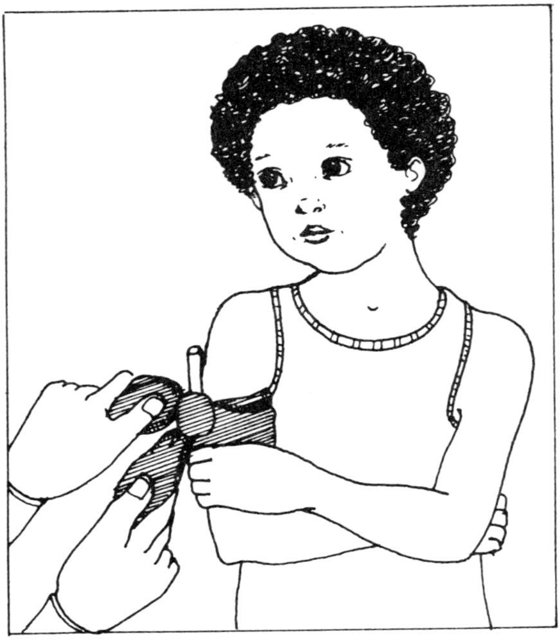

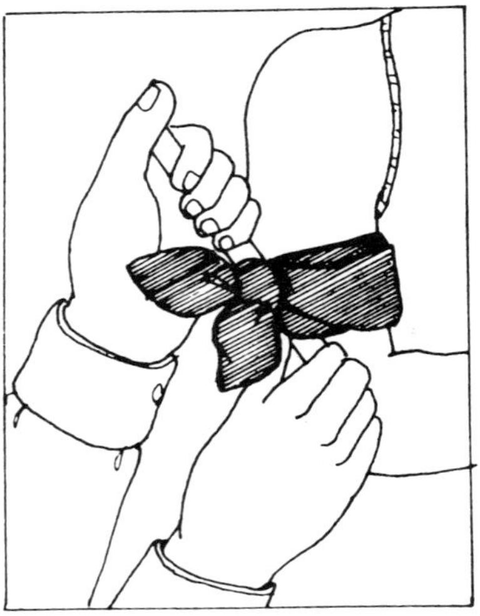

Illustrations show how this method might be used to stem bleeding from a forearm wound (see text for specific instructions). Strip of cloth is tied once around the limb, then again around stick or rod (small sketch); child can hold stick in place while second knot is tied (right). The stick is then twisted (bottom left) to tighten the band.

For a comparison of blepharitis with other inflammations and infections of the eyelids, see CHALAZION; CONJUNCTIVITIS; STYE; TRACHOMA. There is also a congenital condition that may seem to be an eyelid problem but isn't; see TEARDUCT STENOSIS.

blindness: a general term for an inability to see; it may be total or partial, temporary or permanent. Blindness may, rarely, be congenital; it may also be caused by a broad range of things including diseases of the eye, injury, and poisoning of various types.

It is crucial for the parent of a young child who is wholly or partially blind to realize two things. First: the lack of vision will necessarily cause a certain amount of delayed development — the child will not smile as early, sit up as early, and so on — that is no reflection on the child's intelligence, only on his ability to learn by watching, as is normally done; it's important to provide additional stimulation in other ways — touching, talking, music, and so on. Second: it will be helpful to enroll the child, as soon as possible, in a special school that understands the problem and can begin to help the youngster become a fully functioning, self-reliant human being — which an unsighted person *can* be if not treated as a helpless cripple.

blinking: See TIC.

blister: a fluid cushion formed, as a protective mechanism, under the top layer of the skin, when something has irritated or injured that top layer; familiar causes are burns, chemical irritations, allergic reactions, and simple friction (of an ill-fitting shoe, for example). Blisters may also occur at certain stages of rashes (as in chickenpox) or vaccinations (as, smallpox vaccinations). Never deliberately break open or prick a blister; it is best, in fact, to cover it so it won't be broken accidentally (a gauze square held lightly in place by adhesive tape usually works best). New skin is forming underneath, and when it is time, the blister will subside by itself; puncturing prior to that point will expose a raw area that will be not only painful, but open to infection as well.

If a child's blister breaks accidentally, it's best to have the doctor check to make sure there's no infection present or imminent.

Rarely, unexplained blisters can signal some special, unusual skin condition; see PEMPHIGUS.

Block Out: See SUNSCREENS.

blood blister: a small, dark-red formation resulting from a pinch injury. It looks like a blister, but it isn't really; the color is that of a broken blood vessel (the skin itself is unbroken and uninjured) that has formed a tiny clot or beneath-the-skin "scab." Blood blisters are not at all serious and should be left alone to heal by themselves.

blood-brain barrier: a mechanism, not fully understood, that to a great extent (the "barrier" is not a total one) bars the passage of substances from the bloodstream into the cerebrospinal fluid circulation. It is a highly selective mechanism, readily permitting the entry of glucose needed for the brain cells' continuing function, but quite effectively — most of the time, anyway — barring unwanted foes such as bacteria and toxins. Unfortunately the "barrier" also makes the treatment of some conditions involving the brain — such as Tay-Sachs disease — extremely difficult, if not impossible.

blood cells: There are three kinds of cells, sometimes (but now rarely) called corpuscles; each kind has its own special function. All three are continuously formed in the bone marrow and are held in suspension in the plasma, the liquid part of the blood.

Red cells contain a substance called hemoglobin that serves as the vehicle for transporting oxygen from the lungs to the various tissues of the body and carrying away their carbon-dioxide wastes. The red cells, at work around the clock, wear out fairly quickly; those ready to be retired are filtered out and destroyed by the spleen, to be replaced by newly produced cells. Each cell lasts about three months. Red cells are also known as erythrocytes, which means "red cells."

White cells — also known as leukocytes, which means "white cells" — are larger than the red cells, but normally much fewer in number. These are the body's front line of defense against infection, for they can actually attack and destroy invading bacteria. They tend to increase in number in the presence of infection (although their increase can mean other things as well), and this is a handy diagnostic clue for a physician.

Platelets (they are vaguely plate-like in shape) are very tiny, even smaller than the red cells, and are involved in the clotting process. They are sometimes referred to as thrombocytes, which simply means "clotting cells." When there is a wound, contact with the air causes the platelets to break up and put into motion chemical changes that result in the formation, from other elements in the blood, of a clot, or scab.

blood count: an analysis of a small blood sample as to its cell content (see previous entry) and other relevant data such as quality of hemoglobin, distribution of the various kinds of white cells (there are half-a-dozen microscopically distinct ones), and so on — all of which may provide vital clues for the physician in both diagnosis and treatment.

For some examples of the significance of blood counts, see ANEMIA; LEUKEMIA; LEUKOCYTOSIS; LEUKOPENIA; MONONUCLEOSIS.

blood groups: There are a number of methods of grouping (or "typing") blood, all involving factors or qualities that are present (or, as the case may be, absent) normally in the blood of a particular individual. All these factors are hereditary, and most — the M-N-MN groups, the M-N-S-U groups, and a great many more — are of interest only to anthropologists and others specializing in the study of heredity, migration of peoples from one part of the earth to another, intermarriage histories among various groups, and the like, for these breakdowns are very useful in tracing such matters. They can also be helpful in cases of questionable paternity.

Only one grouping system is of practical concern to you, or for that matter to your doctor, and that is the A-B-O system; these are the groups that are critical in blood transfusions, since certain types will prove incompatible with, and reject, certain others.

There are two "factors" and four distinct blood groups in the A-B-O system. Type A blood contains the "A factor," type B blood the "B factor," type AB blood both factors; type O blood contains neither factor. Any type will fight or "reject" — as if they were invading bacteria — factors alien to it; that is, antibodies will be produced.

Thus, a type O person who requires a transfusion needs type O blood, containing none of those alien factors; a type A person's blood will accept either type A or type O, but reject B or AB; a type B person's, similarly, will accept B or O but reject A or AB; while AB blood will accept any other type. Those with type AB are known as "universal recipients," while type O people, since their blood is accepted by all other types, are sometimes referred to as "universal donors" (this statement is not *wholly* true, since there is one other element that must also be considered; for an explanation of that, see RH FACTOR).

In rare instances, these groups and the reactions between them can cause a problem in an unborn child, a situation known as *A-B-O incompatibility.* This can occur only if the mother is type O, her baby is type A or B, *and* an unusually strong rejection mechanism goes into action against the baby's blood. When a mother is type O, the baby's blood group must be determined, and if the child is type A or B, he will be carefully observed for the appearance of jaundice so that treatment, if necessary, may be instituted promptly. The problem is far less serious than the other major mother-baby incompatibility reaction (again, see RH FACTOR).

The possibility of A-B-O incompatibility can be considered in advance by determining the blood groups of both parents, since the relevant factors are hereditary. Such determinations have also been introduced in paternity suits, although the conclusions must necessarily be of a negative nature: the identity of a putative father cannot be firmly established, but in certain instances such a charge can be proved false.

The genes for types A and B are dominant to those for type O, but not to each other. (For a full explanation of those terms, see HEREDITY.) A type O person can pass on only genes for this type. Members of the other groups can relay to their offspring genes for their own factors (meaning A *or* B for a type AB individual), as well as for type O if that recessive gene is present. There are thus a great many possibilities, but some can be readily eliminated. A child of blood group AB, for example, whose mother is type A, must have a type B or AB father; if a man accused of fathering the child is type O, the charge must be false. Further eliminations can be made, too, by using the M-N-MN and other blood groupings.

blood poisoning: See SEPTICEMIA.

blood pressure: the rhythmic pressure of the blood as it is pumped through the arteries, reflecting a number of factors including the strength and speed of the heartbeat, the volume of the blood, the condition of the arteries, and so on. It is expressed in figures — there are two of them — technically representing the height (in millimeters) of a column of mercury that could be supported by the force of the pressure. Actual columns of mercury aren't always used, of course; a sort of "pressure gauge" dial may be used instead (the instrument used is called a sphygmomanometer).

In reading blood pressure, a tight cuff is wrapped around the upper arm, cutting off the blood flow momentarily. The pressure is then gradually released and someone listening through a stethoscope placed below the cuff can hear exactly when the left ventricle of the heart contracts (it is then said to be in a state called *systole*) and when it is at rest *(diastole),* and can note the reading of the gauge at each instant. The two readings are known as the systolic pressure and the diastolic pressure, and together they comprise the blood-pressure reading for the individual, which is written as a fraction with the systolic on the top (as, 120/80) and spoken with the word over ("120 over 80").

Blood pressure normally varies with age and from one individual to another. The average newborn blood pressure is usually 75/40 or even lower; the figure rises to about 105/70 at the age of ten, about 120/80 in the average young adult, and may continue to increase with advancing years.

All of these "average" figures are subject to a great deal of variation from one person to another, and also from time to time within the same individual; among things that can cause a temporary rise in blood pressure are excitement, weight gain, kidney disease, endocrine malfunctions, and a variety of other ailments — while malnutrition, injury, extensive bleeding and a number of illnesses can cause it to fall. Neither an increase nor a decrease is, per se, evidence of illness; the reading will be considered by the physician in relation to other diagnostic factors and also, of course, in relation to the "norm" for the particular patient.

Chronic, or continuing, unusually high blood pressure is called *hypertension.* The opposite condition, blood pressure chronically lower than average, is called *hypotension,* and is not a cause for medical concern unless there are other specific symptoms of illness; it may in fact augur a longer-than-average life expectancy, generally speaking.

Individuals whose blood pressure tends to be lower than average sometimes experience a sudden definite drop — resulting in dizziness that lasts for several seconds and may be coupled with visual disorientation, or even in momentary fainting — on sudden changing of body position from lying down to sitting or from sitting to standing. This phenomenon is called *postural* or *orthostatic* hypotension, and it is caused by a temporary decrease in pressure in the cranial arteries. Even in susceptible people, it occurs only occasionally, and it is nothing to be concerned about; a youngster to whom this has happened should just be reminded not to jump out of bed or a low chair too abruptly.

The foregoing facts, all recounted in the first edition of this book, are still valid. There has been increasing concern, however, about the possibility of hypertension in young people since, if it becomes chronic and remains undetected and untreated, it can be a major factor in subsequent heart disease and shortening of life expectancy. Even children should have their blood pressure checked at regular intervals. It should be added that most cases — perhaps 90 percent — of increased pressure in youngsters under the age of fifteen are not the chronic type but due to a correctable condition such as kidney disease or some obstruction or injury involving the urinary tract.

The chronic, critical kind of hypertension, however, has been known to begin as early as the teens; in a nationwide screening program conducted during the years 1973 through 1975, in which more than a million people were tested, nearly four percent of those under the age of twenty were found to have abnormally elevated pressure. Experts now feel that everyone from high-school age upward should have a blood-pressure check at least once a year.

blood test: any analysis of a blood sample; purposes may include determining the type or composition, judging clotting ability or other characteristics, and/or checking for the presence of such things as bacteria, antibodies, pigments, sugar, cholesterol, etc.

See, for further comment on some types of tests and what they may determine, ACETONES; ACIDOSIS; ANEMIA; BILIRUBIN; BLOOD COUNT; BLOOD GROUPS; CAROTENEMIA; DIABETES MELLITUS; ELECTROLYTES; GLUCOSE TOLERANCE TEST; HYPOGLYCEMIA; LEUKEMIA; LEUKOCYTOSIS; LEUKOPENIA; LIPIDS; RH FACTOR. Blood tests also provide final diagnostic confirmation in a number of infectious diseases.

blood types: See BLOOD GROUPS.

blood vessels: There are three types in the general, or systemic, blood-circulation system (there's another system, and we'll get to it), and each kind has its own function.

Arteries carry oxygenated blood from the heart to the various tissues and organs throughout the body. The arterial flow begins in the left ventricle of the heart (see HEART for discussion of its parts), proceeds through the very large artery called the aorta, thence through a succession of smaller arteries (two middle-sized ones of which you probably have heard are the carotid arteries in the neck, which supply the brain and other structures in the head). Arterial blood is bright red in color, and when an artery is severed, the blood will tend to spurt out of the wound, in time with the rhythmic pumping of the heart.

Capillaries are very small vessels that serve as go-betweens, feeding directly to the outlying tissues from the smallest arteries, and carrying waste materials from the tissues to the veins. Capillaries are the vessels usually cut in small, commonplace wounds.

Veins carry the blood, now deoxygenated and containing waste materials, back to the heart from the various parts of the body (the jugular is the venous counterpart of the carotid artery); the venous flow empties into the heart's right auricle. Venous blood is dark red and seeps out fairly slowly and smoothly if a vein is cut.

The other system is the *pulmonary circulation,* a much smaller system that operates between the heart and the lungs. There are two major vessels. The pulmonary artery, unlike arteries in the systemic circulation, carries deoxygenated blood — from the right ventricle of the heart to the lungs, where it gives up its carbon dioxide and other waste materials and receives a fresh supply of oxygen. The refreshed blood returns to the left auricle of the heart through the pulmonary vein, thence goes on its way into the systemic circulation.

It is obviously crucial that all the vessels in the chain play their parts without interruption of the continuous flow, and it is a source of wonder that they generally do so. Occasionally something can go wrong: see ANEURYSM; COARCTATION OF THE AORTA; FISTULA; HEART DISEASE; PULMONARY STENOSIS; TETRALOGY OF FALLOT.

blotches: They can signify a number of things, including uneven sunburn, allergic reactions, the beginning of a rash of some specific illness; the rubella rash, for one, typically has a blotchy appearance, as does the rash of a mild childhood disease called erythema infectiosum (both are discussed separately under their own entries). Or, it could be simple pressure (as from leaning against something) on skin that's more sensitive than average. There is also a curious condition to which some toddlers are susceptible, sometimes called "Popsicle panniculitis" — a redness (actually of the fatty layer under the skin) that can appear within about 24 hours of contact with something very cold, such as snow, a piece of ice — or a Popsicle; it's not serious, and disappears gradually in four or five weeks. If the reason for the blotchiness is a mystery, and especially if there are other symptoms, the child should be seen by a physician.

"blue angels": a slang term, sometimes used by drug abusers, for amobarbital, a barbiturate; see SEDATIVES.

"blue babies": See TETRALOGY OF FALLOT.

boards: If you hear that a physician is studying for, is taking, or has passed, his or her "boards" (one who has passed may be referred to as "boarded"), the term refers to a qualifying examination in a particular specialty, sometimes in a subspecialty.

The American Medical Association recognizes 22 distinct specialties, including dermatology, family practice, internal medicine, neurology, pediatrics, psychiatry, and others (you'll find them listed under SPECIALTIES, MEDICAL). Boards comprised of distinguished experts in these areas hold periodic examinations for qualifying physicians (those who have served a residency and have had a specified amount of experience). Additionally, certain of the boards give exams testing competence in subspecialties; child neurology and child psychiatry are among these.

A physician who has passed the exam receives a special certificate and is entitled to style himself or herself a *diplomate* of the particular board. Such a physician generally offers above-average competence in his or her field.

boating safety: See ACCIDENTS, PREVENTION OF; DROWNING; FIRST-AID SUPPLIES.

boil: a bacterial (usually staph) infection of the skin, medically termed a *furuncle,* that involves oil glands and hair follicles; it is similar to a pimple, but markedly larger, harder, and redder. Eventually a yellow pus-filled abscess forms at the center, and the child may also experience general malaise and possibly fever. A boil can be a symptom of a generally rundown, low-resistance condition; or, if left untreated, it can help bring about such a condition.

Never treat a boil at home, by squeezing it or by any other means; the infection can easily spread, and serious scarring can result as well. Simply keep the surrounding skin clean and dry, and take the child to the doctor, who will judge the seriousness of the condition and may prescribe various remedies internally and/or externally, including sulfa drugs or antibiotics if necessary. If the youngster is running a fever, bed rest may be recommended for a day or two.

Boils can occur singly, multiply, or in groups (see CARBUNCLE). If they are multiple, or they recur frequently, there may be some other factor involved; diabetes mellitus is one possibility, and another is hypersensitivity to the bacteria normally found on the skin. One preventive, in the latter case, is frequent cleansing with antibacterial soap, such as one containing hexachlorophene, which your doctor can prescribe. Occasionally it is considered advisable to desensitize the child to the bacteria; this is done by a series of injections.

bones, broken: See FRACTURES.

Bonine: a trade name for meclizine; see MOTION SICKNESS.

booboo: an as yet ill-understood phenomenon apparently peculiar to infants and preschoolers, involving a lesion of varying description — but usually acquired under traumatic circumstances — which responds (uniquely) to the incantation, "Let me kiss it and make it well." While few researchers have conducted controlled studies, many clinicians have testified (albeit informally) to the prevalence of the phenomenon and the efficacy of the therapy; a substantial number of parents have volunteered similar observations.

booster shots: See IMMUNIZATION.

boric acid: a highly toxic substance that has no helpful part to play in the care of your baby and should not be kept in the house. It is relatively useless as an antiseptic. An infant can actually be poisoned through ill-advised use of boric acid for the treatment of diaper rash. Any advice you may read or receive advocating its use to rinse diapers, treat burns, apply to scalp infections, or care for an infant's ears is plainly *wrong*.

bottle feeding: There are a number of advantages to bottle-feeding your baby, should you decide to do so (and the decision, of course, is yours); some are obvious, others less so.

Bottle feeding can be done by someone other than the mother — the baby's father, a baby-sitter — and thus offers more coming-and-going freedom for the mother. Your baby receives a standardized, dependably nutritious formula (no matter what the *mother*'s nutritional condition), safely free of any medications it might be necessary for the mother to take. Cow's milk can be further fortified with vitamins if your pediatrician finds it advisable, which human milk can't be.

Aside from the necessity of formula making, there is one disadvantage: infant allergies to formulas are not uncommon; if your baby seems to develop cramps and go on crying jags following feedings, and if a rash appears as well, there's a strong possibility that allergy is the problem. If you suspect an allergy, discuss the question with your pediatrician; the formula can be changed.

The content and preparation of baby's formula — the type of milk, the kind and quantity of sugar — and the feeding schedule itself should be discussed with your pediatrician from the start. There are no generally applicable rules; the doctor's advice will be geared to your own baby's needs. One traditional "rule," incidentally, has now been abandoned: baby's bottles need *not* be warmed; it will do no harm if the formula is at room or even refrigerator temperature.

Nor need you sterilize bottles and nipples, any more than nursing mothers need boil their nipples. It *is* advisable, just for the first couple of weeks, to boil the water you use to mix formula. And it is, and will continue to be, important to wash and rinse feeding utensils and equipment thoroughly, using extremely hot water — and to make sure that you have good refrigeration, which is a continuing need for keeping any food, including formula, reasonably free of bacteria. (Only if you prepare formula as much as 24 hours in advance is sterilizing necessary; that's a long enough period for the accumulation of a significant number of bacteria.)

Do hold your baby in breast-feeding position when you give the bottle, and see that the nipple is full of milk so that a minimum of air is gulped (*some* air will probably be swallowed; see BURPING for what to do about it). The hole in the nipple should be small enough to provide about twenty minutes of sucking at each feeding.

Never prop a bottle for a baby under the age of six months; if the milk begins to come faster than it can be swallowed, it may get into the lungs and choke the child. It is also extremely important for a baby to have the physical and emotional contact with another human being that is part of the early feeding experience, and this is sufficient reason to avoid bottle propping.

There is one other aspect of bottle feeding that is important from a medical viewpoint. Once a child has teeth, allow only one bottle of milk or juice in the crib at night, and remove it promptly when the child falls asleep; for a child who demands several bottles during the night, make the second and subsequent ones water. The reason is that with a series of bottles the lactic acid (in milk) or citric acid (in juice) will accumulate on the teeth and cause decay. (Yes, they're baby teeth — but they are needed for biting and chewing until the permanent teeth arrive.) If plain water meets with resistance, then gradually provide more and more dilute milk or juice over a few days' time, until it is plain water. You will have a soggy baby in the morning — but one with intact teeth.

For comments on the other method, see BREAST FEEDING. Also see WEANING and, for the introduction to solid foods, FOOD, SOLID.

botulism: See FOOD POISONING.

bowel control: See TOILET TRAINING.

bowel movements: The important thing to remember about bowel movements is that, contrary to the thinking in grandmother's day and in spite of advertising stressing the vital nature of something called "regularity," there is no rigid schedule to which everyone must adhere. Each individual establishes his or her own norm, and frequency may vary considerably from one person to another and from one age to another.

Small babies can have up to ten or twelve bowel movements a day, although three or four is the average (and you *should* be concerned, and consult the doctor promptly, if a newborn baby's bowels have not moved at all by the end of the second day). As the child grows, the frequency of movements will generally decrease until, as adulthood approaches, an individual pattern is established — which may vary from two or three a day to one every two or three days. Only a departure from the child's own usual bowel habits, whatever they may be, is a cause for concern; no child should be forced to conform to anyone else's idea of "regularity."

One other fact should be mentioned here, as a guide for you and for children as well, as they are trained. Fecal matter contains bacteria. The bacteria are found there normally and properly. They can, however, cause trouble if they find their way to other places and parts of the body. In wiping a girl after a bowel movement, be sure to wipe in a direction *away* from the vagina and urethra, so no bacteria can get into those tracts; train your daughter, as she begins to handle these things herself, to wipe the right way. For the same reason, be sure to wash your hands — preferably with an antibacterial soap — after wiping a child, and teach your youngsters of both sexes to do the same.

Related subjects, including ills that significantly affect a child's bowel movements, are discussed under a number of entries. See ANAL FISSURE; CATHARTIC; CELIAC DISEASE; CONSTIPATION; CYSTIC FIBROSIS; DIARRHEA; HEMORRHOIDS; HIRSCHSPRUNG'S DISEASE; INTUSSUSCEPTION; MECKEL'S DIVERTICULITIS; MECONIUM; PARASITES; SPRUE; STENOSIS OF THE ANUS; STOOL; TOILET TRAINING; WORMS.

bowlegs: True bowlegs — outward curving of the bones of the legs — are generally symptomatic of rickets, a result of nutritional deficiency (see DEFICIENCY DISEASES).

The *appearance* of bowlegs is a perfectly normal phenomenon in newborn babies, and should not cause any concern; as long as the baby receives sufficient vitamin D, the legs will grow straight. Don't worry, either, if a child looks bowlegged when first beginning to stand alone; that's normal, too, and — again assuming nutritionally sound diet — purely temporary.

brachial paralysis: a condition affecting the upper arm, caused by a birth injury in which certain nerves are torn or bruised; it is also known as Erb's palsy. Such an injury can sometimes occur in a very difficult delivery of an unusually large, broad-shouldered baby, and the symptoms are immediately apparent to the attending physician: the baby is unable to raise his arm and to turn his palm upward, and will typically hold the affected arm in a bent position close to his body; the muscles of the wrist and forearm are usually not involved.

In most cases — the prognosis depends upon the extent of the damage — the condition is not considered at all serious. Often the doctor will simply instruct that the infant's arm be kept in a particular position for a few days; the problem then corrects itself, and by the time the baby is ready to go home, the arm is fine. Rarely is physical therapy, surgery, or any more involved treatment needed.

bradycardia: a pulse rate markedly below the usual for an individual's age and sex; the word derives from the Greek *bradys*, "slow." Bradycardia, like most such terms, is a relative one rather than an absolute; many things, including temperature, can and do affect pulse rate. But this finding will lead the physician to check further.

brain damage: a very general, and widely overused and misused, term for any condition in which the brain's functioning has been physically affected. The phrase itself does not denote either permanence (even if some brain cells have incurred lasting damage, other cells can often readily take over) or the causative factor(s).

It does, basically, describe a *non*-hereditary condition. (Although you will find certain hereditary conditions listed among the references below, they are conditions in which damage to the brain is expected to occur if preventive steps are not, or cannot be, taken; the damage itself is not inherent.) Damage to the brain may occur before or during birth, or later in life; among the many possible causes are serious head injury, major infections (such as meningitis and encephalitis) involving the nervous system, malignancies, certain types of poisoning, nutritional deficiencies, and circulatory ailments interfering with the brain's blood supply.

No inherent lack of intelligence is implied by this term, although — depending upon the exact site of the damage — retardation can be one effect. More commonly, the results include some degree of sensory or coordination difficulties, whether major or minor; it is the former — sensory problems — that have sometimes led to children who do not see (or hear) exactly as others do being classified as uncooperative, stupid, or even psychotic. Both teachers and physicians are more and more aware of these problems, however, and they are more often recognized and dealt with properly than they used to be. How such problems are handled varies, of course, with their precise nature; remedies may involve tutoring, physical therapy, medication, sensory aids, psychological counseling, or a combination of these.

For discussion of various conditions that may involve or relate to brain damage see CEREBRAL PALSY; DEFICIENCY DISEASES; DOWN'S SYNDROME; ENCEPHALITIS; EPILEPSY; HEAD INJURIES; HYDROCEPHALUS; LEAD POISONING; MINIMAL BRAIN DYSFUNCTION; PHENYLKETONURIA; RABIES; RUBELLA; TAY-SACHS DISEASE.

brain tumors: the top-ranking type of solid tumor in children (but not the leading kind of malignancy; see CANCER for further discussion and cross-references), differing usually from those typically found in adults. There has been less progress made in conquering these conditions than in some other types of childhood cancer — partly because of diagnostic difficulties, partly because of problems posed in treatment.

One difficulty is the nature of early symptoms. While they may be evident, they are far from definitive. Seizures, for example, may occur — but brain tumors are the *least* common causes of convulsions in children (who may often go into convulsion simply as the result of high fever). One early symptom may be increase in head size (which would be noticed in a routine checkup by your doctor — but can occur only in infants, in whom the skull is not yet fully fused, and can be caused by many other conditions). Other evident — but certainly equally ambiguous — symptoms may include headache, vomiting, irritability, behavior problems, changes in eating and sleeping patterns, lethargy, and apparent clumsiness. All of these are possible symptoms of many other things, either physical or emotional — and are, in fact, *usually* symptoms of other things.

Another problem in diagnosis is that there may not be any objective evidence at *all.* The effects may be purely subjective, and not at all apparent to anyone else. An infant, for example, may have symptoms that are purely visual and may not interfere with his everyday life to any detectable extent, thus leaving him unaware of the problem. Even if a very small child is conscious of symptoms, he may not be able to report them, simply because he cannot talk or his vocabulary isn't adequate to express his sensations.

That may sound very hopeless. Sometimes, though, a parent may sense something wrong, a vague feeling that something is amiss, and will voice that concern to the physician; that kind of alertness can be extremely helpful. In an older child, there may be such manifestations as headache, temper tantrums (which are normal, basically, only while a child is unable to express anger and frustration verbally), poor school work, lack of coordination, and apathy. The chance of malignancy lying behind any of these is extremely small, but they may of course be indications of other medical problems and should be discussed with the doctor.

If brain tumor is strongly suspected, it must be confirmed by X rays, a special radiovisualization called a brain scan, electroencephalogram, and cerebral arteriography (visualization of the blood vessels within the head). Treatment depends upon the cell characteristics of the tumor and its exact site, and may include surgery, irradiation, or both. Oral drugs cannot be used because they will not reach the trouble site (see BLOOD-BRAIN BARRIER), but in certain brain tumors, injecting drugs directly into the spinal fluid has been found effective.

The prognosis may vary tremendously, not only with speed of diagnosis as in all malignancies, but also with the type and location of the tumor. In many cases, assuming prompt diagnosis and treatment by skilled specialists, there is well over an even chance of full recovery.

breakbone fever: See DENGUE.

breast development: The age at which a girl's breasts begin to develop can vary a good deal; the average is eleven to fourteen, but the process can start as early as eight or as late as sixteen. Essentially, heredity is the determining factor — and it is heredity that determines, as well, the maximum size of the breasts when full development is reached.

Don't be alarmed, or even amazed, if your *son* has some temporary swelling around the nipples (one or both) at the beginning of puberty; it's a fairly common phenomenon, caused by the general hormonal confusion that prevails at this time in life, and it will go away.

Another curious phenomenon is the occasional swelling of an infant's breasts a few days after birth, accompanied by the release of a watery fluid popularly called "witch's milk" from the nipples. It's caused by a small amount of the mother's hormones that have accidentally slipped into the baby's circulation just before birth. Don't worry about it; it too, will go away.

breast feeding: As with bottle feeding, there are distinct advantages to breast feeding; current medical opinion holds that, if the mother herself has no feeling against it, and there are no medical contraindications, it's best to try it (one can always switch to bottle feeding, but the reverse isn't true).

Among the obvious advantages of breast feeding is the fact that milk is always available, at an ideal temperature (although that's no longer considered crucial), and completely sterile; no formulas have to be compounded. Mother's milk is nutritious; it also contains antibodies that help the baby resist minor gastrointestinal infections during the first few months, and it's easy to digest and nonallergenic.

There are even a couple of advantages for mother: breast feeding helps the uterus shrink more quickly, and chances of becoming pregnant while nursing are greatly diminished (though not nil). And if a breast-fed baby spits up after feeding, the material will be odorless.

A mother who has successfully nursed a baby does not need any special advice; she will instinctively make whatever adjustments are necessary with a later child (and there may be some adjustments needed; babies, like older people, are individuals). Following are some hints for the first-timer.

When you begin to nurse, what will be released from your breasts will not be milk but a yellowish, protein-rich fluid called colostrum. The bluish-white milk will appear about the fourth day after delivery.

It may take from two weeks to a month or so to strike a balance between mother's milk supply and baby's demands, and this is perfectly normal. Most babies can pretty easily empty a breast in five to seven minutes of active sucking — and it takes time to replenish the supply. If the baby sucks for 45 minutes and seems to be calling for more an hour later, the mother is likely to be physically exhausted and also worried that the baby is not getting enough milk. Which will probably be the case, since — contrary to old wives' tales — the early milk supply is more likely to be diminished by exhaustion and anxiety than by too little nursing. (Not to mention the cracked and painful nipples that can ensue, particularly if the mother is of fair complexion and the baby very vigorous, if nursing takes place too often and/or too long at one time at the beginning.)

To avoid the foregoing annoyances, it's best — for the first two or three weeks, until mother and baby arrive at a mutually agreeable *modus operandi* — to limit sucking time at each breast to ten minutes (i.e., a total of twenty minutes) and to nurse no more often than every two or three hours. If you have the feeling (and if you do, you will probably be right) that your baby's hungry between nursing sessions, have your pediatrician or family doctor suggest an appropriate formula to offer for those in-between feedings (water isn't nourishment and isn't a substitute).

After a while, mother's milk supply and baby's needs will equalize. Really. Don't worry if, at first, every other feeding is a bottle. Contrary to what you may hear from some quarters, babies do *not* suffer some mysterious deprivation from receiving alternate feedings out of a bottle rather than a breast; they are remarkably adaptable.

So long as food is available and offered, and the child is cradled in loving arms — which can, of course, be those of the father or an older sibling — the baby will be perfectly content. And a balance *will* be struck; after a while, most nourishment will be taken from the breast.

Nevertheless, it's a good idea to substitute an occasional bottle, for a couple of reasons. One is that the baby will become accustomed to the idea; in the event of mother's unexpected absence, a bottle from father, sibling, or sitter will be readily accepted. It is a good idea, too, for parents to have an evening out once in a while, and have the baby-sitter handle a bottle feeding; this tends to relax the mother and relieve tensions, as noted earlier, a good thing all around.

One further note, on shoulds and should-nots for the nursing mother. A number of rumors seem to be still rampant concerning what does or does not encourage a copious milk supply; you may have heard or read a number of them. They include the advocacy of beer, fruits, and a variety of other things. None are true. Milk production is triggered by hormonal processes that occur naturally, without encouragement from any other substances. The nursing mother does need to see that she gets a good, balanced diet — including the equivalent of a quart of milk a day, which can be in the form of calcium pills prescribed by a physician, to be taken with a specified amount of fluids. (This is not for baby, but for mother. If there is not enough calcium in her diet, milk production will continue at the same level, but her own essential supply of this element will be depleted. Skim milk and nonfat dry milk have the same calcium content as whole milk, should undue weight gain be a worry.) Beyond that, her only need is adequate rest, to maintain overall health and energy.

Most babies, no matter how they're fed, swallow a little air during feedings; see BURPING.

For a rundown on the other method, see BOTTLE FEEDING; also see WEANING and, for comment on later feeding, see FOOD, SOLID.

breath-holding: It's a scary experience when your youngster cries and does not take a breath until he loses consciousness, or even starts to go into a convulsion. But don't panic; he *cannot* kill himself, or even create a serious condition. The moment he starts to lose consciousness, the body's own involuntary controls take over automatically; the heightened carbon dioxide level in the blood will instantly trigger deep, rapid breathing in order to restore the normal oxygen–carbon dioxide balance.

In very young children, this phenomenon is usually involuntary, but with increased sophistication, it can be done at will. Your youngster shouldn't be permitted to use it as a weapon. Your best bet is not to overreact. Sometimes a cold cloth on the face or a brief slap will cause an involuntary intake of breath, and that's the end of it.

Brevital: a trade name for methohexital, a barbiturate; see SEDATIVES.

Bright's disease: See NEPHRITIS.

Bristacycline, Bristamycin: trade names for, respectively, tetracycline and erythromycin; see ANTIBIOTICS.

broad-spectrum: as applied to medications, acting against a wide range of infectious organisms. The best-known group of broad-spectrum drugs are the tetracyclines; see ANTIBIOTICS.

broken bones: See FRACTURES.

bromides: toxic compounds that should not be used or kept in the house. The major antacid–pain reliever that featured such a substance no longer includes it, despite the product's name.

Bromo-Seltzer: See PAIN RELIEVERS.

bronchial tubes: the passages that lead from the trachea, or windpipe, to the lungs; they are also called bronchi, and an inflammation of them is called bronchitis.

bronchiectasis: a serious condition in which the bronchial tubes become dilated so that small, tucked-away pockets of infection form; it is now, fortunately, extremely rare. Bronchiectasis can follow an infectious illness such as bronchitis, pneumonia, or whooping cough; if this occurs, the child will usually have great difficulty in breathing, and may spit up — during severe coughing spells that can tear the lining of the bronchial tubes — large quantities of mucus, pus, and even blood. With modern methods of treating, and especially preventing, the prior diseases, bronchiectasis has become uncommon.

If it does occur, treatment will depend upon the severity and extent of the illness; it will certainly include drugs — chiefly antibiotics — to clear up the infection, and may require draining of fluid from the lungs or other measures.

bronchiolitis: an inflammation of the bronchioles, the smallest of the air passages within the lungs, usually caused by a virus and typically affecting babies in the first six months of life. A prominent symptom is wheezing — not, as in asthma, only on exhalation, but on breathing in as well. It is considered quite serious, since it can interfere with the normal delivery of oxygen to the blood, thence to all the tissues of the body. If your doctor has diagnosed this condition, treatment may include antibiotics, and possibly the administration of oxygen and/or placing the child in a croup tent to ease breathing. Hospitalization is often required.

bronchitis: an inflammation of the two bronchial tubes that lead from the trachea, or windpipe, to the lungs; usually, the trachea itself is inflamed as well. It can occur as a complication of a cold or other infection — such as measles, flu, or whooping cough — or can be (and often is) caused by direct invasion by a virus.

The main symptom of bronchitis is a persistent dry cough; there may also be chest pain, poor appetite, difficulty in breathing, and a low fever — plus, if the child is quite young, vomiting and/or diarrhea. If bronchitis is suspected, it's important to call the doctor without delay; infection can easily spread to the ears or the lungs, and a far more serious condition such as bronchiectasis could develop if the bronchitis goes untreated.

Treatment, depending upon the causative agent and the degree of discomfort, may include antibiotics, antihistamines, steam inhalation, and/or expectorants; you can help by keeping the air in the child's room moist and providing warm, mild liquids such as broths to soothe the child's throat. Total defeat of the inflammation, even with careful treatment, may take two to three weeks.

bronchodilator: a medication that acts to relax and dilate constricted bronchial tubes.

bronchopneumonia: See PNEUMONIA.

bronchoscopy: an examination of the interior of the bronchial tubes with a special instrument called a bronchoscope, a procedure that is sometimes called for when a foreign body has lodged in the tubes; a device can be inserted through the bronchoscope for the purpose of removing the object.

brucellosis: a relatively uncommon bacterial infection contracted, directly or indirectly, from infected farm animals. It is also known as undulant fever (for reasons that will soon be apparent) and Malta fever (because it was first pinpointed there, by a physician named David Bruce in 1887); the condition in animals is called Bang's disease. It was unknown in the United States prior to the 1920s, but has since been reported from all states; some 40 percent of all reported cases, however, have occurred in the states of Illinois, Iowa, Minnesota, and Texas. It seems, from reports, to be less frequent in children than in adults —perhaps because children are for some reason less susceptible, perhaps because there is less exposure to possible infection.

Brucellosis is not contagious from one person to another; it can be contracted only from infected animals such as cattle, goats, or pigs, or from their carcasses, or from infected milk or milk products. The first symptoms appear after an incubation period of from five to thirty days, generally averaging about two weeks, and the chief symptom is the undulating fever that gives brucellosis its second name — a fever that rises, to a high of 102° or perhaps 104°F. (39° or 40° C.), for several days, drops off, then rises again. Accompanying the fever (which may also undulate during a 24-hour period, disappearing in the morning and soaring later in the day) are varying manifestations including general aching and weakness, headache, constipation, severe sweating and, rarely, an intermittent rash.

Untreated, brucellosis can continue for weeks or months with its characteristic recurrent pattern. Once diagnosed (the diagnosis must be confirmed by blood test and urinalysis), it can be knocked out fairly swiftly with antibiotics — usually one of the tetracyclines or streptomycin, or a combination thereof — plus bed rest.

The disease can and should be prevented. Although there is no immunization for brucellosis itself, there is a vaccine against Bang's disease, and farm animals should be inoculated. It is vital, too, to make sure that your family consumes only safe, pasteurized milk products, whether or not you live in a rural area.

bruises: Simple bruises are just broken blood vessels under the skin; a fancier word for a bruise is *contusion,* but it is still not serious if there is no other injury such as a cut or fracture. Typically, a bruise is reddish at first; as it heals, it may assume a blue or green tinge. If a bruise is very painful when it first occurs, application of cold cloths or ice usually brings relief; later in the healing process, heat is usually more helpful.

An ordinary bruise doesn't swell. A sharp blow, however, can result in a special kind of bruise called a *hematoma,* in which there is fairly rapid swelling and formation of a palpable lump; there may or may not be broken skin. The discoloration here is much more obvious; the bruise is generally purplish initially, changing over a fairly long healing period to a greenish yellow. And here, it's highly desirable to apply ice quickly to halt the subcutaneous (beneath-the-skin) bleeding; later, as with an ordinary bruise, warm compresses will speed absorption of the coagulated blood.

Neither a hematoma nor an ordinary bruise normally requires medical attention, but there are exceptions to the rule. If there are multiple bruises on the child's body without prior trauma, it may signify a blood disorder, which requires prompt medical diagnosis. A green-stick fracture (see FRACTURES) can appear at first to be just a bad bruise. If an apparent bruise is accompanied or followed by really acute pain, extreme swelling, or fever, there may be — possibly as a result of the injury, possibly not — an infection of the bone. Take the youngster to the doctor; prompt treatment is important. And if a child has had a bad bump on the head, see HEAD INJURIES.

brushburns: See SCRAPES AND SCRATCHES.

bruxism: See TEETH.

Bubartal: a trade name for butabarbital; see SEDATIVES.

bubo: See VENEREAL DISEASES.

bubonic plague: See PLAGUE.

Bufferin: See PAIN RELIEVERS.

bullet wounds: In any accident involving firearms, rush the child to the nearest hospital emergency room, pausing only for sorely needed first-aid measures if extensive hemorrhage is involved (see BLEEDING). If the wound is in the chest, do seal it off by bandaging it securely (use whatever is available, if you have no bandages) in order to prevent air loss from the lungs.

Transport the child lying down, if possible with his head slightly lower than the rest of his body or with his feet slightly raised — unless the wound is in the head or chest, in which case his head should be raised (put a pillow or something else under it). Try, in carrying the child, to limit movement of the wounded part.

The police must always be notified of any gunshot wound, whether or not you have had to call on them for emergency aid.

Home accidents with firearms can be prevented. Guns in the house should be kept unloaded, the ammunition under lock and key.

bumps: See BRUISES. Or, if there is another injury or symptom involved, see the appropriate listing, e.g., CUTS; FRACTURES; HEAD INJURIES; SCRAPES AND SCRATCHES; SWELLING.

BUN: the abbreviation for blood urea nitrogen, a measurement the physician may determine as part of a blood test. Levels markedly higher or lower than normal may indicate a number of inimical conditions, prominently including disturbances in kidney function.

Burkitt's lymphoma: See LYMPHOMA.

burns: Burns are classified according to the extent and nature of the damage, and each type requires different measures. The first three are, specifically, *thermal* burns — burns from fire or heat.

First-degree burns are those involving simple redness (sunburn — discussed separately under its own entry — is usually a first-degree burn). First aid is not, despite what you may have heard, either butter or salt, but simply cold water, which will quickly lower the skin temperature; actually immerse the burned area in a pan or sinkful of water, if possible, for a few moments. Then gently pat the area dry and smooth on a little emollient (if the skin is unbroken) such as a mild hand lotion, to keep the skin lubricated. Don't use burn ointments, sprays, and the like; they can interfere with healing, irritate the skin further, and sometimes cause allergic reactions.

Second-degree burns, also called *partial-thickness burns,* involve damage to the deeper layers of the skin, and are generally more painful than first-degree burns. There is typically blistering, as well as mottled redness; the skin may also appear moist and "weepy," and there is usually some swelling. Most scalds are second-degree burns. A minor second-degree burn, with just one or two blisters, doesn't (with the exceptions in the next paragraph) require medical attention. Again, the immediate remedy is cold water, or an ice pack, applied for twenty or thirty minutes, which will help relieve pain and decrease swelling; then cover the injury with a nonstick adhesive strip bandage or gauze pad.

More extensive second-degree burns require professional medical care, as do even minor first- or second-degree burns if the face, neck, or genitals are involved; if the victim is a small infant or — even if older — suffers from diabetes or another metabolic or circulatory disorder; if the burn was incurred in a building fire and smoke might have been inhaled; if there are any hints of shock (see TRAUMATIC SHOCK).

Third-degree burns, also called *full-thickness burns,* are critical injuries in which damage has been suffered not only by the skin, but by subcutaneous tissues. The skin may be charred and/or discolored and may in fact be broken, exposing underlying tissues; there is usually swelling. There may be little or no pain in the burned area itself, since a severe third-degree burn destroys nerve endings. (Hair roots are also destroyed in a third-degree burn. If you're in doubt as to degree, tug on a hair in the injured area; in a third-degree burn, it will come out easily.)

All third-degree burns require prompt medical attention, which means rushing the child to the nearest hospital or calling for an ambulance to do so. Immediate first-aid measures are minimal and do *not* include treatment of the burned area itself, except covering exposed areas with plastic wrap (if you have none, leave them exposed); *don't* attempt to remove any clothing that may be sticking to the burn. *Do:* keep the child lying down; check for signs of smoke inhalation or carbon monoxide poisoning, if there was a building fire (see GAS POISONING); offer water, or a nourishing liquid such as juice or milk, if the child is conscious and complains of thirst; be alert for signs of shock (see TRAUMATIC SHOCK).

Chemical burns are those caused by powerful acids or caustics; they always require prompt medical attention, whatever the size or location of the injured area. If an eye is involved, turn to EYE INJURIES. For any other area: quickly check the package or container and follow any special emergency instructions you may find; if there are none, immediately flush the area with running water (if a large area is involved, get the victim into a shower or use a hose or spray); then rush the child to the nearest hospital.

Electrical burns are discussed under ELECTRICAL SHOCK.

Burow's solution: a safe and harmless relief for the discomfort of itching, insect bites, poison ivy, and the like; it has a rather unpleasant odor, however, and most physicians feel that calamine lotion is both more pleasant to use and more effective. Burow's solution can be quite helpful, though, as a footbath; see ATHLETE'S FOOT.

burping: Most babies swallow some air from around the nipple along with their milk. There's not very much room in a baby's stomach, and the air can cause colicky pain later, so it's best to help bring up any possible air bubbles right after feeding. Hold the child on your shoulder or upright on your lap and pat the back (some babies need to be burped once or twice during the feeding, as well, and you'll soon find out if yours is one of those). Be patient, and keep patting. If nothing's happened after a full minute, stop, and don't worry about it; there may not be any bubbles to bring up — and a few babies just don't burp at all.

If the baby has a very tight grip on the nipple, the swallowed bubbles may be very small, and it may take an hour or more for them to coalesce into something large enough to burp up. Then, any milk sitting on top of the bubble may come up as well. This is called "spitting up"; it is not vomiting and is not a symptom of illness.

bursitis: an inflammation of a fluid sac near a joint, sometimes also involving calcium deposits. It can occur in any joint, but the ones most often affected are the shoulder, elbow, and knee, in that order. Bursitis can be triggered by severe chilling, by infection, by strain, or by a sharp blow to the joint; the last, incurred in sports activities, is most commonly the cause in teenagers (bursitis is extremely rare in younger children).

Symptoms usually include difficulty in movement, acute pain, a degree of discoloration, and sometimes swelling. The condition can sometimes clear up by itself with rest and applications of heat or cold, but if the symptoms persist for a few days, the youngster should see a doctor; cortisone or other drugs may be needed.

For general anatomical discussion, as well as comment on some other problems, see ARTHRITIS; DISLOCATION; JOINTS; LEGG-PERTHES DISEASE; OSGOOD-SCHLATTER'S DISEASE; SYNOVITIS.

butabarbital (Butisol): a barbiturate drug; see SEDATIVES.

Butazolidin, butazones: See ANTI-INFLAMMATORIES; the first word is a trade name for phenylbutazone, the second the class of drugs to which it belongs.

butterfly bandages: See BANDAGES.

Burping a Baby

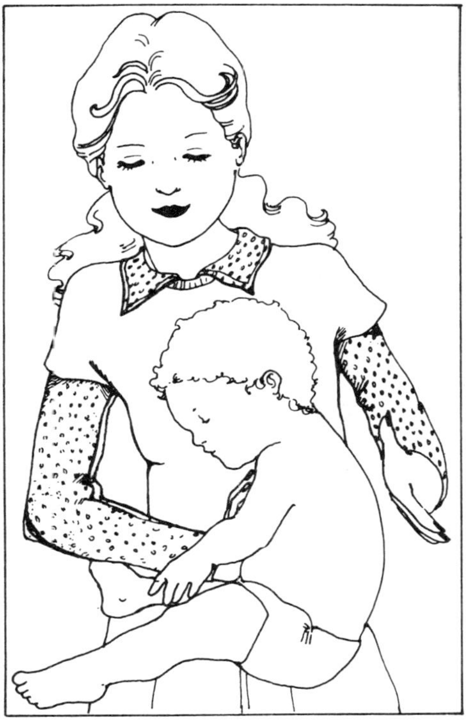

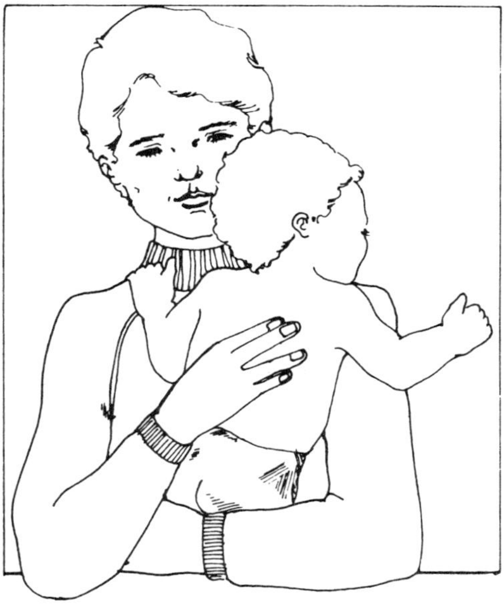

Most infants under the age of about six months swallow air bubbles with their milk and need help in bringing them up. The child can either be placed in a sitting position on your lap with a hand supporting him in front or held against your shoulder, while you pat gently between the shoulder blades.

C

Cafergot: a trade name for a drug used to relieve migraine. *Cafergot P-B* includes phenobarbital, a barbiturate (see SEDATIVES). See MIGRAINE for further comment.

caffeine: a tasteless stimulant that is a natural component of a great many plants and products made from them; the latter include coffee, tea, cocoa, chocolate, and cola drinks. It is also the active ingredient in over-the-counter "wake-up" pills, each of which usually contains the amount of caffeine in a cup of coffee or tea, about 110 milligrams. Caffeine is included, too, in many over-the-counter pain relievers, for reasons that defy rational explanation.

Teens who find themselves feeling jittery may in fact be suffering from what is usually referred to as "coffee nerves." Cola drinks (including the low-calorie kinds) contain anywhere from 20 to 36 mg of caffeine per six ounces. Which isn't much, compared to the amount in coffee — but some teenagers drink a lot of cola.

calamine lotion: a thick, pinkish-white liquid effective in soothing the itching of insect bites, poison ivy, hives, and the like. It's not a cure, but simply a reliever of the symptom; chemically, it is zinc carbonate. There are two kinds available; read the label, and buy the type that doesn't contain phenol, since that ingredient can be irritating to some youngsters. There is also available commercially, under the trade name Caladryl, a combination of calamine lotion with small amounts of camphor, the antihistamine Benadryl, and rubbing alcohol.

calcification: a deposit of calcium in tissue where it is not normal or desirable, usually producing a hardening of a properly soft, flexible area; it may occur as a result of injury or inflammation, and sometimes for reasons unknown. Calcification is not necessarily of serious concern unless there is some interference with normal function of the organ or area involved.

calcium: one of the essential minerals; see NUTRITION.

calcium carbonate: See ANTACIDS.

calculus: a stonelike material formed in the body by deposit of mineral salts; examples are gallstones, kidney stones, and the material that collects on the inner surface of some people's teeth and must be periodically removed by the dentist. Calculus formation is rare in children.

callus: a natural thickening of the skin to protect a much-used area, such as the sole (or the knees of a surfer). Never cut or otherwise try to remove a painful callus yourself; there is always a chance of infection, a possibility that is especially dangerous for a diabetic. If a callus causes discomfort, take the youngster to the doctor. A callus on the sole can also be confused (by a lay person, not by a physician) with a plantar wart; see WARTS.

If your child is recovering from a fracture, and the doctor refers to "callus formation," that's something very different. Here, the term means a substance exuded by the ends of a broken bone in the process of reuniting. There may be a visible lump, usually most noticeable in a broken collarbone. It will disappear eventually and is not a cause for concern.

calomel: a highly toxic compound, chemically mercurous chloride, that should never be used, since it can cause serious malfunction of the adrenal glands; see ACRODYNIA.

calories: units of heat and energy; a calorie is specifically defined as the amount of heat required to raise the temperature of one cubic centimeter of water one degree Celsius. All foods contain calories, although some contain more than others and a few contain little else *but.* Caloric needs vary with the individual and are related to age, height, bone structure, activities, and other factors. In general, a youngster whose weight is right for his or her age and size (in your pediatrician's expert judgment, not yours) is getting the right number of calories; one who's overweight (again, in your doctor's judgment) is getting too many calories, one who's underweight too few.

Only your pediatrician or family physician should decide on changing the caloric intake of an infant. But with older children and teens, you can, with the aid of a pocket calorie counter (there are many available), make some adjustments on your own; it's perfectly possible to offer an overweight child a balanced diet without high-calorie foods. Begin by eliminating extras of little nutritional value: thick gravies on meat, oils added for frying (bake or broil instead), candy and rich desserts.

Then, in doing your shopping and planning your menus, simply select those nutritious foods that fall at the lower end of the calorie scale. Vitamin A, for example, can be obtained from carrots, liver, eggs, fortified skim milk; the B vitamins, from lean meats, milk, greens, enriched breads; vitamin C, from citrus fruits; vitamin D, from eggs, fortified skim milk, leafy vegetables. Protein and the various minerals are similarly available from low-calorie foods — lean meat, fish and poultry, liver, eggs, fortified skim milk, green leafy vegetables.

Also see NUTRITION and, for a discussion of the general problem, OVERWEIGHT.

Calvé-Legg-Perthes Disease: See LEGG-PERTHES DISEASE.

Cama: See PAIN RELIEVERS.

camping: See ACCIDENTS, PREVENTION OF; BITES AND STINGS; FIRST-AID SUPPLIES; IMMUNIZATION; TRAVEL PRECAUTIONS.

cancer: A single word that denotes a plurality — perhaps dozens — of different conditions, affecting the body in different ways and in different locations and perhaps arising from many different causes. The one thing they have in common is the growth and proliferation of cells that are abnormal in form and multiply at an abnormally rapid rate, resulting in disturbance of the body's functioning — whether by the replacement of normal cells by abnormal ones or by the obstruction of other tissues and organs. The aim of treatment in the various types of cancer has, of course, been elimination of these "maverick" cells. Modern therapy may, depending upon the precise nature and location of the problem, employ surgery, irradiation, medication, or a combination of two or more of these.

There have been heartening advances in cancer therapy in recent years, particularly in two areas. One: refinements in X-ray techniques that permit high-dose irradiation of the target cells with considerable precision and avoidance of many of the hazards that once characterized this type of therapy. The second: a vast increase and improvement in drugs that "zero in" on malignant cells and destroy them, with far fewer side effects than earlier medications.

The result has been much increased survival, and sometimes even cure (a word once never even whispered in respectable medical circles in connection with cancer), especially in childhood cancers. Based on present knowledge, there is a two-thirds chance of conquest in most cases of malignancy in children, and in some types the outlook is even better.

That potential is not yet, unfortunately, being realized (cancer still kills more American children than anything else except accidents). In any kind of cancer, successful therapy depends on early diagnosis. Delayed diagnosis typically stems from either fear or ignorance. We hope the first will not deter readers of this book from calling unusual symptoms in their children to the prompt attention of a physician. (The fear is frequently baseless, in any case. Cancer strikes only about five or six children in every fifty thousand. Of every ten youngsters referred to a special cancer treatment center for definitive diagnosis, 80 to 90 percent are found to be suffering from other conditions, including systemic infections, nutritional deficiencies, cysts, and aftereffects of injury).

We hope, too, that the specific references at the end of this entry will help to dispel some ignorance. It must be noted, however, that there can be still another factor in diagnostic delay: the differences between patterns of malignant disease in children and those in adults can be confusing. Symptoms are often different (when in doubt, do see the doctor). And types are different as well.

Seven-eighths of the highly publicized cancers in adults, 87 percent of all cases, are *carcinomas,* malignant growths arising from the epithelial tissues that line the body inside and out. Most cancers of the skin, gastrointestinal tract, lungs, breast, and genital and urinary tracts are in this category. In children, that ratio is nearly reversed: only one in ten diagnosed malignancies is a carcinoma. The other 90 percent usually fall into one of six groups; the nature, symptoms, and treatment of each are discussed under that individual entry. See BRAIN TUMORS; LEUKEMIA; LYMPHOMA (includes Hodgkin's disease); NEUROBLASTOMA; SARCOMA; WILMS' TUMOR. A much rarer type of cancer (rare in both children and adults) is discussed under MELANOMA.

Candeptin, candicidin: See ANTIBIOTICS; the former is a trade name for the latter.

candidiasis: a general term covering any infection caused by the yeastlike organism called *Candida albicans,* also sometimes known as *Monilia albicans.* It may create trouble almost anywhere in the body, but systemic infections are rare. Relatively common are problems in and around the vagina of older girls, and in the mouths and diaper areas of infants; see, respectively, MONILIASIS and THRUSH.

canker sores: These small ulcers, familiar to most of us, that can sometimes occur on the gums, lips, or other mucous membrane inside the mouth, can stem from a variety of causes. Typically, canker sores are due to a virus, the same kind that causes cold sores (herpes simplex); less commonly, they are signs of allergy — to a food, for example, or to material in dental fillings. A canker sore usually indicates that something — a prior general infection or diet imbalance, for instance — has lowered the child's resistance. If one occurs, discuss the question of cause and treatment with your pediatrician or your dentist.

Herpangina is the medical term for a very extensive case of canker sores throughout the mouth and throat; medical treatment is definitely required. The child will usually be in a great deal of pain and will be running a fever, which can shoot up as high as 106°F. (41.1°C.). Your doctor will decide and advise on treatment, which will certainly involve procedures to make the child more comfortable, and may include hospitalization. (Herpangina may also be caused by a different virus known as Coxsackie A, and the condition is then most often limited to the throat; when the gums are involved too, it is typically a herpes infection.) Normally, an individual can have acute, extensive herpangina only once — but having it indicates a residual tendency, and may augur the occurrence of single canker sores, or cold sores, in the future; it also tends to lower resistance in general, so that your doctor will want to be on guard against the possibility of secondary infection.

Also see, for comment on other problems of the soft tissues of the mouth, DEFICIENCY DISEASES; GUM DISORDERS; STOMATITIS; TEETHING; THRUSH.

Cannabis sativa: the botanical name for the plant familiarly known as marijuana; see PSYCHEDELICS.

capillaries: See BLOOD VESSELS.

capillary hemangioma: See BIRTHMARKS.

carbamazepine: an anticonvulsant medication; see EPILEPSY.

carbenicillin: a semisynthetic penicillin; see ANTIBIOTICS.

carbohydrates: See NUTRITION; SWEETENERS.

carbon monoxide poisoning: See GAS POISONING.

carboxyhemoglobin: a chemical compound formed in red blood cells when carbon monoxide binds with hemoglobin; it renders the cells unable to perform their normal function of carrying oxygen to the various parts of the body.

Carbrital: a barbiturate-bromide combination drug; see SEDATIVES.

carbuncle: a serious infection of the skin, essentially a group or cluster of boils. Its appearance at first is similar to that of a boil — a large, painful red lump, but broader and deeper than a boil; subsequently, several openings (as compared with the single opening of a boil) appear. If untreated, there will be massive discharge of pus and other infectious materials, and an open sore that is subject to further infection.

Carbuncles most often occur on the neck, face, or shoulders, but they can appear anywhere on the body. They signal substantially lowered resistance, and may be accompanied by fever, swollen lymph nodes, and other symptoms. If you suspect that your youngster has, or is developing, a carbuncle, it's essential that the doctor be consulted promptly; treatment usually consists of antibiotics administered internally and/or locally, plus hot soaking.

carcinogen: a substance that triggers or encourages the development of cancer (of any type, not limited to carcinomas).

carcinoma: a cancer of epithelial tissues, the most common type of cancer in adults, but rare in children. For a general discussion of childhood malignancies, see CANCER.

cardiac: pertaining to the heart.

cardiologist: See SPECIALTIES, MEDICAL.

carditis: any inflammation involving the heart. You may see or hear the term used alone, or with prefixes that pinpoint the site of the problem more specifically; *peri*carditis, for example, is an inflammation of the pericardium, the membrane *around* the heart. For more on the subject, see HEART DISEASE.

caries: the technical term for decay in teeth; see CAVITIES.

carisoprodol: a muscle relaxant; see SEDATIVES.

carotene: a substance, found in certain foods, which is converted by the body to vitamin A; see NUTRITION for a full discussion.

carotenemia: a condition in which carotene (see preceding) is circulating in the blood. Its only symptom is a yellowish tinge to the skin (but not the eyes, which would be affected by true jaundice), and it results from consuming an extraordinarily large quantity of carrots or other foods containing carotene; it's curious, but not harmful, and of no special medical significance.

carotid: See BLOOD VESSELS.

carpus: the wrist, comprising eight bones; the adjective referring to it is *carpal.*

car seats: See ACCIDENTS, PREVENTION OF.

carsickness: See MOTION SICKNESS.

cartilage: a tough, smooth, plastic connective tissue that covers the ends of the bones where they meet at the joints. It can be torn, occasionally, by extremely violent injury — a not uncommon knee injury among football players; surgery is usually required for correction, but there is generally no permanent crippling.

cascara, castor oil: See CATHARTIC.

CAT: See COMPUTERIZED AXIAL TOMOGRAPHY.

cataract: a clouding of the lens of the eye that reduces vision by preventing sufficient light from reaching the retina. Cataracts can result from disease (usually only in the elderly) or injury; they can also be congenital, and have occurred as one of the tragic results of a mother's contracting rubella during the first three months of pregnancy. Treatment consists of removing the useless lens or lenses and substituting corrective eyeglasses or contact lenses.

cathartic: any substance that induces movement of the bowels; cathartics are also popularly called laxatives, implying (sometimes erroneously) that the substances are milder, gentler, or safer. Some work by irritating the intestinal muscles to stimulate contractions: examples are cascara (which is derived from a specific tree bark), castor oil (made from the seed of the castor bean) and Ex-Lax (the latter very commonly gives rise to side effects, including nausea and allergic skin reactions, in youngsters). Saline preparations such as epsom salts (a particularly powerful cathartic) and milk of magnesia work by drawing fluid into the bowel; simple mineral-oil types act as softening agents; some (such as Haley's M-O) combine the last two types.

Don't give your child cathartics as a regular practice; they can result, eventually, in disrupting the child's normal pattern (see BOWEL MOVEMENTS). Avoid their use entirely, in fact, unless they are specifically advised by your physician — and then use the type and dosage prescribed; use a cathartic made to taste like candy only if your doctor so instructs — and make sure that it is kept locked out of a small child's reach. *Never* give a child a cathartic in the presence of undiagnosed abdominal pain.

Cathartics have a specific purpose, and they are medically useful under certain circumstances. They are emphatically not useful for other, totally unrelated conditions such as colds.

catheterize: to draw off urine from the bladder through the urethra, if the patient is unable to excrete it voluntarily, a procedure that's sometimes necessary after surgery (the difficulty is normally temporary); the instrument used is a catheter. The latter term is also used, less commonly, to apply to the tubing used to extract fluid from, or instill fluid into, other body cavities or organs.

cat-scratch fever: a specific infection transmitted by the scratch or bite of a cat; the exact causative agent is not known but is believed to be a virus. The cat itself is not ill, and can be a household pet; it need not be an alley cat. Not all cat scratches or bites, of course, cause the disease.

The initial wound may, after a day or two, resemble an insect bite or small boil, and apparently heals. After an incubation period that can vary from three to ten days the characteristic symptoms appear, typically very much like a mild case of flu: general malaise, usually mild fever, and swollen lymph nodes, especially those in the neck — plus, possibly, redness and tenderness in the area of the wound, which may seem to have previously healed. Rarely, the infection may spread so that there are also symptoms suggesting encephalitis, such as extreme lethargy and even coma; or, the symptoms may resemble those of viral pneumonia. All this may seem very vague, but the diagnosis can be confirmed by a lymph-node biopsy.

Treatment for cat-scratch fever consists simply of bed rest and drugs such as aspirin to make the child more comfortable; antibiotics will be ineffective. Duration of the illness is from one to three months, and there are no ill effects thereafter. Cat-scratch fever is not contagious, except in the extremely rare instance that the swollen lymph nodes actually abscess and discharge pus — which is infectious and can communicate the illness to others.

caul: the old word for amnion.

cauterize: to dry up fluids exuding from the body, as in a wound or a severe nosebleed; cauterizing is something that's done by a physician, not by you.

cavities: breakdowns of the enamel and dentine of teeth by decay (for which the medical term is caries). What happens is that bacteria normally present on the surface of the teeth pounce gleefully on any carbohydrates (chiefly sugars, but starches as well) that may be left on the teeth; the interaction produces acids that eat through the tooth structure. The dentist, confronted with this situation, removes the decayed part of the tooth and replaces it with some other material, molded to the properly functioning shape of the tooth — gold, silver, plastic, etc. If the decay has progressed too far, it may be necessary to fill the root canals of the tooth, or even to extract the tooth entirely.

Heredity is, it is generally agreed, a factor in the tendency for teeth to decay. It is possible, though, to take some preventive measures. Try to limit the sweets and starches in your child's diet. See that teeth are brushed after each meal or snack — not eventually, but within thirty minutes. Provide a stannous fluoride toothpaste (yes, they really do cut down the incidence of cavities). And, of course, make sure your child sees the dentist regularly — every six months, starting at age three or four.

Additionally, fluoridation of your community water supply is extremely helpful. Addition of a fluoride compound to drinking water has been proved, beyond question, to diminish tooth decay in children; intensive comparative tests have indicated that cavities can be cut by well over 50 percent when fluoridated water is drunk from birth.

The amount used in such community fluoridation is one part per million, a proportion that can do no harm whatever; a certain amount of confusion on this subject has resulted from the fact that in some localities a *higher* proportion occurs *naturally,* and that higher proportion can indeed cause an unsightly (but not toxic or otherwise dangerous) mottling of the surface of the teeth. Nor is there any truth to the briefly circulated rumor that fluoridation is associated with increased incidence of cancer; the National Cancer Institute, whose exhaustive analysis refuted the rumor, in fact noted that — although no cause-and-effect relationship has been suggested — certain cancers appear to occur *less* often in fluoridated areas.

If there is a high incidence of tooth decay in your family, you might also discuss with your dentist a new at-home preventive program involving periodic application of fluorides via a gel provided in a special "tray" that fits over the teeth.

CBC: medical shorthand for "complete blood count"; see BLOOD COUNT.

cc: the abbreviation for cubic centimeter, the unit of liquid measurement usually employed by physicians and other health professionals; it is the same as a milliliter (one-thousandth of a liter) and is equal to a little more than 0.03 ounce.

cecum: See INTESTINES.

Cefadyl, cefazolin: two of the cephalosporins (the first word is a trade name for cephapirin); see ANTIBIOTICS.

celiac disease: a nonspecific term applied to what may be several distinct conditions involving intestinal distress in small children (the word *celiac* is simply derived from the Greek word for "belly"); there is a good deal of confusion on the subject, and current medical thinking is that a diagnosis of "celiac disease" is overly vague and definitely questionable.

Over the age of two years, there is little doubt that what used to be dismissed as celiac disease is probably sprue (you'll find a discussion of that ailment under its own separate entry).

The present confusion centers on the eight-months-to-two-years age group. Typical symptoms of what has been termed celiac disease include abdominal bloating; severe diarrhea with a pale, frothy, and foul-smelling stool; possibly cramps; and usually crankiness and poor appetite (which would be an understandable accompaniment to the other symptoms). All such groups of symptoms were attributed to sensitivity to certain wheat or rye grains in the diet, and treatment of "celiac disease" was always based on this conclusion.

Now, however, it is felt that a number of different problems may give rise to a similar set of symptoms. There may indeed be allergy to wheat or to something else in the diet. There may be some digestive malfunction interfering with normal assimilation of certain foods. And many pediatricians have found that classic "celiac disease" symptoms can appear when an infant is having a difficult time with teething, ceasing after eruption of all the baby teeth. But despite some similarity in symptoms, there is no connection with cystic fibrosis, which is always congenital.

Any such set of symptoms does, of course, require prompt medical attention.

cellulitis: an inflammation of the connective tissues, causing pain, redness, and swelling in the skin, occasionally accompanied by fever; it can be caused by a number of the coccal type of bacteria, including strep, staph, and Pneumococcus. It is treated with antibiotics.

For comment on a similar condition caused specifically by *Streptococcus,* see ERYSIPELAS.

cellulose: a polysaccharide constituent of some plant foods; both natural sugars and synthetic substitutes are discussed under SWEETENERS.

Celontin: a trade name for methsuximide, an antiseizure medication; see EPILEPSY.

Celsius, centigrade: See TEMPERATURE.

centimeter: the unit of length in the metric system, in which heights are likely to be expressed in future; it is equal to 0.3937 inch. To convert inches to centimeters, divide by that figure; to convert centimeters to inches, multiply by it.

cephalalgia: the medical term for headache, derived from the Greek words for "head" and "suffering."

cephalosporins: See ANTIBIOTICS (the group includes a number of drugs, most beginning with "ceph").

cerebellum: the lower, smaller part of the brain, beneath the cerebrum (the "thinking" or "higher" brain) and toward the back, also known as the "hindbrain"; it deals chiefly with such functions as equilibrium and muscle coordination.

cerebral palsy: a condition of defective muscular control resulting from brain damage; it may be more or less serious depending upon what part of the brain (and therefore the body) is affected. Sensory problems (as, with vision) may sometimes be present; mental capacities are affected in only a minority of cases (approximately one-third). The term "palsy," medically, does not mean — as is popularly supposed — spastic or trembling, but simply muscular weakness or lack of control; involuntary trembling may sometimes be present, but not necessarily.

Cerebral palsy is not hereditary, but is specifically caused by physical damage to the brain. It may be congenital, a developmental defect caused by a severe prenatal infection. It can result from an injury during delivery — a risk especially great in premature babies because their skulls are substantially softer; other problems relating to premature birth can also be factors (the general incidence of cerebral palsy has risen as more and more premature infants, with modern medical-care techniques, survive). It can be caused, very rarely, by an infectious disease of the brain such as encephalitis. And it can be the result of a violent head injury, a possibility that decreases with age, as the skull hardens.

Treatment of cerebral palsy is very individual, as is the prognosis; it depends on which functions have been affected, and to what extent. Corrective eyeglasses may be prescribed, for example, if vision is affected. Problems involving the legs and feet may require braces or orthopedic surgery. Speech therapy may in some instances be needed. And in many cases of cerebral palsy, whatever the affected muscles, expert and continuing physical therapy can effect marked — sometimes near-miraculous — improvement.

cerebrum: the upper, larger part of the brain, also known as the "forebrain"; it is concerned with conscious thoughts and actions, and also includes centers dealing with voluntary motor functions.

cerumen: See WAX IN EARS.

cervix: an anatomical term meaning "neck," used in reference to two very different parts of the body. It is that point at the top of the vagina where it opens into the uterus, the "neck" of the uterus. It is also that part of the spine that lies in the neck region, and the vertebrae there are called *cervical* vertebrae.

Cetacillin: a trade name for propicillin, a semisynthetic penicillin; see ANTIBIOTICS.

Chagas' disease: See PARASITES; the other name for this infection is trypanosomiasis.

chalazion: an inflammation of an oil gland on the inside of an eyelid (it may be the upper or lower lid), resulting in an obstruction of the duct of the gland and the formation of a small cyst. It appears as a little red lump, and it can be quite uncomfortable. Don't confuse it with a stye, which involves a lash root and appears on the *outside edge* of the lid.

A chalazion sometimes disappears spontaneously. If it has not done so after a few days, take the child to the doctor, who can prescribe special topical medication that will probably do the trick. If it doesn't, then the cyst may have to be opened, and this must be done by an ophthalmologist; it's minor surgery, usually performed in the doctor's office.

For a comparison with other problems affecting the eyelids, see BLEPHARITIS; CONJUNCTIVITIS; STYE; TEARDUCT STENOSIS; TRACHOMA.

chancre: a symptom of syphilis; see VENEREAL DISEASES.

chapped lips: Sun, wind, cold, licking the lips and continuous breathing through the mouth are the usual causes of chapped lips, and an ordinary chapped-lips problem can be dealt with successfully by a number of things available at your friendly neighborhood drugstore. Simply have the youngster smooth on an emollient such as petroleum jelly, or one of the many effective commercial preparations (BioStik, Blistex, and Chap Stick are among the best known), before going outdoors — and also before bedtime if there's a tendency to breathe through the mouth when sleeping.

A teenage girl whose lips tend to chap should be careful to choose lipsticks with a moist, creamy consistency, and it's wise to apply an antichap preparation under the lipstick as extra insurance. If the chapping continues, especially if there is actual cracking of the lips, she may be allergic to the particular brand or shade of lipstick she's been using, and a switch to another make or color may be in order; choosing from one of the several reputable lines of hypoallergenic cosmetics can save costly and lengthy experimentation.

Rarely, extensive scaling, cracking, and even blistering of the lips can stem from certain vitamin deficiencies, especially of riboflavin; that should be suspected, and discussed with your doctor, if the condition continues despite the measures we've mentioned.

chart: in hospital parlance, not a single graphic depiction, but a complete file on a particular patient giving a detailed record of illness(es), treatments, measurements, observations by medical personnel, symptoms, results of tests, etc.

Ch. B.: the abbreviation for Chirurgiae Baccalaureus, Bachelor of Surgery; it is a British equivalent of the M.D. degree.

checkups: See PHYSICAL EXAMINATIONS.

cheilitis: inflammation and fissuring of the lips, more severe and more painful than simple chapping; it may be caused by certain nutritional deficiencies, as well as by cosmetics allergies.

chemical burns: See BURNS.

chemosurgery: a method of dealing with scarred skin by chemical peeling; an extreme, last-resort method of treatment. It must be done by a qualified physician, or the results could be worse than the original condition.

chemotherapy: a broad term for treatment by the administration of chemical compounds (drugs of any sort) — as opposed to physical therapy, or X-ray therapy, or change-of-diet therapy. Among familiar chemotherapeutic agents are analgesics, antibiotics, antihistamines, sulfa drugs, and synthetic hormones and vitamins.

Cheracol-D: See COUGHS.

chest pain: Like abdominal pain, chest pain can be symptomatic of many different conditions (generally, in children, not including heart attacks). None of these conditions can be diagnosed by you. Chest pain calls for prompt evaluation by a physician.

chickenpox: a highly contagious generalized infection, medically termed *varicella;* it is now the most widespread of the communicable childhood diseases. It is caused by a virus and can be epidemic. It tends to occur mostly in winter and early spring and especially afflicts children in the three- to six-year-old group (although this is one disease for which immunity cannot be passed on to the newborn by the mother, so that a month-old infant is equally susceptible). Its name has nothing to do with chickens, but is connected with chick-peas — which the disease has no relation to either; someone evidently thought the accompanying rash resembled clusters of chick-peas.

The first symptoms, appearing after a ten-day to three-week incubation period, are typically fever — usually a fairly low one (and occasionally none at all), but sometimes running as high as 104°F. (40°C.) — and headache. Within a day or two, the characteristic rash begins to appear in the form of tiny raised pimples that eventually turn into small blisters and form crusts; the eruption occurs gradually over a four-day period, generally beginning on the back, chest, or scalp and ending with the palms and soles (the rash may not reach these areas). The fever, meanwhile, usually disappears by the second or third day.

There are normally no other symptoms — but the rash can be a serious problem, and the older the child, the more so. It is intensely itchy (which doesn't seem to bother children under the age of two or three years), and there is a nearly irresistible impulse to scratch. Scratching can cause secondary infection as well as permanent scarring. You should therefore do everything you can to relieve the itching and prevent scratching.

Keep the child's hands clean, and cut the nails so short that scratching is impossible. Apply calamine lotion, or immerse the child in cornstarch or baking-soda baths, to relieve the itching; if that's not sufficient, ask your doctor to prescribe an antihistamine. As the crusty scabs form (the itching generally subsides then), be sure that the child doesn't pick at them (that can cause scarring, too); let them fall away naturally.

Assuming there are no complications (which occur in only about five percent of all cases), and aside from the problems already mentioned, chickenpox is considered a fairly mild disease, running about a week from start to finish, and there is no other treatment (antibiotics are ineffective). Because of the *possibility* of secondary infection, however, it is important that it be diagnosed by, and the child's condition regularly discussed with, your doctor — and that you keep up the child's resistance by ensuring plenty of rest and a well-balanced diet. And, that you take precautions against spreading the disease to others.

Chickenpox is contagious through two means: contact with pus from any broken blisters, and droplet infection (i.e., coughing, sneezing, or just plain breathing). It can be communicated to others from the day before the rash appears until all the lesions have dried up and formed crusts. If you have other children who have not had or been exposed to the disease, and it's possible to arrange for them to stay elsewhere for a week, do so; the second case in a family is often more severe, probably because the exposure is so much greater.

There is at this writing no immunization against chickenpox. Once a child has had it, he *is* immune and cannot get it again — although he may then be susceptible to another, virally related, ailment in later years; see SHINGLES. (There is a test to determine whether or not a child has had chickenpox.)

An immune globulin, called ZIG (for zoster-immune globulin) is available for chickenpox; it employs serum from adults who have had shingles. Its effectiveness has been questioned, although it seems to work in sufficiently large dosage. It is, in any case, in very short supply and is reserved for instances of extremely high risk — that is, children for whom the disease would pose a special threat, or who lack infection-fighting ability, whether because of a deficiency or as the result of immunosuppressant medication.

Also see REYE'S SYNDROME.

For comment on other communicable "childhood diseases," some of which can now be completely prevented, see COXSACKIE DISEASE; DIPHTHERIA; ERYSIPELAS; ERYTHEMA INFECTIOSUM; IMPETIGO; MEASLES; MUMPS; POLIO; ROSEOLA; RUBELLA; SCARLET FEVER; WHOOPING COUGH.

chigger bites: See the section on insect bites under BITES AND STINGS.

chilblain: a condition involving redness, itchiness, and sometimes ulceration on hands or feet, caused by overexposure to damp cold. The word is used less here than in Great Britain; we would usually call the condition mild frostbite.

chills: If a child is shivering and trembling and complains that he's cold, and he's not outdoors in wintertime, it usually means he has a fever. Take his temperature. If it is elevated, call the doctor and report the child's temperature, along with any other symptoms he may have mentioned or you may have observed. Make the child as comfortable as possible and follow your physician's directions.

If the child is already sick in bed, and severe chills suddenly occur, call the doctor immediately.

chiropodist: See PODIATRIST.

chiropractor: an advocate of the use of mechanical manipulation, chiefly of the spine, to cure ills; such an individual is not a physician, and you should not, in our opinion, seek a chiropractor's advice or treatment for yourself or your family.

chloral betaine, chloral hydrate: potent sleep-inducing drugs; see SEDATIVES.

chlorambucil: an anticancer medication, used especially in treating certain leukemias and lymphomas.

chloramphenicol: See ANTIBIOTICS.

chlordane: See PESTICIDES.

chlordiazepoxide: a tranquilizing drug; see SEDATIVES.

chlormezanone: a "minor" tranquilizer; see SEDATIVES.

Chloromax, Chloromycetin: trade names for chloramphenicol; see ANTIBIOTICS.

chloroxazone, chlorphenesin: muscle-relaxant agents; see SEDATIVES.

chlorpheniramine maleate: See ANTIHISTAMINES.

chlorphentermine: an appetite depressant; see DIET PILLS.

chlorpromazine: a powerful tranquilizer; see SEDATIVES.

chlortetracycline: one of the tetracyclines; see ANTIBIOTICS.

chlorthion: See PESTICIDES.

Chlor-Trimeton: a trade name for chlorpheniramine maleate; see ANTIHISTAMINES.

choking: Often, it means a small piece of food or some other object has stuck in the child's throat. Try to get him to cough it up. If he's quite small, pick him up by the feet and pat him on the back; if he's too big for that, simply clap him smartly on the back while he bends over your lap. Next, if that doesn't work, stick your finger into his mouth and see if you can touch and grab the object; if you can't, tickle the back of his throat to cause vomiting. If

First Aid for Choking

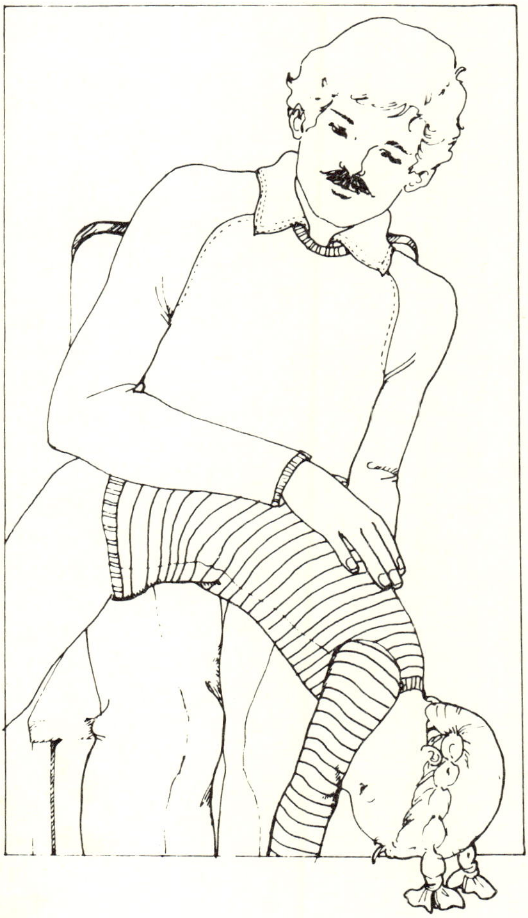

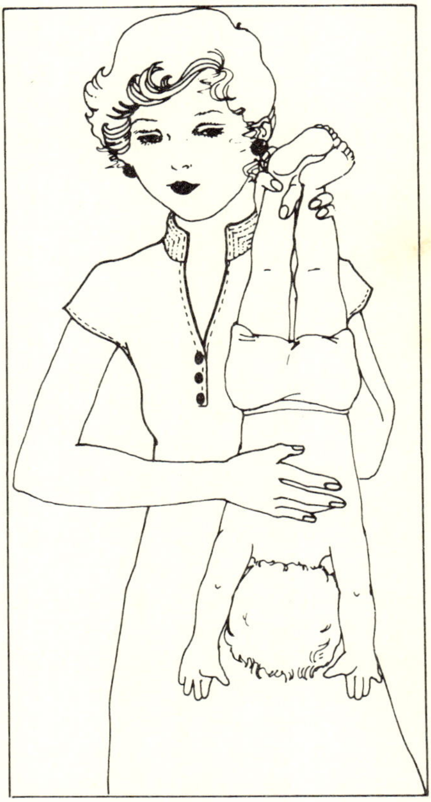

First step in first aid, when food or another object has stuck in a child's throat, is to try to have the child cough it up. A very small child can be grasped firmly by the ankles and held upside down; a larger child can be bent over your lap with head hanging downward. Clapping the youngster smartly between the shoulder blades will often dislodge the object.

none of these measures work, call the emergency squad or rush the child to the nearest hospital, whichever is faster.

In cases where your youngster has, to your knowledge, swallowed a foreign object, but seems perfectly well and *isn't* choking, what to do depends upon the nature of the object. Smooth or round ones, such as marbles, buttons, coins, or prune pits, once they get past the neck (the narrowest part), generally pass through the rest of the alimentary canal without any trouble; do, however, phone your doctor and report the incident, and follow whatever advice you are given. Sharp objects such as pins, nails, screws, or small pieces of jewelry can cause serious problems; take the child to the doctor promptly, and have X rays taken.

A number of other conditions can also cause a sensation of choking. See ASTHMA; CROUP; DIPHTHERIA.

cholecystectomy: removal of the gallbladder.

cholecystitis: inflammation of the gallbladder.

cholecystography: X-ray visualization of the gallbladder.

cholera: a communicable disease that is now virtually nonexistent in the United States, and in fact in the entire Western Hemisphere (although there are occasional fears that it could spread to South America). It has, however, recently been rampant in a number of other areas. In 1973, there were 51,000 reported cases in Asia, chiefly in the Indian subcontinent and in Indonesia; 5700 in Africa, most of these in Senegal, Upper Volta, and Nigeria; and some 300 in Europe, almost all in Italy. It is caused by the kind of bacterium called a spirochete.

Cholera chiefly affects the small intestine. Symptoms, after a one- to three-day incubation period, can range from mild diarrhea to a very serious and potentially lethal condition including extreme diarrhea and dehydration, vomiting, severe abdominal and muscular cramps, and even coma. The disease can be spread by human carriers, by infected feces, food, or water, and by flies — and it can quickly become epidemic when there is a lack of, or breakdown in, sanitation. Antibiotics, especially the tetracyclines, are effective — but proper medical attention can be difficult to obtain in certain areas.

Fortunately for travelers, there is a vaccine against cholera, and anyone in your family who is traveling to an area where it is endemic should be immunized (the destination should be discussed with your physician, who will have up-to-date information on high-risk areas). Immunization consists of two injections (or three, for children under the age of nine years) given a week to ten days apart, the second a full month before departure if possible; it is effective for six months, and a booster shot will be necessary then if there is a continued stay in the area (at this writing an improved, longer-lasting vaccine is under study). Proof of immunization is currently required for entry into many nations of Asia, Africa, and the Middle East; some others demand such proof if the traveler has recently visited a cholera-reporting area.

cholesterol: See LIPIDS.

Choloxin: a trade name for dextrothyroxine, a lipid-lowering agent; see LIPIDS.

chondrodystrophy: See DWARFISM.

chondrosarcoma: See SARCOMA.

Chooz: See ANTACIDS.

chorea: Like rheumatic fever, chorea is now considered a hypersensitivity reaction to strep (or its chemical by-products); it may be associated with rheumatic fever, or may be a separate entity. Prior to the recognition of its infectious origin, it was popularly known as Saint Vitus' Dance.

Typically, the illness afflicts youngsters prior to puberty. The characteristic symptoms — which may at first appear in part to be simple clumsiness — are involuntary twitching and spastic movements of the limbs and facial muscles; these may be accompanied, at the onset of the illness, by various other manifestations including fever, headache, dizziness, weakness, and possibly nausea. The muscular twitching generally involves both sides of the body, but in rare instances occurs only unilaterally. Additionally, speech may be affected in about 25 percent of cases, and there may be extreme irritability and a variety of emotional problems.

The course of treatment is lengthy but eventually successful; parents should know, however, that full recovery may take anywhere from three months to a year or two. There is generally a bed-rest period of at least six weeks, and the doctor will watch the child closely for any complications involving the heart. Convalescence must be gradual, and parental understanding and patience are extremely important.

This condition is sometimes referred to as *Sydenham's chorea;* it is *not* related to *Huntington's* chorea, a hereditary, noninfectious nerve ailment that never appears until middle age.

chromosomes: See HEREDITY; SEX CHROMOSOMES.

chronic: prolonged, persistent, habitual, in referring to an illness or condition; the opposite of *acute.* A chronic illness is one "lived with" over a considerable period of time, usually with no forseeable definite cure, and most such illnesses afflict older people rather than youngsters; among ailments that are or might be termed chronic in children are allergic conditions such as asthma, some forms of arthritis, certain eczemas, and diabetes. A chronic condition can *become* acute if unexpected or unaccustomed symptoms arise, and then requires prompt medical attention.

chrysotherapy: See ARTHRITIS.

ciguatera: See FOOD POISONING.

circumcision: cutting-away of the foreskin of the penis; whether or not the operation is performed on a newborn infant is a matter for the parents to decide, and there are a number of different opinions, medical and other, on the subject.

Certain religions require circumcision, and if yours does, you will presumably want to follow the principles of your faith. Until a couple of generations ago, circumcisions were rarely performed for other than religious reasons.

Then the pendulum swung, and until very recently, *most* newborn boys in the United States were circumcised. The reason was that circumcision was considered a desirable, if not precisely essential, hygienic measure. The area under the foreskin is a site of possible future infection — and such infection occurring later might prevent urination, thus definitely requiring the surgery at that time, perhaps when it would prove a psychological hardship for the boy.

Current medical thinking still leans to that view, but has taken another factor into account: the feelings of the parents, particularly the father of the child. If the father has not been circumcised and feels that the risk of possible physical problems is less important than the boy's physical identification with his father as he matures, the doctor will not usually insist that the operation be performed on the infant. It's best that you and your own physician discuss the question, if you have any doubts.

Circumcision of a newborn boy is minimally painful for the child. Healing takes just a few days. And don't be alarmed if a yellowish membrane appears; that's perfectly normal, and it's the way mucous membrane heals, not with a thick scab as on the skin.

If your baby boy is *not* circumcised, you should gently retract the foreskin daily until it can be retracted completely. It should then continue to be retracted regularly during showers or baths.

"clap": a slang term for gonorrhea; see VENEREAL DISEASES.

clavicle: the anatomical term for the collarbone, actually a *pair* of bones extending from the top of the breastbone to the shoulders; it's very easily broken, and a broken clavicle isn't serious (see FRACTURES).

cleft palate: a congenital malformation in which the roof of the mouth — the soft or hard palate — is not closed completely, and thus opens into the nasal passages; it may sometimes extend to the upper lip (see HARELIP). If the condition exists, it will be discovered without delay; it is one of the things automatically checked for as soon as the baby is born.

The immediate problem is that of nourishment, since food taken into the mouth can go through to the nose. If your child has been born with a cleft palate, your pediatrician will give you advice on feeding procedures (special devices, sealing off the opening to the nasal passages, are available).

The doctor will also judge the best time to schedule corrective surgery, which may, depending upon the physician's judgment, take place at any time from three months to three years; preferably, if there are no contraindications, the operation is performed before the child has begun to talk, since the malformation can and does interfere with speech. The surgery is usually completely successful, and the child recovers rapidly.

Cleft palate occurs at a rate of one in approximately twelve hundred births. It's believed that about 20 percent of the cases are in some way hereditary (the other 80 percent remain a complete mystery), but the mechanism is not yet clear. The probability of bearing a child with cleft palate does seem to increase somewhat with the mother's age.

Cleocin, clindamycin: See ANTIBIOTICS. The former is a trade name for the latter.

clitoris: See SEX ORGANS.

clofibrate: a lipid-lowering agent; see LIPIDS.

clonazepam, Clonopin: an antiseizure medication and its trade name; see EPILEPSY.

clorazepate: one of the benzodiazepine group of "minor" tranquilizers; see SEDATIVES.

clortermine: an appetite suppressant; see DIET PILLS.

Clostridium: a genus of anaerobic bacteria, the best known of which are *C. botulinum* (which causes botulinism) and *C. tetani* (tetanus). The most ubiquitous is probably *C. perfringens;* see FOOD POISONING, PREVENTION OF.

clotrimazole: an antifungal agent; see ANTIBIOTICS.

cloxacillin: a semisynthetic penicillin; see ANTIBIOTICS.

clubfoot: a deformity of the ankle in which the foot is turned in one direction or the other and cannot function properly for walking; it is usually a congenital malformation, although it can occur later in life as a result of injury or disease. Congenitally, clubfoot occurs about once in a thousand births, most of the afflicted babies are male, and in most cases only one foot is affected. The cause is unknown; it is believed not to be hereditary, but due rather to some untoward prenatal condition or event.

The earlier correction of the condition is begun, the better, since a good deal of time and effort is often involved. Depending upon the precise nature of the problem, treatment may include braces, casts or splints, physical therapy, surgery, special corrective shoes, or (frequently) a combination of two or more of these.

clumsiness: What's important, from this book's point of view, is that simple awkwardness, or deliberate carelessness, is not confused with something that might require prompt medical attention. If your youngster obviously can't help or correct apparent clumsiness, don't chastise him; suddenly appearing, unaccustomed clumsiness, in particular, could be a symptom of a number of serious conditions — chorea, cerebral palsy, muscular dystrophy, imbalance resulting from an inner ear infection, and others. The question should be discussed with your physician, and an examination should be scheduled.

CNS: See NERVOUS SYSTEM.

co.: See PRESCRIPTIONS.

coarctation of the aorta: an uncommon congenital problem involving a narrowing of the main artery leading from the heart; it afflicts about twice as many boys as girls. It is usually discovered soon after birth, by the physician's noting abnormal heart sounds; the suspicion can be double-checked by blood-pressure readings (pressure in the upper part of the body is atypically high, that in the legs atypically low), X rays, and other measures. Coarctation of the aorta is completely correctable by surgery.

cobalamin: one of the B vitamins, also known as B_{12}; see NUTRITION.

cocaine: See PSYCHEDELICS.

coccidioidomycosis: See VALLEY FEVER.

coccus: See BACTERIA.

coccyx: the last segment of the vertebral column, the "tailbone."

Coco-Diazine: a trade name for sulfadiazine; see SULFA DRUGS.

codeine: an opium derivative; see NARCOTICS.

cod liver oil: properly, an oil derived from the liver of the codfish, although halibut also serves as a commercial source. It used to be spooned into reluctant children as a regular practice, to provide supplementary quantities of vitamins A and D. *Don't.* If your pediatrician believes your child's diet is deficient in these vitamins, or if you are nursing and such supplements are recommended for you, your doctor can prescribe newer, far more palatable, and usually water-soluble forms.

cold pills: There is, plainly and simply, no cure for the common cold (see the next entry). And there is no over-the-counter medication, beyond ordinary aspirin, that should be given to a child (or taken yourself, for that matter) without a physician's specific instructions. At best, patent preparations promoted for common-cold relief are a waste of money, since many contain unnecessary ingredients; at worst, some ingredients could be, in the long or short run, harmful.

There is no earthly reason why you should give your youngster caffeine, antacids, laxatives, antihistamines, or extra analgesics along with aspirin — yet these are some of the things the advertised cold compounds contain! If the child has something *other* than an ordinary cold, and requires other medications, then your physician will prescribe them.

If the doctor does feel your youngster needs other medication, it is highly unlikely he or she would prescribe any of the astonishing combinations purveyed at the drugstore counter. Quite a number contain chlorpheniramine maleate or other antihistamines, fine for allergies but totally useless for viral or bacterial infections and offering the possibility of undesirable side effects. Some include such far-out ingredients as laxatives, antacids, quinine, or atropine compounds (yes, we do mean major brands). Many contain phenylephrine hydrochloride or phenylpropanolamine hydrochloride, sympathomimetic drugs (see DECONGESTANTS) that can have a number of untoward systemic effects and should not be used without a physician's advice.

For comment on some of the other things manufacturers would like you and your family to take for coping with minor discomforts, also see PAIN RELIEVERS. And for the role of vitamin C, in colds and other conditions, see NUTRITION.

colds: viral infections characterized by symptoms familiar to all of us — sniffling, a runny nose (usually eventually becoming a stuffy nose), coughing, diminished appetite, possibly (though uncommonly) a low fever, and general malaise. Colds, as everyone knows, are very common. And very contagious. And there is *no cure* for a cold, despite the many patent medicines constantly promoted (see the preceding entry).

What causes colds? Not cold weather, contrary to old wives' tales; people tend to get more colds in winter simply because they spend more time together indoors in close quarters. Colds are spread by droplet infection — via coughs, sneezes, or just breathing within a few feet of someone else (the incubation period after exposure is one to three days). The causative agents are viruses; over a hundred of them have been identified as definite culprits, and there may be many more. There is a brief immunity (its exact duration is unknown) following a cold, but it's strictly temporary and applies only to the particular virus that caused that particular cold.

There is no vaccine or other convenient instant immunization, but there are, to an extent, preventive measures. You can keep youngsters' resistance up — to colds or any other infections — by seeing that they get enough rest and a well-balanced, nutritional diet. And — especially in winter — you can see that they avoid enclosed, crowded situations where there are likely to be a number of people dispensing cold viruses.

A "cure" for the common cold will probably continue to be elusive for some time. Even research is difficult. Unlike some other ills — cancer, for instance — most animals cannot be used for experiments; aside from humans, in fact, the only creatures who can be induced to contract a cold are chimpanzees.

Should the usual symptoms appear, the only "treatment" is to relieve the symptoms and make the child as comfortable as possible, while guarding against his contracting other infections. Neither antibiotics nor antihistamines will have any effect.

Simple aspirin, given in whatever dosage your doctor recommends, will help to relieve general discomfort. Use of a vaporizer or humidifier to relieve nasal stuffiness is fine — but use nose drops or other decongestants only if they are prescribed by your physician (see DECONGESTANTS for further comment). Minor throat irritation can be helped by steam inhalation or drinking warm, clear fluids such as broth or tea. Sneezing is actually helpful (it's a natural nose-clearing mechanism), and shouldn't be stifled; if the child is old enough, gentle nose-blowing should be encouraged. And continue to see that the youngster's resistance is kept up.

Do be on the alert for possible complications or secondary bacterial infections of the ears, sinuses, or bronchial tubes; infants and small children are especially susceptible to the latter. An ordinary cold lasts about a week, and its symptoms are normally limited to those we've mentioned; any other symptoms, including the cold's persisting for as long as ten days, mean a call to the doctor is in order.

A so-called "chest cold" is no longer merely a cold; it may be the start of a bronchial infection. Mucus from the nose in an ordinary cold is clear; thick, yellow material sneezed or blown out signals a probable secondary bacterial infection of the nose or sinuses. A lingering low fever combined with a stuffy nose and wet cough hanging on after the cold may also mean sinusitis. The normal cough of the common cold is simply a clearing reaction to material dripped from the nose, and is most noticeable at night and in early morning; if coughing persists throughout the day, or the child complains of severe throat pain, there may be secondary infection in the chest or throat. All of these — plus high fever, chills, chest pain, earache, or gastrointestinal problems — suggest that the condition has gone beyond the common-cold stage, and medical attention is needed.

cold sore: a small cluster-of-blisters sore caused by the herpes simplex virus (*Herpesvirus hominis,* type 1); it's also known as a fever blister, though any connection with either a cold or a fever is purely coincidental, except for the fact that any illness can lower resistance to the virus. A cold sore generally occurs on, or more commonly near, mucous membrane, and the most common site is on the lower part of the face, near the nose or just at the edge of a lip.

Herpes simplex is a hardy, universal virus, always annoying but never really malevolent; it also causes canker sores, possibly herpangina, and a type of stomatitis. It's essentially a parasitic organism, always present but causing little or no trouble for its human host unless said host's resistance drops off suddenly. It's usually picked up in childhood. It's the only known virus, in fact, that a parent can pass on, years after it has caused him or her any trouble, to an offspring without having any signs of illness at the time.

The best treatment for a cold sore is to leave it entirely alone. It's true that there are a few commercial preparations designed to relieve the itching and burning sensations that usually accompany the sore, but it's best not to use them unless you've first discussed the question with your own doctor and one of those medications has been specifically recommended. Within a few days, the sore will usually dry up and form a crust that clings for a week or two, then falls away by itself — and shouldn't be picked at.

If a youngster is subject to frequently recurring cold sores, discuss the problem with your doctor; it's been found that in some cases, for some reason, a series of smallpox vaccinations may raise resistance to attack by the cold-sore virus.

colic: a condition of severe abdominal discomfort common in infants under the age of three months or so; its causes vary and may include swallowed air, excessive gas (a normal product of digestion) in the intestines, allergy to the formula, or residual effects of maternal hormones.

Typically, the baby will fall asleep with no difficulty but will awaken later crying and cranky, in the throes of intense abdominal cramps; he will usually react to the latter by drawing the knees up or, in some cases, extending the legs stiffly. The abdomen may feel rigid.

You should call your physician. While you're waiting for advice, you can make the baby a little more comfortable by turning him onto his stomach, or — preferably — holding him on your lap, face down. Keep him warm. Don't give any medication, or anything else by mouth, until the doctor has specifically instructed you to do so.

Your doctor may prescribe a medication to relax the abdominal spasms, for immediate use and in case of future episodes. Usually, these measures are effective — but if they aren't, don't panic. Colic is a very individual matter, and it's usually self-limited; that is, it will simply taper off by itself when the baby reaches a certain age. The reason may be that as the child — and his digestive tract —grow larger, small air bubbles cause less trouble. And there may very well be emotional factors — on your part, not the infant's — that can cause reflective tension in him; first-time parents are usually somewhat less secure in their roles — and it *has* been observed that colic occurs more often in the first child in a family than in subsequent ones.

If the symptoms we've described are accompanied by vomiting and/or diarrhea, and possibly by a rash, then the condition may very possibly stem from sensitivity to cow's milk. Even this seems to be self-limited, but your pediatrician may feel it advisable to switch the formula, temporarily, to one based on goat's milk, soybean preparations, or meat base.

If your baby has had colic in the past, don't automatically assume that any abdominal problem displaying similar symptoms can be dismissed as simply a recurrence. Your doctor should do the diagnosing; there are other, far more serious conditions that may require fast (even emergency) medical attention. See, for example, APPENDICITIS; INTESTINAL OBSTRUCTION; INTUSSUSCEPTION.

colitis: an inflammation of the lower (large) intestine. The causes can vary considerably, ranging from allergy to psychosomatic factors, from infection to reactions to certain drugs. The term is simply descriptive of a condition. (A diagnosis of *ulcerative* colitis denotes colitis of unknown cause, characterized by ulcerations and bleeding.)

Symptoms may vary considerably and may or may not include pain, diarrhea, constipation, and fever. Treatment of colitis will of course depend upon the physician's determination of the underlying cause and may involve changes in the diet, various medications (including, if there is a definite infection, antibiotics), and other measures, sometimes including surgery.

collagen: a protein substance that forms an important part of connective tissue fibrils, both in the joints and in other parts of the body. Rheumatoid arthritis is sometimes classified as a "collagen disease," but generally is not so categorized, since it attacks the joints almost exclusively. The major collagen diseases, which are discussed separately, are DERMATOMYOSITIS, LUPUS, and SCLERODERMA.

collarbone, broken: See FRACTURES.

colloid cyst: See CYST.

colon: See INTESTINES.

Colorado tick fever: See TICK FEVER.

color blindness: a hereditary vision defect, not generally meaning a complete inability to see any colors at all, but usually an inability to distinguish reds and greens or small tonal variations of other hues; it is much more common in males than in females, but still rare in the general population.

The genetic transmittal of classic red-green color blindness is sex-linked and recessive (see HEREDITY for a full explanation of those terms); the gene is carried on the X chromosome. A boy can inherit the trait only from his mother, and if he does, he will be color-blind; a girl can receive the gene from either parent, and will thereafter be a "carrier" — but she herself can be afflicted only if she receives a "double dose," i.e., from both parents. A color-blind man will pass on the trait to all of his daughters, but to none of his sons. A mother who is carrying the gene but is not herself afflicted has a fifty-fifty chance (the odds remain the same with each child) of passing it to her offspring, whatever their sex —

but if she herself is color-blind, she will transmit it to all her children.

Color blindness occurs more often among those of European or Asian descent than among other peoples. U.S. government estimates, based on national surveys of elementary-school children, suggest that overall, some color vision deficiency afflicts almost seven percent of boys, but only one half of one percent of girls.

colostomy: a surgical procedure in which the large intestine is shifted to empty through an opening made in the abdominal wall; it is performed, usually, when there is some rectal obstruction or other interference with the normal path of elimination. A colostomy may also be performed as a temporary measure (the normal route is later reinstated) in cases of certain congenital rectal malformations.

colostrum: See BREAST FEEDING.

coma: See UNCONSCIOUSNESS.

Combid: a trade name for a medication combining prochlorperazine, a tranquilizer, with isopropamide, an antispasm drug; see SEDATIVES.

Comeback: See PAIN RELIEVERS.

communicable: See CONTAGIOUS.

Compazine: a trade name for prochlorperazine; see SEDATIVES.

Compocillin: a trade name for penicillin V; see ANTIBIOTICS.

compound fracture: See FRACTURES.

Compoz: an over-the-counter "tranquilizer"; see SEDATIVES.

computerized axial tomography: a fairly new diagnostic tool (it was first introduced in England, in 1972) that offers greater specificity than is possible with standard X ray. It utilizes a series of low-dosage X-ray projections — focused on special crystals rather than on photographic plates — which are then combined to form a full cross-sectional image of the area (*tomo-* is from the Greek *tomos*, "section") displaying differentiation of soft tissues as well as bony structures. The technique has proved especially useful in diagnosis of diseases and disorders of the brain, the eye, and various organs in the abdomen. The procedure is completely painless; an infant or very young child may be sedated, simply to prevent motion which would blur the visual image.

Comycin: a medication combining tetracycline and nystatin; see ANTIBIOTICS.

concussion: See HEAD INJURIES.

condom: See CONTRACEPTION.

congenital: present at birth, as opposed to acquired during or subsequent to birth; the term may denote either a hereditary condition or characteristic or one acquired while in the womb, although it often implies the latter.

Congesprin: See PAIN RELIEVERS.

conjunctivitis: any inflammation of the conjunctiva, the mucous membrane lining the eye socket and the inner surface of the lids; it can signal an infection, or it can occur as a result of — or accompany — an allergic reaction, generally to something airborne (including pollen, dust, sprays and scents, various pollutants).

Acute conjunctivitis, popularly called "pink eye," describes a highly contagious infection that may be caused by various bacilli or viruses. Aside from the very noticeable inflammation that gives the condition its popular name, symptoms may include swelling of the eyelids, sticking together of the lids during the night, and itching and burning that a youngster may describe as a feeling of sand in the eyes. See the doctor promptly; pink eye is easily and quickly treatable with medications your physician can prescribe.

If your child has acute conjunctivitis, it's vital to prevent its spread among family members and playmates, and some extra care and supervision is required. The eyes must not be rubbed, or even touched. If they are, the youngster's hands must be washed immediately, since anything touched — books, papers, toys, etc. — can carry the infection. Of course he must not share towels, bed linens, or the like with anyone else while the condition lasts.

For other conditions affecting the eyelids, see BLEPHARITIS; CHALAZION; STYE; TEARDUCT STENOSIS; TRACHOMA. Also see IRITIS and UVEITIS, very different conditions affecting the eyeball itself and requiring the attention of an ophthalmologist.

constipation: a condition involving abnormally hard stools passed less frequently than the child's usual pattern of elimination; both factors — hardness and infrequency — must be present. Note that we haven't used the word "daily"; there is no rule, medical or other, that bowels must be moved every 24 hours like clockwork.

If you do believe that a child is truly constipated, do *not* decide, on your own, to give a laxative, an enema, or any other medication or special food such as bran (which can be quite irritating). Do take the child's temperature, check carefully for other symptoms (involving the abdomen, anus, or any place else), and call your physician; be able to report any recent departures from the child's usual diet. Follow whatever instructions the doctor gives you.

The causes of constipation are many and varied; they include insufficient food or liquid, diet imbalances, muscular weakness, and a number of gastrointestinal problems. If the child is in the learning-to-go stage, there may be deliberate withholding, and the cause may be either physical (as, pain on elimination) or psychological (see TOILET TRAINING).

Also see, for some related comments, ANAL FISSURE; BOWEL MOVEMENTS; CATHARTIC; HIRSCHSPRUNG'S DISEASE; STENOSIS OF THE ANUS.

Contac: See DECONGESTANTS, NASAL.

contact lenses: corrective lenses fitted directly onto the surface of the eyeball, rather than placed in a frame in front of the eye, as with eyeglasses; they are always made for the eyes of the individual patient, so that they fit perfectly. Whether contact lenses are suitable or desirable for a particular child is a decision that must be made by an ophthalmologist (*not* by an optometrist or an optician). Age is not necessarily a factor; contact lenses have sometimes been prescribed for a child as young as four years.

contagious: transmittable directly from one human being to another, as opposed to being transmitted by insects, animals, or other means; a *communicable* disease is one transmittable by *any* means.

Generally speaking, a person cannot transmit a contagious disease unless he or she either is incubating it or actually has it (if your youngster has chickenpox, for example, and you have already had it and are therefore immune, you cannot carry the disease to other people).

There are exceptions to the rule, but they are fairly rare; most familiar to the public have been the occasional discoveries of healthy carriers of diphtheria and typhoid fever. Less well known is the fact that certain strep infections can be carried, to very young and highly susceptible infants, by healthy persons who are caring for them — nurses, baby-sitters, even their own parents and siblings; your doctor may suspect such a situation if a baby who has had very limited contact with strangers has repeated respiratory infections.

All contagious conditions are both communicable and infectious; the reverse is not necessarily true. The common cold, scarlet fever, and syphilis, for example, are both infectious and contagious. Viral encephalitis, typhus, tick fever, and cat-scratch fever are communicable, but not contagious, infections. Acne, tetanus, and warts are all infectious, but not communicable in any way.

contraception: a general term for the use of any devices, drugs, methods, etc., designed to prevent conception — the fertilization of an ovum (egg) by a sperm — or the gestation of a fertilized ovum. There are a number of them, some vastly more efficient than others. Their effectiveness is rated in something called "woman years." If, for example, 1000 women employ a particular system for a period of a year, and 20 of them become pregnant, the system is rated 98 percent effective; for those 20 women, of course, the rating is zero and they are 100 percent pregnant. So much for the curious science of statistics.

The least effective method, but the only one acceptable to those religions that frown on "artificial" means of preventing conception, is the "rhythm" method, which prescribes abstinence from sexual intercourse during those parts of the menstrual cycle when conception is possible — roughly, from day ten to day seventeen (the first day of the menstrual period is called day one). If all females operated internally on an ideal, predictable 28-day cycle, with all events taking place like clockwork, the rhythm system would be fine. Many women, and practically all young women and teenagers, however, do not; "safe" days have frequently proved quite the opposite.

Spermicidal agents — foams, creams, and the like, available without prescription — are a bit more effective, but not much (although they are useful combined with a diaphragm). Dependence on these agents, in the judgment of experts, runs up to a one-in-three risk of pregnancy.

The diaphragm, a circular membrane placed over the cervix (just before sexual relations take place), must be prescribed and fitted by a physician. Its effectiveness is generally rated at about 90 percent — results of various studies have ranged both a bit higher and considerably lower — mainly because sperm can occasionally slip around the barrier. Spermicidal agents employed in conjunction with a diaphragm can apparently increase its effectiveness somewhat.

Condoms are mechanical barriers designed for men, which fit over the penis; they, like the spermicidal agents, can be purchased in drugstores without prescription. They are thus far the only contraceptive designed for use by males. (The reason is not "sexism" but the serious side effects that have appeared with all drugs thus far tested for male use.) Like the diaphragm, they must be put in place just before intercourse. The track record for the condom is not entirely clear, since the device has a history of breakage in use — which of course renders it completely ineffective. Recently, there has been improved quality control in manufacturing, and the possibility of rupture during use is highly unlikely. Condoms have, however, been known to slide off when there is lingering after ejaculation. The potential effectiveness is probably high, although the condom's statistical achievement is — depending upon the authority to whom one listens — perhaps on a par with that of the diaphragm, or even a little lower. It is, however, the *only* contraceptive method that offers at least some protection against venereal disease.

Somewhat more effective are intrauterine devices, or IUDs — variously shaped gadgets that are placed (by a physician) within the womb and act to prevent the implantation there of a fertilized ovum. Their success rate has been variously estimated at 90 to 98 percent, but much seems to depend on the individual woman. They appear, on the whole, to be more effective in women who have previously borne children than in those who have never been pregnant. A significant number of women — as many as two out of ten — develop pain, bleeding, or other complications that necessitate removal of the device; serious infections have also occurred on occasion. An IUD can also fall out. And IUDs have been known simply to fail; sometimes, that failure can result in an ectopic (outside-the-womb) pregnancy.

Oral contraceptives, first approved for use (by prescription) in 1960, have proved pretty successful, and there have been a number of changes in formulation over the years; "the" pill is, at this writing, actually a number of different products. The oral contraceptives are designed to prevent ovulation by altering the menstrual cycle via the use of certain hormones — specifically a progestin (a synthetic much like a naturally occurring hormone called progesterone) and one or another kind of estrogen (a term generally applied to a group of substances produced by the ovaries).

Circulatory and vascular problems that have arisen in a small but significant number of women taking oral contraceptives seem to be related chiefly to the estrogen component; pills with far lower estrogen content are now being marketed — and some have recently appeared ("minipills") that contain only a progestin, no estrogen at all. The last appear to be about 97.5 percent effective, compared with a rate of 98.5 to 99.9 percent for the dual-ingredient products; the "minipills" also sometimes cause unpredictable disturbances in the menstrual cycle affecting both duration of, and intervals between, periods. (The *highest* risk of circulatory problems was associated with the sequential products that consisted of two types of pills, one containing estrogen alone, taken in sequence during the cycle; the sequentials were withdrawn from the market, at the request of the Food and Drug Administration, early in 1976.)

We're not going to list products and ingredients, because they are changing too rapidly; but there are some general guidelines. The estrogen content of the various formulations ranges from .02 to .10 mg. It is now generally felt that a maximum of .05 mg is as effective as, and less risky than, higher amounts. A girl or woman taking oral contraceptives should certainly know what she is taking. Additionally, she should be sure to return to the prescribing physician for regular checkups — which should include blood-pressure readings — and to stop the pill regimen and phone the doctor if any strange symptoms appear; particularly crucial ones are leg cramps, chest pain, headaches, and blurred vision.

Another method that shows promise is a uterine insert called Progestasert, which received marketing clearance from the Food and Drug Administration in 1976; tested in several thousand women, the device — a flexible reservoir that releases progesterone at predetermined dosages over a period of a year and acts only locally, on the uterus itself, to prevent implantation — seems thus far to offer a 97 to 98 percent success rate in preventing pregnancy, along with a fairly low — but not nonexistent — incidence of side effects.

In addition, there are some new directions that are being explored. One: the various possibilities suggested by the group of natural substances that may act, or interact, on a subhormonal level (see PROSTAGLANDINS); thus far, such speculation is entirely theoretical. Another: a pill developed by a Danish physician that uses, instead of female hormones, substances from the agave cactus which seem to have similar chemical actions but fewer side effects. A third, announced in 1976: a device that measures viscosity of cervical mucus, which varies more predictably during ovulatory cycles than temperature does; originally developed as an aid to women who wished to achieve conception, it is obviously potentially useful for avoidance as well, and is expected to be generally available by 1977 or 1978.

There are also three other avenues that might be pursued under certain circumstances.

An injectable contraceptive, medroxyprogesterone (Depo-Provera), has been developed; designed for administration to women on an every-three-months basis, it appears to be almost 100 percent effective. It has not yet, at this writing, been approved by the Food and Drug Administration for general use by physicians. Reported drawbacks include a relatively high incidence of irregular bleeding, and also the possibility of *permanent* inability to bear children.

An "after-the-fact" drug *has* won FDA approval for limited use. That prescription drug, taken by mouth, is diethylstilbestrol (DES), and you may have heard of it in quite another context: during the late 1940s and early 1950s, it was given to some women early in pregnancy to prevent miscarriage (it is no longer used for that purpose), and there have been a number of cases of an unusual kind of vaginal cancer occurring later among daughters of those women. DES appears to be completely effective in preventing pregnancy if institution of medication begins within 72 hours after coitus. There is a very high incidence of severe gastrointestinal reactions, as well as the possibility of other more severe side effects (the drug has not been very widely used). DES is employed only on an emergency basis, such as after a rape.

Finally, there is interference, by surgical means, with the normal route of egg or sperm. In women, this takes the form of cutting or cauterizing, or sometimes simply ligating (tying off) or otherwise mechanically obstructing, the Fallopian tubes through which the eggs travel from the ovaries, so that they cannot reach the uterus (they don't "pile up" in the ovaries, but simply expire uneventfully). In men, it takes the form of *vasectomy* — tying off and cutting the *vas deferens,* the tube that conducts sperm from the testis to the urethra. Neither operation affects hormone production, and menstruation in the woman continues as before.

Unless sterilization — the overall term for these operations — is medically necessary (e.g., if pregnancy would, under any circumstances, pose a threat to life), physicians will not generally perform such surgery except if a patient is a mature individual (it is generally avoided before the 30s or 40s) who has a clear understanding of the procedure and results and is sure that it is what he or she wants. It *is surgery,* which always carries some unpredictable degree of risk, although here it is extremely small. While it is virtually foolproof, some postvasectomy contraceptive protection is needed, since perhaps a dozen ejaculations must take place before the seminal fluid is completely devoid of viable sperm. And it is of course generally permanent (the exception is that in a tiny number of vasectomies, fewer than one percent, there is recanalization that negates the entire procedure): vasectomy can be reversed in something more than half of all cases, via a markedly more complex operation, though even then the ability to father children cannot be guaranteed; in a woman, tubes that have been tied off can occasionally be made functional again, although tubes that have been cut or cauterized cannot. Sterilization, in short, for all practical purposes closes the options.

Increasingly, although state laws vary, physicians may and do advise teenagers on contraception and other sexual matters without the necessity of informing their parents. No reputable physician, of course, would perform nonemergency surgery on a minor without parental consent.

In addition to the contraceptive methods we've mentioned, all of which have drawbacks, a number of others are currently under investigation. They include a variety of male "pills" that might inhibit sperm production without adverse physical or psychological effects; an agent, also administered to men, that acts against the enzyme that is carried by the sperm and enables it to penetrate the egg cell (such an agent has already been proved successful in animal experimentation); and a variety of "just-before" and "just-after" techniques and drugs.

contraindication: a circumstance presenting a reason to the physician for not using a particular medication or treatment otherwise considered desirable for the disease or condition; while penicillin, for example, might otherwise be the most effective treatment for an infection, the patient's allergy to penicillin would be a contraindication.

contralateral: on the opposite side (of the body).

contusions: See BRUISES.

convulsions: violent and uncontrollable multiple muscular spasms. Convulsions can occur, in small children, for a variety of reasons; neither the causes nor the occurrences are necessarily serious or indicative of major disorders. They *are* symptomatic of *something* wrong, and should not be lightly dismissed — but they should *not* be a reason for panic on the part of an adult.

If a child goes into convulsion, it indicates that something is affecting the brain, especially the muscle-coordination centers; that something need not indicate any permanent damage. Among the things that may cause convulsion are epilepsy, head injury, a number of infections, certain deficiency diseases, and — not uncommonly in children under the age of five or six — simply high fever. In general, convulsions are self-limited; their average duration may be anywhere from two to ten minutes.

Symptoms of a convulsion cannot be mistaken for symptoms of anything else. The child becomes unconscious (if he is standing, he may fall to the floor or ground). The limbs stiffen and begin to jerk violently. The eyes may roll upward. Breathing is heavy, and there may be dribbling or frothing from the mouth. Rarely, vomiting, urination, or defecation may occur.

First-aid measures are simple. Place the child on a bed or soft rug — or if that's not possible, put something soft under the head. Loosen clothing, especially anything restrictive such as a collar or belt. Place something soft — a folded handkerchief, a newspaper, a wad of torn clothing — between the teeth to prevent biting of the tongue. If he vomits, turn the child on one side and clean out the mouth to prevent choking. And stay with the youngster; send someone else, if available, to call a doctor — otherwise, the call can wait.

Until the convulsion is over, you should do nothing else. Don't throw cold water in the child's face; neither that nor anything else will stop the convulsion from running its course. Don't even try to hold down or otherwise restrain the child unless it is obviously necessary to prevent serious self-injury.

When the seizure is over, the child will probably be somewhat confused and disoriented and may even fall into a deep sleep; that's normal, and it may last for quite a while. The first thing to do is to see that there is no breathing difficulty. If there is, open the child's mouth and see if the tongue has curled back to block the throat; if it has, roll the child on his side for a moment to let the tongue fall forward. Then keep him lying down, while you quickly consider what to do next, based on the following.

If the child has epilepsy (to your knowledge), the seizure means that medication which generally controls the condition has been omitted or is inadequate, and a call to the doctor is in order.

If the child has a high fever — if he is terribly hot to the touch, it will be obvious; if not, take the temperature — that is probably the cause of the convulsion. It's not at all unusual for convulsion to accompany high fever, especially in small children. If the child indeed has a high fever, turn to HEAT STROKE and take the emergency measures you'll find there. Also notify your physician, who will probably want to confirm the diagnosis of a febrile seizure.

If you have reason to suspect poisoning — if there is an empty container nearby, or if the child admits eating or drinking some toxic substance — turn to POISONING and follow the instructions specified for that substance. Among those that might cause such a reaction are a number of medications, including amphetamines, aspirin, atropine, and others; liquor; DDT, rat poison, and other pesticides; gasoline and kerosene products.

If none of the foregoing apply, have the child seen by a physician without delay; there is no further action that you can or should take without knowing the cause of the event.

Cooley's anemia: See ANEMIA.

Coombs' test: one of a number of blood tests that may be utilized when anemia is evident or suspected, as well as in efforts to determine maternal-fetal incompatibilities. The test reveals the presence of hemolytic (red-blood-cell-destroying) antibody. A positive Coombs' test may suggest a number of conditions, including mother-child blood-group problems, systemic lupus, lymphoma, and hemolytic anemia of unknown cause.

Cope: See PAIN RELIEVERS.

cornea: the transparent membrane on the anterior surface of the eyeball, covering the pupil and iris. A corneal abrasion — a scratch or scrape on the cornea caused by something striking or getting into the eye — can be quite serious, since scar formation directly in front of the pupil can block vision; suspicion of a corneal abrasion calls for immediate consultation with an ophthalmologist. For further comment, see EYE INJURIES.

corns: They're rare in children, but do occur occasionally, usually as the result of improperly fitted or too-small shoes. Don't try to deal with a corn yourself. For one thing, corns can be confused (by you, not by a physician) with warts, and vice versa. For another, commercial corn removers can affect the skin surrounding the corn (if it is a corn) as well as the corn itself, possibly precipitating a nasty infection. Take the youngster to the doctor.

cornstarch: See BABY POWDER. A solution of cornstarch also makes a soothing bath for the relief of extensive itching, as of hives, chickenpox, or poison ivy.

corpuscles: See BLOOD CELLS.

cortex: the outer part of a structure or organ, for example, the cerebral cortex (that layer of the brain) or the adrenal cortex; the latter produces a hormone called cortisol.

corticosteroids: hormones produced by the cortex of the adrenal glands; their full name, which nobody uses, is *adrenocorticosteroids* (sometimes they are referred to simply as "steroids"). In humans, that hormonal substance is cortisol; some other mammals secrete a similar substance called cortisone which, when administered to humans, is converted to cortisol. The "steroid" (sterol-like) part of the term stems from the fact that these substances have a chemical structure (but not effects) similar to that of cholesterol.

A number of versions of these substances have also been synthesized. Generic terms include, in addition to the foregoing, prednisone, prednisolone, methylprednisolone, triamcinolone, and others. Trade names include Aristocort, Cortone, Decadron, Deltasone, Deronil, Gammacorten, Kenacort, Medrol, Meticorten, Paracort, and Sterane — to mention just a very few from a lengthy list.

What cortisone — the popular term, which we use now and henceforth to apply to the entire group of substances — does is help the body withstand various kinds of physical stress, whether caused by injury, toxic substances, infection, extreme temperatures, etc. One reason for giving a substitute for the naturally produced hormone is, of course, failure (or necessary surgical removal) of the adrenal glands. Administered in *addition* to the body's own supply, cortisone helps boost the body's ability to cope; it must be emphasized that these drugs do *not* combat the root cause of the problem, but rather, act to suppress or control reactions to, or symptoms of, the problem. Among the conditions for which they may be administered, whether as an emergency measure or on a long-term basis, are venomous animal bites for which there is no specific antidote, extreme allergic reactions, some conditions involving severe respiratory distress, rheumatoid arthritis, nephrosis, and leukemia.

The results are often dramatic. Unfortunately, adverse effects of long-term administration can be dramatic, too — although these vary considerably with dosage and schedule, as well as with the individual. Among such possible effects are growth retardation (more likely with the synthetics than with the natural substances), slowed hair growth, slowed healing of minor injuries, facial swelling, and others. Physicians, who are very much aware of these possibilities, reserve these drugs for instances in which they are absolutely necessary and keep the dosage as low as possible, often (when the medication is to be taken over a fairly long period) directing that it be taken on an every-other-day basis. The patient is generally taken off the drug as soon as possible — not abruptly, which would prove a shock to the body's hormonal balance, but by a gradual tapering-off.

There are four other facets of long-term cortisone administration of which parents should be aware.

Cortisone can alter the body's ability to cope with carbohydrates. If your child is diabetic and cortisone is prescribed, a change in insulin dosage may be in order; the question should be discussed with the physician(s).

Second, these drugs lower the

body's natural ability to fight off and destroy infectious organisms (they cope, remember, with symptoms, not with causes). Thus the child should be protected, so far as is possible, from exposure to infectious disease. And vaccinations are contraindicated while a child is on cortisone therapy, since there is a risk of overwhelming infection.

Third, a child taking one of these drugs should not be given any *other* medication — especially aspirin or any product including it — unless the drug and dosage have been fully discussed with the doctor.

Finally, a major effect of corticosteroid therapy is the suppression of the body's own *natural* production of cortisol. The result of that phenomenon is that any severe injury — or surgery — could produce a life-threatening situation, unless attending medical personnel are fully informed; replacement therapy is required in such circumstances — both during the period of administration of the drug, *and* for a fairly long "catch-up" period that persists after the drug is withdrawn, before normal function is resumed. After eight or more weeks of cortisone therapy, that catch-up period may last as long as a year. During the course of the drug's administration, then, and for as much as a year thereafter, you should (a) see that the child carries a warning card or other device (see MEDIC ALERT) in case of accident and (b) discuss the situation with the physician beforehand if any surgery is contemplated.

corticotropin: another name for a hormone produced by the pituitary gland; see ACTH.

cortisol, cortisone, Cortone: See CORTICOSTEROIDS.

Coryban-D: See DECONGESTANTS, NASAL.

coryza: one of those wonderfully obscure terms with which your children will no doubt delight in mystifying their friends; it means an acute (not chronic) rhinitis (inflammation of the mucous membranes of the nose). In other words, a cold.

cosmetic surgery: See PLASTIC SURGERY.

costal: relating to a rib (the medical term for which is *costa*) or ribs *(costae).*

coughs: Like many other things, coughing is a symptom of a variety of problems; it certainly indicates that something, major or minor, is amiss in the adenoids, throat, sinuses, bronchial tubes, or lungs.

The nature of a cough due to sticking of food or a foreign object in the throat is fairly obvious; for first-aid measures, see CHOKING.

Other sudden-onset coughs require medical diagnosis. Ask yourself some questions: Is it a dry, hacking cough or a wet one? Is it a continuous cough, or are there spells of coughing with rest periods between? Are there any unusual wheezing or whooping sounds, either on inhalation or exhalation? (See ASTHMA; BRONCHIOLITIS; CROUP; WHOOPING COUGH.) Is the youngster spitting up something when he coughs? If so, what? (See BRONCHIECTASIS.) Are there any other symptoms, such as fever or complaints of pain, anywhere in the body? (See BRONCHITIS.) When you have the answers, call the doctor.

If your child is sick in bed with an illness that involves coughing, your physician will probably have prescribed a remedy; if not, or the coughing becomes markedly worse, phone the doctor.

Ordinary coughs accompanying ordinary colds require ordinary remedies such as warm, soothing broths and steam inhalation (or an electric humidifier; see VAPORIZERS). Over-the-counter cough medicines should be purchased and given to your child only on your doctor's prescription or recommendation, the happy syrup-sipping tots in the TV commercials notwithstanding. Some contain codeine, a narcotic, as a cough suppressant, although most major brands have substituted the somewhat safer suppressant dextromethorphan; others contain antihistamines such as chlorpheniramine maleate (which won't help a cold and may have side effects), or sympathomimetic drugs such as phenylephrine hydrochloride (see DECONGESTANTS, NASAL).

If your physician does recommend that you use one of the patent cough medicines and doesn't suggest a particular brand (naturally, you should follow such a suggestion), it's helpful to understand what these medicines do and under what circumstances they're useful. You do not, as we've pointed out, need extra ingredients. During the day, what's helpful for an ordinary cough due to a cold is an expectorant that loosens and liquefies mucus so it can be coughed up easily. The most effective such substance is glyceryl guaiacolate; among the few preparations that offer it without other, irrelevant ingredients are 2G, Robitussin and GG Tussin (the plain forms with no letters following the names), and Expectran (which has a nicer taste but is less widely distributed). At night, a cough suppressant combined with an expectorant will let the child sleep better and still keep the secretions loose; brands that offer this combination include Cheracol D, Robitussin-DM, 2G/DM, and Romilar Children's Cough Syrup.

Coxsackie disease: an infectious illness vaguely reminiscent of polio or meningitis, but much less serious; it was at first thought to be a form of polio, but the cause has been found to be a different virus — a discovery made in Coxsackie, New York, hence the name.

Typical symptoms, appearing after a two- to fourteen-day incubation period, resemble those of mild, nonparalytic polio or severe intestinal flu, or a combination thereof. They may include headache, nausea and/or vomiting, a fever that may range from low to rather high, possibly stiffness in the back and neck, and sometimes (in about half the cases) a sore throat. The disease runs its course in a few days, and there is no specific treatment — just rest, aspirin, and whatever can be done to make the child more comfortable.

Coxsackie disease is highly contagious, and with a peak incidence in summer and fall it can quickly overrun a children's camp or vacationers' camp site. It can spread by droplet infection, just as colds can, but epidemics have frequently been traced to poor sanitation facilities (feces carry the infection) combined with flies and other insects that carry the virus to inadequately protected food and water. Thus, hygienic measures can usually prevent an extensive outbreak.

Also see VIRUSES.

crab lice: See LICE, BODY.

cradle cap: a condition of early infancy in which greasy, yellowish crusts form on the scalp; if it appears, it's important to take the child to the doctor, who will prescribe a preparation to clear up the condition and prevent secondary infection (which can develop, and spread, if the problem goes untreated).

Cradle cap is caused by inadequate cleansing — and can be prevented by keeping the baby's scalp clean. Soap and water on a soft washcloth, applied once a week, will do it. Don't be afraid you'll hurt that misnamed "soft spot" at the top of the head; it's true that the skull bones haven't fused completely, but nature has provided a tough, leathery membrane to protect the area in the meantime, and simple washing will do no damage whatever.

cramps, abdominal: See ABDOMINAL PAIN.

cramps, feet and legs: They're a common phenomenon in active youngsters, sometimes occurring when a muscle is fatigued or overstretched, sometimes when the child is just sitting still — or even sleeping (and it's no fun to be awakened by a sudden leg cramp). The usual sites are the arch of the foot, the calf of the leg, and the thigh. Rub the area briskly, and if the cramp's in the foot, have the child turn his toes up and bend his foot up as far as possible. If it's the calf muscle that's cramped, have him relax his foot, bend his knee slightly, and stand up (with most of his weight on the other leg) in order to increase the circulation to the lower part of his body, while you continue to massage the calf. If it's the thigh, have the child lie down while you massage the area; application of heat (with a heating pad, for example) may also help to relax the muscle.

cramps, menstrual: They're *not* "normal," and you shouldn't lead your daughter to believe that they are. If mild cramps do occur, though, it's not necessarily a cause for concern; the discomfort may be relieved by taking a little aspirin (avoid the so-called extra-strength and combination-of-ingredients pain relievers) and applying heat to the area in the form of a heating pad or hot-water bottle. But if the cramps are persistent or severe, consult your doctor.

cranium: the anatomical term for the skull.

crawling: See DEVELOPMENT.

cretinism: severe congenital hypothyroidism (see ENDOCRINE GLANDS). It is generally due to underdevelopment of the thyroid, or to failure of the gland to function properly (i.e., to produce the needed hormone). The reasons for these phenomena are not known; iodine deficiency in the mother during pregnancy occurs only very rarely now, except in the world's most primitive areas. The condition is not apparent at birth, but generally manifests itself between the ages of two months and two years.

Typical symptoms include rough, dry skin, distended abdomen, protruding tongue, and general mental dullness. If the condition goes untreated, the result will be a general stunting of the child in all facets of development, including dwarfism and mental retardation; the child will usually not progress beyond a five-year-old mental level.

Cretinism can be treated successfully, by administration of thyroid extract. The treatment must begin early, however, and must generally be continued throughout the patient's life. The earlier treatment is started, the better the outlook for normal mental and physical development.

Since sometimes a degree of retardation has taken place even before symptoms become apparent, it would be advantageous to be able to detect the condition. A special blood test to be performed a few days after birth (it requires only a pinprick of the baby's heel) was introduced early in 1974 for mass screening in Quebec and there has also been experimental use of the test elsewhere in Canada, as well as very limited experimental screening in the United States. Many physicians feel that such a test should be routine and even mandatory, as is the test for phenylketonuria (PKU) throughout most of both countries; the incidence of the two congenital conditions is comparable, about one in ten thousand to twelve thousand.

crib death: See SUDDEN INFANT DEATH SYNDROME.

cromolyn sodium: See ASTHMA.

crossed eyes: Don't worry if your small baby appears cross-eyed some, or even much, of the time; most babies do. One reason is that they can't yet control and coordinate their eye muscles properly. The other is that in babies, the area between the eyes is proportionately wider than that in adults, and a baby can look cross-eyed when he is actually looking straight ahead.

If an infant still seems cross-eyed after the age of six months, however, the question should be discussed with your doctor; there might be an eye-muscle imbalance that, if not corrected, could affect later vision in one or both eyes. Correction may involve eyeglasses, "patching," eye exercises, or surgery for the affected muscle, depending upon the physician's judgment.

croup: a term denoting not a disease, but a symptom — a special sort of harsh, barking cough combined with difficulty in breathing (usually on inhalation, as compared with asthma where the problem is chiefly with *ex*halation); the child may wheeze and gasp for breath, and may even turn blue at intervals. It is serious, but in most cases not as serious as it seems; if the condition is promptly and properly treated, there will usually be no complications.

Croup is also referred to medically as acute obstructive laryngitis, or acute spasmodic laryngitis, and the cause of the characteristic cough is indeed spasm and inflammation of the larynx. Most commonly, the condition stems from a viral infection of the upper respiratory tract; occasionally, the infection is bacterial. Very rarely, there may be a more serious condition such as diphtheria. Prompt medical evaluation is important.

Call the doctor immediately if your youngster has a sudden attack of croup or suspected croup, whether or not fever or any other symptoms are apparent. While you're waiting, keep the child warm and take steps to relieve breathing: get the bathroom steamed up by turning on the hot water in the bath or shower, and keep the child there for twenty to thirty minutes. If, by this time, the child's breathing has not eased, or his temperature has climbed over 103° F. (39.4° C.), take the child to the nearest hospital emergency room.

In most cases, the doctor can prescribe medications that will effectively relieve the congestion and spasms and clear up the infection. Rarely, and only if breathing is critically obstructed and the child's life is in danger, a tracheotomy will be ordered — an emergency incision into the windpipe below the larynx to permit air to reach the child's lungs.

crying: An older child, obviously, can be asked *why* he is crying, and the reason generally involves severe pain or unhappiness. An infant, however, presents a different problem.

Before a child can talk, crying — or some variation of crying — is the only means of communication (actual tears may not be shed until the age of three or four months, or even later). Crying may mean that an infant is hungry, wet, lonely, overtired, too cold, bored — or in pain. Get to know your baby's normal, everyday cries — the usual "I'm wet!" and "Where's my feeding?" ones — and be aware of unusual differences that may mean trouble.

Hoarseness or raspiness in the cry means a possible throat problem, and the doctor should be called. Sharp cries at night may signal sharp pain, and you should look for other symptoms — as of earache (turning the head from side to side) or abdominal distress (drawing legs up or stretching them out stiffly); these, too, of course mean that the doctor should be called immediately. See if the baby is wet or soiled — or needs to be burped. Take a good look; is there anything unusual about the child's appearance? Take the baby's temperature; is there fever?

If you can find no reason for your baby's continued crying, and you have no reason to suspect simple overtiredness — *call the doctor.*

cryotherapy: the use of extreme cold in treatment, especially in surgery. It has been applied, notably, to some neurosurgical procedures, to treatment of certain skin lesions and eye disorders, and to some surgery involving the cervix and the anus (including hemorrhoids).

Crysticillin, Crystifor: trade names for penicillin G; see ANTIBIOTICS.

CT: See COMPUTERIZED AXIAL TOMOGRAPHY.

culture: to place material removed or withdrawn from the body — as sputum, urine, joint fluids, etc. — in or on an appropriate nurturing medium in order to detect the presence and propagation of any infectious organisms therein; a colony of organisms so obtained.

Curads: a trade name for adhesive strip bandages that include a nonstick film over the gauze pad.

curettage: the scraping of the interior of a body cavity in order to remove something — e.g., foreign matter or a growth — or to obtain tissue for analysis.

curvature of the spine: a general term covering many types of misalignment of the spinal column, stemming from a variety of causes — congenital malformation, injury, disease, nutritional deficiency, et al. Correction, which is in the realm of the orthopedist, depends upon the precise condition and its cause. For comment on two major types, see LORDOSIS and SCOLIOSIS.

Cushing's disease: a disorder — characterized by unusual obesity, muscular weakness, facial swelling, and other physical symptoms, as well as detectable metabolic abnormalities — caused by excessive secretion of ACTH (which, in turn, causes excessive secretion of cortisol). The cause may be a growth involving the pituitary gland, a growth elsewhere that is secreting ACTH, or simple hypersecretion of the hormone by the pituitary for no apparent reason; treatment will vary according to the findings.

An array of similar symptoms *not* necessarily including excessive ACTH production is generally termed Cushing's *syndrome,* a broader term meaning excessive production of cortisol by the adrenal glands, whatever the cause — typically, if excess ACTH is not involved, an adrenal growth of one kind or another. Sometimes that broader term is also used to denote the appearance of some of these symptoms as the result of corticosteroid therapy, but the specific and more correct adjective in that case is *Cushingoid,* i.e., "like" the naturally appearing disorder.

cuts: How to handle a cut depends upon its size and nature, and partly its location. Any cut is an invitation to possible infection, so it's important to deal with it quickly and correctly.

A small, uncomplicated cut should simply be washed with soap and running water, then protected with an adhesive strip bandage (as, Band-Aids or Curads). Don't put anything else, such as iodine or any other antiseptic, on it. If the skin is gaping, or there is a loose flap of skin, you can use a butterfly (see BANDAGES) — or take the youngster to the doctor and see if stitching may be needed.

Any large cut requires prompt medical attention; pause only to take emergency first-aid measures if there's a great deal of blood (see BLEEDING). If the cut is in the chest or abdomen, rush the child not to your own doctor, but to the nearest hospital emergency room.

These situations also require an immediate trip to the doctor, whatever the size of the wound: a cut made with glass, if there is any possibility of a fragment remaining in the wound; a cut made with any metal object not definitely clean, especially if outdoors (there is the possibility of tetanus infection); a cut suffered by a child who is diabetic; a cut suffered by a child who has hemophilia or any other serious circulatory problem; any cut from which you cannot stop the bleeding.

Parents of active youngsters should not be alarmed if children cut their tongues or lips in tumbles; it's a rather frequent occurrence in young children. Usually, when the blood is wiped away, the cut will turn out to be smaller than it appeared to be at first. Such a cut needs no special treatment and will heal fairly quickly. A yellowish look to the area is not a cause for concern; that's the way things heal on mucous membrane.

cyanosis: a bluish cast to the skin and mucous membranes, indicating that the body is not receiving enough oxygen. It can be caused by a variety of cardiac and pulmonary problems, and can also occur in such conditions as asthma and croup.

cyclamates: See SWEETENERS.

cyclic AMP: a naturally formed substance in the body, isolated by the distinguished physiologist Earl Sutherland in 1958; the letters stand for adenosine monophosphate, the "cyclic" not for time periods but characterizing its molecular structure. It has proved to be an important part of the biochemical activity that goes on continuously. Dr. Sutherland dubbed it a "second messenger" — an apt term, since it appears, among other things, to "relay" the "messages" of various hormones that influence and regulate bodily functions and processes.

Subsequent research has shown that cyclic AMP also inhibits the growth of certain tumors, triggers the actions of a number of enzymes, and plays a role in regulating fat metabolism and possibly blood pressure. Measurements of cyclic-AMP levels in patients with a variety of disorders suggest, too, that some kidney dysfunctions, asthma, myasthenia gravis, and perhaps certain arthritic conditions may involve disturbances in the activity of this substance.

Researchers are of course pursuing what seems to be a vast therapeutic potential. And cyclic AMP appears to interact, as well, with another set of recently pinpointed substances; see PROSTAGLANDINS.

cyclizine: See MOTION SICKNESS.

Cyclopar: a trade name for tetracycline; see ANTIBIOTICS.

cyclophosphamide: See IMMUNOSUPPRESSANTS.

Cylert: a trade name for the drug pemoline; see HYPERKINESIS.

cyst: an enclosed (limited), benign growth contained (unlike a tumor) in a sac. The interior of a cyst is liquid or semisolid. A cyst is usually not serious and often is not removed unless it is unsightly, causing pain, or creating a problem by pressure on other tissues.

An *adventitious cyst* is one that forms around, and encloses, a foreign object that has entered the body.

A *colloid cyst* is one that contains material jelly-like in consistency.

A *dermoid cyst* is one containing epithelial cells, those that normally constitute skin, hair, and mucous membrane. Dermoid cysts are probably congenital (although they may not become evident for many years) and tend to appear along the midline of the body, over the eyebrows, or in the genitals. One theory postulates that they enclose cells that were originally destined to become a fraternal twin but were accidentally embedded in the body of an already developing embryo. More recently, a second theory has emerged as the result of observing similar phenomena in laboratory animals: that dermoid cysts appearing in the ovaries or related structures of girls and women may be ova that — unfertilized by sperm — have, for reasons unknown, begun to divide and develop spontaneously. A dermoid cyst is removed surgically.

A *ganglion cyst* is a fairly common sort that forms on the sheath of a tendon; the back of the wrist is the most frequent site, but a ganglion can occur at other points as well, such as the back of the knee. It usually begins as a pea-size lump that may get larger and, if it gets large enough, can eventually cause some weakness in the joint as fluid accumulates in the cyst — which is the only serious implication of this kind of cyst. The doctor can remove or destroy a ganglion if it becomes annoying; the means range from simple outside pressure to surgical excision.

A *sebaceous cyst* forms around a blocked oil gland, usually on the scalp, back, or scrotum; consult your doctor, who will judge whether or not removal of the cyst is necessary or desirable.

A *thyroglossal cyst* occurs more often in children than in adults, and involves cells of the type that make up the thyroid gland and the tongue; it is located in the front of the neck. Such a cyst is usually removed, since it can create pressure on vital digestive and respiratory passages.

For another different, misnamed condition, see BARTHOLIN'S CYST.

cystic fibrosis: a hereditary condition involving the combined malfunction of a number of endocrine glands, especially the pancreas (not its insulin-producing cells, but that part of the gland secreting certain digestive juices), resulting in a state of malnutrition; the sweat glands are also involved, with excessive salt loss. It is an autosomal recessive disorder (see HEREDITY) and occurs about once in fifteen hundred to two thousand births, much less commonly among Afro-Americans and extremely rarely among people of Oriental origin. As those carrying the trait grow, with modern medical techniques, to adulthood, it is felt that the incidence of cystic fibrosis may increase. An estimated one in 22 persons of European descent is now a "carrier."

Cystic fibrosis is often discovered immediately after birth by an alert attending physician, since the usual immediate postnatal movement of the bowels (producing meconium) is generally absent. (It cannot yet be detected before birth, nor can "carrier" adults be identified.) In any case, the symptoms will almost always soon be apparent: the infant will appear obviously undernourished; the abdomen will be bloated; stools, containing undigested fats, will be bulky and unusually odorous.

There may also be accompanying bronchitis or pulmonary complications. (Rarely, cystic fibrosis is not diagnosed until later, even as late as the teens, when respiratory problems bring the youngster's condition to light; in these rare instances, the abdominal difficulties in infancy have been atypically mild.) Victims of cystic fibrosis are especially susceptible to bronchial and lung infections, and these used to be — prior to the development of antibiotics — frequent causes of death in infancy. But that's no longer so.

Treatment of cystic fibrosis consists basically of administration of pancreatic extract, plus a special dietary regimen (usually high in protein, low in fat, and including supplementary vitamins to prevent deficiencies). The parents, however, must continue to be on guard against potentially critical pulmonary difficulties; colds, coughs, or other respiratory symptoms must be promptly reported to the doctor, who may prescribe antibiotics or other measures as preventive therapy.

cystitis: an inflammation of the bladder; usually, there is some inflammation of the ureters (above the bladder) and the urethra (the bladder's outlet) as well. It's far more common in females, because of their shorter urethras; it would be hard to give comparative figures for children, but in adults, the average male's urethra measures some eight inches (more than twenty centimeters), that of the average female only about an inch and a half (less than four centimeters).

Symptoms of bladder infection can vary considerably; they usually include more frequent urination than usual, possibly urgency and pain when urinating, occasionally blood or pus in the urine (blood tends simply to make the urine appear dark, while pus is very hard to detect visually), and, rarely, fever. These are also symptoms of other conditions. Your doctor (or a urologist to whom your own physician may refer you) can go beyond by-eye methods with microscopic analysis and culture of the urine and may also employ a cystoscope — a long, thin tube with a light at the end, through which the interior of the bladder can be seen.

Treatment of cystitis usually involves drugs — antibiotics, sulfa drugs, or whatever the physician judges best in the particular situation — to combat the inflammation, plus rest and, possibly, specified changes in the child's diet. The physician will usually also double-check the kidneys to make sure that they haven't been affected by the infection.

cystogram: a procedure, performed by a radiologist or urologist, in which radio-opaque dye is instilled into the bladder and visualized by X ray. It can be helpful in diagnosing conditions affecting the bladder and upper urinary tract.

cytogenetics: the study of chromosomes and their structure (see HEREDITY), primarily with the object of detecting and explaining inherited disorders.

cytology: the study of cell structure, growth, etc.

cytotoxins, Cytoxan: See IMMUNOSUPPRESSANTS. Cytoxan is a trade name for cyclophosphamide, one of the group.

D

d.: See PRESCRIPTIONS.

D and C: See ABORTION.

Dalmane: a trade name for flurazepam; see SEDATIVES.

dandruff: a malfunction of the natural process in which the cells of the scalp surface are continually shed and replaced; a disorder of the sebaceous (oil) glands is usually involved as well. The resultant symptoms are visible flaking and itching of variable intensity. Dandruff's cause has not been specifically pinpointed and has been the subject of considerable speculation; circulatory problems, dietary elements, inadequate cleansing, chemical irritants, bacteria, hormonal disturbances, and emotional factors have all figured prominently among the theories — and it's possible that causes may vary with the individual. The condition doesn't usually appear prior to adolescence.

There is no complete cure, but for most people, one of the commercially available special shampoos or post-shampoo rinses will effect control; it may take a bit of experimentation, and the product should be given a trial of several weeks' use. Bear in mind that if it does work, it must continue to be used, for the tendency is chronic, although for some, the problem is seasonal ("winter dandruff" is a common phenomenon). And be sure that the hair is rinsed very thoroughly after shampooing; soap residue can also give the appearance of dandruff.

If the problem persists or worsens, if it spreads beyond the scalp itself, or if other symptoms such as redness or crusts appear, the youngster should see a dermatologist; another condition, requiring medical diagnosis and treatment, may be involved. (See ALLERGY; DEFICIENCY DISEASES; ECZEMA; PSORIASIS; RINGWORM.)

Darcil: a trade name for phenethicillin, a semisynthetic penicillin; see ANTIBIOTICS.

Darvon: a trade name for propoxyphene; see NARCOTICS.

Datril: a trade name for acetaminophen; see PAIN RELIEVERS.

Dawson's encephalitis: See SSPE.

DDE, DDT: See PESTICIDES.

D.D.S.: The abbreviation for Doctor of Dental Surgery, the degree most commonly held by dentists. Also see SPECIALTIES, DENTAL.

deafness: One of the reasons it is so important that an ear infection, injury, or other problem receive prompt medical attention is that such conditions, if untreated, can cause deafness. It has recently been demonstrated that loud noise, too, can cause deafness — by sudden, violent occurrence (as, an explosion), or by exposure over a long period of time (as to extremely loud music or some types of machinery).

Deafness may also be congenital, sometimes resulting from an infectious disease (especially rubella) contracted by the mother during pregnancy. About one-third of the cases of congenital deafness are hereditary; it is believed that the trait is recessive or, more likely, recessive-plus (see HEREDITY), and there are many instances of children with normal hearing born to parents who have both been deaf from birth.

If you suspect any hearing loss whatever in a child, it is vital to see the doctor and have the child's hearing checked so that therapy, if it proves to be needed, can be instituted promptly; a delay could seriously affect the child's learning and general development.

A child who is totally, or nearly totally, deaf should receive special therapy and other training from the start, in the preschool years (your doctor can advise you on the availability of such therapy in the area where you live); if that's done, the youngster can grow up functioning nearly normally.

debridement: removal of dead tissue from the surface of a wound in order to let the healthy tissue beneath commence the healing process. It is most often needed in cases of severe burns in which extensive tissue destruction has occurred, or in wounds which contain a great deal of foreign matter.

Decadron: See CORTICOSTEROIDS.

Declomycin, Declostatin: See ANTIBIOTICS. The first word is a trade name for demeclocycline, one of the tetracyclines; the second, a trade name for a combination of demeclocycline and nystatin.

decongestants, nasal: preparations designed chiefly to constrict small blood vessels and shrink swollen mucous membranes in the nose in order to permit easier drainage and freer breathing; they may be suggested for colds or for relief of allergic conditions. They should *never* be used without a doctor's specific advice or prescription.

One reason is that a number of the preparations sold over the counter (chiefly drops and sprays, but some in tablet or capsule form) contain other, possibly irrelevant ingredients — which may represent either a waste of money or the possibility of adverse reactions, or both.

Many, for example, include antihistamines — which may be helpful in cases of allergy, but have no effect on a cold (and even an allergic condition may require a different antihistamine). Some of those also contain caffeine, which won't unstuff *anyone's* nose. A few toss in mild analgesics, often inferior to ordinary aspirin for relief of general discomfort.

Certain of these products should, in our opinion, be avoided even if the doctor *does* suggest that an over-the-counter decongestant may be helpful; they contain extra medications that really have no business in any such preparation. These include Contac, which contains belladonna; Dristan tablets and 4-Way tablets, which incorporate antacids; Coryban-D capsules, Sinutab, and Super-Anahist, which contain phenacetin, an analgesic that's a potential cause of kidney trouble.

The second reason that decongestants should not be used without a physician's advice is that they are what are medically called *sympathomimetic* drugs; the ones in widest use are phenylephrine hydrochloride and phenylpropanolamine hydrochloride, and all the products we've mentioned above contain one or the other drug as a major ingredient. Sympathomimetics do indeed act on the small blood vessels to shrink nasal membranes. But they can also act on the system generally — elevating the blood pressure, stimulating the heart (certainly no child who has a heart ailment should use them without medical advice), raising the metabolism, and affecting the nervous system. None of these effects — which are in general fairly mild — are necessarily harmful to a particular individual, but a doctor should do the judging.

If the doctor does suggest a decongestant for your youngster, there are a couple of things you might bear in mind from both economic and physical standpoints.

The doctor may, of course, wish the child to have a combination medication, including antihistamine or some other drug, and, if so, will probably recommend a specific product — or prescribe one, if the desired combination is not available over the counter. But if not, it's certainly wise to buy a preparation containing only the decongestant, and not any other unnecessary ingredients. Phenylephrine is available as Coryban-D spray and as Neo-Synephrine; the latter comes in both drops and spray, and also offers weaker concentrations for small children and infants, in addition to adult strength.

If drops have been recommended, don't buy more than one ounce; within a few days, if the child has a cold, the liquid will have become contaminated by mucus from the child's nose (and leftover drops should be discarded when the cold's over). For that reason, never use a child's drops or spray for another member of the family, even if the doctor has suggested a similar preparation; other patients should have their own drops or spray.

Children under five generally lack the knack of sniffing a spray up into their noses — but if the doctor suggests drops, it's smart to buy the spray version, especially if your child is a violent resister of drops, as many small children are. Held upside down, the squeeze bottle does dispense drops; it's plastic, hence unbreakable; it requires the use of only one hand. All these make holding down and getting drops into a squirming youngster much easier.

Finally, don't let your child get in the habit of using any decongestant on a continuous basis. There is a vicious-cycle "rebound" phenomenon with these drugs which can simply make matters worse: after extended use, the nasal membranes swell even more when the drug wears off, and are eventually unable to shrink without the use of higher and more frequent dosages — which causes them to swell even more each time a dose wears off, and so on and so on. If there's a continuing stuffy-nose problem after a cold or other condition should have ended, the child may have some type of chronic allergic condition; discuss with your pediatrician, or with an ear-nose-and-throat specialist, the possibility of an antihistamine for relief.

deer-fly fever: See TULAREMIA.

defecation: See BOWEL MOVEMENTS.

deficiency diseases: conditions resulting from severe lack of necessary elements in the diet, especially protein or one of the essential vitamins or minerals — or, more rarely, from some glandular or digestive malfunction that keeps the body from assimilating or making use of the element even if it *is* in the diet. These conditions, except in their mildest forms, are uncommon in the United States but are unhappily widespread in some parts of the world.

Protein deficiency in children can cause the tragic disease called kwashiorkor, typified by spindly bodies with bloated bellies. There may be skin manifestations, digestive malfunctions, permanent physical and mental retardation, and eventual death if the condition is not diagnosed and corrected; the degree of stunting of the child depends upon the duration of the disease prior to treatment.

A lack of *vitamin A* can also stunt physical growth if it occurs in a young child. At any age, it can affect the eyes, resulting in "night blindness" (actually inability to see under twilight or dusk conditions) or in xerophthalmia, in which the mucous membranes around the eyes become so thickened that vision is impaired.

Deficiencies in the various *B vitamins* can cause a number of conditions ranging from mild to quite serious, depending upon the degree of deficiency and the vitamin(s) involved. Beriberi, which includes serious nerve inflammation, muscular atrophy, and weakness, is caused by lack of thiamine, or vitamin B_1. Another fairly well-known disease, pellagra, stems from niacin deficiency; it, too, is a serious condition, involving assorted nervous and gastrointestinal manifestations. Too little riboflavin, or vitamin B_2, can result in a number of problems including scaling of the skin, digestive difficulties, and vision impairment. Lack of vitamin B_6 affects both the skin and the nerves. And mild deficiency in the B group or "complex" as a whole, probably the most common of all vitamin deficiencies, will generally result in a chronically edgy or listless state.

Vitamin C deficiency, if it's severe enough, causes the infamous ailment called scurvy that used to afflict sailors on long sea voyages (the problem quickly disappeared when the cause was finally deduced); it's an unpleasant disease involving acute gingivitis, joint pains, and extreme overall weakness. A lesser deficiency will result in similar but milder symptoms — tenderness of the gums, possibly some joint aches and easily fatigued muscles.

Deficiency of *vitamin K* rarely occurs by itself, since only small amounts are needed and they are derived from the same foods as some of the major vitamins; if it does occur along with other nutritional ailments, the telling symptom will be delayed coagulation of the blood (i.e., unusual difficulty in getting a wound to stop bleeding).

A *calcium* deficiency — or lack of *vitamin D,* which is necessary for the assimilation of calcium — is particularly serious in infants and growing children; it can result in rickets, with bowed legs and other malformations of bones and teeth, plus generally weak muscles and joints. This deficiency can also be one cause of an uncommon ailment involving muscular spasm (see TETANY).

Iron deficiency — or deficiency of vitamin B_{12}, a factor in the utilization of iron for blood-cell production — can, as is well known, cause some types of anemia.

Iodine is needed for proper thyroid function (see ENDOCRINE GLANDS), and deficiency of that mineral can cause hypofunction of that organ.

Frightening as some of these conditions are, they are highly unlikely ever to afflict your children. In most parts of the United States, vitamin and/or mineral supplements are totally unnecessary and should not be given to your family, either singly or in multiple-type pills, unless they are prescribed by your doctor to remedy a deficiency or for other valid medical reasons. By and large, all the essentials can be obtained from readily available foods. For a full discussion of the elements and their sources, see NUTRITION.

dehydration: a condition of excessive fluid loss resulting from deprivation of food and drink or from extreme sweating, vomiting, urination, or diarrhea. It is serious, especially in infants, and can cause a critical upset in the body's chemical balance. If any of the foregoing conditions prevail, the doctor will undoubtedly institute measures to guard against dehydration, and it is vital that these directions be followed. If dehydration has occurred, the doctor will probably hospitalize the child for treatment. For tips on preventing dehydration in the most common causative situation, see DIARRHEA.

delirium: a condition of incoherence and possibly hallucinations, indicating, usually, an extremely high fever, a serious head injury, or some type of drug poisoning. It requires immediate medical attention.

Deltasone: See CORTICOSTEROIDS.

deltoid: See MUSCLES.

demeclocycline: one of the tetracyclines; see ANTIBIOTICS.

Demerol: a trade name for meperidine, a morphinelike synthetic drug; see NARCOTICS.

dengue: an infectious tropical and subtropical disease (pronounced *den-gay*) also known, because of the agonizing pain that characterizes it, as breakbone fever. It is caused by a virus, transmitted not person-to-person but via the bite of a particular mosquito found only in the areas where the disease is endemic — so that it can be contracted only by those living in, or traveling to, such areas. These include the Caribbean especially, but other places around the world as well; during recent decades there have been severe outbreaks reported in Australia, Egypt, Greece, Samoa, Polynesia, Southeast Asia (Thailand and Vietnam were especially hard hit) and, uncommonly, the southeastern United States.

Dengue's onset, some three to twelve days after the crucial mosquito bite (the average incubation period is five or six days), is usually quite sudden, with fever, nausea, vomiting, constipation, stiff neck, and the aforementioned almost unbearable pain in bones and joints. The fever is generally quite high, ranging up to 106°F. (41.1°C.), and in a small child may precipitate convulsions. The lymph nodes are usually enlarged, and there may also be a severe headache behind the eyes.

On about the third or fourth day, during a temporary remission of the fever that sometimes occurs, a pale pink rash may appear — typically first on the knees, ankles, and elbows, then spreading to other parts of the body. The disease runs its course in about a week (which generally feels more like a month to the patient), and there is normally full recovery, with no after-effects or complications (except that there is sometimes diarrhea toward the end of the week).

The foregoing describes the usual illness, sometimes called "classic" dengue. There is another, far more critical, form known as dengue hemorrhagic fever in which the virus (the very same virus) attacks the circulatory system and precipitates bleeding from the nose and mouth and other areas; children seem particularly susceptible to it, and it typically proves fatal in some six percent. Serious epidemics of hemorrhagic dengue have occurred more often in Asia than elsewhere (it is the number five cause of death in children in Thailand, which reported nearly twelve thousand cases in 1971).

Why the virus causes these two distinct forms of illness remains somewhat of a mystery. Some researchers have theorized that the more critical form represents a hypersensitive reaction — or something like it — to a reinfection in someone who has previously had the classic form; it appears, if this is so, that the reinfection must take place within five years (U.S. military personnel in Vietnam were *not* attacked by hemorrhagic dengue).

No known drugs are effective against dengue. Once the condition has been diagnosed (the diagnosis can be confirmed by blood tests), treatment is simply to combat symptoms — cool sponging to bring fever down, drugs for relief of pain (potent ones such as codeine may be needed) and, in the hemorrhagic form, adrenalin, blood plasma, and other supportive measures. Nor is there yet a vaccine or other preventive.

dental care: See TEETH.

dental hygienist: See HEALTH PROFESSIONALS.

dental surgeon: See SPECIALTIES, DENTAL.

Depo-Provera: See CONTRACEPTION.

dermabrasion: a method of treating severe scarring, in which the skin is frozen and the top layer planed or abraded off; it is also called skin planing. Dermabrasion must be done by a medical specialist, either a dermatologist or a plastic surgeon.

dermatitis: a general term for any inflammation of the skin, including allergic reactions, eczema, reactions to chemical irritants, conditions such as erysipelas and psoriasis, and the rashes accompanying a great many infectious diseases.

Atopic dermatitis typically refers to an allergic reaction in infants, whether to formula or other food, or to some element in the baby's environment; see ECZEMA for further comment on this condition.

Contact dermatitis specifically means a dermatitis resulting from something coming into direct contact with the affected area (as opposed to something eaten or breathed in); the phrase *allergic contact dermatitis* further specifies that the condition is the result of an allergic reaction (poison ivy is one such condition).

dermatologist: See SPECIALTIES, MEDICAL.

dermatomyositis: one of the major collagen diseases (for the others, see LUPUS and SCLERODERMA) that involve inflammation of various collagen-containing tissues; the cause or causes are unknown. Dermatomyositis specifically affects skin and muscle tissues. (When the skin is not affected, it is sometimes called *polymyositis,* "inflammation of many muscles.") About half of all cases involve some degree of arthritis. It most often appears in middle age, but it has been known, rarely, to occur in childhood.

Initial symptoms usually include low fever, muscular weakness (which may go unnoticed in children), possibly muscle pain. Skin symptoms typically take one of two forms: a pattern of scaly lesions similar to those of psoriasis, often in the vicinity of joints such as elbows or knees, or a purplish discoloration of the eyelids and the area surrounding the eyes. Any of these symptoms can of course suggest other problems, but the diagnosis of dermatomyositis can be established by biopsy of muscle tissue and assessment of certain blood enzyme levels.

In adults, dermatomyositis can be quite a serious condition; a significant proportion do not survive or are disabled. The prognosis appears to be better in youngsters: the condition is typically limited, running about two years, and treatment combining corticosteroids and physical therapy is generally quite successful.

dermoid cyst: See CYST.

Deronil: See CORTICOSTEROIDS.

DES: See CONTRACEPTION.

Desbutal: a trade name for a combination-of-ingredients "diet pill"; see AMPHETAMINES.

Desenex: a trade name for an over-the-counter antifungal preparation; see ATHLETE'S FOOT.

desensitization: a treatment, usually by injection, to reduce severe hypersensitive (allergic) reactions to a known substance; the procedure is used if the problem can be foreseen and the allergen can't be avoided — as in the case of certain pollen allergies, or allergies to everyday airborne substances such as house dust.

For a full discussion of the problem as a whole, see ALLERGY. Also see "Insect Stings" under BITES AND STINGS.

desert fever: See VALLEY FEVER.

desipramine: See ANTIDEPRESSANTS.

Desoxyn: a trade name for methamphetamine; see AMPHETAMINES.

detoxification: the process — sometimes also called *detoxication* — of neutralizing or removing a poison, or the toxic properties thereof, from the body.

development: Naturally, you are concerned not only with your child's physical growth, but with his muscular and mental abilities as well. When will he recognize you? When should he be able to sit up and stand and walk? How long will it be before he'll pick up a spoon or stack his blocks? When can you expect to hear his first word and his first sentence?

There are no flat, pat answers. Every baby is different. Yes, there are some averages, and we're going to mention a few of those landmark achievements in terms of the average. But there are two vital facts you must bear in mind.

First, the word "average" is not synonymous with the word "normal." The average-age figures we present here are medians. If, for example, some babies utter their first word at the age of five months, and other equally healthy, normal, bright babies don't do so until they're a year old, then the "average" figure becomes a bit over eight months — not necessarily a guideline for your baby or any other single baby but merely a statistic showing what has been observed in babies over the years. Don't *ever* measure your baby against such statistics or against the performance of other children you may know. If you have any doubts about your child's progress, discuss them with your own physician.

Second, a baby's muscular control and coordination proceed in a more or less consistent order from head to foot. He must pick up his head before he can sit up, sit before he can stand, and so on. And these basics come before more sophisticated things; it's unreasonable, for example, to expect a child to have bowel or bladder control before he has learned to walk to the bathroom.

With those qualifications, then, here are the average figures — which will reflect your own baby's behavior only if he happens to conform to the statistical median — on vision, movement, hand use, and expression and communication.

VISION

At birth, your child can't see clearly but can perceive the difference between light and dark, can for just a moment follow a moving object if it's very bright, and can distinguish and respond to a human face at a distance of about eight inches (twenty cm). By the age of eight or nine weeks, a baby begins to focus on stationary objects — though only for short periods and possibly with an oddly cross-eyed gaze, since the eye muscles are still wildly uncoordinated.

At about the age of three months a baby may be able to tell one face from another (and may embarrass you by setting up a howl at the sight of your best friends — who are brand-new faces, as far as the infant knows). It will not be until the age of two to six months that the child will have enough eye-muscle control to really look at, and follow, a moving person or object.

Also see CROSSED EYES.

HEAD AND BODY MOVEMENT

A baby can turn his head from side to side at birth; somewhere between one and three months, he will raise it when lying on his back. Next, he'll learn to roll over from his stomach to his back — it's likely to be an accident the first time, and very surprising to him — and the average age for that is quite variable, usually anywhere from two to seven months.

(While a small infant does not yet have the strength to lift himself up on hands and knees, and cannot crawl until he has developed that strength, there is present almost from birth the ability to squirm across a level surface on his stomach. This "creeping reflex" is present well before the feat of rolling over is achieved. Thus a baby of any age can fall from a bed, table, or other above-the-floor surface, and should not be left alone there. For further precautions you should take, both in early infancy and as your baby becomes more mobile, see "Children Under Five" under ACCIDENTS, PREVENTION OF.)

When he first sits up, he'll of course need support; he might be ready to try that at anywhere from five to eight months — and it will probably take him a month or two more to learn to sit up by himself. It's about then that his arms and legs will be strong enough for him to start crawling — perhaps as early as six months, perhaps as late as a year.

After he's been crawling for a little while, he's ready to learn to stand up (though he's likely to prefer crawling for some time, if he's typical). Sometime after *that* — at about one year to fifteen or sixteen months — he'll begin to take a few steps, with help. He will begin to walk without your help any time between twelve and eighteen months, although some do so earlier.

USE OF HANDS

Though even a very tiny baby can and does curl his hand around your finger, it's not really a purposeful action; he won't deliberately touch or grab anything until he's about six weeks old. (Remember that he still can't see very well.) He might begin to actually grope toward things he's interested in at about three or four months, and by the time he's six or eight months old, he may be able to pick up objects awkwardly.

Usually, it's not until about the age of nine or ten months that a child can properly reach out and grasp something — and until that time, there's no point in even trying to teach him to eat by himself. He might begin to stuff food into his mouth with his hands at about a year, or any time after that, and can perhaps be persuaded a few weeks later to start trying to use a spoon (it will take him some time, though, to become accomplished with the spoon).

By about two years, he'll probably have sufficient dexterity to manage simple toys, stack blocks, and the like. And by this time, too, he may begin to show right-hand or left-hand dominance or preference (it's rare for such dominance to appear before the age of two). Do permit him to do as he wishes on this score; it has been proved beyond question that forcing a naturally left-handed child to favor his right hand against his will can do extensive, and permanent, psychological damage.

Girls, for some reason, seem to proceed faster than boys in the area of acquiring dexterity. They can generally manipulate things better earlier, and when they get a little older, they learn button-buttoning and shoelace-tying faster, too.

SELF-EXPRESSION AND SPEECH

Your baby has a voice right from the start — that, you're no doubt very much aware of. All he can do, at first, is cry, whatever need or feeling he wants to express — and it may be difficult to tell if and when he's really unhappy, since most babies can't cry actual tears until they're at least three months old. Which is also, usually, about the time he can smile — an achievement that makes things easier all around. He won't be able to really laugh, though, till he's anywhere from four to six months old.

Even before he begins to laugh, he'll probably start to make other noises — coos, gurgles, and the like (if a three-month-old has made hardly any sounds at all, or has emitted only a monotone, it is a good idea to talk to the doctor about a hearing check). These are the first small attempts to imitate sounds he hears. And it will help if you actually talk to him, since that's the way he learns. After a couple of months, he'll start to make completely unintelligible chattering noises, sounding vaguely like speech in some very obscure foreign language, and you'll wish you had an interpreter. Be patient; he's beginning to get the general inflections of speech, though he doesn't know any words yet.

That momentous first word might be uttered at just a little over eight months, give or take a few weeks in either direction. It is likely to be "da-da" — not because the child prefers his father, but because that seems to be the first syllable all children, all over the world, say first, whatever languages their parents speak (in Russia, of course, a child's first word is thus "yes"). By his first birthday, he'll probably have picked up a few more isolated words (including "ma-ma," which is what babies generally call their mothers in all languages), and when he's perhaps fifteen or sixteen months old, he'll possibly be able to say something meaningful, such as "hi" or "bye-bye."

By the time he's two years old, he may have a vocabulary of some 300 words and be able to put together brief, telegraphic sentences — generally relating to his own wants such as food, drink, toys, and toilet needs (when he's reached this stage, he can probably understand *you* quite well, despite his *own* limited speaking ability). From then on, things usually progress fairly rapidly. By the age of three, he'll know about a thousand words, and he'll increase the list by about five hundred a year from then on.

For further comment on various stages and phases of your child's growth and maturation see (in alphabetical, not chronological, order) ADOLESCENCE; BOTTLE FEEDING; BREAST FEEDING; FOOD, SOLID; GROWTH RATES; PUBERTY; SPEECH DISABILITIES; TEETHING; TOILET TRAINING; WEANING.

deviated septum: See SEPTUM.

Dexamyl: a trade name for an appetite-suppressant drug combining dextroamphetamine with amobarbital; see AMPHETAMINES.

Dexedrine, "dexies," dextroamphetamine: a trade name, a slang term, and the generic word, respectively, for the same substance; see AMPHETAMINES.

dextromethorphan: See COUGHS.

dextrose: another name for glucose; see SWEETENERS.

dextrothyroxine: a lipid-lowering agent; see LIPIDS.

diabetes insipidus: a rather uncommon condition characterized by frequent passing of large amounts of dilute urine; this is not the condition usually meant when the first word is used alone (for that, see the next entry), and the urine does not contain sugar or exhibit other chemical abnormalities.

Normally, among the hormones produced by the pituitary gland (see ENDOCRINE GLANDS) is one called *vasopressin,* also known as "antidiuretic hormone"; this hormone is relayed to the kidneys and acts as an inhibitor of excessive excretion of fluids. Any interference with this process — at either end of the line, or along the way — can give rise to diabetes insipidus.

In a great many cases, no specific cause is found, and the condition is described as *idiopathic;* the only symptoms in these cases are the basic one and concomitant constant thirst (including night waking) because of the fluid loss. This type is usually treated by administration of pituitary extract or a synthetic form of vasopressin and possibly other medications; sometimes it seems to disappear by itself after a few years.

Rarely, that same symptomatic picture signals an X-linked recessive condition (see HEREDITY) called *vasopressin-resistant* diabetes, in which the kidneys fail to respond properly to the hormone. It of course afflicts chiefly males (although their "carrier" mothers may show some signs of it), and is treated by making fluids freely available and sometimes also dietary restrictions and other measures.

In the remaining instances, there *is* a specific cause of the problem, and there are usually additional symptoms of something wrong. There are a great many such possible causes, among them injury at the base of the skull (especially fracture); various kinds of tumors; and a number of infections, including encephalitis, meningitis, syphilis, and tuberculosis. When a specific cause is pinpointed, therapy — surgery, antibiotics, or whatever is indicated — is instituted and, if successful, will eliminate the urinary symptoms as well.

diabetes mellitus: the illness people usually mean when they use the word "diabetes" alone (which is what we shall do here). It is a chronic condition in which the body is unable to utilize sugars properly because of hormonal malfunction(s).

Normally, sugars synthesized from the digestion of carbohydrates are transported to the liver, converted to a substance called glycogen, and stored for later use. This conversion process uses insulin, a hormone secreted by the pancreas (see ENDOCRINE GLANDS); if something — it may be an underproduction of insulin, or it may be some interference with the action by some other hormone — disturbs the process, the sugars stay in the bloodstream and are eventually excreted in the urine, leaving the body's various organs and tissues deprived of needed energy.

Diabetes is a familial ailment. It is not, strictly speaking, hereditary, but the tendency or susceptibility is hereditary, and recessive — that is, a youngster will normally become diabetic only if he has inherited the tendency from both parents (although neither parent need have the disease in order to transmit the susceptibility). Generally, if the ailment afflicts one generation after another, it appears earlier in life with each generation. Given the inheritance, overweight appears to be a precipitating factor, although that's not necessarily true in children (who might even be underweight); about two-thirds of diabetes cases don't appear until after the age of forty. Some researchers believe that while susceptibility is inherited, the cause — at least of the juvenile-onset type — may be a virus.

It's estimated that there may now be ten million diabetics in the United States, and the number is increasing by about 325,000 each year. Prior to the synthesizing of insulin in 1921, diabetes was invariably fatal; since then, it has been effectively controlled (though not *cured,* which would mean somehow restoring or correcting the body's natural hormonal functions), and the life expectancy of a diabetic is now about the same as anyone's, assuming the disease is diagnosed and properly treated. The treatment involves injection of insulin — which must be injected, rather than administered by mouth, because it's a protein substance and would be destroyed by the digestive juices. (There are orally administered drugs, but they are useful only in certain cases of diabetes that begin much later in life.)

There are some key signals of the onset of diabetes, and if there's any history of the disease in your family, it's important for you to be alert to them. The first symptom is typically unusually frequent urination (in a young child who's past the toilet-training age, sudden bed-wetting may be the first clue). Other early symptoms are excessive thirst, and possibly weight loss despite a normally hearty appetite. There may also be some weakness and fatigue. All or any of these may, of course, mean something quite different — but if you observe any of them, a check with your physician is in order; the disease can be diagnosed by simple urine and blood tests. If the diabetes continues untreated, a stress situation (such as a slight infection) could trigger a very critical condition.

Diabetes in children is a little more difficult to control than in adults (not impossible, just difficult) because youngsters' levels of activity are so variable — and they are thus using different amounts of sugar at different times — and also simply because of their smaller size: small under- or over-supplies of insulin can have more noticeable effects. Thus, if your child has diabetes, it is very important that you oversee the management of the disease during the early years.

The doctor's instructions — as to insulin injections, diet, urine testing — must be followed explicitly. The child must see the doctor for checkups periodically (the doctor will say when); of course the doctor must be promptly alerted if any unusual symptoms or reactions develop. It's important, too, that the child learn, as soon as he is able, to manage his condition by himself, since he'll have to do so in later years; he can learn to test his urine at quite an early age, and certainly by the teens he should be giving himself his injections and watching his own diet as well.

All the instructions you receive from the doctor will be geared, essentially, to one thing: maintaining, so far as possible, the child's sugar-insulin balance so that it is close to what it should be. It may take some time to achieve this, especially, as we've noted, in a young child; on a rainy day, for example, or if the child is sick in bed, he'll need more insulin than usual because he's expending less energy and using up less sugar. The crucial point is that any marked deviation from that ideal balance can give rise to either of two dangerous situations — although one is more critical than the other.

Too much insulin can cause an insulin reaction, which can lead fairly quickly to shock; *too little* insulin can lead, not quite so quickly, to coma (the reaction here is usually fairly slow in adults, but somewhat faster in children). The insulin reaction is of course the more serious, and children are more prone to it because of their greater activity and low sugar reserves (it's usually difficult for a child to maintain consistently sugar-free urine without risking such a reaction, and the doctor may tell you it's not necessary to do so).

You should keep an eye on your diabetic youngster and be alert to both types of reactions. The teachers of a school-age child should be alerted as well.

Typically, the onset of an insulin reaction is sudden. The child will feel hungry, the skin will be damp and sweaty, and breathing will be shallow. He may be confused and irritable or behave strangely (in school, he may suddenly become inattentive). If he's under ten, he may vomit (a confusing symptom — but watch for the other factors). The remedy is an immediate something sweet to eat or drink: a piece of candy or some fruit juice, honey, or syrup. After a while, most diabetic children can recognize the start of an insulin reaction, and if the child is school age or even old enough to play away from the house, he should always have a bit of candy (*real* candy, not "diabetic" candy) with him for emergencies. Insulin needs in general rise with age, and if a youngster has frequent insulin reactions, it probably means that he should be getting not less insulin, but more food (he's growing, remember).

The onset of the opposite reaction, caused by a lack of insulin, is generally a bit slower. The child will be thirsty and will urinate often; the skin will be hot and dry, the breathing deep; he may feel drowsy. Vomiting (possibly accompanied by headache) is a more common symptom here, at any age. The remedy, of course, is immediate injection of insulin.

On page 148, for emergency aid, is a quick checklist of key signs of each kind of crisis.

If the child collapses and you're in doubt as to which type of reaction he has had, assume it is an insulin reaction and treat it accordingly; if it's not, the bit of sugar will do little harm — and the opposite course could be extremely dangerous. He should respond within a few minutes; if he doesn't, then you know the reverse situation exists. Because of the possibility of these reactions, every diabetic (child *or* adult) should carry clear identification in order to cope with

	IMPENDING DIABETIC COMA	IMPENDING INSULIN SHOCK
ONSET	*Fairly slow, somewhat faster in younger children*	*Sudden*
HUNGER AND THIRST	*Intense thirst, dry mouth*	*Hunger, no thirst; may drool*
SKIN	*Dry, flushed*	*Damp, sweaty, pale*
BREATHING	*Deep and rapid*	*Shallow or normal*
GASTROINTESTINAL REACTIONS	*Often nausea, vomiting; possibly abdominal pain*	*Seldom nausea or vomiting, except in small children; no pain*
OTHER SYMPTOMS	*Drowsiness; no strange behavior or tremors*	*Possible tremors, confusion, odd behavior or delirium*
REMEDY	*Insulin injection—but only if absolutely sure of condition*	*If conscious: food containing sugar (candy, juice, honey)* *If unconscious: rush to hospital for glucose injection*

away-from-home emergencies; see MEDIC ALERT.

Finally, an additional aspect of diabetes to which you should be alert if you have a toddler in your home and your physician has recommended Clinitest or other tablets for use in testing the urine of a diabetic in your family. These tablets have recently become implicated in a number of cases of poisoning of small children. If they are swallowed — which, of course, they were not meant to be — they can cause serious burns of the esophagus. For that reason, we advise that you treat them as you would any dangerous drug vis-à-vis the potential for accidental poisoning: keep them locked away, well out of the reach of curious tots.

diagnosis: professional medical determination of the existence of an illness or disorder, or of the reason for symptoms or complaints. *Differential* diagnosis refers to the fact that in many cases a variety of problems could give rise to similar symptoms, and the physician who suspects condition A may find it necessary to rule out — via blood tests and/or other means — conditions B, C, and D, since despite similarity of symptoms, treatment may be radically different.

dialysis: See HEMODIALYSIS.

diaper rash: a pimply irritation that may appear on and about the area covered by the infant's diapers. It's caused by a combination of factors, chiefly the chemical action of bacteria on urea (an element in urine), which produces ammonia, which then irritates the child's skin. The condition may be further aggravated by the action of bacteria in the feces, by softening of the skin from rubbing against wet diapers, and by blocking of the sweat ducts.

Diaper rash generally doesn't appear until after the baby's second month and may appear as late as the tenth or eleventh month; some children seem to be more susceptible to it than others.

It's best to prevent the problem in the first place, if you can. Change diapers often, to keep your baby as dry as possible. Smooth a protective film of petroleum jelly or zinc oxide on the area to protect the skin from potential irritation (they're just as effective as expensive baby lotions). Don't overdress your youngster or let him get overheated.

Laundering of diapers can be a factor, too; harsh soap residue remaining on them can act as a further irritant. If you have a diaper service, you can generally depend on having thoroughly clean and trouble-free diapers. But if you wash them yourself, there are a couple of precautions you should take. Before washing them, it's helpful to take the extra step of soaking them for half an hour or so in a borax solution — a teaspoonful to a gallon of water. Do the washing itself with a *mild soap,* and, very importantly, be sure to *rinse thoroughly* — not with any special solutions, which would add chemicals at this stage, but with plain water.

If, despite your efforts, the rash does appear, certainly continue all the measures we've already mentioned. Cleanse the area with soap and water. Treat the rash itself by exposing it to the air as much as possible and by applying a zinc oxide ointment, such as Lazar's paste. (Do *not* use boric acid on this or any other ailment your child may have; it is a highly toxic substance, through the skin as well as if it's swallowed.) In addition, leave the child's diapers off for as long as you can whenever you can, and use an air conditioner or fan to draw off perspiration. And avoid the use of plastic pants as long as the rash remains.

Should the condition worsen or spread to adjacent areas of the baby's body, or if there are any other symptoms such as fever, take the child to the doctor promptly; the problem — which can sometimes be a fungal infection — may require medical attention and treatment.

diaphragm: the muscular partition between the thorax (chest cavity) and the abdomen, just under the ribs, that moves up and down in breathing. For another use of the term, see CONTRACEPTION.

diaphragmatic hernia: See HERNIA.

diaphysis: the shaft of a long bone, as of the arm or leg. For the other major parts, see APOPHYSIS and EPIPHYSIS.

diarrhea: a condition of frequent, watery stools in a child who also shows other symptoms of not feeling well. That is to say: neither an occasional loose stool nor several movements (of normal consistency) during the day is a matter of concern — unless there are other symptoms as well.

Diarrhea can indeed be a serious symptom, especially in a small infant, since there can be a dangerous amount of fluid loss in a short time. If an infant has even three or four such stools, combined with any listlessness or even a vague not-quite-himself look, you should call your doctor promptly — and give the baby absolutely nothing by mouth. You should not even wait for more than one stool if there are also other symptoms from the start, such as vomiting, fever, a rigid or bloated abdomen, or a peculiar color or odor to the baby's stool. If that last symptom exists, save the stool for the doctor to examine.

After infancy, the situation is a little different. Ask the child how he feels. Take his temperature. Check the stool to make sure that it is not bloody, or another unusual color. If it's just diarrhea and a general malaise, with no fever or just a degree or two, simply have the child stay home and rest quietly. Feed him very little; limit food to such mild things as bouillon, tea and toast. (Don't give anything fatty, such as eggs, butter, whole milk, or fried foods. If you decide to try skim milk, do *not* boil it; it becomes too concentrated and places an undue burden upon the kidneys.) If those things don't appeal to the youngster, you might — *if* your physician approves — put him on a short-term Gatorade diet. This soft drink will serve to prevent dehydration (it should be diluted for a child under two years) and is readily absorbed so that the intestines need do little work; it should be continued for no more than 24 hours. If there isn't any improvement by then, the doctor should be called.

Even in an older child, though, the doctor should be called immediately if there are any other accompanying symptoms — vomiting, pain, high fever, rigidity or bloating in the abdomen, anything strange about the stool other than its looseness (and again, save it for examination). And if there are any of these symptoms, give the child *nothing at all* by mouth until the doctor has advised you.

(There is one other condition that should be mentioned that occurs, though rarely, in toddlers of two or three, or even older. A more or less continuous "trickle diarrhea" — small, almost wholly liquid stools — may signify not diarrhea, but the presence of impacted feces in the rectum which the child may, for one reason or another, be unable or unwilling to pass. Movements may be painful [see ANAL FISSURE]. Or perhaps the child has simply not learned bowel control and is not aware of the impacted feces — for emotional reasons, because of some physical malfunction, or because he had been ill during the normal toilet-training period. If you suspect this problem, discuss it with your doctor; it can be corrected, and the child can and should be trained to control the situation, which could cause continuing embarrassment and psychological damage if it's permitted to continue.)

There are various drugs that may be prescribed in cases of simple diarrhea such as that resulting from a short-lived intestinal viral infection. One of the most widely used is Lomotil, a prescription medication combining a chemical called diphenoxylate with a small quantity of atropine; there is, however, a fine line between helpful and potentially dangerous doses, and it is definitely not recommended for very small children (nor should adult doses be given to older children or teenagers). Or the doctor may specify paregoric (camphorated tincture of opium), which is one of the safest and most effective antidiarrheals if used as prescribed — but bear in mind that it is a narcotic, follow instructions exactly, and keep it locked away.

Diarrhea is a rather frequent occurrence in foreign travel, and it may or may not signal a serious disorder. For further comment, see TRAVEL PRECAUTIONS.

diastolic: See BLOOD PRESSURE.

diazepam: a tranquilizer and muscle relaxant; see SEDATIVES.

dicloxacillin: a semisynthetic penicillin; see ANTIBIOTICS.

Didrex, diethylpropion: See DIET PILLS; the latter is a generic term, the former a trade name for benzphetamine.

dieldrin: See PESTICIDES.

diethylstilbestrol: See CONTRACEPTION.

diet pills: There are two types, one essentially worthless and the other potentially dangerous, and both are best avoided.

Over-the-counter reducing aids, whether in pill or "candy" form, don't do much of anything. Generally the product is accompanied by a detailed diet or diet-and-exercise plan that is perfectly valid but has nothing to do with the pills themselves — which are generally mild analgesics (they act as mild "tranquilizers," as aspirin does, and might temper "nervous nibbling") or just low-calorie snacks meant to substitute for higher-calorie ones (but low-calorie snacks are available much more cheaply at any corner grocery).

Prescription pills are something else again. They are often quite powerful drugs, some of which are indeed properly used medically for a variety of other purposes. By far the greatest number of practitioners dispensing these pills, however, are the so-called "diet doctors" or "fat doctors," some 75 percent of whom are not even Doctors of Medicine but chiropractors, homeopaths, and the like. Many such people dispense the pills (often they're doled out right in the office) without adequate testing, examination, investigation of patients' histories, or consideration of side effects. There have been deaths and near-deaths documented as a result, including some among college students. They have also figured in the drug-abuse problem.

Most of the drugs misused in this manner have been the extremely dangerous "pep pills" (see AMPHETAMINES). There have also been, in recent years, a number of nonamphetamine (but chemically related) drugs introduced for this purpose, in a markedly *un*successful attempt to achieve the hoped-for results with lower risk; these include, prominently, benzphetamine (Didrex), chlorphentermine (Pre-Sate), clortermine (Voranil), diethylpropion (Tenuate, Tepanil), mazindol (Sanorex), phendimetrazine (Plegine), phenmetrazine (Preludin), and phentermine (Ionamin, Wilpo). Sometimes those unscrupulous practitioners include in the regimen such addictive substances as barbiturates, in an effort to counter the effects of the foregoing drugs. And they have also been known to throw in such irrelevant things as diuretics, cathartics, heart stimulants, and a variety of hormones.

Toxic as these substances are for adults, you may imagine what perils they pose in a household with small children who are wont to pick up, and pop into their mouths, almost anything they find. Many drugs suitable for — and sometimes necessary for — teenagers and adults are potentially hazardous to toddlers, and of course we are not suggesting that older folks forgo needed therapy (although the medications should be kept safely locked away). But it does seem both cruel and foolish to subject oneself and one's family to clearly *un*necessary risks.

For advice on sensible methods of weight reduction, see OVERWEIGHT.

digestion: the process of breaking down ingested food substances into forms that can be used by the body, largely via enzymes (chemical catalysts) that change the foods into amino acids (the "building blocks" of protein), sugars, storable fats, and other useful components.

The process starts in the mouth, where saliva begins to break down some starches. Further breakdown, especially of proteins, by the gastric juices of the stomach takes two to four hours. A great deal of the activity goes on in the small intestine, where enzymes from the pancreas, bile from the liver and gallbladder, and many small glands in the intestinal wall are involved. By the large-intestine stage, only water and indigestible residues remain, the former to be absorbed, the latter excreted. The total time required, from start to finish, is 24 hours or more.

You need not worry about this process, which normally takes place smoothly and automatically, except for one thing: vigorous exercise or extreme cold (as, swimming) immediately following a meal isn't a good idea, as it can interfere with some of the early stages of the digestive process.

digitalis: a medication derived from the herb called foxglove; its action is to regularize and strengthen the heartbeat, and it is prescribed or administered especially when the problem is an irregular heartbeat, weakness of the heart muscle, or heart failure. *Digitoxin,* a purified form of the active ingredient in digitalis, or *digoxin,* a drug with a different period of action derived from a related plant, may also be prescribed for similar purposes.

These are extremely powerful drugs; it is vital to follow the prescribed dosage exactly. An overdose can in fact be *cumulatively* toxic. Symptoms of digitalis poisoning are palpitations and difficulty in breathing; if you suspect this condition in a patient who has been receiving the medication, call your physician immediately, and if you cannot reach the doctor, take the patient to the nearest hospital emergency room.

Dilantin: a trade name for the drug phenytoin, an anticonvulsant used to control epilepsy and other conditions; it is chemically similar to phenobarbital but more effective, less sedative, and nonaddictive.

There are, however, some side effects that may occur, to which parents should be alert. Muscle weakness or lack of coordination and visual peculiarities are often hints that the dosage should be reduced. Overgrowth of the gums is a fairly common side effect but sometimes can be prevented via oral hygiene (and if it does develop, it's correctable); if your youngster takes this medication, it would be a good idea to discuss prophylactic measures with the dentist, even if no apparent problems have yet developed. Rashes occasionally occur, but are usually not considered serious. And there are some other, fortunately quite rare, reactions that may indeed be serious. *Any* untoward manifestation, even if it seems minor, should be promptly discussed with the prescribing physician.

Dilaudid: a trade name for hydromorphone, a semisynthetic morphine derivative; see NARCOTICS.

dimenhydrinate: See MOTION SICKNESS.

dimethyl sulfoxide: See DMSO.

diphenhydramine: See ANTIHISTAMINES; MOTION SICKNESS.

diphenylhydantoin: the former generic name for phenytoin, an anticonvulsant; it is discussed under the prominent trade name, DILANTIN.

diphtheria: a contagious disease caused by the bacillus *Corynebacterium diphtheriae,* which primarily infects the throat but also releases a toxin that affects the nervous and circulatory systems and the heart. It is transmitted via droplet infection.

The first symptom, after an incubation period of two to seven days (occasionally longer), is generally a sore throat accompanied by low fever, and possibly vomiting. A grayish membrane soon forms in the throat, posing a serious obstruction to breathing; it is this membrane formation and the effects of the toxin that are the most critical aspects of the disease.

Treatment must be prompt and requires hospitalization. There is an antitoxin, which is administered immediately; several of the antibiotics are effective against the bacillus itself. There is a 99 percent recovery rate when treatment is instituted early; the rate drops to 75 percent if the condition goes untreated for as long as five days, and there may be heart complications from the effect of the toxin.

If there is a diagnosis of diphtheria, everyone in the family should have a *Schick test* for immunity to the disease, since it is contagious from 24 hours before the first symptoms appear and for two weeks thereafter. This test consists of injecting a minute amount of the diphtheria toxin. An immune person has no local reaction at the site of injection (although allergy to the solution may cause redness and swelling within minutes or hours, which disappears within three days). If the subject is *not* immune, there will be a large red swelling within 24 hours, persisting for four to five days, with a brownish spot remaining for several more days.

We hope that none of this will ever be necessary for anyone in your family. There is an effective vaccine against diphtheria, and the first shot should be given to your baby at the age of two or three months (immunity derived from an immune mother lasts about three months); this is customarily in the form of a DPT (diphtheria-pertussis-tetanus) shot that protects simultaneously against all three infections. The injection is repeated twice more, usually at about one- to two-month intervals; these are followed by booster shots at the age of about a year and a half and again at five years. After that, your own physician should be the judge. Most pediatricians feel that a DT (diphtheria-tetanus) shot is advisable at the age of fifteen; whether the schedule goes beyond that will depend upon the risk in your area.

It must be emphasized that diphtheria is an extremely serious, potentially fatal infection (one in six child victims dies), and that the Center for Disease Control (CDC) has been warning Americans for the last several years that a frightening proportion of our children lack protection against it; estimates have varied from one in five to three out of ten. There have been recent epidemics, including outbreaks in Miami, Phoenix, and San Antonio in 1970; CDC investigation revealed that immunization levels there were no lower than those in other major cities — so any community could be next.

For full discussion of protection your children should have, see IMMUNIZATION.

diplomate: See BOARDS.

diplopia: See DOUBLE VISION.

disaccharides: a classification of sugars; see SWEETENERS.

discoid lupus erythematosus: See LUPUS.

dislocation: a displacement of the bone or cartilage at a joint, usually resulting from violent stress or injury; it generally involves a good deal of pain and swelling.

Never try to correct a dislocation by yourself. If you are quite sure the shoulder, hip, or any joint is dislocated, get the child to a doctor or hospital emergency room as quickly as you can, and with as little movement of the affected joint as possible. If a long or rough trip is necessary, it's best to gently tie the leg — if a hip or knee is injured — to the other leg, or an arm to the chest: not tightly, just enough to keep the limb from shifting around.

Dislocations in children, in particular, require prompt professional treatment, because otherwise the injury could affect bone growth. Dislocated shoulders, elbows, and wrists are common injuries among toddlers who have been swung or lifted by one arm; such an injury should be suspected if, after such an event, the child suddenly begins to cry, is obviously in pain, and refuses to use that arm.

It is often difficult for someone without medical training to distinguish a dislocation from a fracture. If you are in any doubt at all, assume there is a broken bone and turn to FRACTURES. You will also find there some precautions to follow if a cast has been applied; they apply to dislocations, as well.

Congenital dislocation of the hip is an uncommon affliction of the newborn, affecting about three thousand babies each year, six or seven times as many girls as boys; it's due to a failure of the hip joint to develop properly, so that the upper end of the femur (thigh bone) slips out easily, and both legs are often affected. Although it's not provably hereditary, the incidence of the condition does seem to differ among certain peoples; it is most common (though still fairly rare) among American Indians and in northern Italy, where it occurs in about nineteen of every thousand births (in Sweden, by comparison, the rate per thousand births is fewer than five).

Early diagnosis of this condition is quite important, and major hospitals now check for it routinely; if it is discovered in a newborn child, it can generally be corrected by keeping her in a particular position for a certain length of time, and there will be no further problems. If the diagnosis is not made until later (one leg will typically seem shorter and be turned out), or even after the child has learned to walk (the child will likely limp or waddle), correction will require casts, splinting, or perhaps surgery to remove overgrown cartilage that has filled in the bone sockets.

distal: farthest from the torso, or farther in that direction relative to something else. Thus, of the two joints in a finger, the one closer to the end of the finger is the *distal interphalangeal* (between finger bones) joint; an injury on the forearm might be described as "distal to the elbow." The word is a lot more precise than the subjective terms "first," "second," "above," or "below"; its opposite is *proximal.*

diuretic: a drug given to stimulate urination, used in some kidney disorders that involve excess fluid accumulation (notably in association with hypertension) and in certain cardiac and liver impairments. Such a drug is *not* properly used as an aid to weight reduction.

diverticulitis: See MECKEL'S DIVERTICULITIS, the only type that is likely to afflict a child or young adult.

dizziness: a vague word meaning something a little different to everyone who uses it, and likely to mean something quite different to a child who complains of it. It may or may not be a symptom of something serious, and you have to exercise some judgment.

If the child has been running around in circles (literally), the cause — and the remedy — are obvious.

If the child has been lying down or sitting down and complains of dizziness when he stands up suddenly, it's probably postural hypotension (see BLOOD PRESSURE), not a serious problem.

If he's on a boat or in a car or some other vehicle, and the dizziness accompanies a feeling of nausea, see MOTION SICKNESS.

Vertigo is the sensation that the world is spinning around; it usually indicates some disturbance in the semicircular canals of the inner ear, which govern the sense of balance — due possibly to an infection there or in the eustachian tube between the nose-throat area and the ear. Of course it requires prompt medical attention.

A sensation a child may describe as "dizziness" may also result from a number of other things including epilepsy, head injury, and poisoning. If the cause is not apparent, take the child to the doctor without delay.

DLE: short for discoid lupus erythematosus; see LUPUS.

D.M.D.: the abbreviation for Doctor of Dental Medicine, a degree held by some dentists.

Also see SPECIALTIES, DENTAL.

DMSO: short for dimethyl sulfoxide, a substance that has long been in use as a veterinary medicine and as an industrial solvent, and since the mid-1960s has been hailed in some quarters as a true "miracle" drug for humans. A better word is "mystery."

Its advocates have urged its use for a host of ills ranging from mental retardation to arthritis, from ulcers to fungal infections — and have labeled the federal hesitation to make the drug generally available "persecution." It is true that limited studies have shown that the drug has some remarkable properties, including the ability to affect internal conditions via absorption through the skin. On the other hand, there have been reports of side effects that include serious blood abnormalities, visual difficulties, and nerve damage.

We feel the Food and Drug Administration has been wise to require broader and more definitive research experience before releasing the drug for widespread use; many apparent panaceas of the past have later proved to be perilous. Carefully controlled investigation of DMSO and its properties continues.

"DMT": See PSYCHEDELICS.

DNA: the familiar short form for deoxyribonucleic acid, the material of which genes — those elements in the chromosomes that carry hereditary traits — are made; chemically, it is composed of sugars and phosphates.

For more about the results of what DNA does, see HEREDITY.

D.O.: the abbreviation for Doctor of Osteopathy; see OSTEOPATH. Don't confuse this abbreviation with O.D., which stands for Doctor of Optometry.

dog bites: See the appropriate section under BITES AND STINGS.

dominant: See HEREDITY.

Donnatal: a trade name for a drug combining phenobarbital, a barbiturate, with other ingredients; see SEDATIVES.

"dope": a slang term formerly used for heroin, now frequently for marijuana, occasionally for mood-altering drugs in general.

Doriden: a trade name for the sleep-inducing drug glutethimide; see SEDATIVES.

Dormin: an over-the-counter "sleeping aid"; see SEDATIVES.

dorsal: toward the back of the body; the opposite of *ventral.* The word may refer to the back itself (one can't get farther back than that), in locating a condition — as a dorsal cyst. It is also used to locate a part of the body in relation to another; the anus is dorsal to the vagina, for example, and the spleen is dorsal to the stomach.

double-blind: describing a study, as of a new medication, in which neither researchers nor patients know to whom the drug under study is being administered. If, for example, a new pain reliever is being tested, half the patients in the study might receive that drug, the other half a placebo — an inert substance designed to look and taste exactly like the real medication; or the patient group may be broken down still further, one group receiving the new drug, another a placebo, a third an established remedy (as, aspirin). The drugs dispensed are coded; only when the study is completed and the results have been recorded is the code "broken" and the data translated into terms of the actual substances. In this way, neither patient nor physician has any preconceived notion about what the medication is "supposed" to do, and results and observations can be recorded objectively.

double pneumonia: See PNEUMONIA.

double vision: "seeing double," as the phrase implies; the medical term is *diplopia.* It can be a symptom of a number of serious things, including botulism (see FOOD POISONING) and severe head injury; if it occurs, the child should be seen by a physician quickly.

Down's syndrome: a congenital condition combining a variety of defects, including epicanthic folds of the eyelids that create a vaguely Oriental look (hence its other name, mongolism). Generally the infant will have unusually flat facial features, a stubby nose, somewhat deformed ears, and weak muscles, and will hold the mouth open with the tongue protruding; there may also be other physical defects including impaired sight, congenital heart disease, cleft lip or palate, strictures in the intestinal tract, and a variety of skeletal abnormalities. The child's intelligence will be below average, perhaps markedly so; mongoloid children often, though, have pleasant and affectionate personali ties.

Although a number of specific physical defects can and should be treated or corrected (e.g., cleft palate, heart defects, vision problems), there is no overall remedy. A mongoloid child, because of low intelligence, will be slow in all areas of development and functioning, including speech. Physical growth will generally be stunted as well, and it is unlikely that the child will ever grow beyond the height and appearance of a normal twelve-year-old. Additionally, mongolism often involves underdevelopment, and high susceptibility to infection, of the lungs, kidneys, and other organs.

Although these children may often be best cared for at home, parents may choose to place such a child in a special institution where his needs can be met with expertise and understanding, particularly if the demands of his care interfere with normal family functioning.

That is, of course, the parents' own decision, and one that should be made after careful thought that takes into account a number of factors including the abilities (both physical and emotional) of the parents to offer needed care and protection, effects on siblings, the family's general circumstances — and discussion with trusted friends, physician, clergyman, etc. Whatever the parents decide, they deserve understanding, help, and emotional support. There is no reason whatever for parents who choose to institutionalize the child to feel guilty about that decision; it may be the kindest one for the child and for the entire family.

A great deal of study has been devoted to Down's syndrome — it is the most common autosomal (genetic, nonsex-linked) abnormality known, affecting over five thousand newborn babies yearly in the United States alone — and much is now known about its causes. The condition now has, among physicians, a third name: trisomy-21 — meaning a defect in a specific chromosome (see HEREDITY) known as number 21. In 95 percent of all cases, this is accidental and involves an egg or sperm (more often the former) that is carrying an extra number 21 chromosome, so that the resulting embryo has three instead of the normal two. The possibility is statistically related to the mother's age: the chance of having a mongoloid child is less than one in two thousand in teenagers, more than one in a hundred in a prospective mother who is over forty.

In the remainder of cases, a phenomenon called *translocation* is involved: the breakage of two chromosomes which then rejoin and, in the process, "exchange" some parts. In some cases, an extra number 21 chromosome (mainly 21, anyway) may "stick to" that hybrid, creating the same trisomy situation. In other cases, it doesn't, so that the egg or sperm cell will have a perfectly normal amount of genetic material, and the baby born will be outwardly normal — but will grow up to be a "carrier," with a risk of producing unbalanced eggs or sperm. The risk varies with the specific details of the translocation, including what other chromosome is involved. This can now be determined by a process called *karyotyping* — an analysis of an individual's chromosomes. Chromosomal analysis can be done in an adult, in an infant, or — during the twelfth to fourteenth week of pregnancy — in an unborn child (see AMNIOCENTESIS).

The "odds" of having a child with Down's syndrome are, overall, statistically one in six hundred. (That, at least, is about how often it has occurred, over the years, in the total number of births. With increased knowledge of fetal defects, and an increasing number of mothers opting for abortion upon discovery of such defects, the number of mongoloid children may decrease. Probably three out of four mongoloid fetuses, incidentally, are lost via miscarriage.) As we noted previously, the odds are greater the older the mother — and whatever the mother's age, they are multiplied by a factor of three if she has had a prior child with Down's syndrome; that is, a woman over forty who has given birth to one such child runs a one-in-thirty risk of bearing another.

Those risks are substantially higher — we are talking now about the five percent, the translocations — if the mother or father is a "carrier"; they range from one in twenty to certainty, depending upon both the exact nature of the translocation and which parent carries it. Certainly a parent— or sibling — of an affected child would do well to seek genetic counseling and, if pregnant, fetal karyotyping.

We might add, for the sake of completeness, that there occurs, very rarely, a condition called *mosaic* mongolism. Such children have some cells with the chromosomal abnormality and others without it. As they grow older, the proportion of normal cells appears to increase, physical appearance tends to improve, and the children often do better mentally than had been expected.

"downs" or "downers": slang terms sometimes used to refer to drugs, especially barbiturates, that have a depressant or sedative effect; see SEDATIVES.

doxepin: See ANTIDEPRESSANTS.

doxycycline, Doxychel, Doxy-II: one of the tetracyclines and two trade names for it; see ANTIBIOTICS.

D.P.M.: the abbreviation for Doctor of Podiatric Medicine; see PODIATRIST.

DPT: a combination vaccine giving protection against diphtheria, pertussis (whooping cough), and tetanus. For guidance on the scheduling of this and other shots, see IMMUNIZATION.

Dramamine: a trade name for dimenhydrinate; see MOTION SICKNESS.

Dramcillin: a trade name for penicillin G; see ANTIBIOTICS.

drinking: It's not our province to advise whether or when you permit your teenagers to consume alcoholic beverages; we simply suggest that you make your own attitudes on the subject, whatever they may be, known clearly and early. For your information and theirs, we present here a few physical facts.

Alcohol has little or no value as a food; it is relatively high in calories but not in any nutritional elements. It can irritate and cause inflammation in the stomach, throat, and intestines; continued and excessive drinking can also cause permanent damage to the heart, liver, kidneys, and central nervous system.

On a less lasting basis alcohol afflicts the drinker temporarily with (depending upon the amount consumed) lack of coordination, thickened speech, an impaired sense of balance, decreased judgment and perception, and a variety of mental difficulties. Two or three ounces will have a measurable impact on the brain, affecting the higher mental processes first. Five or six ounces begin to affect the motor areas of the brain, ten ounces emotional centers, sixteen ounces sensory mechanisms (vision, etc.).

Also see, for comment on other escape devices in which young people may evidence interest, AEROSOL-SNIFFING; AMPHETAMINES; DIET PILLS; GLUE-SNIFFING; NARCOTICS; PSYCHEDELICS; SEDATIVES.

Dristan: See DECONGESTANTS, NASAL.

droplet infection: the spreading of a contagious disease by exhalations of the infected person. The "droplets" need not be visible globs of coughed-up or sneezed-out material, but are often fine, airborne particles that can travel for several feet; they need not result from coughs or sneezes, but can be transmitted simply by ordinary breathing.

dropsy: an obsolete term for edema.

drowning: Take precautions to prevent the occurrence of such a tragic accident. Never leave a toddler alone in the bathtub; a small child can easily drown in two inches of water. As to recreational situations, see the section on "Swimming and Boating" under ACCIDENTS, PREVENTION OF.

EMERGENCY PROCEDURE

Pull the child out of the water as fast as you can. Don't leave him; if there is another person present, send that person to call for an ambulance, the Coast Guard, etc. Place the child face down to allow water to drain out; if he is breathing and sputtering, he'll be able to eject the rest of the water, and he'll be all right. If he isn't breathing — or if you're not *sure* he's breathing — give him immediate resuscitation (see RESPIRATORY RESUSCITATION) and continue until he is breathing normally or medical help arrives.

Even if the resuscitation is successful and the victim has apparently recovered fully, get him to a hospital as soon as you can. There is a possibility that, despite appearances, pulmonary function has in fact been impaired. Only thorough professional examination, including X rays, can reveal the true situation and determine whether further treatment is needed.

drug abuse: See AEROSOL-SNIFFING; AMPHETAMINES; DIET PILLS; DRINKING; GLUE-SNIFFING; NARCOTICS; PSYCHEDELICS; SEDATIVES.

"drug fever": the term generally applied to fever that can occur, though rarely, as a hypersensitive reaction to a variety of medications, in particular phenothiazines, epinephrine, and some anesthetics. Drug fever usually vanishes quickly when the agent causing it is discontinued.

DTP: See DPT; "DTP" is simply a variation used by some physicians.

duct: a tube leading from a gland or other organ, serving to conduct fluids. The common bile duct, for example, leads from the liver and gallbladder into the intestine; many small ducts in the breast, called mammary ducts, carry milk to the nipple.

ductless glands: See ENDOCRINE GLANDS.

duodenal ulcer: See PEPTIC ULCER.

duodenum: See INTESTINES.

Duodex: a trade name for a combination-of-ingredients "diet pill"; see AMPHETAMINES.

Duracillin: a trade name for penicillin G; see ANTIBIOTICS.

dur. dol.: See PRESCRIPTIONS.

D.V.M.: the abbreviation for Doctor of Veterinary Medicine.

dwarfism: There are a number of conditions classified as dwarfism; they all have to do with physical stunting due to congenital or otherwise intrinsic traits or malfunctions, rather than malnutrition. The three types you are most likely to hear or read about affect neither mental abilities nor life expectancy.

Achondroplastic dwarfism, also medically termed achondroplasia or chondrodystrophy, is a hereditary condition involving malformation of the bones of the limbs; the head and torso are normal, but the arms and legs will never grow to normal proportions. Genetically, the trait is apparently generally dominant, but is believed to be sometimes the result of an accidental mutation (see HEREDITY for an explanation of those terms). Thus if one parent is an achondroplastic dwarf there is a fifty-fifty chance that the children will be, and if both parents have the condition it will be passed on to a majority of their children; occasionally, though, an achondroplastic dwarf is born to normal-size parents.

There is a familiar example of consistently inbred achondroplasia in the animal world: the dachshund.

Hypopituitary dwarfism results from a lack of one of the hormones normally secreted by the pituitary gland (see ENDOCRINE GLANDS). It can be corrected to some degree by administration of the missing hormone (see GROWTH HORMONE).

Midgets, unlike achondroplastic dwarfs, have normal proportions, but will simply never grow to normal size; their full adult height is generally defined as varying from 21 to 42 inches (that is, an adult of 45 inches is unusually short, but is not a midget). The condition is hereditary, but the genetic mechanism is not completely clear; it is possible for normal parents to produce a midget.

Dynapen: a trade name for dicloxacillin, a semisynthetic penicillin; see ANTIBIOTICS.

dyscrasia: a term deriving from the Greek for "bad temperament," formerly used broadly to mean just about any kind of disease (generally preceded by an adjective indicating the site). It is now used solely to refer to abnormal conditions in the bloodstream (and may be preceded by the word "blood"); it's still nonspecific and does not denote a particular kind of abnormality or its cause.

dysentery: a term covering two types of infections affecting the colon (large intestine), both endemic in certain tropical areas. Symptoms of both usually include severe diarrhea (although in rare cases, this is not so), abdominal cramps, and possibly blood or mucus in the stool; if dysentery is even suspected, the stool should be saved for analysis.

Since the symptoms can result from a number of other conditions as well, careful diagnosis is important, as is prompt treatment; if it's untreated, the infection can spread to other organs, especially the liver and lungs. Treatment depends upon the exact cause, which can be determined by laboratory tests of the blood and the stool.

Both kinds of dysentery are transmitted by infected fruit, vegetables, and water (which should be avoided in endemic areas), and by contaminated feces (via insects, especially flies), and both are capable of reaching epidemic proportions. The problem can and should be prevented by insect control, correction of water pollution, and proper sewage facilities.

Amebic dysentery, or amebiasis, is caused by a protozoan invasion of the digestive tract, and has an incubation period varying from three days to several months. Typically — but not necessarily — there is only very slight fever or none at all. It is treated by the administration of various antibiotics.

Bacillary dysentery is caused by a bacillus; it is sometimes called shigellosis, after the Japanese scientist named Shiga who discovered the infectious agent. Its incubation period is more specific and shorter — from one to eight days and typically two to four. High fever is common. Treatment is usually with sulfa drugs or antibiotics, especially the tetracyclines. At this writing, there is hope for an eventual protective vaccine (for the bacillary type of dysentery only).

dyslexia: difficulty in reading or, more specifically, in understanding the printed word; there is no particular correlation with intelligence or the lack of it. (It has been reported that Nelson A. Rockefeller suffered from this handicap as a child.)

dysmenorrhea: See MENSTRUATION.

dyspepsia: an old term, no longer in use, for indigestion or "upset stomach."

dysphagia: difficulty in swallowing — a symptom, not a disease.

dysplasia: a general term for any abnormality in growth or physical development.

dyspnea: the medical term for difficulty in breathing.

dystrophy: See MUSCULAR DYSTROPHY, to which this term nearly always refers.

E

earache: a symptom of a number of things including potentially quite serious infection (see OTITIS). The child should be seen promptly by a physician and in the meantime should be given no medication except possibly aspirin to relieve pain; *don't* put or poke *anything* into the ear.

ear, discharge from: a sign of infection whether the discharge is pus, blood, or some other fluid. Put a plug of absorbent cotton in the ear, very gently. Then take the child to the doctor.

ear, insect or other object in: Don't try to get it out by poking, pouring in fluids, or any other means; take the child to the doctor without delay.

ear, water in: a fairly common occurrence in swimming, and one that usually doesn't require medical attention. First, have the child try shaking his head vigorously toward the side of the affected ear; hopping up and down at the same time is sometimes helpful. If that doesn't seem to work, have the child yawn widely several times. If the problem still persists, then do consult the doctor.

ears, protruding: They can be corrected, and probably should be if they're sufficiently unsightly or embarrassing to the child; see PLASTIC SURGERY. Neither taping nor binding will help.

EB virus: short for Epstein-Barr virus; see VIRUSES.

ecchymosis: a fancy word for a black-and-blue appearance of the skin, resulting usually (though not always) from a bruise; the plural is *ecchymoses.*

ECG: See ELECTROCARDIOGRAM.

ECHO viruses: See VIRUSES.

ecology: in medical terms, a couple of things in addition to the familiar meaning of the word: (1) the relationships of human beings to their environment, both physical and social; (2) the balance of life *within* a human being, which naturally and normally includes many microorganisms that are harmless or even beneficial.

Ecotrin: See PAIN RELIEVERS.

ectopic: a direct translation from the Greek, meaning "out of place." It is most often heard in reference to pregnancy, and it means that the fertilized egg has not become implanted in the uterus, as it normally is, but is developing elsewhere — as in a Fallopian tube.

eczema: a general, nonspecific word used to describe various skin conditions. It may refer to any rash of unknown cause. It may refer to a condition involving two or more of a group of symptoms — stemming from almost any cause — such as redness, scaling, fissures, or blisters; it's often used in this sense to refer to an adult dermatitis of more or less chronic nature due to allergy or psychosomatic factors.

Atopic eczema in infants means something a little more specific — a dermatitis (it may be pimply, blistery, or nodular) due to hypersensitivity. The allergen is something in the baby's immediate environment (such as soap), or something in the diet; most common among the latter are certain proteins in wheat, eggs, or milk.

edema: a medical term meaning swelling due to accumulated fluid, whether in the skin or elsewhere; it's a symptom or condition, not a disease. The term *pitting edema,* which means that finger pressure on the swollen area produces an indentation that persists, generally indicates a somewhat more serious condition.

EEG: See ELECTROENCEPHALOGRAM.

efferent: See NERVOUS SYSTEM.

EKG: See ELECTROCARDIOGRAM.

Elavil: a trade name for amitriptyline; see ANTIDEPRESSANTS.

electrical shock: If your child has been obviously injured, or become unconscious, while playing with — or near — an electrical appliance, cord, or wall plug, assume that electrical shock has occurred. And, that the child is in an extremely critical state. (The most dangerous of all types of commonly available electrical power are low-voltage alternating currents, the kind most of us have in our homes.) The child may well be unconscious, respiration may have ceased or almost ceased, and the pulse will likely be weakly fluttering.

Begin resuscitation (see RESPIRATORY RESUSCITATION) at once, and at the same time send for medical or other professional help. (Some electric and telephone companies have crews trained in handling such emergencies; if you are reading this ahead of time, before any emergency has occurred, it would be well to query local utility companies and make appropriate notes in the emergency-number section at the end of the book.) Continue giving resuscitation until professional help arrives, or the victim has recovered and is breathing spontaneously and normally; until he is fully alert, don't give him anything to eat or drink.

Even if there is apparent recovery without professional aid, the child should be taken to a hospital for medical examination. There is a very real possibility of burn damage. Electrical burns do not look like ordinary thermal (heat or fire) burns, and may well be overlooked. External evidence of such a burn — at the entry point of the current, and at the often ignored exit point as well — usually appears as a small, sharply defined round or oval discoloration, seemingly not very serious; but damage to underlying tissues may be quite deep, and may include — among other things — critical blood-vessel injury.

electrocardiogram: a graphic picture or tracing of the heartbeat by a stylus connected to electrodes placed at various points on the body, thus moved by electrical impulses from the beat itself. Technically, what's recorded is the electrical potential at those selected points; these reflect electrical charges developed (normally) by the heartbeat. The device used for this procedure is an electrocardio*graph;*

the tracing is usually referred to by medical personnel as an ECG or EKG.

An EKG is often used to detect certain irregularities in the heartbeat, but if the doctor orders this procedure for your child, it doesn't necessarily mean a heart problem is suspected; it's sometimes included routinely as part of a general examination, to round out the physician's picture of the patient's complete condition and functions at that time. There is, incidentally, no pain or even discomfort involved; the patient doesn't feel any electricity.

electroencephalogram: a graphic picture of the brain's electrical activity ("brain waves"), often called an EEG for short. It's helpful to the physician in diagnosing epilepsy, possible damage from a head injury, or an infection or disease that may be affecting the brain.

electrolytes: certain substances — sodium, potassium, chlorides, and carbon dioxide — found in the blood. Tests to determine their concentration, especially in conditions involving dehydration, can give the physician clues as to the cause and severity of the disturbance.

electroshock: See SHOCK THERAPY.

elimination diet: See ALLERGY TEST.

embolism: the obstruction of a blood vessel, whether by a clot or some other entity. An *air* embolism is specifically one that is caused by an air bubble; a *pulmonary* embolism is one that occurs in a pulmonary artery.

embryo: a potential living entity in the very earliest stages of cellular development. In humans, that is generally considered to be the first two months after conception; during this period, it cannot be clearly distinguished as a potential human being. Also see FETUS.

embryology: the study of the developing being from conception until the moment of birth. Yes, this term seems to contradict the preceding definition, and there are those who would either call it "embryology and fetology" or would coin a new word ("prenatology" would seem a good choice). But that, at the moment, is what it means.

emetic: an agent used to induce vomiting — as when a child has swallowed something he shouldn't have, and it's important to get it out of the stomach quickly. The best and handiest emetic in an emergency is your finger, stuck far into the child's mouth and used to tickle the back of the throat; it often works like magic. If it doesn't, he must be given something to swallow that will provoke the reaction.

The best thing is syrup of ipecac (which you should have on hand; see MEDICINE CHEST): two teaspoonfuls for a child under three, a tablespoonful for an older youngster.

If you have no syrup of ipecac, there are other effective but somewhat unpleasant solutions that must nevertheless be given if vomiting is necessary: warm mustard water (a teaspoonful of dry mustard in eight ounces of water), or warm salt water (again, a teaspoonful in eight ounces of water), or warm baking-soda water (the same proportions).

Vomiting is not always desirable when a child has swallowed something toxic; nor, even if desirable, should emetics be given in unlimited quantities or over long periods of time. For detailed first-aid measures concerning dozens of specific swallowables, see POISONING, HOUSEHOLD SUBSTANCES AND MEDICATIONS.

e.m.p.: See PRESCRIPTIONS.

emphysema: a difficulty in breathing caused by air spaces around the bronchioles, the smallest of the network of air conduits in the lungs. Essentially an ailment of older people, emphysema can, rarely, occur in youngsters as a serious complication of asthma.

Empirin: See PAIN RELIEVERS.

empyema: a condition — from whatever cause — involving an accumulation of pus within the body; used without further qualification, the word usually refers to the chest cavity.

E-Mycin: a trade name for erythromycin; see ANTIBIOTICS.

encephalitis: an inflammation of the brain, whether occurring as a result of the action of a toxic agent (as in lead poisoning), as a complication of some other illness (such as meningitis), or caused by a direct attack by a virus or other infectious agent. Whatever the cause (which must of course be determined in order to treat the illness properly), it is typically characterized by fever, headache, and drowsiness, and possibly nausea and muscular weakness as well; in severe forms, symptoms may include paralysis, convulsions, or coma. It is not contagious from one person to another.

All this aside, when you hear about encephalitis it is likely to be either "sleeping sickness" or one of the viral kinds of encephalitis found, in varying forms, throughout the world. African "sleeping sickness" is a special form of encephalitis peculiar to parts of that continent; as its name suggests, extreme drowsiness is its most pronounced symptom, and it is caused not by a virus but by a parasite carried by a particular insect, the tsetse fly.

In the United States, there are four known types of direct-attack encephalitis (i.e., not connected with or following another illness), each caused by a distinct virus. Although they are named for the areas where they were first isolated, they are not necessarily limited to those areas; in all of them, the infection is carried by certain kinds of mosquitoes that have previously bitten infected animals or persons. Incubation periods, after bites by mosquito vectors, may vary from three days to three weeks; treatment requires hospitalization and expert care for a week or two followed by complete recovery in most cases, but there have been a significant number of fatalities in most recent outbreaks, and those who survive may suffer physical and mental aftereffects.

The four U.S. types are: *Eastern equine,* carried chiefly from infected horses, mules, and other farm animals, but sometimes from birds; *Western equine,* also carried chiefly from infected horses, etc., as well as from birds; *California,* carried chiefly from wild rabbits and other rodents; and *St. Louis,* most prevalent in the central and western part of the country but found as far east as Florida, carried chiefly from infected birds. (There was a severe outbreak of the last in 1975: almost fifteen hundred cases, with more than ninety deaths, were reported, with the heaviest concentration of cases in Illinois, Indiana, Mississippi, and Ohio.) In 1971 a fifth type, *Venezuelan equine,* invaded the southwestern United States via Central America and Mexico.

All types can become epidemic, and prevention hinges mainly on control and elimination of the insect vectors, the mosquitoes that transmit the disease from one animal to another. Sensible personal precautions include insect repellents and staying indoors at night when the mosquitoes are active. Additionally, there is a vaccine available for animals — and horses, mules, and other farm animals in areas where equine encephalitis has been found should be vaccinated; the vaccine is not recommended for human beings.

Once a person has had one type of viral encephalitis, there is an immunity, but only to that specific virus; there is still susceptibility to the other types.

encephalogram: an X ray of the brain.

endemic: typical of a particular locale, and always present there to some degree; used in reference to a disease or condition (don't confuse this word with *epidemic).* Cholera, for example, is endemic in certain parts of the Orient; dengue, in the Caribbean islands; histoplasmosis, in the central United States; sinusitis, in many metropolitan areas with a high level of air pollution. An endemic ailment need not be contagious, or even infectious.

Enderin: See PAIN RELIEVERS.

endocarditis: See HEART DISEASE.

endocrine glands: glands that secrete their products, called hormones, directly into the bloodstream (unlike, for example, the liver); they are also called ductless glands. The various hormones have specific jobs, and also work together for the general continued normal functioning of the body. There are seven major glands or pairs of glands in this category.

The adrenals, located in the upper abdomen just above the kidneys, produce a number of hormones essential to life, and their malfunction is quite serious (see ACRODYNIA; ADDISON'S DISEASE).

One of these hormones is adrenalin, also called epinephrine, which is produced in great amounts under conditions of external stress. It increases the heart rate — thus rushing more oxygen to the muscles for greater efficiency — and slows down the digestive process, and also speeds coagulation of blood in case of a wound. Because it has the effect of relaxing bronchial spasms, it is sometimes administered for the relief of asthma and other respiratory allergies; it may also be injected when fast overall stimulation is needed, as in anaphylactic shock.

Another is cortisol (so called because it is secreted by the outer part or cortex of the gland), a hormone that enables the body to cope with a variety of internal stress situations such as infection, severe burns, and toxic reactions. (See CORTICOSTEROIDS for further comment.)

Other hormones produced by the adrenals function in the utilization of various minerals and other food elements and in the workings of hormones secreted by some of the other glands.

The gonads or sex glands, of course, are the basic organs of reproduction; the ovaries release eggs, the testes sperm. In addition, they secrete a number of hormones that affect the development of secondary sex characteristics — estrogens in the case of the ovaries, androgens (notably one called testosterone) in the case of the testes (or testicles). It's believed that estrogens may also protect females, to a degree, against certain ailments — especially heart problems — that seem to be more prevalent among men.

The pancreas, located behind the stomach near the liver, secretes insulin, a hormone that regulates the use of starches and sugars; it also produces a number of digestive juices. An adequate supply of insulin is essential to life (see DIABETES MELLITUS).

The parathyroids are in the neck, near the thyroid gland; their main role is in helping to regulate the body's use of certain minerals, especially calcium and phosphorus. Underactivity of these glands can result in muscular cramps and spasms (see TETANY); overactivity can cause calcium deposits in various places, including the bloodstream (a means of diagnosing the condition), and weakness and fragility of the bones.

The pituitary, located at the base of the brain, is an extremely vital organ. It produces many and varied hormones that affect metabolism of fats and carbohydrates, stimulate the activity of the adrenal cortex (see ACTH and CUSHING'S DISEASE), control physical growth and the achievement of normal stature (see GROWTH HORMONE), influence kidney function (see DIABETES INSIPIDUS), and trigger the productive activities of the gonads and thyroid. Because the pituitary influences the action of so many of the other endocrines, it has been nicknamed the "master gland."

The thymus, located in infants in the upper part of the chest, was for many years a mystery organ, with the question of its precise function — and even whether or not it *was* an endocrine gland — in hot dispute. It is present in the newborn, but atrophies after the first couple of years of life. In the past few years, strong evidence has been presented suggesting that the thymus is probably an endocrine gland, and that it plays a particular role in the body's ability to combat foreign invaders, including disease-causing organisms.

A substance — named *thymosin* — has in fact been found in humans, has been extracted from calf thymus, and has been successfully used in clinical trials to treat congenital lack of immunity associated with underdevelopment of the thymus. While final conclusions have not been drawn (and research continues) the current theory postulates that thymosin is responsible for setting into motion the manufacture of certain lymphocytes, of which there are two main types. Those called B-cells are primarily engaged in making antibodies against specific bacteria; the others, tentatively called T-cells (for thymus-dependent, because they do pass through that organ), cluster around, and directly attack, cells of foreign invaders, and are believed to constitute the front line of defense against viruses, fungi, foreign (including transplanted) tissue, and malignant growths. It is also hypothesized that they may play a role in controlling or regulating the activities of B-cells.

It is not yet known what role thymosin may play in therapy, but it is currently speculated (we emphasize that it *is* speculation; the hormone is in short supply even for investigation) that many conditions, in addition to immune deficiencies in the newborn, could be treated with it. These conditions include cancer, transplant surgery (in which a period of "anti-thymosin" treatment might decrease the possibility of rejection), and the so-called "autoimmune" disorders — including lupus, rheumatoid arthritis, and others — in which antibodies are produced, presumably by B-cells, against the body's own tissues, conceivably because of lack of T-cell "control."

The thyroid, located in the neck, controls metabolism of the body's cells — their rate of activity and use of oxygen and foods. Overactivity of the thyroid (hyperthyroidism) can cause a variety of conditions including weight loss, increase in heart rate, and hair loss; it is treated by drugs or by removal of part of the gland. Underactivity (hypothyroidism) can cause the opposite of these conditions, plus extreme skin dryness — and a number of other serious results if the condition is congenital (see CRETINISM); it is treated by administration of thyroid extract, or by remedying an iodine deficiency if that is the cause. Either condition can result in enlargement of the gland (goiter).

endodontist: See SPECIALTIES, DENTAL.

endometrium: the inner lining of the uterus; the latter part of the word comes from the Greek *metra,* "uterus."

endrin: See PESTICIDES.

enema: an introduction of fluid into the lower intestine via the rectum; it may be given for various reasons — to stimulate defecation, to prepare the youngster for special examination or for surgery, to permit X rays involving that part of the digestive tract (see BARIUM ENEMA).

Never give a child an enema unless you are specifically directed to do so by the doctor, who will instruct you as to what to use — and never give an enema with ordinary tap water, which can deplete the body of vital minerals and cause the child to go into shock.

enteritis: a general term for any inflammation of the small intestine, no matter what the cause.

Entero-Vioform: See TRAVEL PRECAUTIONS.

enterovirus: See VIRUSES.

ENT specialist: See SPECIALTIES, MEDICAL.

enuresis: See BED-WETTING.

enzymes: catalysts of various biological processes that "activate" certain substances chemically (specific enzymes act on specific substances) or trigger actions or interactions. Most well known are the enzymes that play a part in the digestive process: some help to turn foods into materials the body can use, others are prominent in breaking down waste products into forms suitable for elimination.

It is becoming increasingly apparent, however, that enzymes have many other roles to play. Some interact with secretions of the endocrine glands, one, for example, hexokinase (all enzyme names end in -ase), with hormones from the pituitary and the pancreas in maintaining blood-sugar levels. Others are crucial factors in such matters as reproduction; it's an enzyme carried by the sperm that breaks down the coating of the egg cell to permit the sperm to penetrate it (and the lack of that enzyme that may possibly cause some cases of sterility).

Not all enzymes are beneficial, however. The venom of some poisonous snakes, for example, contains an enzyme called lecithinase that shatters red blood cells by attacking a crucial part of their structure. And more and more, researchers are turning up proof or high probability that enzymes (whether by their absence or by their too-eager activity) are implicated in certain previously perplexing disorders. See, for example, ALCAPTONURIA; AUTISM; FABRY'S DISEASE; FAVISM; GAUCHER'S DISEASE; MIGRAINE; NIEMANN-PICK DISEASE; PHENYLKETONURIA; TAY-SACHS DISEASE.

ephedrine: a synthetic drug similar in action to adrenalin (see ENDOCRINE GLANDS); it may be administered, by mouth or injection, in a variety of conditions including asthma, shock, and severe hemorrhage (it constricts small blood vessels and elevates blood pressure).

epidemic: a (temporarily) widespread occurrence of a particular communicable disease (don't confuse this word with *endemic). When* the occurrence is to be termed an epidemic, and what special protective or other measures are to be taken for control, are matters for decision by public health authorities in the area, since it is essentially a community problem. General coordination of information on actual and potential epidemics in the United States is handled by the Center for Disease Control (formerly the National Communicable Disease Center) in Atlanta, Georgia, an arm of the U.S. Public Health Service.

epidemiology: not, as the word seems to suggest, the study of epidemics, but the study of the geographical distributions and patterns of diseases (which can of course *include* epidemics) and the factors contributing thereto.

epidermis: the outermost layer of the skin.

epididymis: a portion of the excretory channel of the testis, through which the sperm pass.

epiglottis: the elastic cartilage that automatically closes off the windpipe during swallowing, so that food will go into the esophagus and not into the trachea.

epilepsy: a condition involving sudden, recurring brief disturbances in brain function. It may be caused by a severe head injury (at birth, or later in life), by a tumor, or by infectious disease; often there is *no* known cause, and it is termed *idiopathic.* It is not hereditary, although there is some indication that there may be a familial predisposition; that is, should one of the causative factors occur, some youngsters may be more susceptible to the resulting condition than others. Epilepsy resulting from a birth injury is more likely to be a permanent condition than epilepsy caused by injury later; the latter is usually temporary.

The estimated incidence of epilepsy in the United States is at least two percent — meaning some twenty persons for every thousand in population or a total, based on a nationwide population of over 210,000,000, of at least four million. There is no evidence that epilepsy has any effect on intelligence; records show that one-third of its victims are of average intelligence, one-third below average, and one-third above — by definition, precisely the proportions found in the population as a whole.

Epileptic seizures may range in severity from very minor to major. A number of terms, not necessarily mutually exclusive, may be used to describe them.

Petit mal ("little sickness" in French) seizures, also called "absence seizures," involve very brief "blankness" or loss of awareness, with little loss of motor function; the only visible symptom may be a momentary dazed look, with inability to pick up the thread of a conversation.

Grand mal seizures are generalized and convulsive (see CONVULSIONS for a full description).

Jacksonian seizures are basically convulsive, but they are limited to one part or one side of the body, and the child is usually not unconscious. They represent one type of *focal* seizure, in which the abnormal electrical activity in the brain can be traced to a small area or to several small areas.

Psychomotor epilepsy is also manifested by focal seizures, which are typically not convulsive (although they may include unusual muscle movements) but are characterized by a moment or two of odd or irrational behavior combined with apparent confusion; that behavior, by the way, is not generally violent or destructive, just strange.

Myoclonic may describe any seizure involving muscle spasm.

Other symptoms are beginning to be considered by many physicians (though not all; there is still some controversy) as atypical manifestations of epilepsy. Among them are a number of syndromes in which certain events seem to occur on a periodic basis with no apparent cause — brief headaches, stomach pains ("abdominal epilepsy"), temper outbursts, and others.

In many cases, epileptic conditions can be mostly, or even completely, controlled by the regular administration of medication(s); since epilepsy is often a very individual matter, an extended trial-and-error period may be necessary. Among the most widely used are phenytoin (Dilantin) and certain barbiturates, especially mephobarbital (Mebaral) and phenobarbital. A new anti-epileptic drug called carbamazepine (Tegretol), which is related to the tricyclic antidepressants, was approved by the Food and Drug Administration in 1974; it is effective in grand-mal and psychomotor epilepsy, though not in petit mal. Certain tranquilizers, in particular diazepam (Valium) and clorazepate (Tranxene), have been reported to exhibit anticonvulsive properties in some patients. Mephenytoin (Mesantoin) and primidone (Mysoline), chemically related, respectively, to phenytoin and the barbiturates, are alternatives for major seizures. In petit mal, a group of drugs called succinimides — they include ethosuximide (Zarontin), methsuximide (Celontin), and phensuximide (Milontin) — are often effective, as are two other agents, paramethadione (Paradione) and trimethadione (Tridione); the succinimides are particularly low in undesirable side effects. The latest (1975) addition to the antiseizure pharmacopoeia, as this is written, is clonazepam (Clonopin), a drug related to the benzodiazepine tranquilizers, which has been found effective in petit mal and may be useful in other types of seizures as well.

It is important for parents of an epileptic child to follow the doctor's instructions carefully (*never* omit, or change the dosage of, medication without medical consultation); to realize that it is purely a physical, not a mental, problem; to be patient and understanding; and, in our opinion, to do everything you can to dispel the totally unreasoning prejudices that have prevailed concerning this condition (that includes being entirely open about the problem — with the child, and with teachers, baby-sitters, and others involved in the child's care).

Parents should also, as far as possible, help the youngster avoid events or conditions which have been observed to precipitate seizures; these vary from one individual to another and may include both physical and emotional stimuli, among the latter undue stress. It has recently been observed that epileptic seizures may also be triggered by light patterns or flashes, including "light shows," some television images, light-and-shade patterns beneath trees, and the flickery effect of moving past a picket fence on a sunny day. Most of this special photosensitivity has been noted during adolescence, and it is twice as prevalent among girls (about two-thirds of epileptic girls evidence it during this period, only about one-third of the boys).

There is, by the way, no reason to automatically forbid a youngster with epilepsy to participate in sports and other physical activities. A particular individual's condition may call for some such restriction, but don't automatically assume so; discuss the question with your physician. (A number of professional athletes, past and present, have been epileptics — as have many other noted individuals, from poets to prime ministers.)

It is a good idea for anyone with any form of epilepsy to carry away-from-home identification; see MEDIC ALERT.

epinephrine: another name for the hormone adrenalin; see ENDOCRINE GLANDS.

epiphysis: the growing end of a bone; an inflammation of it is called *epiphysitis.*

epistaxis: the medical term for nosebleed; it comes from a Greek verb, which in turn derives from a root meaning "to fall in drops."

epithelium: the covering and lining tissue of the body — the skin and mucous membranes, including those membranes lining passages inside the body.

eponym: a name for a condition, disease, structure, or symptom that includes the name of the person who first described or discovered it or is most prominently associated with it; there is often an alternate name as well. Well-known examples are Cooley's anemia (thalassemia), Down's syndrome (mongolism), Hansen's disease (leprosy), shigellosis (bacillary dysentery), and Wilms' tumor (congenital tumor of the kidney).

epsom salts: a very powerful purgative that should never be used unless it is specifically advised by the doctor; see CATHARTIC.

This substance is also sometimes

recommended for use in solution as a bath to relieve the discomfort of muscle strains or aches; it is actually no more effective for this purpose than plain hot water.

Epstein-Barr virus: See VIRUSES.

Equagesic: a combination-of-ingredients analgesic containing ethoheptazine (see NARCOTICS), aspirin, and the tranquilizer meprobamate.

Equanil: a trade name for meprobamate, a tranquilizer and muscle relaxant; see SEDATIVES.

equine encephalitis: See ENCEPHALITIS.

Erb's palsy: See BRACHIAL PARALYSIS.

Ergomar, ergotamine: See MIGRAINE; the terms are respectively a trade name and the generic for a medication used in that condition.

Erypar: a trade name for erythromycin; see ANTIBIOTICS.

erysipelas: a skin infection caused by *Streptococcus*, the same type of ubiquitous bacterium that causes scarlet fever, strep throat, and a number of other serious and unpleasant conditions. Because rheumatic fever, chorea, and nephritis can result from an untreated case of erysipelas, prompt diagnosis and treatment are vital, especially in an infant (for whom an overwhelming untreated strep infection could be fatal).

Frequently, in erysipelas, the organism enters via a wound or small abrasion (there needn't be an obvious cut; a diaper rash involving a little broken skin could provide the entryway). After a two- to five-day incubation period, typical symptoms appear: the skin is red, shiny, and swollen; the baby obviously feels ill; there is fever, which may climb quite high.

The doctor should be called immediately. With swift administration of antibiotics or sulfa drugs, the infection will be banished within one or two days; the swelling will go down, and the skin will usually peel. There will be no scarring unless delayed treatment has permitted an abscess to form.

Erysipelas is contagious if there is broken skin that's easily touchable by another child; to be on the safe side, siblings should be kept away from the patient until recovery.

erythema: the medical term for visible redness — not, despite its ominous-sounding name, a disease, but a symptom; it could describe sunburn, most rashes, etc.

erythema infectiosum: a mild but highly contagious childhood disease chiefly afflicting children between three and twelve. The main — usually, the only — symptom is a rash; rarely, there are other, somewhat flulike, symptoms as well. Its cause is unknown and is presumed to be a virus.

Sometimes this infection can be confused with rubella, scarlet fever, or hives. But the pattern of erythema infectiosum is distinctive. After an incubation period of a few days to two weeks, a rash appears — specifically on the cheeks, which become bright red and remain so for several days. Then, the redness disappears. A day or two later, a spotty rash appears on arms and legs — perhaps parts of the torso, too — and may itch. This rash comes and goes unpredictably for about two or three weeks, tending to reappear especially when the child becomes warm, as during exercise or in sunlight. It finally vanishes completely.

This condition is, of course, nothing to worry about. It is frequently overlooked by physicians and parents alike, tending to be diagnosed only when there is an obvious outbreak in a neighborhood.

Erythema infectiosum is also sometimes known as "fifth disease," resulting from someone's penchant for list-making; it is not clear exactly whose. Some sources attribute the appellation to one Nil Filatov, a nineteenth-century Russian pediatrician who had set about numbering the known red-rash diseases; his first was purportedly scarlet fever, the second measles, the third rubella, the fourth possibly roseola — and then he encountered this fifth one. Other medical-history buffs postulate that someone, whether individual or committee, sat down to draw up a schedule of diseases with measles-like rashes caused by viruses — with measles itself in first place, rubella second, chickenpox probably third, roseola fourth, and erythema infectiosum in the fifth slot. Take your pick.

erythroblastosis fetalis: a form of hemolytic anemia in the newborn in which jaundice is a typical symptom ("yellow babies"); see RH FACTOR for a full discussion of when and why it occurs, what can be done about it, and how it can be prevented.

Erythrocin: a trade name for erythromycin; see ANTIBIOTICS.

erythrocytes: See BLOOD CELLS.

erythrocyte sedimentation rate: See SED RATE.

erythromycin: See ANTIBIOTICS.

Eskabarb: a trade name for phenobarbital; see SEDATIVES.

Eskatrol: a trade name for a combination-of-ingredients "diet pill"; see AMPHETAMINES.

esophagus: the gullet; the food passageway between the throat and the stomach.

ESR: the abbreviation for erythrocyte sedimentation rate; see SED RATE.

Estrafon: a medication combining amitriptyline (see ANTIDEPRESSANTS) with the potent tranquilizer perphenazine.

estrogens: a group of hormones, the chief one of which is estradiol, produced by the ovaries (see ENDOCRINE GLANDS).

ethchlorvynol, ethinamate: See SEDATIVES.

ethmoid sinuses: See SINUSES.

Ethobral: a combination of three barbiturates; see SEDATIVES.

ethoheptazine: a potentially habit-forming analgesic; see NARCOTICS.

ethosuximide: a drug used in the control of petit mal seizures; see EPILEPSY.

Ethril: a trade name for erythromycin; see ANTIBIOTICS.

etiology: the cause of a disease, also the study of the general causation of diseases. The word implies more than simply an organism, for example, found to give rise to a particular illness; it includes, too, the mode of transmission, other conditions favoring the development of the illness, predisposing factors, etc.

eustachian tubes: the passages that lead from the back of the nose-throat area to each ear. It is the temporary blocking of these tubes by a change in air pressure that causes the familiar "funny feeling" in the ears that can occur in a plane or in an elevator in a tall building.

*Un*funny conditions can also occur via the eustachian tubes. An infection or other type of blockage in them can affect hearing, and a nose or throat infection can travel through them to the middle ears. Both these things happen more easily in small children, because their eustachian tubes are shorter and straighter.

evacuation: in medical terminology, the elimination of waste material from the gut — a bowel movement.

exanthem subitum: See ROSEOLA.

Excedrin: See PAIN RELIEVERS.

excretion: the elimination from the body of waste materials; there are three normal methods — defecation, perspiration, and urination. Don't confuse this word with *secretion,* which is the production of a substance by an organ, for example, a hormone by an endocrine gland.

exfoliation: scaling of the skin, whether occurring spontaneously or done deliberately.

Ex-Lax: See CATHARTICS.

exodontist: See SPECIALTIES, DENTAL.

expectorant: a medication given, usually in liquid form, to loosen congested material clogging the throat, bronchial tubes, or lungs and make it easier for the child to cough it up. It is generally the single most effective remedy for an ordinary cough connected with an ordinary cold, since the basic cause of such a cough is congestion resulting from material dripped from the back of the nose — but it, like any medication, should be given only on doctor's instructions.

Your doctor may prescribe an expectorant or suggest that you buy one of the over-the-counter preparations, generally known as "cough medicines" or "cough syrups." For comments and specific suggestions on these products, see COUGHS.

expiration: medically, not an ending as of a magazine subscription, but simply meaning "breathing out"; its opposite is *inspiration.*

exposure: a word meaning just what it says, used medically without further qualification to mean two different things. It can mean exposure to a specific communicable disease by contact with an individual who has it, with infectious material, etc., as in "symptoms appear five days after exposure"; the time between exposure and onset of illness is the *incubation period.*

Exposure in such a phrase as "suffering from exposure" means a condition resulting from prolonged exposure to extreme cold, and first-aid procedure is as follows. Get the child into a warm place and immediately wrap him in blankets or whatever is available. If breathing is extremely weak, take resuscitative measures (see RESPIRATORY RESUSCITATION). If — or when — breathing is normal, immerse the child in a tub of warm (not hot) water until he begins to feel a bit better (if there's no tub available, just keep him snugly wrapped up). Then dry thoroughly, wrap in blankets again, and offer something hot to drink. If, at any point, there is no satisfactory response to these measures, call a doctor immediately.

If you find a child completely unconscious and apparently totally unresponsive following such exposure, *don't* assume he's dead — even if you can't detect a heartbeat; simply rush him to the hospital. When internal temperature has dropped, the body adjusts to that lowered temperature, and normal criteria don't necessarily apply. Heart sounds may not be audible if internal temperature has dropped to 86°F. (30°C.). No response to light by the pupil of the eye will be evident at an internal temperature of less than 77°F. (25°C.). But people have been known to survive even after chilling to temperatures below 65°F. (18.3°C.) — partly because even the brain adjusts to lack of oxygen in lower temperatures: while at normal temperatures reduced oxygen will cause irreversible damage after four or five minutes, at 68°F. (20°C.) the brain can survive with diminished oxygen for as long as 25 minutes.

Also see FROSTBITE.

extensor: See MUSCLES.

eye injuries: Any violent injury to an eye or eyelid, including a cut or tear of the latter, requires immediate medical care — which means either a hospital emergency room or an ophthalmologist (M.D. specializing in treatment of the eyes). The latter is the person to whom we refer in the specifics that follow — *not* an optometrist or optician, and *not* a nonspecialist physician, who will not have the necessary instruments for examination.

Corneal abrasions — scrapes or scratches of the cornea, the transparent membrane over the front of the eyeball — typically occur when something, such as a tree branch or twig, brushes across the eye. They can be quite serious, since scarring directly in front of the pupil could block vision. But even a minor corneal abrasion is usually extremely painful, often far out of proportion to the degree of actual injury. There are no first-aid measures you can or should take; if you suspect such an injury, simply get the child to medical care quickly.

Chemical burns of the eye most commonly result from splattering of window-cleaning fluid or other detergent solutions. Burned conjunctiva (the mucous membranes around the eye) may appear watery and reddened or, if the damage is more severe, whitish; a burned cornea is a dull white.

Immediate first aid is irrigation with water — ordinary tap water, at room temperature — to dilute the chemical. The most effective method is to fill a sink, or large basin or dishpan, with water; immerse the top of the child's head, including the injured eye(s), and have the child blink rapidly (or, if necessary, move the lids up and down with your fingers) in order to circulate the water around all adjacent tissues. Continue the irrigation for two to three minutes. Then cover the injured eye with sterile gauze — or a clean handkerchief or other cloth — and rush the child to the doctor or hospital.

A small cinder or "speck" in the eye can usually be coped with at home. Typically, it's on the surface of the eye or on the inside of a lid. Don't let the child rub the affected eye. Wash your hands with soap and water.

If the speck is on the lower lid, pull the lid downward by tugging gently on the lower lashes and remove the speck with the moistened corner of a clean handkerchief. If it's on the upper lid, pull the lid downward as far as possible and move it gently from side to side (the speck may slide downward and the lower lashes will act as a "brush" and catch it); if that doesn't work, pull the lid outward and slightly upward, and see if you can catch the speck with the handkerchief corner. A speck on the surface of the eyeball can usually be transferred to the lid by blinking — or can be picked up with the moistened handkerchief corner (be very, very gentle).

If these efforts do not work and the speck remains stubbornly stuck on the lid or on the eyeball (in the latter case, it may be embedded), professional help is needed.

A large fragment or splinter in the eye is an altogether different matter. Make no attempt to remove it yourself. The eyelid's up-and-down motion could drive the object in deeper or otherwise make the situation worse, and the lids tend to move in sympathy with each other. To prevent that, cover the injured eye with sterile gauze or a clean handkerchief, then tie something — roller bandage, scarf, or whatever is handy — around the child's head, covering *both* eyes; not tightly, just to keep him from blinking. Then get him to medical care, transporting him in a lying-down position if possible. Bear in mind that, unable to see, the child probably will be quite frightened; someone should stay close, and provide reassurance, on the way to the hospital or ophthalmologist.

Sunburn of the eyes can occur after overexposure to strong sunlight or — more likely in teenagers than in younger children — unwise lack of protection (or reading, with the light reflecting from the pages) under a sunlamp. Often, symptoms do not appear for several hours. They consist mainly of a painful sensation of grittiness, as if there were sand under the lids, and intensification of the discomfort upon exposure to any light. The only first aid is application of cold, which may dull the pain; professional treatment is needed.

eye, redness in: What to do, and what the redness may signify, depends on just where it is.

Redness of the mucous membranes inside the lids and around the eye may stem from a number of different conditions, some serious and contagious (see CONJUNCTIVITIS), and the child should be taken to the doctor.

A "bloodshot" look is not normal in children or teenagers and shouldn't be dismissed; it may signify varying conditions from eyestrain, to nutritional deficiency, to drug usage, to the beginning of a contagious illness (it can, for example, be an early symptom of measles). Nor should you use any patent medicines to remedy the condition. Take the youngster to the doctor.

A bright red patch on the white of the eye, without any accompanying pain, discomfort, or interference with vision, looks very alarming, but probably isn't at all serious. It's a sign of subconjunctival hemorrhage, which sounds scary but just means a cluster of tiny broken blood vessels; it usually results from a self-inflicted injury, such as the child's accidentally poking a finger in the eye. It can also occasionally appear after an episode of violent coughing or sneezing. And sometimes it's observed in a newborn baby, due to rupture of some of those tiny vessels as the baby's head pushes through the birth canal.

As with any bruise, initial applications of cold may be helpful to a degree. Even without such ministrations, the patch will grow duller in color and gradually diminish and disappear in a week or two.

eyelid ills: See BLEPHARITIS; CHALAZION; CONJUNCTIVITIS; STYE; TEARDUCT STENOSIS; TRACHOMA.

eyes, crossed: See CROSSED EYES.

eyesight: See VISION.

eyes, yellow in: See JAUNDICE.

F

F.A.A. . . .: You may sometimes see a set of letters starting this way following a physician's name and degree; it means that the physician is a Fellow (sometimes a higher ranking than mere "member") of one specialty organization or another. F.A.A.P., for example, means Fellow of the American Academy of Pediatrics; F.A.A.F.P. stands for Fellow of the American Academy of Family Physicians. Almost invariably, you may assume such a physician is certified in the specialty (see BOARDS).

Fabry's disease: a relatively rare hereditary condition (only a few hundred cases have been reported), transmitted by classic X-chromosome inheritance (see HEREDITY); it afflicts only boys. We include it in this new edition — in contrast to a number of other rare hereditary disorders — because in just the past few years, a therapeutic approach has been developed. Actually, it may be more widespread than statistics indicate: the rarer a condition, the more likely it is to be misdiagnosed and thus underreported; this particular condition offers many possibilities for misdiagnosis.

Fabry's typically manifests itself during the teen years. The first symptom may be a purplish rash on the lower abdomen and the genital and anal areas. Or, pain and/or swelling in hands and feet — sometimes misdiagnosed as an arthritic disorder. Later in life, there is kidney failure. All of these are caused by the same phenomenon: lipid (fatlike) deposits; *they* are caused by the hereditary absence of a particular enzyme called alphagalactosidase. (There are a number of other hereditary disorders with similar causes. See, for example, GAUCHER'S DISEASE and TAY-SACHS DISEASE.) Until 1973, kidney transplant appeared to be the sole means of treating the condition. Now, replacement therapy may be possible.

Because of the small number of identified patients, there have been few clinical trials of enzyme replacement. It appears that therapy — as with diabetics who lack insulin — must be given on a continuous basis. It is not, at this writing, known whether early therapy would prevent later development of problems (therapeutic trials have involved men in their twenties and thirties). Nor has the enzyme been synthetically produced; the supply thus far depends upon extraction from human placentas (animal tissue, used to produce insulin and some other substances used therapeutically in humans, has been judged to pose a rather large risk of allergic reaction).

Fabry's is one of the handful of congenital disorders that can at present be detected by prenatal cell sampling; see AMNIOCENTESIS and GENETIC COUNSELING.

facial palsy: a paralysis due to disease of, or injury to, the nerves of facial muscles. *Bell's palsy* is a specific type involving one side of the face only; characteristically, one eyelid and one side of the mouth will droop visibly. Treatment and prognosis depend upon the extent and cause of the problem.

F.A.C. . . .: a designation very similar to the first entry under this letter. The "C" stands for "college" in this case — no more tangible buildings than the "academies" previously mentioned. They are, like the academies, professional organizations. Among the designations you are most likely to see are F.A.C.O.G., Fellow of the American College of Obstetricians and Gynecologists; F.A.C.P., Fellow of the American College of Physicians (basically, internists); and F.A.C.S., Fellow of the American College of Surgeons.

fainting: See UNCONSCIOUSNESS.

fallopian tubes: See SEX ORGANS.

Fallot's tetralogy: See TETRALOGY OF FALLOT.

falls: A fall may or may not be a cause for concern. If the child has obviously been injured, determine the extent and nature of the injury and refer, for first-aid measures, to the appropriate listing, e.g., BACK AND NECK INJURIES; BLEEDING; BRUISES; CUTS: DISLOCATION; FRACTURES (actual or suspected); HEAD INJURIES; KNEE INJURIES; SCRAPES AND SCRATCHES; SPRAINS; UNCONSCIOUSNESS. If the child isn't moving, don't attempt to move him until you know exactly what's wrong.

Even if there is no apparent injury, keep a careful eye on the child for a while to watch for any delayed symptoms that may appear — headache, dizziness, repeated vomiting (if he fell on his head), soreness, limping, and so on.

familial: tending to recur within a particular family — as a familial trait or a familial illness; the word is not necessarily synonymous with *hereditary* (all hereditary conditions are by definition familial, but not all familial conditions are hereditary).

The word may indeed characterize a hereditary physical trait such as albinism. It may denote an illness in which there is known to be hereditary predisposition, as in the phrase, "there is a familial history of diabetes." It may also describe a condition in which the hereditary factor has not been proved but is only suspected; psoriasis, for example, can be said to display a "familial pattern." Or, less commonly, it may be used to describe a condition resulting from environmental factors; tooth decay, for instance, can be a familial affliction in a household where tooth-brushing and visits to the dentist are unknown.

family doctor: in the most broadly used sense of the term, a qualified physician who cares for all the members (or all the children) of a particular family and is familiar with their lives, general activities, medical histories, and so on. He or she may be a general practitioner or a pediatrician or an internist; the phrase does not describe training or special qualifications, but the doctor's role in relation to the patient.

There is now, additionally, a recognized specialty, involving special training, called "Family Practice" (the practitioner is a *family physician*); see SPECIALTIES, MEDICAL.

farsightedness: a vision defect in which sight is normal at a distance but nearby objects are blurred; the medical term is *hyperopia.* It is much more common than nearsightedness; its incidence tends to increase with age, but it is not unknown among children.

Farsightedness, since it is a focusing defect in the lens of the eye, can occur without the individual's being aware of it. The muscles controlling the lens strain to correct the focus, and there may be no apparent difficulty with vision itself; but the result may very well be severe eyestrain, with eye fatigue and headache.

The condition may be hereditary, but the mechanism is unclear. It is, at any rate, easily correctable with proper eyeglasses or contact lenses.

fatigue: in terms of symptomatic significance, *unusual* tiredness that occurs persistently and under unexpected conditions. If a child is unusually tired after a day of hard work or play or unaccustomed strenuous activity, or if he has not had enough sleep the night before, that's perfectly normal. But tiredness that persists day after day, or tiredness following some activity that never tired the child before, may be the first symptom of a number of ills, some of them serious; take the youngster to the doctor.

fats: See NUTRITION.

favism: a hereditary enzyme defect in the red blood cells, also known as primaquine sensitivity; the gene for it is recessive (see HEREDITY), so that a child can inherit the trait only if it is carried by both parents (who need not have the defect themselves). The trait has been reported only among inhabitants of Mediterranean countries, North Africa, the Near East, and parts of Southeast Asia, and individuals descended from those peoples — although because of its peculiar nature, it may simply never have come to light in other groups and other parts of the world.

In those who have favism, there is an extreme sensitivity to fava beans, whether they are eaten or their dust or pollen is inhaled, and to certain antimalarial drugs derived from the beans; additionally, the same sensitivity applies to primaquine, another antimalarial drug. (Obviously, someone who never encounters these substances will never have a problem, whether or not he has the enzyme defect.) The reaction is a sudden hemolytic anemia or widespread destruction of red blood cells; among the usual outward symptoms are jaundice and a reddish color to the urine.

Treatment of the anemia is the first order of business, if such a reaction occurs, but diagnosis of the underlying cause is extremely important so that the child will be able to avoid the potentially lethal substances in future.

favus: See RINGWORM.

febrile: characterized by fever (not feebleness, despite the confusing appearance of the word). A febrile disease is one normally or typically accompanied by fever; if a child's condition is described as febrile, he's running a fever.

feces: the material excreted in bowel movements.

feeding: See APPETITE; BOTTLE FEEDING; BREAST FEEDING; FOOD, SOLID; NUTRITION; WEANING.

Femicin: See PAIN RELIEVERS.

feminine hygiene sprays: See VAGINAL SPRAYS.

femur: the anatomical term for the thighbone.

fentanyl: a morphinelike synthetic analgesic; see NARCOTICS.

fetus: generally understood to mean a developing child in the uterus after the eighth week of pregnancy; the study thereof is called *fetology* (but see the further comment under EMBRYOLOGY).

fever: a temperature more than two degrees Fahrenheit (or one degree Celsius) above whatever is normal for the individual child. It usually indicates infection (fever is a defense by the body, since many disease-causing organisms are killed by heat) but there are other things, notably vigorous exercise, that can cause a rise in temperature; a youngster should rest for half an hour before his temperature is taken.

The degree of fever does not necessarily indicate the seriousness of a child's condition; a high fever need not mean a critical illness — nor is a slight fever necessarily a reason for complacency. Generally speaking, a fever (including one that occurs during teething; it's not "normal") should be promptly reported to your physician, along with any other symptoms the child may have.

For a discussion of normal ranges, thermometer-handling, and so on, see TEMPERATURE.

fever blister: See COLD SORE.

"fiber": See ROUGHAGE.

fibrin, fibrinogen: elements in blood clotting. The first is the material formed when blood coagulates; it is formed, by chemical conversion, from fibrinogen, an essential "clotting factor" present in normal blood.

fibroid: a small, noncancerous tumor containing fibrous connective tissues; fibroids tend to occur especially in the wall of the uterus.

fibroma: a benign fibrous-tissue growth, often occurring just under the skin.

fibrositis: literally, inflammation of fibrous (connective) tissue, but usually used nonspecifically to describe general aching and/or stiffness, especially as associated with systemic infections such as flu.

fibula: the smaller of the two bones in the lower part of the leg, positioned to the outside of and slightly behind the shinbone; the lower end of it is that knob at the outside of the ankle.

"fifth disease": See ERYTHEMA INFECTIOSUM.

filariasis: See PARASITES.

finger injuries: See AMPUTATION, ACCIDENTAL; DISLOCATION; FRACTURES; NAIL INJURIES.

Fiorinal: a combination-of-ingredients product including a barbiturate; see SEDATIVES.

fire extinguishers: While this topic is not, strictly speaking, a medical one, we include it because it (and the next entry, too) could well play an important part in preserving your children's well-being and possibly their lives.

Your home should have not just one fire extinguisher, but several, selected to reflect your needs. There should be one in, or immediately adjacent to, the kitchen; another in, or convenient to, the living room; a third, in the bedroom area. If you have a separate workshop, laundry room, or the like, that too should have its own extinguisher, as should any other buildings or structures on your property. In short, have an extinguisher handy.

There are three classes of home fires and four types of extinguishers.

Water-type extinguishers are not very practical purchases, for a number of reasons. They are effective only against Class A fires — those involving ordinary combustibles such as paper, wood, fabrics, and common plastics — and are not only useless against other fires, but may even make them worse. They are also extremely heavy and difficult to use, and the contents will freeze in low temperatures.

Standard dry-chemical extinguishers use sodium bicarbonate, and are designed to fight Class B fires — involving flammable liquids such as paints, solvents, and grease — and Class C (electrical) fires. *Purple K dry-chemical extinguishers* serve the same purpose; these employ potassium bicarbonate and have a somewhat greater initial fire-stopping power. It is one of these two types that should be in a kitchen and in a garage (and in some workrooms, as well), where the dangers are mostly from Class B and Class C fires.

Multipurpose dry-chemical extinguishers use ammonium phosphates and are effective against all types of fires; they are the best bets for living and sleeping areas.

There are several factors you should look for when buying fire extinguishers. Number One is an indication of listing or approval by Underwriters Laboratories. There should be clear operating instructions on the front of the extinguisher, as well as advice on maintenance (pressure testing or other procedures) and on how to restore the extinguisher to functioning condition after use. Finally, compare ratings. There should be letters and numbers on the extinguisher, looking something like this: *6–B:C,* or *2–A:10–B:C.* The letters tell you what classes of fires the extinguisher is designed to deal with. The numbers give relative ratings of fire-fighting ability for Class A and Class B fires; a 10–B rating, for example, means the extinguisher can put out a Class B fire about twice the size of one with which a 5–B extinguisher can cope.

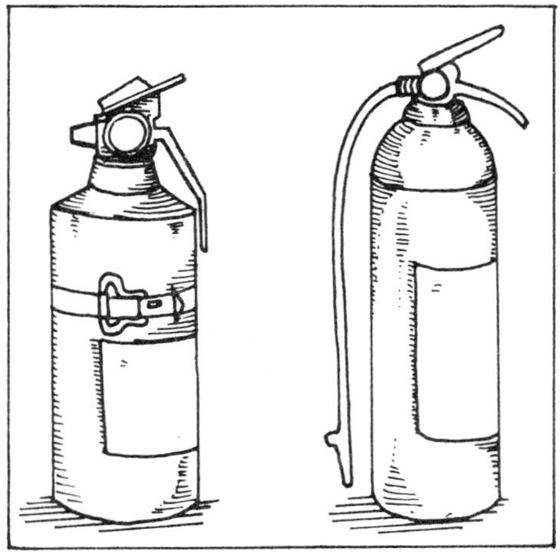

Fire Extinguishers
Your home should be equipped with several extinguishers, carefully chosen. Dry-chemical types (left) are preferable to those using water (right); the latter are of limited utility and can even make some fires worse. See text.

Obviously, the finest extinguisher will function merely as a useless wall decoration if no one knows how to use it. Not only you, but baby-sitters and your children of teen age as well, should be fully familiar with the location and use of extinguishers in your home.

fire-retardant clothing: Children's

sleepwear, in particular, has frequently contributed to severe injury and death in fires. Since mid-1973, federal law has required that all such sleepwear (robes, gowns, pajamas) in sizes 0 to 6x be made of flame-resistant fabrics, and extension of the requirement to sizes 7 to 14 took place in 1975 (ideally, that protection will one day cover all clothing).

Certainly parents should read labels carefully and make sure that covered clothing does offer flame resistance. Laundering must also be done carefully; otherwise, the flame-resistant finish may be damaged. And it should be done at home; the strong chemicals used by commercial laundries can definitely damage the finish. *Don't* use bleach, fabric softeners, soap, soap powder, very hot water, or a standard nonphosphate detergent. *Do* use a phosphate-based detergent; or, if those are not sold in your area, use a citrate-based, heavy-duty liquid detergent (Dynamo and Cold-Water Liquid All are examples, and others are available under supermarket brand names). Water temperature should be between 105° and 120° F. (40.5° and 48.9° C.). If you use a dryer, tumble-dry at low heat.

Quite a few fibers can now be treated to give them flame-resistant properties they would not have otherwise; they include cotton, linen, and cellulose synthetics (rayon, acetate). Nylon, polyesters, acrylics, and the like are relatively flammable, but there is a special high-temperature-resistant nylon (so labeled) that is fire retardant. Silk is less flammable but often contains dyes that are highly so. Wool is naturally somewhat flame resistant; it can be ignited, but it burns very slowly. Modacrylics and glass-fiber fabrics are synthetics with flame resistance built in.

first-aid rules: The first rule, if you will forgive the authors' immodesty, is to keep this book handy at all times, both at home and away; it covers virtually every emergency situation you are likely to encounter. If you leave your children with anyone, such as a baby-sitter, be sure she or he knows where to find it.

Second, be sure to fill in the appropriate emergency-use information on the pages provided in the back of the book — phone numbers for the police, your doctor, the nearest hospital, and so on, plus the special data concerning your children.

Third, be familiar ahead of time with the basic emergency procedures (see ACCIDENTS, FIRST-AID MEASURES, and other specific listings mentioned there); don't wait for an emergency to occur. See that teenage youngsters are familiar with these procedures, too.

Fourth, be prepared with the supplies you may need in case of emergency — both in your home (see MEDICINE CHEST) and outside and away from home (see FIRST-AID SUPPLIES, following).

first-aid supplies: You'll find a list of those you should have in your home, along with some comments and suggestions on their keeping and storage, under MEDICINE CHEST. Here are the minimum essentials you should have to be prepared for away-from-home emergencies.

YOUR GARAGE OR BARN

Any building on your property not directly connected with your house should have its own small stock of first-aid materials for dealing with the kind of emergency in which running back and forth could waste precious time. These should include:

- at least one of each type of bandaging material (see BANDAGES);
- something — a strip of cloth, a belt — to use as a tourniquet;
- pieces of wood in various sizes or other items suitable for use as splints;
- two or three clean handkerchiefs or other pieces of clean cloth (old sheets, diapers, or any rags, as long as they're clean) kept sealed in a plastic bag;
- a piece of candy or other sweet food if there is a diabetic in the family;
- a small amount (at least one dose) of any medication that has been prescribed for any chronic condition in which there is potential for an emergency situation.

Should any of these things be used, they should of course be replaced promptly.

TRAVEL BY CAR

All the things just listed as essentials for your garage or barn should go with you on family car trips. In addition, it's a good idea to have:

- a pair of scissors to cut cloths or bandages;
- a scarf or something else from which a sling can be made;
- aspirin (including the children's type if you have small children) and a container of fresh water;
- a fire extinguisher of the B:C type (see FIRE EXTINGUISHERS);
- a signal flare for use in pull-off-the-road emergencies;
- data on your family's hospital and medical insurance;
- if it's a first-time long car trip for a child, or you know that your child is susceptible to carsickness, appropriate medication (see MOTION SICKNESS);
- supplies of current prescriptions sufficient to see you through the trip;
- in very hot weather, some salty snacks;
- in very cold weather, blankets in case of breakdown;
- this book.

BOATING

If you're fortunate enough to own a boat on which you can get away for vacation, a weekend, or even a day, it's vital to realize that you're on your own, medically speaking. You should be prepared to cope with almost any eventuality.

Your boat should be equipped with fire extinguishers (those approved by the Coast Guard are so labeled), a radio with which to summon the Coast Guard or other assistance, and appropriate lights and signal flags for conveying distress messages visually. There should also be Coast Guard-approved flotation devices for everyone on board. And your set of medical supplies should be fairly extensive:

- all the basic at-home essentials (see MEDICINE CHEST);
- medication for motion sickness;
- materials that could serve as splints and slings (at least two of each);
- scissors to cut cloths or bandages;
- a generous supply of fresh water;
- an oral airway (see RESPIRATORY RESUSCITATION);
- calamine lotion, the type that doesn't contain phenol;

• insect repellent in liquid form (the aerosol types are mostly gas);

• a sunscreen preparation;

• a two-ounce bottle of syrup of ipecac (*not* the powder) to induce vomiting in case of poisoning;

• salty snacks;

• sufficient quantities of current prescriptions to see you through the trip and then some, plus anything — such as remedies for life-threatening allergy — that has been prescribed for emergency use;

• if you'll be doing any fishing, wirecutters in case of fishhook injury;

• if you'll be swimming in salt water off the boat, spirits of ammonia or alcohol in case of Portuguese man-of-war sting;

• this book.

CAMPING TRIPS

Your first step should be to learn all you can about the area you're headed for, including information about the climate and any poisonous snakes or other dangerous animals. Make it your business, too, to find out exactly how near or far help will be in the event of emergency; know the location of the nearest doctor or professional first-aid or rescue team, the nearest hospital, the nearest rangers — and the best and fastest way of signaling for help.

Everything listed for boat trips should go with you when you camp out (including the spirits of ammonia or alcohol if you are likely to encounter any stinging caterpillars). Additionally, you should carry in your backpacks:

• whistles or other loud signals (each person should have one) to call for help or warn of danger;

• a sharp knife;

• plenty of matches, kept waterproof;

• at least two flashlights or battery-powered lanterns;

• snakebite serum and equipment for injecting it;

• anything else authorities in the area may suggest.

For guidelines on out-of-the-country trips or forays off the beaten path within our borders, see TRAVEL PRECAUTIONS.

fishhook injuries: If in the eye, see EYE INJURIES; if elsewhere, see PUNCTURE WOUNDS.

fissure: a cleft or crack; for discussion of a common kind, see ANAL FISSURE.

fistula: an opening or passageway that shouldn't be there; it can be congenital, or can result from such mishaps as injury or the blockage of a normal duct. A fistula can occur almost anywhere — between the vagina and an excretory passage, for example, or between an artery and a vein, or from the lining of the rectum to the skin near the anus. It is corrected by surgery.

"fits": See CONVULSIONS.

flat feet: a lack of the normal arches in the feet; it's often a familial trait. Flat feet are not necessarily weak, painful, or in any way incapacitating; whether any treatment is needed is up to the physician.

flea bites: See the appropriate section under BITES AND STINGS.

flexor: See MUSCLES.

floxacillin, Floxapen: a semisynthetic penicillin (the second word is a trade name for the first); see ANTIBIOTICS.

flu: See INFLUENZA.

flu, intestinal: See INTESTINAL FLU.

fluoridation: See CAVITIES.

fluoroscope: a diagnostic device that

provides a picture similar to that of an X ray, except that it is not quite as precise and is projected on a screen instead of recorded on film. There is less radiation involved than with X ray, so the physician may choose to fluoroscope if a permanent record is not needed; or fluoroscoping may be done prior to a series of X rays to establish (and thus limit) the number and type or angle of the X rays needed. Additionally, fluoroscopy may be called for if the doctor wishes to see a part of the body in action or while it is being treated — as a limb in motion, or in setting a fracture, or in the removal of a foreign object.

fluphenazine: a major tranquilizer that also has antinauseant properties; see NAUSEA and SEDATIVES.

flurazepam: a nonbarbiturate hypnotic; see SEDATIVES.

folic acid: one of the B-complex vitamins; see NUTRITION.

follicle: the small sac from which a hair grows; an inflammation of it is called folliculitis. A *Graafian* follicle is that which forms around a maturing ovum within the ovary; its development is triggered by follicle-stimulating hormone, produced by the pituitary gland.

fontanel: the so-called "soft spot" on an infant's head where the bones of the skull have not yet fused firmly; there are actually several spots, and they are far from soft. The total is, in fact, six — although four are so unobtrusive that they're usually not noticed. They permit slight flexibility so that the skull — the largest part of a newborn baby — can pass through the birth canal. Additionally, this cranial flexibility accommodates

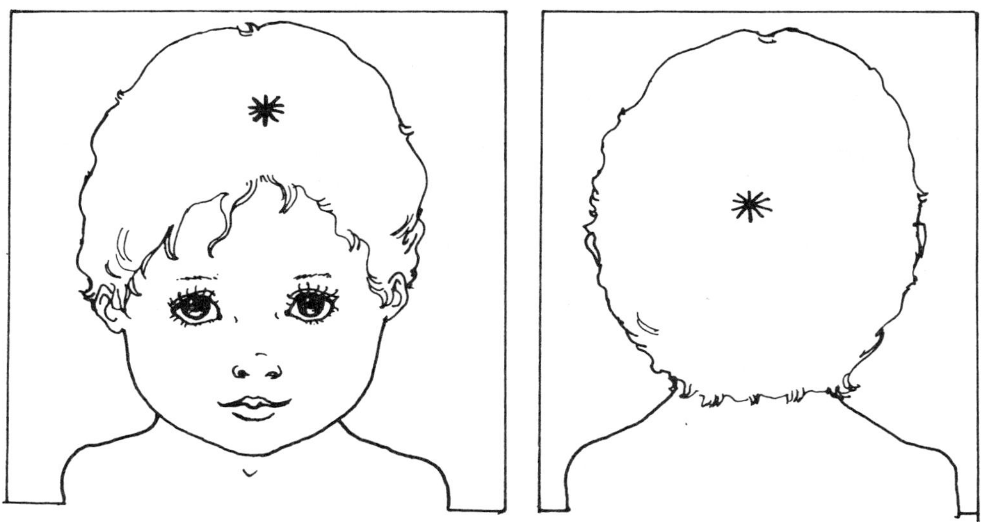

Fontanels
The two major fontanels, junctures where an infant's skull bones have not yet fused, are indicated by the asterisks; they mark the ends of a central division called the sagittal suture. The posterior fontanel (right) closes by the approximate age of four months; the anterior (left), largest of the fontanels and the one usually denoted by the phrase "the soft spot," is closed by the age of 18 to 24 months.

growth of the brain; although the spots close while the child is still a toddler, ossification isn't completed until maturity.

There are two main spots that you'll probably be aware of. One, toward the back of the baby's skull, will be closed by about the age of four months. The other, at the top of the head, is the largest of all and the one usually meant when *the* "soft spot" is mentioned; it will close by the time the child is a year and a half or two years old.

Don't be afraid to touch — or wash — the "soft spot"; it's well protected by a very tough membrane under the skin. Too-gingerly handling can, as a matter of fact, cause problems; see CRADLE CAP.

food poisoning: This entry deals with symptoms and emergency (or other) action. If prevention is what you have in mind, see the main entry that follows.

Food poisoning should be suspected if several persons become ill simultaneously, or nearly simultaneously, and exhibit the same symptoms after eating the same food. It should also be suspected if someone becomes ill after eating something no one else has consumed.

All types of food poisoning can be serious. Some can be fatal. Prompt action is needed. The various types are covered here roughly in order of seriousness, from most to least; the most critical kinds are, happily, the rarest.

BOTULISM

If the food was fresh, forget about botulism. The culprit is typically nonacidic canned food, especially home-canned or -preserved vegetables, meats, or poultry, but occasionally commercially processed foods. The toxin cannot develop in tomatoes — except for the low-acid type — fruits, or pickles.

Symptoms usually appear some 18 to 48 hours after eating the poisoned food. There may be mild stomach upset and general malaise, but the chief symptoms are neurological and muscular and tend to appear in the following order: dizziness and headache, with blurred or double vision; general muscular weakness; difficulty in swallowing and speaking; respiratory failure and coma, with death by respiratory paralysis. There is a two-to-one possibility of death; the odds depend upon the amount of poison ingested vis-à-vis body weight and how fast treatment is obtained.

Immediate hospitalization is needed; antitoxin is required, plus other measures that must be carried out professionally. If botulism is suspected, the victim should simply be rushed to the hospital — and given *absolutely nothing* by mouth.

Antitoxin is not available at all hospitals but is stocked at key points around the country. If you are reading this after you have called a doctor to your home, have the physician phone the 24-hour botulism "hot line" at the Center for Disease Control in Atlanta for medical guidance and information on the nearest supply of antitoxin. The line is for use *only by physicians* who have diagnosed a case of suspected botulism. Numbers are (404) 633–3311 during the day, (404) 633–2176 at night and on Sundays and holidays, or dial Atlanta information, (404) 555–1212.

The CDC, on receiving the physician's report, will also take any other indicated measures: notifying local health authorities, locating and confiscating contaminated food, issuing warnings to the public if the suspected food is on store shelves, etc.

SEAFOOD POISONING

There are two types, both resulting almost invariably from seafood caught or gathered by individuals for their own consumption; there is strict and continuous surveillance of commercial fisheries.

Mytilotoxism results from eating mollusks — prominently, mussels, clams, oysters, or abalone — that have fed on certain toxic micro-organisms; most cases have occurred on the Pacific coast during summer and early fall.

Symptoms appear very quickly, usually within half an hour. They generally include nausea, vomiting, and abdominal cramps, followed by paralysis that begins in the hands and feet and spreads to the rest of the body; eventual death is by respiratory failure. In the absence of prompt treatment, there is a high fatality rate.

If vomiting has not already occurred, *induce* it (see EMETIC) at the *same time* that the victim is being rushed to the nearest hospital. If more than one person has eaten the suspicious shellfish, do exactly the same with all members of the group, whether or not any symptoms have yet appeared.

Ciguatera poisoning may result from eating any contaminated seafood — shellfish or other fish — and occurs only in tropical and subtropical areas.

Symptoms, which usually take three to five hours to develop (although the time may be a little shorter or a little longer), at first include headache, nausea, fatigue, giddiness, and outpouring of fluids — increased salivation, watering of the eyes, sweating. As the effects of the toxin increase, the headache and dizziness grow worse, vision dims, and the pupils contract. Difficulty in breathing follows and can progress to respiratory failure.

Rush the victim to the hospital; don't stop to do anything else. If there is another person available, that person should — on the way to the hospital — assist the victim's breathing if it becomes necessary (see RESPIRATORY RESUSCITATION).

MUSHROOM POISONING

Suspect poisoning only if the mushrooms eaten were found growing wild; fresh mushrooms sold in stores are perfectly safe. (*Note:* If the mushrooms eaten were canned, what should be suspected is the much more serious botulism, discussed earlier in this entry.)

Symptoms vary with the type of mushroom and generally assume one of two characteristic patterns; first-aid measures are the same for both.

Both the bright "fly agaric" found across the United States and a related flat-topped species of mushroom native to the northwest contain a toxic chemical called muscarine. Symptoms of muscarine poisoning appear rapidly, often within minutes; they typically include abdominal pain, vomiting, diarrhea, difficulty in breathing, and outpouring of fluids — sweating, salivation, tears.

A third species of mushroom, a tall, broad kind found in many wooded areas, contains a different toxin. Symptoms of poisoning may not appear for six hours or more, perhaps as long as a full day. The first sign is usually sudden, severe abdominal pain. It may be accompanied or followed by nausea, vomiting, diarrhea, and extreme weakness; the vomited material and/or the stool may contain blood.

In either case, get the victim to medical care immediately and on the way, take two first-aid measures: keep the victim resting quietly; induce vomiting if it is not already taking place (see EMETIC) — and save the vomited material, so that the toxin can be identified and proper treatment given.

JIMSONWEED POISONING VIA TOMATOES

As with mushrooms, store-bought produce is safe. The problem has arisen — particularly in the Midwest — only from home-grown tomatoes, specifically those grown by grafting to jimsonweed roots; other, local, names for jimsonweed are stinkweed, thorn apple, and devil's apple. The poison attacks the nervous system.

Symptoms appear fairly quickly. Initially, they include dryness of the mouth, difficulty in swallowing, fever, a flushed appearance, blurred or double vision, and dizziness; there may or may not be headache or nausea. Physical weakness and mental confusion follow, and there may also be delirium and/or hallucinations.

Take the same measures as for mushroom poisoning (see the section immediately preceding this one), and also wrap the victim in cold, wet cloths to reduce fever.

SALMONELLA POISONING

This lower-intestinal infection should be suspected if typical symptoms appear after eating fresh food that may have been contaminated. Most often implicated are eggs or other dairy products, poultry, raw or rare meat; uncommonly, fruits or vegetables.

Symptoms take six or more hours to develop; if the contaminated food was eaten at an evening meal, symptoms generally appear during the night or early the following morning. They usually include abdominal cramps, watery diarrhea, chills with fever as high as 102° F. (39° C.), headache, and extreme weakness.

Call a physician immediately; the infection is a serious one, especially in an infant or in a child whose resistance is low. The diagnosis is established by stool culture. Antibiotics or other medications may be needed — although they are *not* advised for an otherwise healthy child; nor should anything be given to stop the diarrhea, since it represents a "cleansing" process. (Discuss with your doctor measures to prevent dehydration; see DIARRHEA.) Full recovery may take up to a week.

"ORDINARY" FOOD POISONING

There are a number of common bacteria that cause it — particularly in warm weather, when foods have not been properly refrigerated. It's generally not critical but should be watched closely.

Symptoms vary depending upon

the exact organism involved, and can appear anywhere from two to twenty hours after the questionable food was eaten. They generally include a sick-to-the-stomach feeling, nausea, overall malaise, and possibly vomiting and/or diarrhea.

At the first sign of symptoms, get the child off his feet; a very small child should be put to bed. Vomiting need not be induced, but don't discourage it, either. Don't give the child anything by mouth until the initial symptoms subside; at that point, offer warm, mild fluids such as broth or tea. Over the next couple of days, keep the child's diet on the bland, easily digestible side: nothing fried, heavily spiced, etc. No medications should be given unless a physician has so instructed.

In most instances, that is sufficient, and medical treatment is not needed. You should, however, call the doctor: if the child gets worse rather than better; if the initial, acute symptoms, even though mild, persist for more than twelve hours; if there is severe abdominal pain; if there is fever, which is not a typical symptom of this mild type of food poisoning; if there are any symptoms whatever beyond those we have mentioned.

food poisoning, prevention of: Here, we discuss the ways and means of avoiding emergency situations. If there is already an emergency and you seek first-aid advice, see the main entry immediately preceding this one.

In almost all cases, food poisoning can be prevented by taking a few simple precautions. It is helpful, in the first place, to understand the causes. They do not include ptomaines; whatever you may have heard, there is no such thing as "ptomaine poisoning." Ptomaines do exist, but they are simply normal by-products of decay; they are destroyed in the normal process of digestion, and they are not toxic. The actual causes of food poisoning are bacteria and a variety of naturally occurring toxins.

Botulism is, as you doubtless know, the most lethal kind of food poisoning; happily, it is also the rarest. Its cause is a bacterium called *Clostridium botulinum* or, more accurately, a toxin (botulin) the bacteria produce in the course of propagation. That process can take place only in the absence of oxygen; a sealed container such as a can or jar thus provides ideal conditions and conversely, open air discourages bacterial activity. Acids also inhibit the toxin-producing process. You will never get botulism from fresh foods or from acidic food products such as orange juice, tomatoes (exception: the special low-acid type), pickles, and the like.

The key to keeping *C. botulinum* out of canned and preserved foods is proper cooking during the canning process, which destroys the organism. Generally, commercially processed food is safe; the exceptions are what make headlines. Because there have been instances of such foods causing outbreaks (in botulism, one case constitutes an official outbreak), you should be alert to signs of possibly toxic contents in canned foods. The main one is an ominous bulge or swelling at the end of the can, since toxin production creates gases that expand the contents. Don't just leave such a can on the store shelf; it should be promptly reported to the management. Even if there is no bulge apparent, be suspicious — and call the situation to the attention of both the store and local health authorities — if the contents spurt out explosively when you open the can, which is another sign of internal pressure.

Most outbreaks of botulism can be traced to home canning and preserving. During the years 1970–73, there were thirty outbreaks reported to the Center for Disease Control; they involved a total of 91 cases and included 21 deaths. Only three — 10 percent — of those outbreaks stemmed from commercially processed foods; the foods involved were soup, mushrooms, and peppers. As the popularity of home canning increases, so do botulism outbreaks; twenty were reported in 1974 alone, all but one traceable to home-canned foods. The obviously higher risk of botulism from home-preserved foods can be avoided by not eating, or permitting your children to eat, such foods unless you are positive they were properly processed or have so processed them yourself. Acidic foods can be safely processed in a boiling-water bath. But with nonacidic vegetables, meats, and poultry, such baths, ovens, open kettles, or unpressurized steamers do not produce enough heat to kill the organisms; to put up these foods safely, a pressure canner must be used, and it must be used correctly. Appendix C at the back of this book lists some helpful literature on the subject.

Natural plant toxins include, prominently, those found in certain wild-growing mushrooms, and a chemical component of jimsonweed that has been known to find its way into tomatoes that have been grown by grafting onto jimsonweed roots. If you limit the mushrooms and tomatoes on your family's menu to those purchased at groceries and supermarkets — which is what we strongly advise — you will never have to worry about this kind of food poisoning.

Seafood poisoning, similarly, usually stems not from commercially available fish and shellfish, but from that gathered by individuals for their own consumption, at times and places (see the preceding entry) when the animals have been feeding on certain microorganisms that may contain the toxins. If digging clams and similar activities are among the great joys of your life, certainly limit them to the sites and seasons when risks are low.

Salmonella includes over a thousand varieties of bacteria (one causes typhoid fever); they are responsible for the second most serious kind of bacterial food poisoning. The ills they cause are not, strictly speaking, cases of poisoning — since there is no toxin involved — but systemic infections caused by the bacteria themselves; they can be quite severe and even fatal. Food-borne salmonella cases in the United States have more than doubled over the last three decades, with about three hundred outbreaks reported annually (experts believe the real figure may be ten times that); the phenomenon can only be attributed to human carelessness.

Typically, the foods involved are fresh ones that have been contaminated with the bacteria through unsanitary handling or fouling by animals. The most frequent ones are eggs, cheeses, and other dairy products; poultry; and meats eaten raw or rare. Occasionally, though uncommonly, fruits or vegetables may be contaminated.

Your best protection against salmonella is to buy food only from establishments that handle it properly: frozen foods should be solidly frozen, meats and dairy products refrigerated, and fruits and vegetables should appear clean and fresh. It is also wise to buy only government-inspected meats and poultry, to cook meats adequately, and to clean fruits and vegetables well before you use them.

Common, widespread bacteria are behind the great mass of food poisonings, which may include many outbreaks of "intestinal flu." The American Public Health Association has in fact estimated that such ills may well total ten million cases a year, making food poisoning possibly second in incidence only to the common cold.

Probably the most prevalent of these bacteria is *Staphylococcus aureus* ("staph"), which, like the botulism organism, does its dirty work via a toxin — albeit a far less nasty one. Other food-borne bacteria causing gastrointestinal problems include *Clostridium perfringens* (a less virulent cousin of *C. botulinum,* it may be, in the opinion of some authorities, more widespread than "staph"), *Escherichia coli, Bacillus subtilis, Streptococcus fecalis,* and more. While the ills they cause are usually mild, why subject yourself and your children to them at all?

These bacteria are indeed ubiquitous — they live in the air around us, on human skin, and almost anywhere else you can think of — and most of the time do no harm whatever. It's only when they manage to contaminate and multiply in food that they pose a threat. The following routine precautions can do much to diminish that threat:

• See that food is kept and stored properly, both in the store and in your home. The danger zone for fast bacterial growth is from 60° to 120° F. (approximately 16° to 49° C.), which includes ordinary room temperatures as well as usual warm-weather outdoor temperatures. Spoilable food, cooked or uncooked, should not be left in this range for any length of time.

Refrigerate foods that need it as soon as you get them home from the store. This of course includes all meats, fish, poultry, eggs, dairy products, and many fruits and vegetables (when in doubt, refrigerate), as well as any foods, cooked or uncooked, containing eggs (custards, pies, cakes, salad dressings, etc.).

Hot, cooked foods should be served and eaten immediately or else refrigerated (a cooling-off period is not necessary). Leftover meat, fish, and poultry should be refrigerated for use within a few days, otherwise frozen.

Refrigerator and freezer temperatures are important for safe food storage. Refrigerator temperature should be below 40° F. (4.4° C.), preferably between 33° and 37° F. (under 3° C.); your freezer should be kept at 0° F. (−18° C.). In the event of power failure, assume that an unopened refrigerator will keep food safe for only a few hours. A fully loaded, unopened freezer will safeguard food for at least two days; the length of time is diminished in direct proportion to the amount of unoccupied freezer space. If a more prolonged problem is anticipated, use dry ice; 25 pounds of it will maintain a fully loaded ten-cubic-foot freezer at below freezing temperatures for at least three or four days. Thawed foods may be safely refrozen (there may be some flavor loss) only if they are still very cold; otherwise, use them immediately or discard them.

• Be sure hands are washed thoroughly after going to the bathroom, changing a baby's diaper, or disposing of pet stool or droppings. Many of these mischief-making bacteria are found in feces, both human and animal. As we noted earlier, they are also present to some degree on all human skin; for that reason, thorough hand-washing before meals should be a house rule, as it should before preparing food — especially food that requires direct handling, such as sandwiches, salads, meat patties, and so on.

• Never eat, or permit your children to eat, any food — fresh, canned, frozen, or leftover — that looks or smells the least bit odd. And that means don't even *taste* it.

• See that all kitchen utensils and implements that come in contact with food are kept scrupulously clean; food residue at room temperature provides a highly congenial climate for the rapid growth and proliferation of bacteria. One oft-overlooked source of contamination is the can opener: the cutting blade always touches the can's contents, and so picks up some food — at the same time contaminating those contents if any prior residue has fostered bacterial growth on the blade.

• Do everything you can to discourage household pests — insects and rodents — which can and do carry many of the troublemaking bacteria.

• *When in doubt, throw it out.* If there is the least question in your mind about a food's freshness, cleanness, or safety, discard it. That should include any food with even the least bit of mold showing; visible signs of mold mean that there is considerable growth in the invisible part as well, and the entire item should be thrown out. This last precaution does not apply to cheeses, on which mold is a normal surface growth; the moldy portion can simply be cut away, and the rest is safely edible.

food, solid: Your own pediatrician or family physician will advise you on the introduction of various solid foods in your baby's diet; you should follow this advice, since your doctor knows your child best.

As a general guideline, the approximate schedule is usually: puréed fruits and cereals at fourteen to sixteen weeks; gelatins, puddings, and the like at four or five months; potatoes, strained vegetables, noodles, and such at six to nine months; "real" food, cut up very small, at nine months to one year.

Store-bought baby cereals offer a specific nutritional benefit: they are fortified with iron, which a baby does need by the age of four to six months (prior to that time, an infant is "tided over" by iron stored in the liver during the prenatal period). But cooked fruits can be puréed in a blender —

and later, when your baby's diet becomes more varied, you can also prepare an expanded menu at home. Simply combine leftovers in a refrigerated container; save, too, leftover gravy, meat juices, and pot liquors (liquids in which vegetables have been cooked, which contain many nutrients). Then, a couple of times a week, toss an appropriate mixture in the blender, using the liquids to bring the mixture to proper blending consistency. Pour the resulting purée into an ice-cube tray; when it's solidly frozen, place the cubes in a plastic bag in your freezer, labeled with date and contents. Frozen leftovers will keep four to six months, so you can remove and thaw one or several cubes as needed, and there's always baby food on hand. This economical system also avoids compulsive "empty-your-plate" eating for the rest of the family and accustoms your baby to parental cooking.

Many parents have found that early spoon-feeding mess can be minimized — assuming baby's a capable grasper — by offering items, such as whole carrots or broccoli stalks, that are cooked to the point where they're still solid enough for a small hand to hold, but soft enough to turn to mush in the mouth as they're nibbled; this technique works with hamburger and other soft foods as well. But never turn your back during such a self-feeding session; you want to be able to act promptly if the child bites off more than he can handle and starts to choke (see CHOKING).

foot, broken: See FRACTURES.

forceps: tongs of various shapes and sizes used for grabbing and pulling or holding various things; among the procedures that employ the use of forceps are extracting teeth, helping a baby's head through the birth canal, clamping blood vessels during surgery, removing bullets, and many more.

foreign object, swallowed: See CHOKING.

foreskin: See CIRCUMCISION; PARAPHIMOSIS.

formula: See BOTTLE FEEDING.

fractures: There are over two hundred separate bones in the human body, and anyone who can avoid breaking even one leads a charmed life indeed. Children of the active-outdoor-play age are especially susceptible to such mishaps; most fractures are not serious and heal very quickly in youngsters. We'll come, in a moment, to emergency first-aid procedures, which differ depending upon the part of the body involved. First, some categories of fractures you may hear your doctor mention, which can be useful for description if you're phoning for medical help. We list them in order of their seriousness, from least to most.

- *Green-stick fractures* are breaks that do not go all the way through the bone. This type of fracture can occur only in young children (generally under the age of ten) whose bones are not yet rigid; its name reflects the difficulty in snapping a young, green twig. It may at first appear to be no more than a sprain or severe bruise, but mounting pain and discoloration will occur. The fracture must be confirmed by X ray.

- *Closed (simple) fractures* involve a

break through the bone; the skin is unbroken.

• *Open (compound) fractures* involve both a break through the bone and broken skin; the latter may be due either to injury from without or to piercing of the skin by a jagged piece of the bone.

• *Comminuted fractures* involve multiple lines of breakage in a bone; they may be either open or closed.

EMERGENCY PROCEDURES

Any fracture or suspected fracture requires medical attention: X ray to determine the precise nature of the injury, and expert setting (realigning) of the bone if it is indeed a fracture. You should get the victim to a hospital as quickly as possible, with minimal movement of the injured part; the latter often requires a degree of immobilization, both to avoid further injury and to prevent extra pain. Generally, immobilization should include the joints close to a suspected fracture.

Here is what you should do, *in this order:*

1. Make sure the child is breathing. If not — or if you're not sure — see RESPIRATORY RESUSCITATION.
2. Take precautions against the all-too-frequent aftermath of severe injury; see TRAUMATIC SHOCK.
3. If there is, as far as you can see, a possibility of skull fracture, turn immediately to HEAD INJURIES. If you think there may be a fracture involving the spine (the backbone), turn to BACK AND NECK INJURIES. These involve — or potentially involve — the nervous system, with the possibility of permanent impairment, and need a special sort of approach. Otherwise, keep reading.
4. If there is an open fracture, *gently* apply any available clean cloths to cope with bleeding. Do *not* attempt to push back or realign any protruding bone. Usually, extensive bleeding will not be a problem in such an injury; if there seems to be such a problem, turn to BLEEDING and take the measures indicated there — very carefully.
5. Get professional medical help quickly. Meanwhile, try to keep the child calm — meaning, stay with him, and don't move him unless it's necessary to save his life and/or yours.
6. Don't give the child anything whatever by mouth — food, drink, water, aspirin, *anything.*
7. If you are in the position of transporting the child to medical care — rather than vice versa — the fractured (or possibly fractured) part should be immobilized as completely as possible. Do so, if circumstances permit, according to the list that follows. Take the child to the emergency room of the nearest hospital. Splinting — see the accompanying illustrations — should be done especially carefully if there is an open fracture.

Ankle — Splint the lower part of the leg, including the foot.

Arm — Splint whatever part of the arm is involved — including, if possible, the joints above and below the fracture — and also put the arm in a sling, if this can be accomplished without increasing the pain.

Cheekbone — See facial bones.

Collarbone — Put the arm on the

injured side in a sling. Although there may be a great deal of pain in the shoulder and arm, this is one of the least serious of all fractures.

Facial bones — Fracture should be suspected — and X ray is necessary to confirm or disprove it — if any of the following signs are evident around jaw, cheekbone, orbit (surrounding bony structure) of the eye, or nose: obvious swelling, marked discoloration, depression or other distortion of the area, numbness, extreme tenderness. Fracture of the orbital area may also include eyesight disturbances. Fracture of the nose may cause difficulty in breathing through it. Don't attempt any bandaging; simply get the child to the hospital.

Finger — The child will instinctively keep the finger in a fixed position; splinting is normally not necessary. Do put the hand in a sling to further reduce the possibility of movement.

Foot — Loosen the child's shoe (it's not necessary to remove it) and be sure no weight is placed on the foot on the way to the hospital.

Hand — Splint the hand and wrist and put it in a sling.

Hip — If the victim is an infant, or a child so small you can carry him without permitting any leg movement, do so. In an older child, treat the injury the same way as an actual or suspected fracture of the spine, since any untoward movement of torso or legs could cause serious internal injury, as well as considerable pain; see BACK AND NECK INJURIES.

Jaw — See facial bones. Keep the victim sitting up on the way to the hospital, and don't let him try to talk. (*Note:* A dentist specializing in oral surgery is also capable of dealing with a fractured jaw.)

Kneecap — See leg, following.

Leg — Splint the leg. If the knee or thigh is involved, the entire leg should be splinted; if the fracture is below the knee, include both knee and ankle in the splinting. If possible, transport the child lying down; certainly permit no weight to be placed on the injured leg.

Nose — See facial bones.

Rib(s) — If there is an open fracture, simply cover the wound securely to prevent air from being sucked into the chest cavity. If it's a closed fracture, wind an elastic bandage lightly around the child's chest, which will help to relieve pain a little. A rib fracture can be extremely painful; the physician will probably prescribe a potent painkiller. After the child is treated, keep an eye on him and inquire frequently how he feels; if there is shortness of breath or increased pain, take him back to the hospital emergency room *immediately.*

Toe — Relieve pressure on it by cutting a hole in the child's shoe or by removing the shoe altogether. Splinting isn't necessary, but of course no weight should be placed on the toes of that foot.

Wrist — See arm.

FRACTURE FOLLOW-UP

Additional X rays should be taken in order to be sure the bones are correctly positioned and are healing properly. Their frequency depends upon the exact nature and site of the fracture; follow the advice of the physician who treats it in the first place.

After a cast has been applied and the child is home, be alert for any complications that might arise from a too-tight cast (the reason a cast might become too tight is that swelling — the degree of which is unpredictable — may occur). To help prevent or at least minimize this problem, a casted

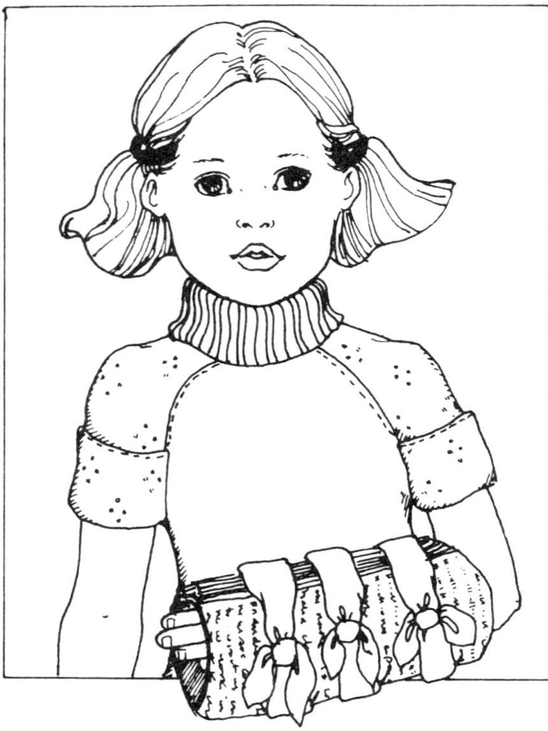

Splinting
A fracture or suspected fracture should be immobilized in order to minimize pain and to prevent further injury. Anything that's handy and fairly rigid can be used: newspapers wrapped around the limb, sticks cushioned by whatever soft materials are available, etc. Shown, possible makeshift splints for a wrist fracture and for a fracture involving the lower part of the leg (note that knee and ankle are included). Not all fractures require splinting; see text for details.

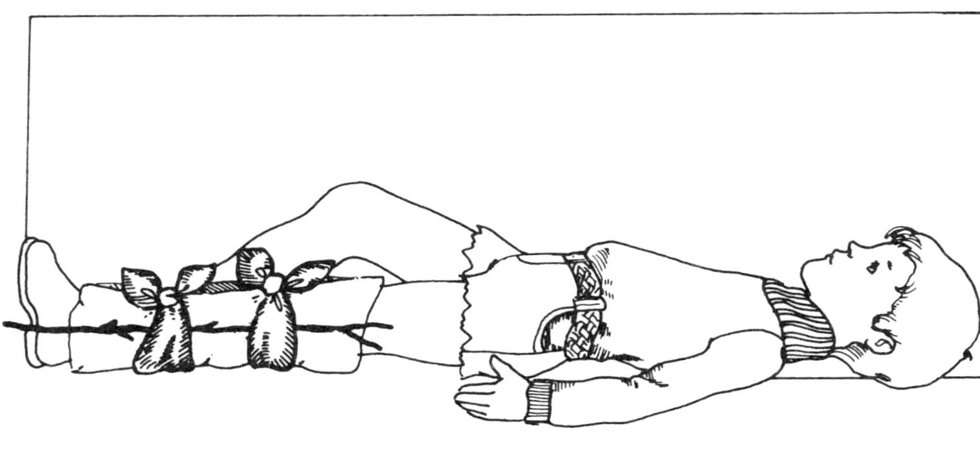

arm or leg should be kept elevated; sometimes this may involve continuous elevation, even bed rest (do as the doctor advises). If the affected part, or the area adjacent to it, becomes cold, discolored, or numb — or there is increased pain — take the child back to the hospital *immediately.*

Away-from-home casting (e.g., on a ski trip) suggests an extra precaution. If the physician applying the cast is not necessarily the one who will oversee subsequent treatment, it is a good idea to ask the cast-applier to draw a picture of the injury directly on the cast, showing exactly where the break or breaks occurred — along with a verbal description of the fracture (open or closed, etc.) and the date the cast was applied.

F.R.C.P., F.R.C.S.: the British counterparts of the U.S. designations F.A.C.P. and F.A.C.S.; the "R" is for "Royal." Another letter, such as C, E, or I, may follow these four; they stand, respectively, for Canada, Edinburgh, and Ireland.

frenum: an anatomical term for any band of mucous membrane connecting a movable part to a relatively fixed part. It can refer to a number of such structures in the body, but is most widely applied to the one under the tongue and the one between the upper lip and the gum.

frostbite: sufficient exposure to cold of a part of the body — typically an extremity such as a hand or foot, less commonly the nose or chin — to actually freeze the tissues and markedly impair circulation. The affected part will feel stiff, numb, possibly stinging (with thawing, there may be burning pain); it may appear unusually light in color, and there may be blistering or fissuring.

Frostbite is a critical matter; there is a very real danger of gangrene. Arrange for medical aid or transportation to a hospital, fast. If it is not immediately available, start to take first-aid measures. There has been a good deal of misinformation on that score; what *not* to do is as important as what to *do.*

Do NOT rub, or put any pressure on, the injured area or expose it to dry heat, as of a fire or stove or electrical heater; do NOT break any blisters that may be present or apply any medication, dressing, or the like; do NOT let the child walk if feet or toes are involved or give the child any alcoholic beverage.

DO begin to gently thaw the frostbitten area. Immerse it in — or apply to it, if it's a nose or chin — water in the temperature range from 107°to 112°F. (41.7°to 44.4°C.). If you have a thermometer, check the water temperature; if you haven't, use water that feels just a *little* hot to your own hand. Continue for twenty minutes or until medical aid is available.

As the injured area thaws it is likely to become extremely painful (it's fine to give the youngster some aspirin); nevertheless, slow movement of the injured part should be encouraged, to help restore circulation. And when the child is up to it, give something warm to drink, such as soup, tea, or cocoa.

fructose: a natural sugar; see SWEETENERS.

FTA test: a highly specific test for syphilis; see VENEREAL DISEASES.

fulminant or fulminating: occurring

or progressing rapidly, for the worse — as fever, pain, or a particular illness.

Fulvicin: a trade name for griseofulvin; see ANTIBIOTICS.

functional: describing a symptom or condition for which no organic cause can be found — as a "functional heart murmur" or "functional diarrhea."

Fungizone: a trade name for amphotericin B; see ANTIBIOTICS.

fungus: a low form of plant life; the mushroom is a familiar example, and some mushrooms can cause trouble (see FOOD POISONING). Some fungi — lower-ranking and smaller than mushrooms — can cause infections, usually on the skin (most often on warm, moist sites such as the feet) but also on mucous membranes and in the respiratory system; these vary considerably in symptoms and treatment.

For some examples of ills caused by fungus infections, see ATHLETE'S FOOT; CANDIDIASIS; HISTOPLASMOSIS; MONILIASIS; PARONYCHIA; RINGWORM; THRUSH; VALLEY FEVER.

furuncle: See BOIL.

G

gagging: usually, the first sign of impending vomiting; see VOMITING for a discussion of that subject. If the child is gagging on something swallowed, whether food or a foreign object, see CHOKING.

galactose: one of the three basic sugars; see SWEETENERS.

gallbladder: a small gland just below the liver; it condenses and stores bile from the liver and discharges it (as does the liver, too) into the small intestine, where bile plays a part in digestion. If the gallbladder is diseased — a situation rare, but not unknown, in children — it can be removed without ill effect.

Gammacorten: See CORTICOSTEROIDS.

gamma globulin: the substance in blood that contains infection-fighting antibodies; it may be extracted from the blood of one person and given to another, generally in an instance where the second person has been or may be exposed to a particular disease, has no self-protection against it, and to whom such protection is critical. It thus confers a short-lived immunity when such immunity is necessary — although for general immunization purposes, vaccines are longer-lasting and more effective.

Gamma globulins are available for, and may be used to protect against, a number of ills including chickenpox, type A hepatitis, measles, tetanus, and whooping cough. One has also been employed against mumps but has not been proved effective, and rubella gamma globulin is not considered especially dependable. The amount of gamma globulin given depends upon the weight of the individual, plus the duration of immunity desired — and when given as pretravel protection, should be given as closely as possible to the day of departure.

Gamma globulin is also used in the rare instance that a child lacks all natural protection; see AGAMMAGLOBULINEMIA.

For discussion of the various types of natural and acquired protection against infection, see IMMUNITY.

ganglion cyst: See CYST.

gangrene: the death of body tissue in a particular area, caused by severe impairment of circulation over a period of time; without a supply of oxygen and a means of waste disposal, tissues cannot survive. Gangrenous tissue will appear swollen and blistery, greenish or black in color.

There is danger of gangrene in any situation that cuts off blood flow to an area, including frostbite, a crushing injury, a severe burn, disease that damages the blood vessels, a strangulated hernia, and continued mechanical pressure such as a too-tight tourniquet.

Gantanol, Gantrisin: trade names for, respectively, sulfamethoxazole and sulfisoxazole; see SULFA DRUGS.

Garamycin: a trade name for gentamicin; see ANTIBIOTICS.

gasping for breath: There could be various causes, including croup, asthma, and the swallowing of a foreign object. If it is the last, turn to CHOKING for first-aid procedures. If you know that there has been gas or smoke inhaled, see the next entry. If the cause is unknown, call the doctor immediately — unless the child is losing consciousness or turning blue, in which case rush him to the nearest hospital emergency room.

gas poisoning: In any instance of gas poisoning — including smoke inhalation in a fire — the first and most important step is to get the child into fresh air: shut off the gas source if possible, open windows, take the child outdoors. If someone else is present, have that person call the police or fire department while you aid the child's breathing (see RESPIRATORY RESUSCITATION). If there is no one else, continue resuscitation until the child can breathe alone; keep him lying down, and warm, while you make the call.

Carbon monoxide poisoning is a particularly insidious condition. The gas itself is invisible and odorless, so that poisoning can begin before the victim is aware of it. Typical symptoms, in the approximate order in which they occur, are: yawning, headache, nausea, dizziness, and ringing in the ears, followed by gasping for breath and eventual unconsciousness. The mucous membranes — and the skin, if it is naturally light in tone — will be a bright cherry red.

Any gas poisoning, and carbon monoxide in particular, attacks the bloodstream by replacing the oxygen it normally carries, and can conceivably thus cause temporary, or even permanent, brain damage. Even if breathing has resumed and is apparently completely normal, the child should be rushed to a hospital; if sufficient carbon monoxide remains in the blood, transfusion may be necessary.

gastric ulcer: See PEPTIC ULCER.

gastritis: an inflammation of the stomach; the causes may include infection, food poisoning, poisoning resulting from swallowing a toxic substance, etc. Typical symptoms may consist of loss of appetite, nausea, vomiting, headache, upper abdominal pain, and fever. If you suspect gastritis, call the doctor promptly.

gastrocnemius: See MUSCLES.

gastroenteritis: a general term meaning inflammation of both the stomach and the intestines, whether due to infection, food poisoning, allergy, etc. It is usually characterized by cramps, possibly also nausea, vomiting, or diarrhea. If you suspect gastroenteritis, the doctor should be called.

gastroenterologist: See SPECIALTIES, MEDICAL.

Gaucher's disease: a fairly rare hereditary disorder (the inheritance is straight recessive; see HEREDITY) involving deficiency of an enzyme called glucocerebrosidase. Like Fabry's and Tay-Sachs diseases, Gaucher's is classed as a lipid-metabolism disorder; the enzyme deficiency results in accumulation of fatty deposits —

here, mainly in the liver, spleen and bones, although a few cases have involved the nervous system. Symptoms, depending upon the sites affected as well as the degree of deficiency, may include anemia, bone fracture, muscle pain, lack of coordination, and — in those few instances in which the central nervous system is involved — mental retardation.

In late 1974, scientists at the National Institute of Neurological and Communicative Disorders and Stroke, who have been concentrating on this entire spectrum of disorders and who had previously developed the treatment for Fabry's disease, announced successful treatment of two Gaucher's patients — one a teenage boy, the other an older woman — with injection of the missing enzyme. The material for injection, like that used in Fabry's, is thus far obtained only from human placentas, but from early indications may be needed far less frequently, perhaps only every few months.

Gaucher's disease is one of the increasing number of disorders that can be pinpointed prenatally, and "carrier" parents can also be identified; see AMNIOCENTESIS and GENETIC COUNSELING for further comment.

general practitioner: a qualified Doctor of Medicine not specializing in some particular part of the body, kind of service, or category of patients.

For the titles of those who *do* specialize, see SPECIALTIES, MEDICAL.

generic drugs: drugs sold under their descriptive or chemical names rather than by brand name. Many such drugs, both prescription and nonprescription, are available and often cost far less than the same medication sold under a trade name, since the latter is usually advertised, either to the public or to the medical profession. You'll find some advice on this subject in various parts of this book, especially as relating to nonprescription medications.

As far as prescribed drugs are concerned, the question should be discussed with your doctor, who may agree in some cases to prescribe a drug by its generic name as a help to your budget — especially useful if the medication is to be taken over a long period. In others, the physician may feel — possibly based on personal experience or special knowledge about certain manufacturers — that a brand-name prescription is necessary or desirable in order to assure purity or effectiveness of the particular drug (or acceptable taste, in the case of medications for children).

genes: See HEREDITY.

genetic counseling: advice given by a qualified physician — either your own personal physician, or a specialist in genetics — regarding the possibility of having a subsequent child with the same congenital condition found in an earlier child. Parents still have to make the ultimate decision whether or not to have another child, but this advice may help them to arrive at their decision. In a number of such conditions, it is now possible to check the developing fetus (see AMNIOCENTESIS), and in some that are hereditary, "carrier" states can be identified in the parents, so that the odds of producing an afflicted child can be reliably estimated. (Once the genetic pattern of inheritance has been determined and parental pedigree established, the risks and probabilities can be calculated with accuracy. For details, see HEREDITY.)

genitalia, genitals: the external reproductive organs; see SEX ORGANS.

gentamicin: See ANTIBIOTICS.

Geocillin, Geopen: trade names for carbenicillin, a semisynthetic penicillin; see ANTIBIOTICS.

germ: formerly, a word denoting a disease-causing organism. More specific terms — bacterium, virus, etc. — are now used and "germ" is correctly reserved, medically, to denote the basic components from which the embryo develops, i.e., the egg cell and the sperm cell.

German measles: See RUBELLA.

giantism: a condition of overgrowth characterized by enlargement of the pituitary gland and directly caused by an oversupply of a particular pituitary hormone; if it occurs after normal growth has ceased, it is known medically as acromegaly. For an explanation of the function and malfunction of the substance, see GROWTH HORMONE.

giardiasis: See PARASITES.

gingivitis: See GUM DISORDERS.

GI series: a series of X rays following the progress of an ingested opaque substance — generally barium sulfate — over a period of time in order to diagnose a possible problem in the upper gastrointestinal tract.

The procedure isn't painful or unpleasant. Barium sulfate is a tasteless white powder; it's usually flavored with vanilla, chocolate, or mint (sometimes a choice is offered). There may be slight temporary constipation or (rarely) diarrhea afterward, and your doctor will advise you on what, if anything, to do about it.

gland: any organ that secretes an identifiable substance or substances.

glands, endocrine (ductless): See ENDOCRINE GLANDS.

"glands," lymph: See LYMPH NODES.

"glandular fever": See MONONUCLEOSIS.

glans: the head of the penis.

glaucoma: a condition involving fluid accumulation within the eyeball which can, with increasing pressure, damage the retina and optic nerve. It may be congenital (but there are rarely hereditary factors) or can appear later in life, and there may or may not be any apparent symptoms such as blurred vision or loss of peripheral (corner-of-the-eye) vision. An ophthalmologist can, however, spot the condition early, and looks for it as part of the standard examination — which is another reason for your family to have regular eye checkups. Glaucoma cannot be corrected by eyeglasses, but can be treated with drugs and/or by surgery, and blindness (which may follow if the condition goes untreated) can be prevented.

glomerulonephritis: See NEPHRITIS.

glucose tolerance test: a test to determine the body's ability to cope with ingested sugar; it may or may not be related to a suspicion of possible diabetes mellitus. The usual method is to give the patient a measured amount of sugar — as via heavily sugared tea or a supersweet soft drink devised for such testing — and then to take both blood samples and urine specimens at specified intervals. For a full discussion of glucose and other sugars, plus synthetic substitutes, see SWEETENERS.

glue-sniffing: Parents of children who develop a sudden interest in model-airplane building, and who seem to "lose" the glue or for some reason never complete the models, should be alert to this extremely dangerous kind of "kick" that developed among youngsters in recent years.

The children usually place the glue in a paper or plastic bag and sniff the fumes, which contain a variety of intoxicants. Asthmatic symptoms, red nostrils, swollen lips, bloodshot eyes, and staggering are among immediate manifestations of glue intoxication; it may also produce hallucinations. Much more critical are the longer range results, which may include permanent brain, lung, and liver damage, anemia, and death. If you suspect a youngster has been fooling with glue, get him to the doctor promptly.

For other thrill-seeking activities to which parents must unfortunately be alert, see DRUG ABUSE.

glutethimide: See SEDATIVES.

gluteus: See MUSCLES.

goiter: an enlargement of the thyroid; see ENDOCRINE GLANDS.

gonads: See ENDOCRINE GLANDS; SEX ORGANS.

gonorrhea: See VENEREAL DISEASES.

graft: the transplanting of tissue from one site or person to another; the word usually refers specifically to the transplanting of bone or skin, frequently within or on the same individual.

Also see TRANSPLANTS.

grain: an apothecary measure, abbreviated *gr;* a grain is equal to 65 milligrams *(mg).*

gramicidin: See ANTIBIOTICS.

Gram-negative, Gram-positive: These are terms you may hear in descriptions of infections or the organisms that cause them. "Gram" refers not to a metric unit but to Hans C. J. Gram, a Danish bacteriologist who devised a technique — called Gram's stain — for differential identification and structural analysis of two groups of bacteria, bacilli and cocci. Establishing the category of an organism as Gram-negative or -positive is also helpful in treatment, since some antibiotics are active against only one type or the other.

Gram-positive bacilli, few in number, include *Cornybacterium diphtheriae* and *Clostridium tetani;* cocci in this class include strep, staph, and the pneumococcus *Diplococcus pneumoniae.* Penicillin G is the antibiotic of choice in the treatment of all Gram-positive infections, as well as those caused by Gram-negative cocci; the major organisms in the latter group are the gonococcus (*Neisseria gonorrhoeae)* and the meningococcus *(N. meningitidis).* Most other bacilli — including the various *Salmonella* and the organisms that cause brucellosis, tularemia, cholera, whooping cough, and bacillary dysentery — are Gram-negative, and most do not respond to penicillin (although a number of them can be successfully treated with ampicillin and the other semisynthetic penicillins, as well as with other antibiotics).

grand mal: See EPILEPSY.

G-Recillin: a trade name for penicillin G; see ANTIBIOTICS.

green-stick fracture: See FRACTURES.

Grifulvin: a trade name for griseofulvin; see ANTIBIOTICS.

"grippe": See INFLUENZA.

Grisactin, griseofulvin: See ANTIBIOT-

ICS; the former is a trade name for the latter.

"growing pains": an old-wives'-tale phrase dismissing pains in a child's limbs or joints as "normal." They are not. They may be symptomatic of a variety of otherwise inapparent ills or injuries, and the child should be seen by a physician.

Muscle or joint pains in a physically active youngster may occur at night when he is resting; these are due to muscle fatigue and can be relieved by heat, massage, and/or aspirin. They are generally not serious — but let your doctor make the diagnosis.

growth hormone: one of several critical hormones produced by the pituitary (see ENDOCRINE GLANDS); its secretion in correct amounts controls continuing growth and development of normal stature (which, of course, may vary from short to tall, depending upon the individual's genetic inheritance).

In growing children, cartilage separates the epiphysis, or growing end, of the long bones from the main shaft of the bone. The shaft lays down hard material, growing toward the ends; the cartilage grows too, pushing the end away — thus, the bone grows longer. In the mid or late teens, the bone "catches up" and replaces the cartilage, ossification is complete, and growth stops. It is growth hormone that keeps the cartilage going; pituitary malfunction producing an incorrect amount of the hormone (the cause is unknown; it is not hereditary) will thus interfere with the normal growing process.

An *under*supply will mean too-rapid ossification and cessation of growth before normal stature is reached. It can be remedied by administration of the hormone, which is unfortunately very scarce and therefore very expensive. Hormone derived from animals simply doesn't work. It's necessary to use human hormone, extracted after death, and there is a central agency, located in Baltimore, Maryland, that coordinates this activity.

(In 1971, medical headlines were made by the announcement that human growth hormone, after long years of study, had finally been broken down in the laboratory; it will be several years, however, before supplies of a synthesized hormone are widely available. Late in 1973, further findings on the action of the pituitary hormone were revealed: it has been found that it acts not directly but — like a number of pituitary hormones — indirectly, in this case by stimulating secretion by the liver of another hormone called somatomedin. This second hormone thus offers another potential for therapy. It is extracted from blood plasma, but only a minuscule amount can be obtained from huge quantities of plasma, so the natural substance is not considered remotely feasible for therapeutic use. Investigators are presently attempting to analyze somatomedin's chemical structure, with the hope that it, too, may eventually be synthesized.)

An *over*supply of the hormone will let the cartilage progress too fast, not permitting the bone shaft to catch up when it should, so that giantism, or growth beyond the norm, occurs. Sometimes oversupply occurs after ossification has been completed and normal stature has been reached, a condition medically termed acromegaly; the result is then new growth at the ends of the limbs and at the end of the lower jaw. It can sometimes, though not always, be successfully treated.

growth rates: The rates at which your children gain height and weight will depend upon (assuming no malfunction or illness affecting either) two factors: heredity (tendencies and final statures inherited from their parents) and environment (circumstances — chiefly diet, and whether it's balanced to provide all the essential nutrients — which can modify inherited tendencies and traits). Overfeeding, incidentally, will make a child overweight; it will not make him grow faster or taller.

Bear in mind that the figures we present here are simply *averages* — statistical results of observations of a great many children — and don't include the upper and lower limits of the normal and healthy range; nor do they represent goals or guidelines for *your* child, which can be defined only by your own doctor.

HEIGHT

At birth, the average baby measures 18 to 21 inches (45 to 53 centimeters) from head to heel; the legs account for about one-third of the body length, a proportion that will change to about one-half by adulthood.

During the first two years, growth is usually quite rapid. Height increases by about 50 percent — that is, by about nine to twelve inches (23 to 30 cm) — during the first year, so that by one year, a baby measures about 27 to 33 inches (68 to 84 cm). Growth is generally about four inches (10 cm) during the second year, so that height at age two averages 31 to 37 inches (79 to 94 cm). There are theories that multiplying the two-year figure by two, or by two and a fraction, will give an approximation of the future adult height, but whether this really works is highly questionable; the child's own bone structure and heredity are probably better guidelines.

From the age of two onward, the rate of height increase becomes a very individual matter. In general, growth is fairly fast — though less so than during the first two years — up to the age of six, somewhat slower during the preteen years, then slightly speedier during adolescence; there is usually a final spurt between the ages of ten and fifteen in girls, between thirteen and eighteen in boys. On the average, girls reach their full adult height at fourteen or fifteen, boys at sixteen to eighteen.

WEIGHT

The average newborn baby weighs about seven pounds (3.2 kilograms) — a little weight is lost during the first week, regained during the second — a figure that usually doubles during the first four or five months and increases again by 50 percent during the next six months or so. Thus, a baby who weighs seven pounds at birth will weigh about 21 pounds (9.5 kg) by the first birthday, a gain of about 200 percent for the full year. During the second year, weight gain is usually about half a pound (0.2 kg) a month, so that a baby whose birth weight was average will generally weigh 26 to 28 pounds (12 or 13 kg) by two years of age.

There are no figures after that; the situation is so individual and so variable that statistical averages would be meaningless. Both the child's height (and rate of height increase) and bone structure are factors; your own physician will advise you, at the time of the youngster's regular checkups, if the child's weight is more or less than it should be and, if so, what should be done about it.

For discussion of some other aspects of growing up, see ADOLESCENCE; DEVELOPMENT; FOOD, SOLID; PUBERTY; TEETHING; TOILET TRAINING; WEANING.

gtt.: See PRESCRIPTIONS.

gum disorders: The gums, like other body tissues, are subject to a variety of afflictions. *Gingivitis* is the term for any inflammation of the gums, whatever its cause or degree of severity. Gingivitis may appear as a primary ailment, can sometimes reflect nutritional problems, can be a secondary symptom of a systemic ailment, and may sometimes appear in reaction to drugs (e.g., see DILANTIN).

The most common form of acute gingivitis in young children is called *primary herpetic gingivo-stomatitis*. As its name implies, it is an infection caused by the Herpes simplex virus (see COLD SORES and CANKER SORES); it is highly contagious, and may involve other soft tissues in the mouth besides the gums. Often, there is fever and a great deal of pain. There is no specific treatment, and the child will usually be ill for about a week. Because of the acute discomfort, the child is typically reluctant to eat or drink — but it is important, in order to prevent dehydration, to encourage liquids and soft, bland foods that are least likely to irritate the inflamed tissues. Your physician may also prescribe aspirin or other medication to help relieve pain and reduce fever. Call the doctor if you suspect this condition.

Other types of acute gingivitis, not characterized by systemic symptoms such as fever, are often due to underlying factors within the mouth, such as poor hygiene (resulting in plaque and calculus formation) and overcrowding of teeth. Secondary infection by bacteria and viruses normally present in the mouth may aggravate such conditions, leading to swelling, redness, pain, and possibly bleeding from the gums. Your dentist should be consulted regarding causes and therapy.

There are additional terms you may hear, and they are not always used consistently, even by physicians and dentists. *Vincent's disease* (or *Vincent's angina*) and *trench mouth* are used more or less interchangeably to denote what is technically *acute necrotizing ulcerative gingivitis*. Signs and symptoms may include pain, bleeding, ulceration, and marked swelling of the gums; if the disease has spread to other soft tissues of the mouth, which is relatively uncommon, there may also be fever and general malaise. This type of gingivitis often stems from generally low resistance combined with a precipitating stress factor (which may be physical or emotional), and is much less common in young children than among teenagers and college students. Treatment may include systemic antibiotics (the organisms involved are typically bacteria) and other medications, as well as local therapy by the dentist. At the same time, efforts should be made to improve general nutrition, assure adequate rest, and alleviate stress.

Once a youngster has had any kind of gingivitis, there seems to be increased susceptibility. It becomes particularly important to keep up the child's resistance to infection and to see that there are regular dental visits so that future problems can be avoided; follow your dentist's recommendation on the frequency of checkups.

Also see, for some other conditions affecting the gums and other soft tissues of the mouth, DEFICIENCY DISEASES; STOMATITIS; TEETHING; THRUSH.

gunshot wounds: See BULLET WOUNDS.

gynecologist: See SPECIALTIES, MEDICAL.

Gynergen: a trade name for ergotamine; see MIGRAINE.

H

hair, falling: Don't be alarmed if your newborn baby seems to be losing his hair; it's perfectly normal. The hair is gradually lost over the first three months and is replaced — possibly by hair of a different color.

If there seems to be undue hair loss in an older youngster, see BALDNESS.

hair growth, shade, and texture: As mentioned above, your child's hair color at birth is not necessarily what it will be later — nor, for that matter, is eye color; while the color of the eyes will be "set" at about six months, the shade and texture of the hair will not be established until the age of two years, or even later — and even after that, it will often tend to darken with age, especially if it is blond.

The color and texture of a child's hair depend entirely upon heredity. In general (there are isolated exceptions), the hair will eventually be no darker than that of the darker-haired parent, and no curlier than that of the curlier-haired parent — and may very well be considerably lighter or straighter, since those are genetically recessive traits (see HEREDITY) that can be carried, though not manifest in the parents. Red hair color is a special trait that will "show" as red only if it is combined with hereditary hair lightness; otherwise, it will simply bestow a warm tone on darker hair.

Parents anxious for their children to acquire long, luxurious locks should know that hair grows, on the average, a little less than half an inch a month — and nothing you can do (assuming there is no nutritional deficiency to be corrected) can change your child's individual rate. Similarly, the straightness or curliness of hair is, as we've said, a matter of heredity, and that can't be changed either; permanents — whether for waving or straightening — contain powerful and potentially injurious chemicals, and aren't recommended for use on the tender scalps of preadolescents.

Haley's M-O: See CATHARTIC.

hamstrings: See TENDONS.

hand, broken: See FRACTURES.

hands, use of: See DEVELOPMENT.

hanging, emergency procedure for: Don't panic if a cowboys- and-Indians game has somehow gotten out of hand; be calm, and move fast. Cut the child down, being careful to support the body while you untie or sever the rope or other material by which he's suspended. Lay him gently on the ground or floor, and loosen his collar. Give immediate respiratory assistance (see RESPIRATORY RESUSCITATION), while someone else calls for an ambulance; continue the resuscitation until the ambulance arrives or the child is breathing normally, whichever happens first.

hangnails: They should be carefully cut, as close as possible, with cuticle clippers. Don't let a child pick at hangnails, which can cause infection (see PARONYCHIA); if there is continued picking at the area, cover the site with a small adhesive-strip bandage. If you suspect there's already an infection, don't put any medication on it; take the child to the doctor.

Hansen's disease: a tropical infection caused by a bacillus similar to, and related to, the one that causes tuberculosis; it is named after the physician who discovered the infectious agent in the 1870s. It is also known as leprosy. There has been much confusion and misunderstanding about Hansen's disease. Although the odds against your encountering it, unless you live in certain areas, are great, we here present some air-clearing facts.

The Biblical "leper" was most likely not a victim of the disease known as leprosy today; the term used then probably referred to an indistinct grouping of virulent and highly contagious afflictions. Hansen's disease *is* contagious, but only through long and intimate contact with someone who has it (that is, in fact, the only way to contract it, although the method of communication is unknown); even under those conditions, only about three to five percent of all people are even susceptible, and these seem to be concentrated in areas in which leprosy is endemic — giving rise to the suspicion that the susceptibility may be inherited. Hansen's is thus probably the least contagious of all communicable diseases.

Where is it found, and how many people are afflicted with it? The first question is easier to answer than the second. It has been reported in all but seven states of the United States and in all races except the American Indian, and isolated cases have been found almost everywhere; most victims, however, are natives of parts of Asia (there are at least seventy thousand cases in Vietnam), Africa, and South America. In the United States the highest incidence is in the states of California, Florida, Hawaii, Louisiana, and Texas.

The number of persons who have Hansen's disease is difficult to say, since it is estimated that only 20 to 25 percent of its victims are being treated (yes, there is treatment, of which more in a moment). It is difficult to diagnose and easily confused with other ailments; most physicians in areas where it is rare have never seen it and are simply mystified by the symptoms. Many of its victims, because of fear of the misguided social prejudice prevalent in the past, have not sought treatment for themselves — or even for their children. Some twelve million cases are known throughout the world; the total may be closer to twenty million. There are over two thousand known cases in the United States; expert estimates place the true figure at anywhere from four thousand to ten thousand.

Hansen's disease is a systemic illness that chiefly affects skin and mucous membranes and their peripheral nerves. The first symptoms, after an incubation period that may be up to two or more years (it cannot be diagnosed before symptoms appear), are usually a loss of sensation and a change in skin color, often in the extremities such as hands or feet; eventually, other nerves are also attacked, and there can be muscular atrophy.

It cannot be *cured,* but Hansen's disease *can* be *controlled* and rendered inactive with sulfones, a type of sulfa drug; at least several months of treatment are generally needed. After it has been arrested, the disease is no longer contagious and the patient need not be hospitalized; the patient does return for periodic checkups to make sure the disease stays under control.

Early diagnosis and treatment can also avoid the deformities so long associated with leprosy — deformities not usually resulting from the disease itself, but from the anesthetic effect of nerve destruction; if the ailment persists untreated, loss of the sense of pain can cause the victim to injure himself inadvertently and to ignore minor wounds that can become seriously infected — and it is thus that loss of fingers and toes has occurred.

There is continuing research, directed toward both a cure and effective prevention. Among those few who are susceptible to the disease, resistance seems to increase with age; both BCG vaccine and the administration of sulfones at an early age offer some protection to children, and these methods are now used, in areas where Hansen's disease is endemic, for children believed to be at risk and who have close relatives with the disease.

harelip: a congenital malformation involving incomplete joining near the center of the upper lip; it may or may not be associated with a similar malformation of the roof of the mouth (see CLEFT PALATE).

Harelip can be successfully corrected by plastic surgery, which is usually performed shortly after birth unless there is some special medical reason to defer the operation until later.

Haverhill fever: See RAT-BITE FEVER.

hay fever: a condition caused by allergy to pollen — not usually to hay, and normally not involving fever. Hay fever is seasonal, coinciding with the appearance of the particular pollen to which the individual is allergic; among the culprits are ragweed, timothy, roses and other flowering plants (it then occurs in spring and is often called "rose fever"), many grasses, and several varieties of trees.

Hay fever most often first appears between the ages of four and eight, but it has been known to make its initial appearance at ages ranging from two to seventy. Typical symptoms include a runny nose, itching of the mucous membranes of the nose accompanied by frequent sneezing, and watery eyes (the mucous membranes there are often affected too).

If your youngster has — or you suspect he has — hay fever, don't treat it with over-the-counter remedies. Discuss the problem with your doctor or with a recommended allergist. Prescribed antihistamines taken throughout the season may help a good deal. In some cases, perennial desensitization treatments are successful in minimizing the allergic reaction.

It's helpful, too, to have an air conditioner or air-purifying device in the room where the child sleeps. Coat the filter with a light film of oil to help it trap pollen particles more effectively; wash and recoat it frequently.

For a discussion of the problem as a whole, see ALLERGY.

headache: Like fever, headache can be a symptom of a large and varied assortment of ills including eyestrain, respiratory infections both mild and serious, tension, tumors, allergy, and many more. If you know the cause (if, for instance, the child has a cold, or a chronic sinus problem), and the child is over ten, a little aspirin (plain aspirin, not one of the extra-strength or multiple-ingredients products) is fine — but the child should see a doctor if the headache is very severe or persists more than a few hours. A child under ten should not be given anything; just call the doctor.

Whatever the child's age, don't give aspirin or anything else, and see the doctor without delay if the headache is accompanied by pain in the eyes or ears, follows a head injury, seems to be localized on one side of the head, is connected with dizziness or loss of consciousness, is accompanied by fever, follows a convulsion, is sudden and very severe, or is mild but recurrent.

For discussion of a special sort of headache, see MIGRAINE.

head-banging: This peculiar activity sometimes appears toward the end of an infant's first year; it's by no means uncommon, usually occurs in the crib, and isn't a cause for alarm. It's true that the child may keep it up long enough and hard enough to cause a few bruises, or even to rub a bit of hair off, but serious injury is practically unknown; the child seems to instinctively stop short of that point. (To be on the safe side, however, put some padding or quilting around the sides and ends of the crib.)

No one knows what causes an infant to carry on in this manner. It's *not* any kind of mental illness, nor is it usually connected with any physical ailment. Speculation includes the theory that the child just likes it because it's rhythmic, or that it serves as some kind of tension reliever (you might try a warm bath and some extra cuddling before bedtime, with the aim of relaxing the child).

Do, nevertheless, discuss the problem, if it arises, with your doctor.

head injuries: Probably every single child, at one time or another, falls on his head; the younger the child, the softer the skull, and the less the possibility of fracture or other serious injury. Toddlers who are just learning to walk tumble to the floor repeatedly; they don't, after all, have far to fall, and they instinctively relax as they go, usually picking themselves up in a few seconds.

You should, nevertheless, consider any blow to the head a potentially serious matter, especially if the child fell from a height (as, a ladder or tree) or has been hit on the head by something fallen from a height or thrown from a distance. Serious damage may include concussion (a "jarring" of the brain, with temporary functional disturbance), skull fracture, injuries to major blood vessels, and combinations of these. It is difficult, if not impossible, for a nonphysician to sort out specific symptoms. The advice that follows takes all possibilities into account.

FIRST-AID PROCEDURE

What to do depends upon the victim's condition.

If the child is unconscious, check first to see if he is breathing. If breathing is absent or very weak, turn to RESPIRATORY RESUSCITATION and follow the instructions there; have someone else, if available, summon medical aid.

When — or if — the child is breathing normally, check quickly for the following key signs: evidence of shock (see TRAUMATIC SHOCK); external evidence of definite injury (a cut, swelling, depression, bleeding from mouth, nose, or ears); other immediately observable signs of brain injury, particularly unequal pupils (pull up the child's eyelids and look) or deep coma (clue: firm rubbing of the child's breastbone will fail to elicit any response). Then call for an ambulance, reporting what you have observed.

Don't do anything else, except to gently apply clean cloths if there is extensive bleeding, and to cover the child if the accident took place outdoors and the weather is chilly. Don't attempt to give him *anything whatever* by mouth. Don't move him, unless there is an immediate threat to life, such as an advancing fire; if the child must be moved, follow the special procedure shown under BACK AND NECK INJURIES.

If the child has lost consciousness but awakens spontaneously, he must nevertheless be taken to the hospital immediately for examination and X rays, whether or not there is evidence of injury or any other unusual symptom. Don't give the child *anything* by mouth prior to the hospital visit.

If the child has not lost consciousness, check for signs of injury. Small cuts and bruises (the latter may sometimes produce large lumps) are common and are usually not cause for concern; it will be helpful to apply ice to a bruise. If, however, you find a dent or depression, a prompt trip to the hospital is in order. Even if you find no injury, you should be alert for delayed symptoms, as detailed next.

FOLLOW-UP

Although the incident may have seemed minor at the time, you should be alert for any delayed symptoms that suggest more serious injury.

Some clues that immediate medical attention is necessary may appear within hours and generally involve weakened vital functions and/or a change in appearance. Rush the child to the hospital if any of these occur shortly after the incident: a weakened pulse, or any change in pulse rate; difficulty or change in breathing; convulsion or loss of consciousness; a "sick look." It must be added that a small child who has had a bump on the head may naturally and normally want to nap; such sleepiness, which might be considered unusual in relation to the youngster's customary habits, need be considered an alarm signal only if the child can't be roused (try every fifteen minutes).

Other signs of serious injury may not appear until 24 hours, several days, or even weeks later. (An injury to an artery in the membrane surrounding the brain, for example, may result in gradual development of a clot.) When a child has had a recent head injury, consult the doctor without delay if any of the following occur:

- bleeding — or any other unusual fluid — from mouth, nose, or ears;
- repeated vomiting (within a day or two);
- any disturbance of vision or change in appearance of the eyes;
- headache (its severity may not necessarily be related to the seriousness of the injury);
- convulsions or "blanking-out" episodes or complaints of dizziness (may be quite a few weeks after the injury);
- restlessness, bizarre behavior, changes in personality or in mental abilities;
- speech difficulties;
- muscular weakness, numbness, or paralysis in any part of the body.

Heaf test: one of several skin tests for tuberculosis. A positive result indicates to the doctor that the child either has TB, *or* has had the infection at some time in the past, and that further testing or treatment is called for. (If a child has received BCG vaccine, however, Heaf tests will often be positive for several years thereafter; this is perfectly normal, and not a sign of trouble.)

"health foods": Advocates of these foods generally promote them as being superior on the basis that they are "organically grown," or have not been commercially processed, or have not had substances added to them.

Organic growing (i.e., without the use of synthetic fertilizers) may influence the yield per acre; it has no bearing on quality. Special processing, such as pasteurization, may indeed remove some nutrients (pasteurized milk, for example, has no vitamin C, but it also no longer contains disease-causing bacteria); those same nutrients, however, are readily obtainable from other foods (see NUTRITION).

Sometimes foods sold in establishments that specialize in these products have been simply dishonestly promoted or deceptively labeled. Some grown with chemical fertilizers have been sold as "organic." Expensive "raw" sugar has been purchased by people somehow under the impression that ordinary sugar is harmful; in fact, raw sugar is sold nowhere in the United States. What is so described is partially refined, and the only difference is that its mineral content is a tiny bit higher than that of white sugar (as is brown sugar's). Speaking of sugar, it constitutes 20 percent of one of the widely promoted "natural" cereals — less than the 35 to 50 percent found in the glazed cereals touted on TV, true, but far more than the average person would spoon on a bowl of unsugared cereal.

Other items in "health food" stores tend to be out-of-the-way or unfamiliar foods offering, it is implied, mysterious benefits hitherto unavailable — often based on the usually unproved, frequently fanciful theories of writers of popular "diet books." Many of these sprouts, seeds, grains, etc., are in fact organically grown in small quantities — which makes them a lot more expensive; they are in no way superior nutritionally to foods at your supermarket, and they are certainly not the remedies for disease that some of their less scrupulous advocates have suggested.

Additives may be another matter. Although the Food and Drug Administration must approve all preservatives, colorings, and so on, and most of them are perfectly safe (*none* interfere with, or cancel, any inherent nutritional values in the food), some legitimate questions have recently been raised about a few. You'll find some of these disputed additives discussed separately under SWEETENERS. Also very questionable are the nitrites used in frankfurters, salami, sausage, and other cured meats both as a colorant and to discourage certain harmful bacterial growth. (These types of meats are not particularly nutritious anyway, and they contain substantially less protein, ounce for ounce, than beef, poultry, and other fresh meats; if you'd like to avoid possibly harmful additives, it will not hurt your children to go without hot dogs.)

Your best course as a parent is probably to be as well informed as possible, and to read labels, in order to see that your youngsters receive the most in food value, and the least potential harm, for your food dollar. (See some pertinent pointers in Appendix C.) In our view, it is perfectly possible to accomplish that at your supermarket or corner grocery, without contributing to the rapidly growing coffers of the "health food" industry.

See also, for some related comment, VEGETARIANISM.

health insurance: We recommend that your family, whatever your means, have such insurance; the most serious accidents and illnesses are precisely those that tend to strike most unexpectedly — and can, as hospital care becomes more and more expensive, deal an irreversible blow to your family's finances.

There are various types of health insurance, often offering a choice of plans that generally include total or partial costs of hospitalization, and sometimes surgery, doctors' bills, medications, and so on. Group plans, such as those offered through an employer, are usually the most economical. But if you are self-employed, or neither your nor your spouse's employer offers such a plan, it's wise to check into several plans to find the one that will best suit your family's needs; talk to the person or company who handles other insurance for you, as well as to your friends, and compare both costs and benefits to be sure what each kind of plan entails and covers.

It's especially vital to have adequate major medical coverage, the type that pays a good part of the bills for serious accidents, prolonged illnesses, and unexpected major operations that often prove devastating. This insurance commonly includes a deductible amount — a sum you must pay in full — beyond which the policy typically covers a fixed percentage of costs, perhaps 75 or 80 percent. Usually, the lower the deductible, the higher the cost of the insurance. If it seems financially feasible, it is often wisest to set cash aside for relatively minor medical expenses and to buy high-deductible "catastrophe" insurance at a low premium.

Do, before you buy, read the policy carefully (a sample should be available). Ask questions about anything you don't understand (answers should be forthcoming and should make sense). Renewability is important: will the policy last for life, or will it be cut off at a certain point? At what age, or under what circumstances, will your children cease to be covered? Are benefits stated in terms of fixed "schedules" that may fall far behind reality should there be substantial increases in hospital-room costs or special medical fees?

And do be sure to tell your doctor exactly what services are covered, so necessary paperwork can be properly done.

health professionals: There are a number of people you may encounter from time to time — possibly at your physician's office, more likely in a hospital or by referral from your physician — who may play an active part in your children's health care. We offer, here, a brief rundown of their responsibilities and qualifications. None of the people listed here is a medical doctor or a dentist (for a list of those, see SPECIALTIES, MEDICAL, and SPECIALTIES, DENTAL); all carry out their work under the direction of, or at the recommendation of, a physician or dentist.

Audiologist — a specialist to whom your pediatrician or family physician, or an otologist, may refer your child if there are special hearing problems; such a person may be on a hospital staff or in private practice. An audiologist has a master's degree and may have a doctorate as well (a Ph.D. rather than an M.D.), and is qualified to measure and analyze your child's hearing and its limitations, and to work with the child in a program of corrective hearing and speech therapy.

Nurse's aide — someone your child may encounter in a hospital, not a nurse but a person who has been trained — usually at the hospital itself — to assist the nurses, specifically in nonmedical tasks. A nurse's aide is not qualified to administer medications or otherwise treat a patient, but may bring meals, freshen beds, assist the child in going to and from the bathroom, and otherwise help in making the patient comfortable.

Nurse-midwife — a registered nurse who is a college graduate and has, in addition, received about a year's special training in obstetrics. A nurse-midwife works under the aegis of a hospital obstetrics department, and is qualified to assume full charge of — and to advise a woman throughout — normal, uneventful pregnancy and childbirth; should any complications or difficulties arise, a physician must be called in.

Oral hygienist — a dental assistant who acts as the dentist's aide and also is qualified to do surface cleaning and polishing of the teeth (but may not work beyond the gum line) and to advise patients on at-home dental care and hygiene.

Physical therapist (or *physiotherapist*) — an individual who works under a physician's immediate direction or supervision, and is specially trained in rehabilitative techniques to help a patient recover or attain normal function following illness, surgery, or injury, or in case of some physical deformity or malfunction; the techniques may include heat or electrical treatments, special exercises, and other measures. A physical therapist may or may not be a registered nurse as well.

Physician's assistant — a relatively new category of professional, whom you may increasingly encounter in the offices of family physicians, general practitioners, and pediatricians, particularly in smaller communities, rural areas, and some urban areas with a low physician-to-population ratio. A PA — as the title has become abbreviated — has at least a high-school diploma and may have a college degree as well; has usually previously qualified as a nurse, military medical aide, physical therapist, or the like; has taken certain college-level science courses; and has been certified after completion of a two-year PA curriculum that includes both academic and clinical training in the medical sciences. The PA may carry out either a narrow or wide range of duties and activities, as required and directed by the supervising physician. These typically include performing routine physical examinations, taking histories, carrying out diagnostic and therapeutic programs ordered by the doctor, treating minor wounds, and dealing with common minor systemic infections. A few PAs have chosen, even as have physicians and nurses, to specialize in certain types of patients or ills, but by and large, the role of the PA is envisioned as that of a "right hand" to overloaded primary-care physicians.

Practical nurse — an individual who has usually had about a year of special training in nursing, holds a certificate attesting to that fact, and is qualified to perform many — though not all — of the functions of a registered nurse, including general patient care (under the supervision of a physician), observation of a patient, and dispensing of medication. A practical nurse has narrower theoretical training and academic background than a registered nurse, and is not qualified to assume care of someone who is critically ill. (Many women have turned to practical nursing, after raising children, as a second occupation; such a woman may be especially well suited to assuming responsibility for a child who needs nursing care for a time but is not seriously ill.) A qualified practical nurse is identified by the letters *L.P.N.* (Licensed Practical Nurse) following the individual's name.

Registered nurse — a graduate of an accredited nursing school, who is entitled to place the letters *R.N.* after her or his name, who is at least a high-school graduate prior to nursing training and may be a college graduate as well. A registered nurse works — as does a practical nurse — under the direction of the patient's physician, but has deeper and broader medical knowledge, and is qualified to exercise greater judgment, as well as to care for a patient who is critically ill. Some nurses choose to specialize, because of special talents and interests, so that there are pediatrics nurses, surgical nurses, and so on, who have additional training and experience in the particular area.

Speech therapist — a professional with special training in speech problems, including — but not only — those of children with hearing impairments. A speech therapist is a college graduate, may also have advanced degrees, and may be a psychologist as well.

Student nurse — someone your child

may encounter in a hospital situation, who is studying to become a registered nurse and has already had at least one year of training before being permitted to deal with patients. A student nurse is qualified only to carry out instructions and works always under the supervision of a registered nurse.

Technician — an individual your child may encounter in a hospital, a laboratory where you may be sent for special tests, or possibly in the physician's office. Such an individual typically has a background of laboratory training; is primarily engaged in chemical analysis, the compilation and/or recording of data, and the like; and has contact with patients limited to association with these activities. A technician may draw blood for laboratory tests, measure and record blood pressure, take X rays, take an electrocardiogram, and so on.

Therapist — a term that, broadly, denotes anyone who is involved in treating any ailment, thus includes physicians, but is commonly used to mean someone who works under a physician's guidance in a directly helpful, but paramedical, way — i.e., audiologists, physiotherapists, psychotherapists, etc.

Also see, for others potentially involved in dealing with your child's physical and emotional problems, INTERN; OPTICIAN; OPTOMETRIST; PHARMACIST; PSYCHOLOGIST; RESIDENT.

hearing: Since this faculty is so integral a part of your child's learning process, and thus overall development, it's vital to have hearing tested as part of all regular physical examinations. The Children's Bureau of the U.S. Department of Health, Education, and Welfare has stated that at least six out of every thousand children under the age of sixteen have some degree of hearing impairment; this figure is a minimum one, since it is based only on reported cases. Even a small, easily correctable, impairment could have a lasting effect on your youngster's future.

A hearing loss need not, of course, be permanent; it can result from an infection (and could *become* permanent if the infection's left untreated), from wax in the ears, and other conditions. If you even suspect your child may have any loss of hearing, lose no time in consulting your doctor.

Also see DEAFNESS.

heart: a four-chambered muscle in the chest, more or less centered behind the breastbone but tilted slightly to the left, so that its beat is felt more strongly there; it acts as a pump to circulate blood throughout the body. The heart sends blood through the lungs to pick up fresh oxygen, then out again through the arteries (see BLOOD VESSELS) to all the body's cells and organs. It contracts rhythmically in so doing; this contraction (heartbeat) is detectable at various points on the body (see PULSE).

The flow of blood through and within the heart is very carefully regulated, and follows — except if something goes wrong — a specific pattern. There are two upper chambers, called *auricles,* which are not connected with each other; each, however, is connected through a one-way valve with a lower chamber called a *ventricle.* If all goes well, each contraction of the heart will send the blood on its way in precisely the right direction: from the left auricle to the left ventricle, thence out to the rest of the body; back to the right auricle and through the right ventricle to the lungs for a new supply of oxygen; then back to the left auricle.

Occasionally, though rarely, something does go wrong. See HEART DISEASE; PULMONARY STENOSIS; TETRALOGY OF FALLOT.

heart disease: a general term that can cover many different kinds of conditions, all of them relatively serious, but hardly any of them now fatal or even permanently damaging to children, thanks to modern surgical and therapeutic techniques.

Congenital heart disease means that the child was born with the condition, generally a malformation of some sort (see, for example, TETRALOGY OF FALLOT, perhaps the best known); such conditions may be caused by, among other things, maternal rubella during early pregnancy — which can now be prevented (see RUBELLA). In almost all cases, congenital heart malformations can, if deemed necessary, be corrected by surgery; the youngster is unlikely to become a professional athlete but can otherwise look forward to a normal life.

Later in life, heart disease can be caused by a variety of infections, nutritional problems, toxic reactions, and so on. Among the infectious problems, the one you are most likely to hear about is *rheumatic heart disease,* usually a complication of rheumatic fever following a strep infection, and now rare because the primary infection is generally effectively treated; if the heart complication does occur, it can still usually be treated with antibiotics or other drugs — and isn't likely to result in permanent damage to the heart, as it did a generation or two ago.

You may also hear a number of terms denoting specific inflammations: *carditis,* an inflammation of any part of the heart; *endocarditis,* an inflammation of the membranes lining the chambers of the heart; *myocarditis,* an inflammation of the heart muscle itself; *pericarditis,* an inflammation of the membrane around the outside of the heart. You're unlikely to hear much about *occlusion,* the closure of a coronary artery; it's extremely rare in children.

heart murmur: an abnormal heart sound heard through a stethoscope; it doesn't necessarily indicate disease or even a condition that should cause the least concern. About 75 percent of all youngsters have, at one time or other, what physicians call a *functional* or *innocent* murmur — an aberrant sound signifying absolutely nothing, generally vanishing with adolescence.

If such a sound is heard, though, the doctor will probably check further, just to make sure it doesn't signal a less common but more serious condition such as congenital heart disease or acute rheumatic fever. Another may be slight heart damage resulting from a past infection, and in such a case the doctor may prescribe protective medication to prevent future infections. In any event, the physician will probably order an electrocardiogram, and perhaps blood tests, in order to pinpoint the diagnosis.

Other problems may also cause a discernible abnormality in the heartbeat; see the previous entry, HEART DISEASE.

heat exhaustion: a condition also called heat prostration, usually not a critical matter and — assuming proper measures are taken — not likely to require medical attention. It is extremely important to differentiate between this condition and another that *is* quite serious; see HEAT STROKE. They can occur under similar conditions and need not include exposure to direct sunlight. Typically, heat exhaustion occurs with high humidity as well.

Symptoms generally include weakness, dizziness, and possibly headache; the child's vision may also be a bit blurry. Loss of consciousness is unlikely. The child's skin is characteristically cool, clammy (a "cold sweat"), and pale; there may or may not be nausea or a fluttery pulse. The child's temperature will be normal or just slightly elevated. (*Important:* If key symptoms — skin condition, sweating, and body temperature — do not dovetail with this description, turn immediately to HEAT STROKE.)

Get the child into the coolest available place, and do whatever you can to lower humidity and encourage evaporation of sweat: air conditioning, a fan, someone waving newspapers back and forth. The child should be lying down, and restrictive clothing should be loosened.

Part of the problem is that there has been extreme loss, through perspiration, of salt as well as fluids. Which means that *both* need to be replaced. If the child is nauseated, don't insist on getting anything into him — but keep offering, and do insist that something be taken as soon as nausea begins to subside.

Some things to offer, in order to achieve replacement of both salt and fluids: salt tablets, if you have them, combined with cool fluid such as juice or soda; or salty foods (pretzels, potato chips, salty crackers) along with a cool, salty fluid such as tomato juice; or — if none of the preceding are available — salt water (one teaspoonful of table salt plus one-half teaspoonful of baking soda combined in four cups — one quart, 32 ounces — of water), followed by other cool fluids. If the child's pulse seems very weak, include some strong iced coffee or tea.

Don't give the child anything else; *no* medication — aspirin, "stomach-settler," or anything else — is needed.

If there's no improvement within an hour, the child should be taken to the hospital. If the child is diabetic, don't even wait that long; fifteen minutes is an outside limit.

heat rash: a rash caused by clogging of sweat glands, also known as "prickly heat"; the heat refers to the temperature of the child's skin, not necessarily the atmosphere, and the rash can occur in winter as well as in summer, although the latter is more common. It can be prevented by dressing children lightly in hot weather (and not overdressing them in winter), and being sure that perspiration is carried off the skin — by breezes or air conditioning, by occasional sponging of the skin. And in hot weather, it is best to stick to pure cotton clothing and avoid synthetic blends.

The condition is typified by small red pinpoints and a generally flushed appearance of the area — which is often the back of the neck, the folds under the arms or in the groin, although it can occur anywhere on the body. An older child who can describe the symptoms will usually complain of an itching, burning, prickly sensation; a younger child will be uncomfortable but may or may not whine or otherwise protest audibly.

Relief can usually be achieved by getting the child into a breezy place, sponging the area with cool water, then dusting it with cornstarch. Don't let the youngster scratch the rash, since that can (though rarely) cause an infection; nails should be cut short if necessary. If the condition still persists, the child should be seen by a physician.

heat stroke: an extremely serious condition, popularly called "sunstroke" (although the victim need not have been in direct sunlight) and medically termed *accidental hyperpyrexia*; the second word means very high fever, which is one of the characteristic symptoms.

The child suffering from heat stroke has invariably been in a situation involving very high temperatures; frequently, there has been a great deal of physical exertion.

Symptoms are distinctive, and it is important to distinguish them from those of heat exhaustion, a far less critical condition. They appear, for one thing, far more quickly. (The child may suddenly keel over, unconscious.) The child's skin will be hot and dry, possibly flushed; the pulse will be weak and unusually rapid. There may be visual disturbances, twitching, and convulsion. Nausea may be present, but it's uncommon.

Some of the symptoms may also be characteristic of heat exhaustion, but the key points are three in number: (1) the skin is hot and dry, rather than cool and moist; (2) the child will not be sweating (sweating is a key symptom of heat exhaustion); (3) there will be definitely high fever — possibly 106° F. (41° C.) or higher — and the temperature elevation occurs quite rapidly.

Heat stroke is a threat to life; such high temperatures can be rapidly fatal: the higher the temperature, the lower the body's ability to maintain vital functions such as breathing.

Lose no time. Call for an ambulance, or — if you have transportation immediately available — take the child to the nearest hospital. If you are waiting for an ambulance or other transportation to arrive (or on the way to the hospital, if it is practical), take first-aid measures aimed at reducing body temperature. Remove the child's clothes. If the temperature — oral, axillary, or rectal — is 105° F. (40.5° C.) or higher, immerse the victim in cold water or apply ice packs. If it is not quite that high, sprinkle the child with cold water and get him near an air conditioner or fan to encourage evaporation. Give the child only *one* kind of medication, if it's available: rectal aspirin suppositories; don't give *anything* by mouth.

Even if the child has apparently recovered before you reach medical aid (or medical aid reaches you), hospitalization is nonetheless vital; professional examination and monitoring are necessary for a period of time.

height: See GROWTH RATES; HEREDITY.

hemangioma: See BIRTHMARKS.

hematocrit: one of the measurements usually obtained in a complete blood count; it is a determination of the proportion of cells to fluid volume after separation by centrifuge. If the values are not within normal ranges, the physician will generally undertake further analysis of cell type and content to determine the cause (causes may include anemia and a number of other conditions).

hematologist: See SPECIALTIES, MEDICAL.

hematoma: See BRUISES.

hematuria: the medical term for blood in the urine. It can be a symptom of a number of different conditions, including infections of the kidney, bladder, or other parts of the urinary tract; tumors; reactions to medications; and others. It's important, if hematuria is suspected in a girl, to make sure that the blood is indeed being excreted with the urine, and is not normal urine mixing with blood from the vulva or vagina.

A not uncommon hereditary condition can result in what *appears* to be blood in the urine; see URINATION.

hemodialysis: the removal of waste products from the blood by circulating it through a machine that filters them out, acting essentially as an "artificial kidney" when an individual's own kidneys are unable to perform that necessary function.

hemoglobin: the substance in red blood cells that carries oxygen from the lungs to the various parts of the body, and also transports carbon dioxide and other waste products of cell metabolism back to the lungs for exhalation.

See, for further discussion of the circulatory mechanism, ANEMIA; BLOOD CELLS; BLOOD VESSELS; HEART.

hemolytic: causing the destruction of red blood cells.

hemolytic anemia: See ANEMIA.

hemophilia: a hereditary inability of the blood to clot properly; the trait is recessive and sex-linked (see HEREDITY), and is passed on in the same way as color blindness (see the explanation under that entry), thus affecting chiefly males — although fortunately, it is even more rare than color blindness (in the United States there is less than one hemophiliac for every hundred color-blind persons).

Normally, blood clots and seals a small wound within five minutes or so. The blood of a hemophiliac will simply keep flowing; there is thus danger of severe blood loss from even the tiniest cut. The condition is generally discovered early — at the time of a boy's circumcision, or with the occurrence of a small scratch or scrape, or perhaps via a sudden and persistent nosebleed.

There *are* measures that can be taken to remedy the situation if a hemophiliac is wounded, including transfusions of normally clotting blood, and the administration of drugs that act as clotting agents; regular injections of clotting agents — whether at home or in a hospital — may also be used as a preventive measure. Nevertheless, if it has been established that a child has hemophilia, it's wise to avoid activities and circumstances that might lead to serious injury involving a break in the skin. And every physician and dentist called upon to treat the child must be forewarned.

As with any other potentially lethal condition, any youngster afflicted with hemophilia should be so identified in case of away-from-home emergencies; see MEDIC ALERT.

Hemophilus influenzae: a bacterium (it has no connection with the illness called influenza) that is responsible for perhaps three out of five cases of meningitis in the United States; it can also cause a number of other serious and unpleasant ills, including ear infections, infectious arthritis, and pneumonia. A vaccine has been developed which appears to be effective in preliminary trials but has not yet been approved for general use.

hemorrhage: a word literally meaning any discharge of blood from blood vessels but usually used more subjectively to connote a *great deal* of blood or a flow that's especially difficult to control.

For first-aid measures, see BLEEDING.

hemorrhoids: swollen veins in the rectum very close to the anus, also called piles; they are rare, though not unknown, in children. They are not dangerous or serious, although they may be painful and quite annoying.

Sometimes hemorrhoids are first noticed because there are traces of blood in the stool or on the toilet paper. Don't assume hemorrhoids, however; other things can cause bleeding from the anus, including anal fissure and problems within the intestines. In short, if you suspect your youngster may have hemorrhoids, *don't* use patent medicines or any kind of suppository; *do* consult the doctor. Even if that is the problem, the highly touted patent preparations are far less effective than medications the physician can prescribe.

heparin: an anticoagulant factor occurring naturally in the liver and other tissues, and that also may be administered when it is deemed advisable; its role is to prevent the formation of blood clots.

hepatitis: an inflammation of the liver, which occurs in at least two forms. It is caused by two or more distinct viruses, which differ in their means of transmission and in their incubation periods, although symptoms and duration of the illnesses are generally similar. Hepatitis now ranks second in prevalence to chickenpox among the reportable diseases in our country (not counting venereal diseases); some sixty thousand cases a year have been reported, and the actual figure may be far higher, perhaps five times as high.

"Infectious" hepatitis — more accurately termed Type A, since both are infectious — is contracted directly or indirectly from others (contaminated food and water and substandard sewage have often been implicated), and can be epidemic; it is known to be endemic in a number of parts of the world, prominently Africa, most of Asia, Central and South America, rural sections of Mexico, the Philippines, and the South Pacific. There is a two- to eight-week incubation period. The organism involved is believed to be an enterovirus (see VIRUSES).

"Serum" or Type B hepatitis virus was once believed always to enter directly into the bloodstream — as via nonsterile hypodermic needles or transfusions, probably by insect bite as well (there is strong circumstantial evidence for the latter in certain parts of Africa where epidemics have recurred seasonally and have been most common in areas with large mosquito populations); it has also been shown to be transmitted venereally and by human bite. The incubation period is six weeks to as long as six months. (There may also be a "Type C," causing a proportion of posttransfusion cases, having a slightly shorter incubation period than Type B.)

Both types of hepatitis are characterized by loss of appetite, fever, body aches, frequently nausea, vomiting and diarrhea, and arthritis (which may be the first symptom.) There may or may not be abdominal pain. Perhaps half of all cases involve jaundice, which may appear about two weeks after the initial symptoms. Treatment consists mainly of rest and carefully controlled diet; in some instances, certain drugs may also be used — but not antibiotics, which are ineffective. The illness generally runs its course in about six weeks (but Type A can be transmitted as long as the virus remains in the stool, which may be up to six months). It is believed that having Type A hepatitis bestows lasting immunity to that type, but that it is possible to contract Type B more than once.

There is no vaccine yet generally available against either type, although several formulations are under study. There is an immune serum globulin (gamma globulin) that protects against Type A, to which two-thirds to three-quarters of Americans are believed susceptible; it is recommended for travelers whose itineraries will take them to areas where the disease is endemic. It is rated at least 87 percent effective and protects for one to six months, depending upon the dose given. A gamma globulin against Type B has been tested, seems promising, and may soon be available for those at especially high risk.

Type A hepatitis, seafood devotees should be aware, can also be contracted from eating marine mollusks that may harbor the virus because offshore waters have become contaminated by sewage. A number of Cape Cod vacationers fell ill in 1971 after feasting on inadequately steamed clams, and there were several 1973 outbreaks in the Gulf states that resulted from eating raw infected oysters. The Center for Disease Control advises that steaming clams until the shells open — approximately one minute — is not sufficient; it takes four to six minutes for the clams themselves to reach a temperature high enough to destroy any hepatitis virus they may contain.

heptachlor: See PESTICIDES.

heredity: Hereditary characteristics and traits are those you, as parents, passed on to your offspring at the very moment of conception (see, for comparison, the definitions of CONGENITAL and FAMILIAL). And, unless there is a *mutation* after that — an accidental change in the genetic structure of your developing baby's cells — the traits that can be passed on to your grandchildren by that child have *also* been determined.

Each egg produced by the mother, and each sperm produced by the father, is in a manner of speaking half a cell; each contains precisely 23 chromosomes, each chromosome carrying anywhere from 10,000 to 45,000 genes — the "message units" of heredity that carry the information needed to create the new human being that is your child. The egg and sperm combine to form the fertilized cell, now containing 23 pairs of chromosomes, for a total of 46; this is the cell that carries your child's complete genetic pattern, a pattern ultimately repeated in all cells of the body.

Among the 23 pairs of chromosomes in the cell is a pair you've probably heard of: the *sex chromosomes.* Normal females have two X chromosomes; normal males have one X and one Y. The mother can contribute only an X chromosome to each egg cell; the father's sperm cells each carry *either* an X or a Y, and thus are the determining factor in the sex of the child. There are rare aberrant fertilized cells that apparently contain an extra X or Y. The significance of the phenomenon in XXX girls or XYY boys has not, at this writing, been fully explored (see SEX CHROMOSOMES); see KLINEFELTER'S SYNDROME and TURNER'S SYNDROME for two other wrong-number conditions. None of these variations is hereditary; all are accidental. The X chromosome is also the site of *sex-linked* genetic traits, of which more shortly. The 22 pairs of nonsex chromosomes are called *autosomes.*

What follows is a brief, general, and necessarily oversimplified explanation of the major hereditary mechanisms. It's a highly complex subject, about which entire volumes have been written, but we hope our discussion here will simply serve to clarify some of the references in other parts of this book.

DOMINANTS AND RECESSIVES

You'll find these words mentioned a number of times. Although there are exceptions, in general a dominant characteristic or trait is one that "shows" even if it is inherited from only one parent; it "dominates" other, or opposite, hereditary information. A recessive gene, on the other hand, won't be operative unless the characteristic is received from both parents — although an individual can still pass it on to his or her offspring. A number of traits are decided on such a dominant-recessive basis.

DOMINANT INHERITANCE

(one parent has dominant characteristic; both parents are of unmixed heredity)

Parents: DD rr

Possibilities: Dr Dr Dr Dr

Result: All children will display dominant characteristic, but will carry recessive gene, which may be passed on to their offspring.

Eye color is one example. Let's say that *B* represents dark eyes, and *b* light eyes; *B* is dominant. Each parent will have received one gene for this trait (there may actually be more than one, but let's assume one) from each of his or her parents — so that an individual may be characterized, genetically, as *BB* (dark eyed), *Bb* (also dark eyed, since the dominant inheritance will show), or *bb* (light eyed). A *BB* parent can transmit to children only the gene for dark eyes, a *bb* parent only a gene for light eyes; a *Bb* parent, however, might pass on either gene.

Thus if one parent's inheritance is wholly dark eyed *(BB)*, all children will be dark eyed, no matter what the other parent's hereditary background; if both parents are entirely of light-eyed inheritance, all their children will be light eyed as well (the probability is actually about 98 percent). But if both parents are dark eyed but are carrying recessive genes for light eyes (that is, they are genetically *Bb*), each can pass on either gene to their children, and the possible combinations are: *B+B, B+b, b+B,* and *b+b.* Those possibilities are true for each child; thus there is a 25 percent chance that each child will have light eyes, and a 75 percent chance for each child to inherit at least one gene for light eyes, whether or not the child's own eyes are light.

DOMINANT INHERITANCE
(one parent has dominant characteristic; that parent is of mixed heredity)
Parents: Dr rr
Possibilities: Dr Dr rr rr
Result: Each child has 50% chance of displaying dominant characteristic and, if so, will also carry recessive gene, which may be passed on to offspring.

We have, as we've said, oversimplified to an extent, and it should be noted that there are exceptions to this pattern. Some characteristics are, for instance, believed to be *dominant-qualified* or *recessive-qualified* — meaning that they generally perform in the classic pattern, but sometimes not, and there appear to be certain factors, hereditary or otherwise, modifying the genetic effects; others are believed to be *recessive-plus,* meaning that they are not only recessive but must be combined with still other genes to produce the condition (midgets are thought to be, possibly, one example).

It should also be noted, in connection with the particular example we chose for our probability example, that there are minute shadings of eye colors, and that a light brown can appear optically to be gray or blue — so that making confident predictions can be a risky business.

Among traits generally believed to be dominant, in addition to dark eyes, are dark hair, prominent facial features (such as a large nose or a broad jaw), dimples, curly hair and coarse-textured hair, and long eyelashes. There are also over 940 known defects or disorders — many, such as extra fingers or toes, are comparatively trivial and do not really interfere with physical or mental functioning — that are known to follow dominant inheritance. Among the major ones are achondroplastic dwarfism, one form of porphyria, and some types of tendencies to develop high blood cholesterol.

In general, serious hereditary defects and disorders tend to be recessive. (Among all congenital defects, incidentally, only about five percent are hereditary.) More than 780 conditions are now known to be transmitted by autosomal (nonsex-linked) reces-

"Throwback" Inheritance

Recessive genes may be passed on from generation to generation, emerging as visible traits only when chance combination with a like recessive occurs. In our fanciful yet theoretically possible illustration, the child displays four recessive characteristics — hair that is both light and straight, light eyes, and short eyelashes — seen in neither parent and in none of the four grandparents; each one of these traits appeared in just one member of each pair of the eight great-grandparents (marked by asterisks). All the child's grandparents, in this hypothetical scheme, carried recessive genes for both blond hair and pale eyes; their offspring, in turn, each received such a gene from one parent. Both paternal grandparents, and the maternal grandmother, carried straight-hair recessives; two grandparents — the paternal grandmother and the maternal grandfather — received, and passed on, recessive genes for short lashes. Thus it came to pass that both parents carried genes for all four recessive traits and, against overwhelming odds (but fortunately for illustrative purposes) — the mathematical probability is actually one chance in 128 — the child has inherited them all.

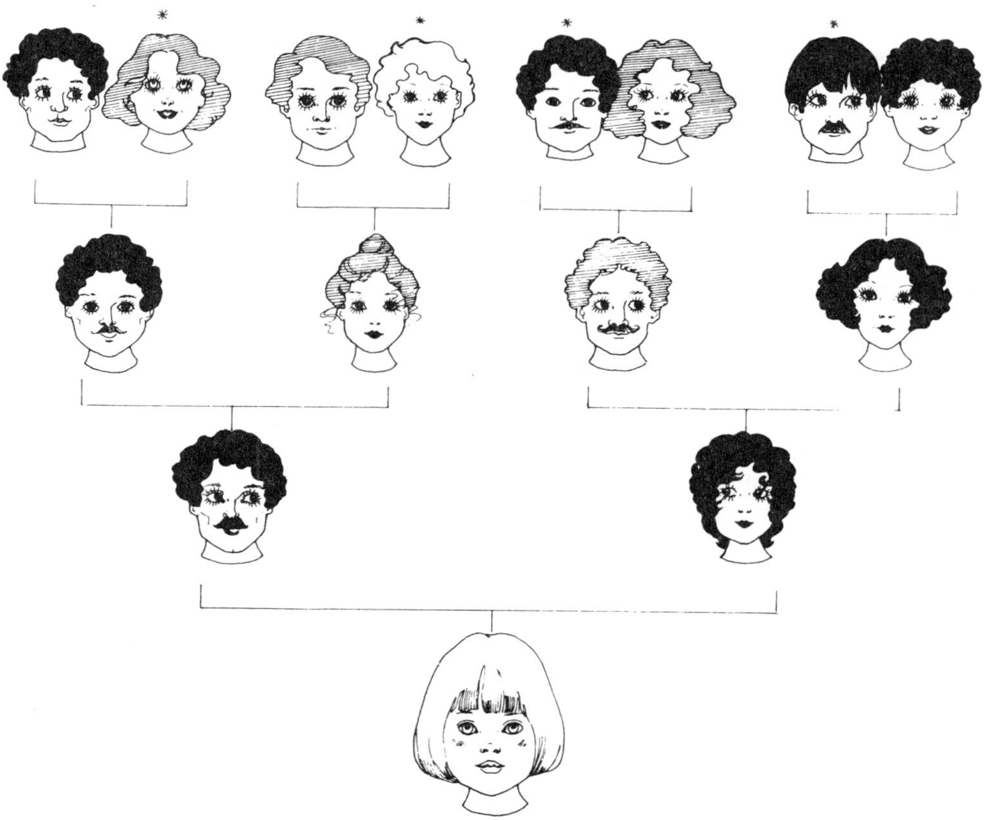

sive inheritance; they include phenylketonuria, Tay-Sachs disease, the hereditary anemias (sicklemia, thalassemia), Gaucher's disease, Niemann-Pick disease, albinism, and cystic fibrosis.

AUTOSOMAL RECESSIVE INHERITANCE
(neither parent displays characteristic, but both carry the gene for recessive trait)
Parents: Dr Dr
Possibilities: DD Dr Dr rr
Result: Each child has 25% chance of displaying recessive characteristic (of being afflicted, if it is a disorder), plus 50% chance of carrying recessive gene for trait.

There are an additional 150 or so known disorders called *X-linked recessive.* In these conditions, the recessive gene can be carried only by an X chromosome; it is recessive, specifically, to a normal X chromosome that is not bearing the gene. Thus, for a woman, the possibility of having one of these conditions exists only if she inherits the gene from both parents — which means that her father must be afflicted with the disorder (he has, remember, contributed one X chromosome to a daughter) and her mother must be at least a carrier of the trait.

The problem in X-linked recessive disorders arises with "hidden" carriers of the inimical genes, who are invariably women. The conditions that are known to be transmitted by X-linked recessive inheritance include classic red-green color blindness, hemophilia, Fabry's disease, and agammaglobulinemia. (It should be noted that, as in some of the autosomal recessive conditions, a carrier may show evidence of some partial physical problems, but the impact by no means approaches that of straight inheritance.)

X-LINKED RECESSIVE INHERITANCE
(neither parent displays characteristic, but mother carries gene on one X chromosome, indicated by a small "x")
Parents: Xx XY
Possibilities: XX XY Xx xY
Result: By rules of probability, chances of male or female offspring are 50–50. With male offspring, there is 50% chance of affliction (nonafflicted male cannot even, by definition, be carrier). Assuming, as in postulated example, that mother is simply carrier of trait in question, there is 50% chance for each daughter to carry trait as well. In brief, each child, boy or girl, stands 50–50 chance of inheriting particular gene.

The nature of so-called "throwback" inheritance should at this point be apparent. It is perfectly possible for a child — via a chance combination of recessive genes — to display a trait that hasn't appeared on either side of the family for a number of generations.

DETECTION AND PREDICTION

Over the past few years, there has been vastly increased interest in family planning. Accordingly, there is more concern on the part of parents about predicting the likelihood of congenital problems, both hereditary and nonhereditary, in their offspring and identifying possible problems in each pregnancy. If such problems are found, the pregnancy can be terminated, thus preventing some heartbreaking eventualities. It is now possible to determine a forthcoming baby's sex, as well, and in situations where one sex is more likely to enter life as the victim of an uncomfortable and incurable disorder, it seems wise to seek that information.

Since we have voiced an opinion, we should append a bit of explanation. We have made every effort to include the latest knowledge and information. We feel that you, our readers, deserve that; your decisions, based upon that information, are of course entirely your own. We feel strongly that as a fully informed parent, you will do better by your children.

We urge you to make every effort to learn your, and your spouse's, pedigrees from a medical viewpoint. That effort may lead you to terminate some pregnancies that are highly likely to result in the birth of a seriously afflicted child.

A number of serious conditions we have mentioned can now be detected in an unborn baby (see AMNIOCENTESIS). They include Fabry's disease, Gaucher's disease, porphyria, Tay-Sachs disease, and Turner's and Klinefelter's syndromes, as well as such congenital problems as Down's syndrome and Rh reactions; assessment of fetal age and development can also be made. It is hoped that the list will soon include PKU, cystic fibrosis, and the hereditary anemias. (Sickle-cell anemia was detected in a fetus for the first time in 1976. The procedure is considered risky, however, since a blood specimen must be obtained; it is hoped that a way may be found to diagnose the condition from a sample of amniotic fluid.) Additionally, the "carrier" state — i.e., the presence of the recessive gene — for an increasing number of conditions can be detected in prospective parents by analysis of blood samples or other tissues; sicklemia, thalassemia, Tay-Sachs, Gaucher's, PKU, and porphyria are among those, and at this writing, researchers appear close to developing a detection test for carriers of the recessive gene for cystic fibrosis, the most widespread of these disorders.

Genetic counseling is the term for advice given to parents and prospective parents on these matters. It may be available from your pediatrician or family physician, or from persons specializing in that subject; there are also centers devoted to providing such guidance.

COMBINATIONS AND VARIABLES

Some hereditary characteristics are combinations, representing compromises between hereditary factors derived from the parents, rather than either-or choices. A number of different genes are involved in determination of skin color, for example. A very dark person and a very light one are likely to have offspring whose skin color is somewhere in between; while two parents of medium skin shade but of mixed heredity may have children lighter or darker than they are, or about the same.

Similarly, such variable characteristics as intelligence and stature are likely to be combinations of multiple genetic traits inherited from both parents — and such traits as physical stature are even further modified by the child's environment; a well-nourished child is likely to be taller and stronger than a child with deficiencies in the diet. A child's genetic potential in such variable areas will be affected by environment — although that environment won't affect future *offspring;* if, for example, malnutrition causes stunted physical growth in a youngster, he or she may still, as an adult, pass on a genetic potential for above-average height.

There are a number of disorders we have not mentioned that may be due, at least in part, to hereditary factors. No clear pattern of dominance or recession has emerged, and it is felt that combinations of genes — perhaps affected by environmental factors — may be responsible. Geneticists call this mode of transmission "multifactorial inheritance"; some conditions that may fit into this category are pyloric stenosis, cleft palate, clubfoot, spina bifida, and congenital dislocation of the hip. The probability of having two or more children with the same multifactorial-inheritance disorder or defect is quite low, less than five percent.

hermaphroditism: a condition in which a child appears to be neither male nor female, but ostensibly has physical traits of both. Many plants, and some lower animals, are normally hermaphrodites; mammals, including human beings, are not — so it's important both to determine the nature of the problem and to take corrective steps. There are two distinct types.

True hermaphroditism describes a situation in which, through some prenatal accident, both male and female sex organs have developed internally and externally. The genetic situation must definitely be analyzed (see the immediately preceding entry), and corrective surgery must be performed — again, both internally and externally — to eliminate the incorrect organs. It's quite important that surgery be performed as early as possible in order to avoid psychosexual problems.

Pseudohermaphroditism denotes, specifically, a situation in which the external sexual organs, only, seem doubtful or inconclusive; the internal organs are intact and definitive. What is done in such a case depends upon the individual situation and the extent of under- or overdevelopment of the external organs. Creating a functional penis when none exists is virtually impossible surgically, while it is far less difficult to turn inconclusive external genitalia into those of a functional female, whatever chromosomal analysis may reveal (if the baby is XY, administration of female hormones will of course be necessary at puberty if that route is taken — and the individual will not be able to bear children, but will have definite psychosexual identity). Clitoral overdevelopment in a baby who is otherwise clearly female may be treated by surgery, the administration of hormones, or both. Again, early treatment is vital and should certainly take place by the age of two years — before that, if possible.

hernia: the protrusion of an organ or passageway through the wall of the abdominal cavity — causing, depending upon the nature of the situation, either a condition of mild concern, an emergency situation, or something in between. All hernias are secondary to some congenital structural weakness.

Inguinal hernia is what is generally meant when the word hernia (or, sometimes, rupture) is used without further qualification, and about 85 percent of all hernias are this type; it is a loop of intestine protruding through the lower part of the abdominal wall into the scrotum (most victims are boys) — or, if it is a girl, into the thigh. If this type of hernia has been diagnosed in your youngster, surgical correction should be scheduled as soon as possible — not because the hernia itself is dangerous, but because there is the possibility of strangulation, an extremely critical condition.

If a hernia becomes strangulated — that is, if by a sudden strain or twist the blood supply to the herniated tissue is cut off — it must be considered a medical emergency because of the possibility of gangrene. The child will be in severe pain, and there is often nausea and possibly vomiting. Should this occur, don't wait for a physician to come to your house. Rush your child to the nearest hospital, and telephone your doctor to meet you there.

Diaphragmatic hernia involves, as you might suspect, the diaphragm; it is a protrusion of part of the stomach upward through what has become a too-wide gap (there is, of course, normally an opening in the diaphragm, through which the esophagus passes), and is also sometimes known as a *hiatal hernia.* This type of hernia is more common in infants than in older children. It, too, can and should be corrected by surgery. When this type of hernia is large and congenital, prompt diagnosis and surgery are necessary to save the life of the newborn baby.

Umbilical hernia occurs in infants and small children; it is a protrusion of a piece of omentum, the membrane at the front of the abdomen, into the navel, which has failed to close properly. It is not painful to the child, and usually the only symptom is a small lump at the navel that becomes larger when the child cries. An umbilical hernia is not serious; 99 percent of them disappear as the infant gets older. Only one percent are large enough to require surgery. Your physician will make the decision.

heroin: an opium derivative; see NARCOTICS.

herpangina: See CANKER SORES.

herpes simplex: See CANKER SORES; COLD SORE; GUM DISORDERS; VENEREAL DISEASES; VIRUSES.

herpes zoster: See CHICKENPOX; SHINGLES; VIRUSES.

hetacillin: a semisynthetic penicillin; see ANTIBIOTICS.

heterozygous: having different hereditary information (for a particular trait) at corresponding sites on chromosomes received from the two parents. Someone having brown eyes (dominant) but carrying a recessive gene for light eyes is said to be heterozygous as to eye color. The opposite is *homozygous.*

hexachlorophene: an antibacterial agent available in a three percent liquid solution called pHisoHex, and formerly incorporated, as well, in a large number of antibacterial soaps. In late 1972, the Food and Drug Administration directed that hexachlorophene-containing soaps, as well as the liquid solution, be withdrawn from over-the-counter sale, after it was determined that there was some potential for harm to newborn infants (although later studies have suggested that probably only unusually small premature babies are at risk). The liquid is still available by prescription, and many physicians find it useful for skin cleansing in teenage acne and in cases of impetigo and other skin infections. Do, if your doctor recommends this product, be sure to follow directions; the liquid should be diluted and rinsed off thoroughly and should never be applied to open wounds or severely burned skin.

hiatal hernia: See HERNIA.

hiccough: a disturbance in the phrenic nerves regulating movement of the diaphragm, the muscle at the bottom of the chest cavity that goes up and down when we breathe; the result is the sudden noisy intake of breath familiar to us all. Hiccough is very common in small infants and isn't really bothersome to the baby; it can simply be ignored.

An older child is likely to be annoyed by his hiccoughing and ask for your help in bringing it to a halt. Many remedies have been proposed over the years, including holding the breath for a few seconds, drinking a glass of water without stopping, gargling, and having someone startle the victim; we can't endorse or condemn any of them. We do suggest that the operative factor when one of them works is that the child is focusing his attention on the procedure rather than the problem; often, if the child is distracted and begins to concentrate on some other topic, the hiccoughs will simply vanish without his being aware of their departure.

There are, it's true, rare instances in which nothing works. If hiccoughing persists for more than a couple of hours, and the youngster is definitely uncomfortable, do call your doctor.

hip, broken: See FRACTURES.

Hirschsprung's disease: a congenital condition involving constipation from birth; it's uncommon, and especially rare in girls. In Hirschsprung's disease, the colon, or large intestine, is dilated, while there is extreme constriction at the junction of the colon and rectum or within the rectum itself; it is caused by an incomplete nerve supply to the rectal area. The result is that fecal material is not normally excreted, but accumulates in the rectum; the baby's abdomen is visibly distended, and there are noticeably odorous gases arising from decomposition of the material in the rectum (there may be a very few, very hard occasional stools). Treatment is surgical, and the prognosis for complete correction of the condition is usually good.

The cause of Hirschsprung's, technically termed *congenital megacolon,* is not known; there may or may not be hereditary factors. It has been noted that, statistically, the chances of having a second child born with the condition are quite low, only about one in sixty (about 1.5 percent), one in twenty (5.0 percent) — still very low risk — if the second child is a boy.

Histaspan: a trade name for chlorpheniramine maleate; see ANTIHISTAMINES.

histoplasmosis: an increasingly common fungus infection that attacks the respiratory tract; it is found in various parts of the world, but is now considered endemic in the eastern and central United States, with some five hundred thousand cases annually, chiefly among children.

Much like the valley fever found farther west, histoplasmosis ranges from the Dakotas east to New York in the north and Florida on the south, but is concentrated in the Mississippi River states and especially in the area from Missouri to Ohio. It is not contagious but is contracted by breathing the airborne spores of the particular fungus, which thrives in moderate heat (temperatures generally in the 70s and low 80s) and high humidity, and tends to lurk in such spots as river banks, caves, old stumps, chicken houses, and silos; the spores may also be present in bird droppings and can be released into the air when old droppings are scraped from buildings and other structures. The incubation period is usually five to eighteen days.

Histoplasmosis may be difficult to diagnose. There is one very rare form that is serious, producing emaciation and anemia. The usual, common form is not considered serious, but it can be quite painful and can sometimes be confused with a number of other things; symptoms, generally similar to those of pneumonia, tuberculosis, or psittacosis, may (or may not) include high fever ranging to 106° F. (41.1° C.), chest pain, difficulty in breathing, cough, and nausea. The diagnosis of histoplasmosis is confirmed, however, by a skin test, which reveals antibodies to a current or recent attack, and a blood test, which shows the presence of active disease.

It is treated with various drugs, including sulfas and fungicidal antibiotics.

hives: a rash specifically due to hypersensitivity (see ALLERGY), most often due to food allergy. It usually takes the form of itchy welts, and there may also be swelling in various areas such as hands and feet and tissues around the eyes. The medical term for hives is *urticaria*.

Typically, hives appear and disappear within hours after the child's encounter with the allergen. Depending upon the severity of the reaction, especially if there is extensive swelling or difficulty in breathing, the doctor may administer drugs such as adrenalin, cortisone, or ACTH — or, if the problem is essentially itchiness, an antihistamine.

If you're familiar with the cause and reaction, and it's not the first time, follow whatever instructions your physician has previously given you. If you suspect this kind of reaction and it's never happened before, it's important that the doctor see the child promptly, since some allergic reactions can be quite serious.

As in asthma and other allergic conditions, there may be an emotional component — not as a cause, but as an aggravating factor — and if you have noted that your youngster's hives bear a distinct relationship to possibly disturbing incidents, you should mention it to your doctor.

hoarseness: a symptom of a number of different conditions ranging from serious infections to simple irritation from yelling. If there are other symptoms as well — such as fever or sniffles — call the doctor. Even if there are no other symptoms, as far as you can determine, the doctor should see the child if the hoarseness persists for a week.

Hodgkin's disease: See LYMPHOMA.

homeopath: an adherent of an obsolete and totally disproved theory of curing disease by administering minute doses of substances that produce, in a healthy person, symptoms similar to those of the disease itself. A homeopath is not an accredited physician and should not be consulted for treatment or for medical advice. But don't confuse this word with another that *does* denote an accredited professional; see OSTEOPATH.

homograft: a transplant of tissue from one person to another (or from one animal to another of the same species) who is not an identical twin; the word is synonymous with *allograft.*

homosexuality: orientation toward, and preference for, one's own sex rather than the opposite sex in the matter of sexual relations. Parents may become interested in, or concerned about, this subject in relation to their children at three different stages. We present, here, the consensus of current medical thinking — of which you should be aware, whatever your personal views or inclinations.

Homosexuality as a conscious choice by an individual old enough to make a decision — which includes a significant proportion of teenagers — is no longer considered an aberration or disorder, per se, by a 1974 decision of the American Psychiatric Association, which defines and classifies mental and emotional illnesses for the U.S. medical community. Only if the individual is disturbed by, or feels unhappy with, that orientation is special counseling or therapy recommended. Thoughtful persons in medicine, law, and other fields agree that discrimination against individuals based on their sexual orientation is wrong.

Such discrimination, of course, still exists among many people, in many places; a realistic decision to follow any pursuit or life style must take that fact into account. If you, as a parent, feel that your son or daughter is acting without clear understanding of the societal stigma that is sometimes still encountered, it is certainly a good idea to discuss your concern with your family doctor, who can give you objective advice and guidance.

It should be mentioned, before we leave the subject of chosen orientation, that innumerable studies have been made to determine if homosexuality is correlated with any particular psychological problems (as perceived by homosexuals themselves or by others). Findings indicate that homosexuals in general are neither more nor less unhappy, anxious, maladjusted, etc., than heterosexuals in general. Obviously, if an individual is forced or coerced into a relationship, of whatever sexual orientation, that person is not going to be very happy. Ideally, all such decisions should be made thoughtfully and maturely; in practice, of course, many are not — witness the high divorce rate in our nation.

Decisions about sexual activities cannot, by definition, be made until sexual maturity, which typically develops some time during the teen years. (And teenagers, it must be noted, are wont to engage, often, in sexual experimentation that may have nothing to do with their ultimate choice of orientation; parents are sometimes unaware of that fact — or have conveniently forgotten their own teen years.) Prior to that time, stronger interest in one's own sex — including "crushes" on adults, and even great hostility toward the opposite sex — is commonplace and not in the least suggestive of future predilections.

The third circumstance that may arouse parental concern — and rightly so — is apparent homosexual activity involving a child and a teenager, or a child (or young teen) and an adult. It is a proper matter for concern not because of its homosexual nature, but because it constitutes assault, both physical and emotional. Sexual activity between consenting adults, be they eighteen or eighty, is something radically different from sexual coercion on the part of an adult (of either sex) toward a child (of either sex). Should something of this nature befall a child, it is best, we think, if — assuming out-and-out force was not used — the guilty individual be characterized as emotionally ill or disturbed, rather than "criminal," since the former is the truth. A youngster will generally accept such an explanation, without your going into further detail.

A final comment. In our opinion, it is extremely unfortunate that individuals who associate with children, youth leaders and teachers in particular, have been singled out for harassment because they are homosexuals. A homosexual in such a position is no more likely than a heterosexual to assault his or her young charges. Nor is such an individual especially inclined — any more than a heterosexual — to go about describing and advocating particular sexual activities. Those, whatever you may have heard, are the facts.

homozygous: having the same kind of genes at paired sites on the chromosomes received from each parent. A person who receives genes for blue eyes, for instance, from both parents is homozygous for eye color. The opposite situation, in which one or the other inheritance is dominant, is called *heterozygous.* See HEREDITY.

honey: See SWEETENERS.

hookworms: See WORMS.

hormones: substances secreted by various structures and organs, primarily serving to set other processes into motion. Some, for example, are produced in the gastrointestinal tract and act to stimulate digestion via the release of certain enzymes. The majority are created by specialized organs that do nothing else; see ENDOCRINE GLANDS.

hornet stings: See BITES AND STINGS.

h.s.: See PRESCRIPTIONS.

humerus: the anatomical term for the bone of the upper arm.

humidifier: See VAPORIZER.

humor: a word chiefly — though not entirely — of historical interest, so far as medicine is concerned. The word itself derives from the Latin for "fluid," and referred originally to a group of liquids coursing through the body and believed by early physicians to be responsible for health (or lack of it). They were related to astrology and to "primary elements" theories that have figured prominently in folk medicine, and included blood (related to air, described as hot and wet), phlegm (water, wet and cold), yellow bile (fire, hot and dry), and black bile (earth, dry and cold). These characterizations came to be analogous to various moods and temperaments, hence the popular meanings of the word.

Medically, the word survives as the root term in "rheumatism" and in a small number of anatomical designations; among the latter is the *aqueous humor* — literally, waterlike fluid — that fills the eyeball. (The name of the upper-arm bone, *humerus,* comes to us from a different linguistic source.)

hyaline membrane disease: a lung affliction chiefly, though not exclusively, affecting premature babies; it involves the formation of a glassy membrane in the lungs, preventing proper oxygenation of the blood. Its cause is completely unknown, but there is a great deal of research being done, for this disease is responsible for the death of thousands of infants in the United States each year (President John F. Kennedy's son Patrick was one of its victims).

Hyaline membrane disease is not, however, consistently fatal; most infants afflicted with it, in fact, now survive. Treatment may include placing the baby in an incubator, the administration of certain drugs, and other measures. It is best treated in the neonatal intensive care unit of a hospital.

Hyasorb: a trade name for penicillin G; see ANTIBIOTICS.

hydrocele: an accumulation of fluid in the scrotum that is often present at birth and disappears gradually; it sometimes occurs later in infancy. It's not serious and usually goes away by itself. It can, however, easily be confused with a hernia by a lay person, so your doctor should promptly see and diagnose the problem.

hydrocephalus (or hydrocephaly): an accumulation of intracranial fluid; "water on the brain" is the somewhat inaccurate popular phrase. It is caused by blockage of the normal circulation of cerebrospinal fluid, due to infection, tumor, injury, or congenital malformation (it's not hereditary).

The chief symptom is enlargement of the infant's head, which is fortunately possible, since the skull bones are not yet fused; the enlargement may be too small for you to notice, but your pediatrician is alert to such things and automatically looks for them — which is one very good reason to take your baby for regular checkups. Surgery is required to correct the condition.

hydrocortisone: See CORTICOSTEROIDS.

hydrogen peroxide: If your doctor has suggested you purchase some of this — it may sometimes be recommended for use in treating certain wounds, and it is also an efficient loosener of ear wax — what is meant is the three percent medicinal type, *not* the twenty-volume bleaching solution. Use peroxide in the situations mentioned only when your physician so advises.

hydromorphone: a semisynthetic morphine derivative; see NARCOTICS.

hydronephrosis: an excessive accumulation of urine in a kidney, accompanied by enlargement of the kidney; it is usually caused by blockage of the ureter, the tube leading from the kidney to the bladder. If the condition is caught early, the ureter can in most cases be unblocked; sometimes, removal of the kidney is necessary.

hydrophobia: See RABIES.

hydroxyzine: an antianxiety agent that also acts against motion sickness; see MOTION SICKNESS and SEDATIVES.

hygienist, oral: See HEALTH PROFESSIONALS.

hyoscine: an alternate name for

scopolamine, a belladonna alkaloid that is included in a number of over-the-counter "sleep aids"; see SEDATIVES.

hyperglycemia: an acute condition involving an excess of sugar in the blood; it is the situation that prevails in diabetic coma (see DIABETES MELLITUS).

hyperkinesis: hyperactivity; excessive motion or activity. That's the literal meaning — obviously a subjective one (what is "excessive"?). The word has been variously used — and misused — probably because its ordinary meaning and its medical meaning have sometimes become confused. A sedentary adult — parent, teacher, or anyone — might consider a normally active, curious youngster "hyperkinetic." Medically, however, hyperkinesis involves not only a great deal of random activity, but a constellation of characteristics including a certain intensity, difficulty in adapting to new situations, and, prominently, inability to concentrate on one subject or activity for the normal period of time. (That last ability is age-related and increases as people grow older. No small child is expected to have the capacity for concentration of an older child, let alone that of an adult; any such behavior must be evaluated in its own context, not judged by adult norms.)

The diagnosis is not always easy, even for physicians; yet a surprising number of nonphysicians have leaped to it with ease. In one reported study, nearly half of a group of young boys were labeled hyperkinetic — by their teachers. The actual incidence is perhaps two or three percent.

In most instances of hyperkinesis, the pediatrician or family physician is qualified to diagnose and treat the condition. Sometimes, the child's problems are largely emotional and require therapy in that area. Occasionally, organic dysfunction is great enough to call for consultation with a pediatric neurologist.

When deemed advisable by the doctor, certain medications may be prescribed. A word about those, since this has been another area of widespread misunderstanding.

The medications commonly used are the amphetamines or, more likely, a nonamphetamine drug with similar properties called methylphenidate (Ritalin). These are basically stimulants; if given to an adult — or, for that matter, to a child who does not have this particular problem — they will have the effect described under AMPHETAMINES. In a truly hyperkinetic child, however, there is (for reasons not clearly understood) a paradoxical effect: the youngster is calmed, develops an ability to concentrate better, and on the whole functions much more effectively. Properly used in such a situation, such drugs carry no risk of habituation or dependence, and are discontinued after a time with no ill effects. It should be added that a child who is truly hyperkinetic *may* benefit from emotional counseling as *well* — of the child, parents, or both.

Recently, a new drug called pemoline (Cylert) has been introduced, offering the advantage of once-a-day administration, which eliminates the necessity for remembering a midday dose during school hours. Pemoline is also believed to be devoid of any potential for abuse by others who may have access to it.

If you suspect your child may have this difficulty, the question should be discussed with your pediatrician or family physician. The child may need treatment of one kind or another, but this is a *medical* judgment.

hyperlipidemia, hyperlipoproteinemia: See LIPIDS.

hyperopia: See FARSIGHTEDNESS.

hyperpyrexia: the medical term for extremely high fever; *accidental hyperpyrexia* is synonymous with *heat stroke*.

hypersensitivity: See ALLERGY.

hypertension: See BLOOD PRESSURE.

hyperthyroidism: See ENDOCRINE GLANDS.

hyperuricemia: an excess of uric acid in the blood, whether because too much is produced by the body (it is a by-product of the breakdown of certain food substances) or because there is underexcretion by the kidneys. Hyperuricemia is found in many more males than females (it is believed to involve hereditary factors, although the mechanism is unclear), and is one of the operative elements in gout — although only about one in ten males with hyperuricemia actually develops gouty arthritis. This finding is also associated with a very rare type of mental retardation in children, again predominantly afflicting boys. In the vast majority of people who have it, hyperuricemia is simply an interesting laboratory finding and is not associated with any problems.

hypervitaminosis: a condition brought about by toxic overdose of a vitamin, almost invariably due to inordinate pill-popping. A letter following the word denotes the particular vitamin involved, as in *hypervitaminosis A.* See the section on vitamins under NUTRITION for discussion of such conditions.

hypnosis: a technique of inducing a particular type of suggestible state (it is not sleep), used for various purposes including assisting memory, treating psychosomatic problems, relieving pain by inducing partial anesthesia, preparing a patient for treatment (as, children for surgery), etc. It is a valid device when it is used by a qualified practitioner — physician, dentist, or psychologist specially trained in the technique.

Some people can be more easily hypnotized than others, and about one in five cannot be hypnotized at all.

hypnotic: as an adjective, relating to hypnosis; as a noun, a sedative to induce sleep. See SEDATIVES.

hypoglobulinemia: see AGAMMAGLOBULINEMIA.

hypoglycemia: an abnormally low sugar level in the blood, determined by a blood test. What the physician decides to do about it depends upon the cause and other factors. Hypoglycemia is generally an indication of lack of food. It may occur in a small child who for some reason has had no food for many hours, and is also under tension — and may cause the child to go into convulsions. It can occur as a result of a teenager's starving herself on a self-prescribed "diet." In a diabetic youngster, it can signal impending insulin shock (see DIABETES MELLITUS). It may be associated with a pancreatic or other endocrine problem causing overproduction of insulin. And it occurs, but very rarely, as a chronic condition due to an inherent defect of carbohydrate metabolism.

hypophysis: an alternate, now little used, term for the pituitary; see ENDOCRINE GLANDS.

hypospadias: a congenital malformation of the urethra, in which this excretory passageway from the bladder is too short — thus discharging (in boys, by far the most common victims of the condition) slightly short of the tip of the penis or (in girls, in whom the condition rarely occurs) into the vagina. The condition is classified according to its severity: *first-degree* hypospadias, in which the opening is very close to where it should be, may not require any corrective measures; *second degree* indicates a more serious departure, requiring surgical correction; *third-degree,* severe hypospadias may require more than one surgical procedure in order to correct it.

Hypospadias is sometimes associated with a not uncommon chromosomal disorder in boys; see KLINEFELTER'S SYNDROME.

hypotension: See BLOOD PRESSURE.

hypothermia: extremely low body temperature; *accidental hypothermia* describes such a condition that has resulted from overexposure to the elements.

hypothyroidism: See CRETINISM; ENDOCRINE GLANDS.

Hyzyd: a trade name for isoniazid, an antituberculosis drug.

I

iatrogenic: describing a state or condition caused by a physician through careless or erroneous treatment; the first part of the word derives from the Greek *iatros*, "physician."

ichthyosis: a congenital defect of the outer layer of the skin, primarily involving deficient oil secretion, with resultant dryness and scaliness. There are a number of types, categorized by the area affected and by the severity of the condition, which can range from very slight, with minimal scaling, to quite marked; the latter is extremely rare.

icterus: See JAUNDICE.

idiopathic: a word used to characterize a condition for which the cause is, at that point, unknown — as "idiopathic hypertension" or "idiopathic eczema." It's one of those made-up medical terms, made up in this case from two Greek words meaning, simply, "peculiar (to the individual) suffering."

ileitis: an inflammation of the lower part of the small intestine. Typical symptoms are cramps or colic following meals, and sometimes fever, diarrhea, weakness, or weight loss. Treatment will depend upon the doctor's judgment of the cause and severity of the inflammation and usually includes both medications and dietary measures.

ileum: See INTESTINES.

ileus: intestinal obstruction accompanied by colicky pain, vomiting, and possibly fever, also sometimes called "intestinal colic"; it may be caused by a variety of things, including gallstones, parasitic infestations, and postoperative complications of abdominal surgery.

Ilosone, Ilotycin: trade names for erythromycin; see ANTIBIOTICS.

imipramine: See ANTIDEPRESSANTS.

immune deficiency disease: See AGAMMAGLOBULINEMIA.

immunity: successful resistance to an invading infection, so that the disease or illness is not contracted. There are some diseases — common colds, fungus infections, strep infections, venereal diseases, and many others — to which immunity does not occur as far as is known. When immunity is possible it can be achieved in several different ways.

Natural immunity is immunity that exists from the moment of conception, usually by virtue of being the type of creature one is. Just as fish don't get measles, humans don't get mange. Most animals aren't susceptible to most human diseases, and vice versa, although there are exceptions (see ZOONOSES). There are also rare instances of apparent natural immunity to purely human afflictions; 95 to 97 percent of people, for example, seem to be naturally immune to Hansen's disease.

Acquired immunity can be attained actively or passively — that is, by developing one's own antibodies, or by using antibodies developed by another. There are, generally speaking, three classifications:

1) *Having the disease* bestows a kind of active immunity, since in the case of diseases that work this way, one develops one's own antibodies — which may or may not last forever. Once someone has measles or chickenpox, he can never contract it again; having whooping cough, on the other hand, gives long, but not lifelong, immunity.

2) *Having a mother who's immune* to certain diseases will give the baby (via the mother's antibodies, which makes it a kind of passive immunity) an immunity that lasts, depending upon the disease, for three to nine months after birth. Most major contagious diseases are in this category, except chickenpox.

3) *Deliberate immunization* may take place two ways. *Gamma globulin* (serum containing antibodies — thus passive) is little used, except in certain cases of exposure to infectious hepatitis and a few of the childhood diseases. This kind of immunity is quickly effective, but lasts for a limited time. *Vaccination* introduces a small amount of the particular antigen (bacteria or virus), thus stimulating the body to make its own antibodies (an active type); the protection takes longer to develop, but lasts longer — in some cases, permanently. See the next entry for the many ills for which vaccination is used.

immunization: the deliberate administration of a substance in order to prevent the individual from contracting a particular disease or infection, one way to achieve acquired immunity (see the preceding entry). Immunization against some diseases is now routine and should be given to every child; for other diseases, immunization is necessary only if there is exposure, or potential exposure, to the particular illness.

Your own physician may differ with some of the schedules presented in the listing that follows; there are legitimate differences of opinion among pediatricians and others in the field regarding some optimum intervals between vaccinations, and these should be taken simply as approximate guidelines. Your doctor may also advise postponing certain shots when your child is ill, and that is in fact usual; there are exceptions, though, depending upon what the shot is and what the child has, so let your doctor decide.

When your child, or your family, travels, the question of whether and what immunization measures are needed should be discussed with your physician. Patterns of disease do shift, and what we state here could change; your doctor will have up-to-date data on any new areas in which diseases may have appeared. Do check with your doctor well in advance of the trip, since some shots need a certain amount of time to take effect.

We urge you to see that your child receives at least all the necessary basic immunizations, and that the schedule is started early; these visits to the pediatrician or family physician are also good opportunities for the child to get to know the doctor as a friend who not only *treats* illness but also can *prevent* illness. And a reminder: be sure to record your child's immunizations, routine and otherwise, in the pages provided at the back of this book.

Following are the ailments for which immunization of some sort is currently available; those marked with an asterisk (*) are now considered routine protection that all children should have. You'll find more details about each disease elsewhere in the book, under its own entry.

Brucellosis (undulant fever) — There's no immunization for human beings, but brucellosis is always contracted from animals infected with Bang's disease, for which there is a vaccine, and susceptible farm animals should be inoculated.

Chickenpox (varicella) — No vaccine is yet available, although researchers have been working to develop one for some time and continue to do so. There is a gamma globulin; see CHICKENPOX for details.

Cholera — Vaccination should be given when traveling to areas where the disease is endemic. It consists of two injections given a week to ten days apart, and the second should be given a full month before departure; immunity lasts for six months, when a booster shot will be needed if there is a continued stay in the area. (In babies and children under the age of nine, the original series is divided into three doses rather than two.)

**Diphtheria* — Vaccination is commonly in the form of DPT (diphtheria-pertussis-tetanus) shots that protect simultaneously against diphtheria, whooping cough, and tetanus. The initial series consists of three shots, the first generally given at the age of two or three months, the second a month or so later and the third a month or two after that, followed by boosters at about eighteen months and at five years (a total of five shots). A DT shot should be given at about the age of fifteen, and possibly one in between — at about nine or ten — if your doctor feels it's advisable, as far as the "D" component is concerned. (See *Tetanus* for further comment on protection against that infection. See *Whooping cough* for comment on DPT versus DT.) Whether or not diphtheria vaccination is to be continued after that is a matter for your doctor to judge; the disease is considered endemic in some areas but not in others.

If, incidentally, your child has a mild fever after a DPT or DT shot, don't be alarmed; it happens not infrequently. If the reaction is severe, however, your doctor may find it advisable to change the schedule and/or the dosage for future shots. Also, occasionally a lump develops at the site of the injection and may persist for weeks or even months; this is not an infection, but simply a reaction to the material in which the vaccine is precipitated, and it will eventually go away by itself.

Encephalitis — The vaccine is not recommended for humans, but in an area where equine encephalitis occurs, horses, mules, and other farm animals which are potential sources of infection should be vaccinated.

Hansen's disease — Vaccination with BCG vaccine is recommended only for children who live in areas in which the disease is endemic; it is not necessary for travel to such an area, since some 95 percent of the U.S. population is naturally immune, and even the remaining five percent require long and intimate contact with an infected individual in order to contract the disease.

Hepatitis (Type A) — There is as yet no vaccine, but gamma globulin is available and is recommended if a person is exposed or is traveling to an area or community where the disease is known to be prevalent. The protection lasts up to five or six months, depending upon the dosage, and gamma globulin is then repeated if necessary.

Influenza — Your youngster can be immunized if a vaccine is available for the virus causing a particular wave or epidemic, and should be if your own doctor feels it's advisable.

Malaria — There is no vaccine at this writing (the possibility is under study), but certain preventive drugs can be given before travel to an area where malaria is endemic and insect control may be inadequate.

**Measles* (rubeola) — Vaccination should take place at the age of one year and is usually given in the form of MMR (measles-mumps-rubella) vaccine, which protects against all three diseases, it is believed for life. A child who was vaccinated prior to the age of one year should be revaccinated; it is now known that there is not enough antibody-making ability before that age to provide lasting protection. (The three vaccines are available separately, and there are also measles-rubella and mumps-rubella combinations.) There is also a gamma globulin for measles, which should be promptly given to an unvaccinated child if a sibling contracts the disease.

Meningitis — The vaccines are not yet routinely recommended at this writing, but see the comments under HEMOPHILUS INFLUENZAE and MENINGITIS.

**Mumps* (epidemic parotitis) — The vaccination is usually given at the age of one year as part of the MMR shot (see *Measles*), although some doctors believe that it should not be given until the child is approaching adolescence, since it is only then that the disease is likely to be serious. Mumps gamma globulin has not proved effective.

Paratyphoid fever — There is a combination typhoid-paratyphoid vaccine, which should be given before a trip to areas where the two infections are endemic (they tend to be the same areas; see *Typhoid fever*).

Plague — A vaccine is available, administered in a series of three injections, that gives protection for four to six months; vaccination is considered essential, now, only for travel to Southeast Asia, but may also be advisable preceding camping trips to some parts of the United States (see PLAGUE).

Pneumonia — a vaccine may soon be generally available, against pneumococcal infections only; see the comments under PNEUMONIA.

**Polio* — All three viral strains that can cause this disease are covered by TOPV, which stands for trivalent oral polio vaccine (the injected vaccine is no longer used), which all children should have at the times of the five DPT shots (see *Diphtheria*). Boosters are given every three or four years thereafter, and many physicians feel they should be continued indefinitely; booster doses should certainly precede travel to areas where polio is still endemic.

Rabies — Vaccination is necessary and recommended for human beings only if they are bitten by an animal known to be rabid, or by a possibly rabid animal unavailable for examination. There is, however, an effective vaccine for animals, and dogs should be vaccinated every three years.

**Rubella* (German measles) — Vaccination is usually part of the MMR shot (see *Measles*), and all children of one year or older who are susceptible should be vaccinated; a past diagnosis may be questionable, but there is a blood test to determine whether or not an individual is immune. It's believed — although there's no final confirmation — that one shot will protect the child for life. Vaccination is not recommended for anyone who is pregnant, or who may become pregnant within three months. There is a rubella gamma globulin, but it is not considered dependable.

Scarlet fever — There is neither vaccine nor a gamma globulin, but a susceptible child *or* adult who is exposed to the disease should have a three-day course of preventive antibiotic therapy, which is effective.

Smallpox (variola) — Vaccination is no longer routine in this country but is still required for entry into many parts of Africa, Asia, and Central and South America (it is also required for reentry into the United States if the traveler has been in a nation reporting cases of smallpox within the past two weeks). The certificate of vaccination is valid for three years.

**Tetanus* — The vaccine is incorporated in the five DPT shots (see *Diphtheria*), and should thereafter be continued for life at minimum intervals of ten years; the recommended American Academy of Pediatrics schedule retains this gap between the DPT and DT shots at ages five and fifteen. Many physicians feel that five-year intervals are safer. Many pediatricians, in particular, feel that the likelihood of injury in active children is far too great to permit a lapse of ten years, and that smaller doses at two- or three-year intervals are preferable in order to maintain adequate antibody levels. In the event of serious injury requiring emergency treatment, tetanus-immune globulin is generally given routinely if there is uncertainty about prior immunization.

Tick fever (Rocky Mountain spotted fever, Colorado tick fever) — A series-of-injections vaccine is available, and is recommended if the child will be spending time outdoors in a tick-infested area. Protection lasts for a year.

Tuberculosis — BCG vaccine is given routinely in some countries, but it is not used in the United States except if TB is considered a public health problem in a particular area, or under special circumstances; the vaccine is not available to, or through, private physicians in this country.

Typhoid fever — Your child should be vaccinated prior to travel to an area considered risky (the destination should be discussed with your doctor). Mass vaccination is also recommended in the event of a flood or other disaster that threatens contamination of a community water supply. The vaccine is effective for one to three years.

Typhus fever — Vaccination is available, but is considered unnecessary unless a lengthy stay in an extremely high-risk area is in the offing; such areas are limited to those with crowded living conditions and a high level of lice infestation, plus a few temperate-to-tropical waterfronts swarming with a great many rats. Again, discuss the destination with your doctor. Protection lasts for a year.

**Whooping cough* (pertussis) — The vaccine is generally given as part of the standard schedule of DPT shots (see *Diphtheria*); the whooping cough vaccine is usually discontinued after the age of five, since the disease is far less serious in older children, and they tend to have more extreme reactions to the vaccine itself. There is also a gamma globulin that can be given if a nonimmune youngster is exposed to the disease.

Yellow fever — Vaccination is recommended if there's a scheduled trip to one of the areas where yellow fever is still considered endemic, including parts of Central and South America as well as the central part of Africa (a number of African nations *require* evidence of vaccination for entry into the country); it's extremely effective, lasts ten years. In the United States, the vaccine is available only through designated Public Health Service vaccination centers.

immunology: the study of the mechanisms of immunity, allergy, and antigen-antibody reactions in general.

immunosuppressants: agents also called cytotoxins (literally, "cell-killers"); they include azathioprine (Imuran), cyclophosphamide (Cytoxan), methotrexate, and others. They are used medically for three distinct purposes.

They are employed, as their class name implies, to suppress the "immune reaction" that triggers rejection of transplanted organs or tissue and that treats such grafts as "foreign matter"; these drugs help to mute such reactions, to enable the transplant to "take hold." They are also used (but not in young children) in certain of the so-called "auto-immune" diseases — prominently, dermatomyositis and lupus — to counteract the production of antibodies that act against the body itself. And third, their propensity for attacking rapidly proliferating cells has made them useful in the treatment of some malignancies, since cells of cancerous growths tend to multiply more rapidly than normal cells.

Since these medications behave quite indiscriminately, they are used with great care and continued for no longer than absolutely necessary. And because they tend to inactivate the body's natural defenses against infection, the health of a patient receiving any of these drugs is guarded assiduously; an otherwise routine immunization might be postponed, for example, since under some circumstances vaccination could trigger a fullblown systemic infection.

impetigo: a contagious skin infection, caused variously by staph or strep bacteria, usually the latter; anyone is susceptible (including parents of youngsters who have it), but it's most prevalent among small children, probably because of their extensive physical contact in play. It often follows a minor wound or insect bite that's scratched and becomes infected.

The most common sites for infection are the face, hands and arms, legs, and buttocks — but it can appear anywhere on the body, including the scalp. Characteristic symptoms, which appear after an incubation period of two to five days, are red spots that gradually change to pustules, then rupture and form honey-colored or light brown crusts. It should be noted, too, that the rash is sometimes atypical in appearance, resembling an abrasion or a cluster of insect bites.

If you suspect that your child has impetigo, the doctor should be consulted promptly, since secondary infections of a far more serious nature can develop if the condition goes untreated. Don't apply over-the-counter preparations; prescription medications are needed, usually antibiotics applied topically and/or given internally. The condition can be cleared up in a week or two with proper treatment. You can help prevent complications by cutting the child's fingernails down to the quick to make scratching impossible.

In the meantime, take measures to prevent the infection from spreading through the family and the neighborhood. The possibility of contagion involves not only skin-to-skin contact (unlike a strep throat, there is no droplet transmission from nose or mouth), but anything that might come in contact with infectious material from the sores and then be touched by someone else: clothing, towels, toys, furniture, bicycles, the edges of swimming pools, etc. If the affected area cannot be easily covered, it is best to keep the child in the house or out of contact with others until there has been at least 48 hours of antibiotic therapy and the lesions are no longer discharging infectious material. Your doctor may want to prescribe an antibacterial liquid cleansing agent for family use, as an extra prophylactic measure. There is, incidentally, no such thing as immunity to impetigo; another child can catch it even if that child has had it before.

Impetigo is a nasty business, best prevented by general cleanliness, warnings about sharing such things as towels, and proper care of such potential trouble sites as scrapes, scratches, small cuts, and insect bites.

Imuran: a trade name for azathioprine; see IMMUNOSUPPRESSANTS.

incubation period: the period between exposure to an infection and development of the first symptoms; such periods can vary, depending upon the particular infection, from hours to weeks, or even months, and can also vary with the individual. Incubation periods are helpful to know if you're aware of the existence of, or your child's exposure to, a particular infection in your area; for quick reference, here is a checklist of some major and/or common ones (we have not included smallpox since, for all practical purposes, it no longer exists in most of the world):

Brucellosis — 5 to 30 days
Cat-Scratch Fever — 3 to 10 days

Chickenpox — 10 days to 3 weeks
Cholera — 1 to 3 days
Colds — 1 to 3 days
Coxsackie Disease — 2 to 14 days, usually 3 to 5
Dengue — 3 to 15 days, usually 5 or 6
Diphtheria — 2 to 7 days, possibly longer
Dysentery, Amebic — 3 days to several months
Dysentery, Bacillary — 1 to 8 days, usually 2 to 4
Encephalitis (viral) — 3 to 21 days, varying with the virus
Erysipelas — 2 to 5 days
Erythema Infectiosum — 4 to 14 days
Food Poisoning, Botulism — 18 to 48 hours, rarely a week
Food Poisoning, Salmonella — 6 hours or more
Food Poisoning, various common bacteria — 2 to 20 hours
Giardiasis — 1 to 3 weeks, occasionally longer
Gonorrhea — 1 to 14 days, usually 3 to 5
Hepatitis, Type A — 2 to 8 weeks, usually 3 to 4
Hepatitis, Type B — 2 to 6 months
Histoplasmosis — 5 to 18 days
Impetigo — 2 to 5 days
Influenza — 1 to 3 days
Malaria — 5 days to several weeks
Measles — 10 to 14 days
Meningitis — 1 to 7 days, varying with the cause of infection
Mononucleosis — at least a week, perhaps as many as 6
Mumps — 2 to 3 weeks, averaging about 18 days
Paratyphoid Fever — 1 to 10 days
Plague — 2 to 8 days
Pneumonia, Bacterial — 2 to 5 days
Pneumonia, Viral — 1 to 2 weeks
Polio — 1 to 2 weeks, occasionally as many as 5
Psittacosis (parrot fever) — 4 to 15 days, usually about 10
Q Fever — 14 to 26 days
Rabies — usually 2 to 6 weeks, or longer, in humans; 3 to 5 days in other mammals
Rat-Bite Fever — 3 to 30 days, depending on type
Rickettsialpox — 7 to 10 days
Rubella (German measles) — 2 to 3 weeks
Scarlet Fever — 2 to 5 days
Shingles — 2 to 3 weeks, usually closer to 2
Strep Infections — 2 to 5 days
Syphilis — 10 days to 3 months, usually about 3 weeks
Tick Fever (Rocky Mountain spotted fever) — 2 to 12 days
Tonsillitis — 1 to 5 days, depending upon the cause of infection
Toxoplasmosis — up to 2 weeks
Tuberculosis — 2 to 10 weeks
Tularemia (rabbit fever) — 1 to 10 days
Typhoid Fever — 1 to 3 weeks
Typhus Fever — 5 to 15 days
Valley Fever — 1 to 3 weeks
Whooping Cough — 5 to 21 days, but usually fewer than 10
Yellow Fever — 3 to 6 days

incubator: a controlled-environment device designed to maintain stable temperature, humidity, oxygen, etc. — usually for a premature infant — and often equipped to monitor the child's vital functions; essentially, such a device is employed to tide the infant over until the baby is sufficiently developed to cope with the outside environment.

indication: a circumstance suggesting to the physician that a particular diagnostic or therapeutic procedure is required. Also see CONTRAINDICATION.

indigestion: See the specific symptom(s), as ABDOMINAL PAIN; DIARRHEA; etc.

Indocin, indomethacin: See ANTI-INFLAMMATORIES; the former is a trade name for the latter.

infantile paralysis: See POLIO.

infection: a condition caused by any of a number of microscopic organisms — bacteria, rickettsiae, viruses, fungi, protozoan parasites. A *local infection* is one involving only a small part of the body, such as a small cut, a tooth, a fingernail, or the outer ear. A *general,* or *systemic, infection* is one affecting several or many parts of the body, such as a cold or any of the infectious diseases. A local infection that goes untreated can *become* a general infection.

Warning signals of possible spreading infection in a wound or other apparently minor injury are redness or swelling; fever; and/or red or pink streaks radiating from the site of injury toward the center of the body (if, for example, it is a wrist injury, the streaks would be in the direction of the elbow, not toward the fingers).

infectious: describing diseases or other conditions stemming from infection (see the preceding entry), as opposed to some other cause such as heredity, structural malformation, glandular malfunction, nutritional deficiency, etc. An infectious disease or condition is not necessarily catching (see CONTAGIOUS).

infectious hepatitis: See HEPATITIS.

infectious mononucleosis: See MONONUCLEOSIS.

inferior: medically, not a quality judgment but an anatomical term meaning "lower," i.e., below or toward the feet.

inflammation: a term describing a condition, not the cause of the condition — which might be infection, injury, allergic reaction, etc. The tissue involved usually exhibits redness (from an influx of blood to the area) and swelling (from increased amounts of blood and lymph), and often there is pain (from the swollen tissue's pressure on nerve endings).

Most, though not all, words denoting inflammation end in *-itis,* and the first part of the word generally specifies the type of tissue or part of the body involved. Familiar examples are bronchitis (the bronchi, or bronchial tubes), colitis (the colon or large intestine), dermatitis (the skin), gastritis (the stomach), laryngitis (the larynx), otitis (the ear), tonsillitis (the tonsils).

influenza: that scourge we have all come to know and loathe, known familiarly as flu. The single word actually denotes a variety of ills, caused by two distinct viral strains that have been labeled A and B. (A now-outdated term, "grippe," was the same thing, generally implying a milder case.) Epidemics of the A strain seem — for unknown reasons — to stem primarily from the Orient; their appearances are highly unpredictable. The B strains — symptoms seem to vary a great deal, and in children may include a measles-like rash — typically attack every two to four years. Both strains have a nasty habit of mutating: undergoing structural changes that cancel out previously acquired immunity and send the virologists scurrying back to the labs to break down the new chemical structure — necessary for formulation of an effective vaccine.

HISTORY AND PEDIGREE

The first A-strain virus was isolated in 1933. A variant that caused the 1946–47 epidemic was designated A_1; another mutation appeared in the winter of 1957–58 and was dubbed A_2. The "Hong Kong" flu — so-called because that's where the virus was first identified — appeared in the winter of 1968–69; it struck at least one in four Americans and was responsible for some ten thousand deaths (chiefly indirectly — due not to the flu itself but to secondary infections).

Early in 1972, another A-strain mutation was discovered, this time a minor one. Like its predecessors, it first appeared in the Far East; but because it was isolated in Great Britain, it was named A/England/72. It arrived here in October of that year and by January had been officially declared epidemic. But there had been a breakthrough; a vaccine had been prepared. For that reason, and because the viral mutation was minor (many who had suffered through A/HK/68 were apparently immune), the "London flu" epidemic was far less severe than the outbreak of 1968–69.

Meanwhile, 1970–71 had seen sporadic outbreaks of the other flu strain in the northeast; the isolated virus was coded B/Mass./71. Early in 1973 still another B strain was reported, this time from Hong Kong, and labeled B/HK/72; pharmaceutical firms rushed to incorporate that strain in vaccines already in production. Vaccines including it were in short supply, and B-strain outbreaks were reported in at least twenty states.

In the interim, a new A wave had hit New Zealand and Australia, with isolated cases elsewhere; the new mutant strain was ultimately designated A/-Port Chalmers/73 and was incorporated in 1974 vaccines in this country. Another, A/Scotland/74, was isolated a year later, and still another, A/Victoria/75, the year after that. The latter arrived in this country, as expected, the following winter (1975–76); it caused sufficiently widespread illness to be termed epidemic in fifteen states. Two other minor variants, A/England/75 and A/Tokyo/75, failed to make significant inroads in the United States.

We've summed up, briefly, the pattern of flu attacks over a period of just a few years; it's typical. Each new variation demands new vaccine — which, in turn, raises new questions each year.

"SWINE FLU"

In 1976 an unexpected and disturbing event occurred, complicating the already complex flu situation: the discovery of a new — or, possibly, old — A-strain variant. It was isolated not in Australia or in some teeming Oriental seaport, but at a U.S. Army post in New Jersey. During the ensuing months, the press — both lay and medical — was filled with argument and speculation, much of it based on inaccurate and misleading information.

What happened, in brief: In early

February 1976, a young soldier at Fort Dix, believed suffering from "ordinary" flu (i.e., A/Victoria/75), collapsed and died of fulminating viral pneumonia. Routine investigation disclosed that the virus involved was not the Victoria strain, but a different one; it was subsequently isolated in eleven other sick soldiers, and shortly thereafter there was serological confirmation of exposure to the same mysterious virus in five hundred additional recruits.

Within weeks, the question of mass immunization was under intensive study by the Food and Drug Administration, the Center for Disease Control, and the National Institute of Allergy and Infectious Diseases, and the nation's leading virologists had been called into consultation. In late March, President Ford announced plans to begin immediate production of vaccine. By mid-April, clinical testing — necessary to establish effective dosages, responses, and reactions — had begun. Some writers observed pointedly and skeptically that it was, after all, an election year; they suggested that the expressed concern was cynical at best. They were mistaken. The worry was real.

The virus isolated at Fort Dix had not been seen before. It was, however, evidently more than "just another" A-strain variant.

For one thing, it was structurally similar to — though *not* identical with — a virus that causes a respiratory illness, much like human flu (but never fatal), in pigs; the latter is commonly known as "swine flu," hence the popular misnomer applied to the new human-flu virus. A few rare cases of flu transmitted from swine to humans had been reported. (It should be added that these have all involved human contact with live or just-slaughtered animals. The virus is found only in the respiratory tract, not in muscle tissue; pork products sold for human consumption cannot carry it.) But never before had there been person-to-person transmission of a virus contracted from an animal — *if* indeed the original source of the Fort Dix virus, officially designated A/New Jersey/76, *was* an infected pig.

Another fact, too, contributed heavily to the official concern. It had long been known that many Americans have antibodies to the "swine flu" virus, which had been isolated in the 1930s; these individuals were, almost invariably, born before 1925. There was a devastating influenza pandemic — tagged, at the time, "Spanish flu" — the winter of 1918–19; twenty million people died, including more than five hundred thousand Americans. No one knows what virus caused that worldwide catastrophe. But if it was something like the "swine flu" organism, that would explain the antibodies in older persons who had survived the 1918–19 pandemic, as well as the lack of immunity in those born later. Further, there was something special about that pandemic, unlike the situation in most flu epidemics: there was an extraordinarily high mortality rate among those between the ages of fifteen and fifty.

Experts concluded that there were four likely possibilities: A/New Jersey/76 (1) just happened, by sheer coincidence, to resemble the "swine flu" virus; (2) represented a mutation of that virus, with new characteristics that made possible person-to-person contagion; (3) was in fact the same virus responsible for the 1918–19 pandemic, dormant for nearly sixty years and suddenly, for unknown reasons, reactivated; or (4) was a hybrid, a genetic combination of the "swine flu" virus with the A/Victoria/75 strain. Whatever the explanation, one fact was clear: with so many unprotected, there existed the potential for an extremely critical situation the following winter. Hence, the decision to launch a nationwide campaign for mass immunization. (The vaccine decided upon was bivalent, combining A/Victoria/75 and A/New Jersey/76.)

No one can be sure, as this book goes to press, whether or not the threatened epidemic of 1976–77 will come to pass. But given the foregoing facts, there is no doubt that the decision to anticipate the possibility was wholly justified.

SHOTS: IF AND WHO

A problem for many people is the difference of opinion among physicians regarding use of flu vaccines (which are, according to various estimates, 70 to 90 percent effective). Some feel that only those at high risk of complications should receive vaccine: certain infants, persons suffering from chronic problems, those in constant contact with such individuals, and the aged; these doctors generally discourage shots for healthy people not in those categories. Other physicians, while giving high-risk patients priority, will provide vaccination for anyone who wants it. Both viewpoints are valid, and no binding consensus has been arrived at. Don't wait till December to discuss the question with your doctor; flu shots should be given by early November.

It should be added that there is one other protection, a prescription drug called amantadine. It is taken — at the first sign of an outbreak, if a nonimmunized person is at special risk — on a regular regimen which is continued for the duration of the epidemic; it is, however, specifically not considered desirable for small children.

IF/WHEN FLU STRIKES

The television commercials are, for once, reasonably accurate, at least in their depiction of symptoms. Flu may resemble a cold (and has a similar incubation period, from one to three days), with stuffy nose and sore throat, but may also include — depending upon the particular virus — fever, severe headache, and/or muscular pains. If your child contracts flu, the important thing is to keep resistance up and protect the child from other, more serious problems — secondary bacterial infections such as bronchitis or pneumonia. The child should be kept home and warm, fed a light but balanced diet, and given aspirin for general discomfort. Bed rest isn't essential, unless the child feels more comfortable there or has fairly high fever. Assuming there are no complications, the illness should be over in a few days, at most a week or two.

The foregoing advice is based on your certainty that flu is in fact what the child has; if you're in the least doubt, the doctor should be called to make the diagnosis. Additionally — even if you're positive it's flu — the doctor should be promptly consulted if the child has a fever of more than two degrees F. (one degree C.) or is in severe pain, if there are any symptoms whatever other than those we've mentioned, or if the youngster has a history of recurrent respiratory problems.

Antibiotics will have no effect against any flu virus. They may, however, be given if the doctor has determined that there is a secondary bacterial infection or if, in the physician's judgment in a particular case, it is advisable to anticipate such infection.

Also see REYE'S SYNDROME.

inguinal hernia: See HERNIA.

injection: the introduction of a substance — a vaccine, medication, or anesthetic — into the body via a hypodermic needle rather than by mouth or some other method. Sometimes this is done because immediate action is needed, and the substance can thus reach the bloodstream quickly — as, to counteract poison from a snakebite. Sometimes it is done not because there is a rush, but in order to avoid the digestive juices, which would dissolve the particular substance before it could get into the system. Sometimes, a medication is injected because the physician wants to be positive it gets into the patient, rather than counting on a prescription's being filled and the medication later administered at home. And sometimes, that's the only form in which the medication is available.

injuries: See the specific type, as BURNS; CUTS; FRACTURES; HEAD INJURIES; etc.

inoculations: See IMMUNIZATION.

insect bites: See the appropriate section under BITES AND STINGS.

insecticides: See PESTICIDES.

in situ: a Latin phrase literally meaning "in position," which by implication means *original* position; medically, it may be used two ways. One is in denoting the restoration to position of something that has been displaced (e.g., a dislocated bone or knocked-out tooth) or the placement of something (e.g., a pin holding broken bone ends together) in proper position. The phrase may also describe a condition or lesion that is confined to its initial site and has not spread to other areas — as a malignant growth that has not metastasized.

insomnia: If a child can't seem to fall asleep — or complains of being unable to sleep — there could be any number of causes; we suggest here just some that you should check for before you call the doctor.

The child — especially a very young one — might be overtired, a keyed-up state resulting from a full and exciting day plus staying up past the usual bedtime. There might be some unusual condition — the temperature in the room, or lightness or darkness — that is disturbing. Children do tend to need less sleep as they get older; perhaps it's time to stop afternoon naps, or to set the youngster's bedtime a little later. Do try to determine if the child has any discomfort or pain; if so, turn to the appropriate listing to see what can or should be done about it. If the child is a teenager, consider the possibility of experimentation with some stimulant type of drug (see AMPHETAMINES; DIET PILLS; PSYCHEDELICS).

Should the insomnia persist all night, or should the child have difficulty falling asleep night after night (and you've eliminated the possibilities suggested), then do consult your physician. If the doctor feels a sedative is advisable, be sure to follow the prescribed dosage exactly, and do *not* continue the medication for more than a week without further discussion with the doctor.

inspiration: medically, simply the act of breathing in; its opposite is *expiration.*

insulin: a hormone, necessary for the utilization of carbohydrates, secreted by part of the pancreas. It is also manufactured and used in the treatment of glandular malfunction involving carbohydrate metabolism; see DIABETES MELLITUS.

insulin shock: See DIABETES MELLITUS; SHOCK THERAPY.

insurance, health: See HEALTH INSURANCE.

Intal: a trade name for cromolyn sodium; see ASTHMA.

intelligence testing: It should not be taken to heart. The results tend to be, in children, extremely misleading, since they can vary depending upon the books the child has read, his mood of the moment, whether or not he has a cold in the nose, and so on. There is, in fact, no real "intelligence test" in existence; all such tests, while their intentions are perfectly good, of necessity measure knowledge, and reasoning power based on command of language and certain abstract concepts, against a pre-established "average."

We hope that someday a true intelligence test may be devised. You should know, as a parent, that none now exists — and that while high scores on present tests probably indicate high intelligence (i.e., ability to accumulate knowledge and to follow prescribed reasoning methods), low scores do not necessarily indicate low intelligence or lack of potential. *No* child's intelligence can ever be *lower* than such a test score indicates, but it may quite possibly be *higher.*

IQ figures — the letters stand for intelligence quotient — do not denote quantitative measures of intelligence but rank relative to a hypothetical "average." The latter is arbitrarily assigned the number 100. Thus, a child whose IQ is judged on the basis of the aforementioned testing to be, for example, 110 is deemed somewhat more intelligent than average.

intensive care: super-specialized, constant nursing and medical care for a hospitalized patient who is seriously ill or is recovering from major surgery. The patient's condition is carefully and continuously monitored, and all the latest medical and nursing techniques are instantly available.

interferon: a protein substance produced by the body in response to viral attack; its potential to prevent and/or treat such attack, and to prevent complications of viral infections, is presently being explored.

intern: an individual you may meet in a hospital. He or she is an M.D., having graduated from an accredited medical school, and is now acquiring practical experience, under the direction of higher-ranking physicians, in the various facets of medical care. For the next step in medical training, see RESIDENT.

internist: a physician specializing in the practice of *internal medicine;* see SPECIALTIES, MEDICAL.

intertrigo: probably the most widespread skin disorder occurring in infants and very small children, according to published estimates by dermatological authorities; the rest of us know it as diaper rash. See that entry for full discussion.

intestinal flu: a general phrase for a viral infection of the stomach and/or intestines. Like "regular" flu, this kind of infection can occur in waves — not sufficient to be termed epidemics, but enough for physicians and lay people alike to conclude, at those times, that it's "going around." It's definitely spread by omitting thorough handwashing after bowel movements, and many physicians now feel that it may be transmitted by droplet infection as well.

The infection typically lasts a day or two, whence its popular characterizations as the "24-hour virus" or "48-hour virus." Symptoms may vary somewhat but usually include nausea and/or vomiting, diarrhea, and cramps, any one of which may be the first symptom; the onset is usually quite sudden. Sometimes there are headache and slight fever, as well.

Do notify the doctor if you suspect intestinal flu. It's true that antibiotics and similar drugs won't work, but the doctor *can* prescribe medications that will make the child feel a good deal better, such as relaxants to stop painful cramps. Your doctor will advise you, too, about the child's diet, and may want you to limit it to certain foods until the problem clears up, or even to withhold food entirely for a brief period.

intestinal obstruction: the prevention of normal passage of material through the intestine. If a physician uses this term, it does *not* necessarily mean that some object or growth is causing the obstruction; there are a number of other possibilities including adhesions, kinked intestinal muscle, hernia, worms, etc. Symptoms may vary considerably, as may treatment, depending upon the doctor's determination of the cause.

A *volvulus* is a specific type of obstruction involving a twist in the intestine; why it occurs is generally unknown, but when it does, it is considered an emergency situation and usually requires surgery.

A special, critical type of intestinal obstruction that can afflict infants is discussed separately; see INTUSSUSCEPTION.

intestines: the flexible tube — or, more accurately, series of tubes — through which food passes, and is processed, between the stomach and the rectum. The small intestine, the first part of the passageway, includes the duodenum, the jejunum, and the ileum; the large intestine or colon includes the cecum, ascending, transverse, and descending segments, and the sigmoid (S-shaped) final section.

Peristalsis is the medical term for the normal contractions of the intestines that push food through the passageway. If the movement of the intestines is visible through the skin of a child's abdomen, it often indicates something is wrong, and you should call the doctor; this is especially so if there are other symptoms such as vomiting, diarrhea, constipation, or apparent pain.

intravenous feeding: feeding by injecting a solution of nutrients directly into the bloodstream. This technique is employed when a patient is unconscious or unable to eat by mouth, or when the physician decides it is inadvisable (because of some problem in the digestive tract, for example) to feed the patient by mouth.

intussusception: a particular type of intestinal obstruction in which part of the passage — usually at the junction of the small and large intestines — suddenly collapses and telescopes into the following section, thus blocking the intestine and causing a great deal of pain. Sometimes a definite reason, such as a rupture or sudden strain, can be pinpointed, but in most cases there seems to be no determinable cause.

The afflicted infant (it occurs chiefly in children under a year of age) will be in obvious distress, howling and drawing the knees up; the abdomen will be distended; there may be vomiting and a discharge of blood-stained mucus from the rectum. Intussusception is an acute medical emergency. If you suspect this condition and you cannot reach your own doctor immediately, the baby should be rushed to the nearest hospital. In some instances, the intussusception can be corrected by a barium enema; if not, prompt surgery is essential.

iodine: an essential mineral in the diet; see NUTRITION.

iodine, tincture of: an antiseptic, but not a particularly good one; furthermore, it burns the skin and is toxic if accidentally swallowed. Don't have it in your home.

Ionamin: a trade name for phentermine; see DIET PILLS.

ipecac: See EMETIC.

Ipral: a trade name for probarbital; see SEDATIVES.

ipsilateral: on the same side (of the body).

IQ: short for intelligence quotient; see INTELLIGENCE TESTING.

iridocyclitis: an eye disorder occasionally accompanying juvenile rheumatoid arthritis; see ARTHRITIS.

iritis: an inflammation of the iris of the eye; it's quite rare. If your regular doctor finds this condition, you will doubtless be referred to an ophthalmologist, who must treat it.

iron: one of the essential minerals in the diet. See ANEMIA; NUTRITION.

irradiation: the use of rays — X rays are often implied, but the word may refer to light or heat rays as well — in diagnosis or therapy, especially the latter.

irrigation: washing out of an area (e.g., a wound or a body cavity) with flowing water or other liquid.

isocarboxazid: See ANTIDEPRESSANTS.

isoniazid: an antituberculosis drug.

itching: a minor symptom of a number of things; the medical term for it is pruritus. The first thing to do is to try to find the cause, if it's not already apparent.

Itching typically accompanies a number of skin problems (see the cross-references at the end of this entry), as well as the rash of such diseases as chickenpox, and certain vaccinations, notably that for smallpox; in the latter instances, where the cause can't be eliminated, discuss with your doctor the possibility of giving the child antihistamines to temper the reaction.

A small child's itching in the vicinity of the anus — or, in a girl, the vagina — may signal the existence of pinworms, especially if the itching consistently occurs at night; see WORMS. Vaginal itch in a girl who has passed puberty can signal another kind of difficulty; see MONILIASIS.

All-over itching may sometimes result from a simple lack of humidity in the air; this kind of itching can usually be relieved by immersing the child for a while in a cool-to-lukewarm tub of water with enough cornstarch or baking soda to cloud the water noticeably.

Some people tend to have mild itching around the site of a nearly healed wound in the process of scar formation; a little calamine lotion usually relieves it.

The most important thing to remember about any itching, whatever the cause, is: *don't let the child scratch.* Scratching can, and often does, cause serious infection. In addition to doing whatever you can to relieve the itch, cut the child's fingernails as short as possible.

If you can't either relieve or determine the cause of persistent itching, take the child to the doctor.

For some common causes of itching, see ALLERGY; ATHLETE'S FOOT; BITES AND STINGS; COLD SORE; CONJUNCTIVITIS; DANDRUFF; HEAT RASH; IMPETIGO; LICE; PITYRIASIS; POISON IVY; RINGWORM; SCABIES.

IUD: See CONTRACEPTION.

IVP: short for intravenous pyelogram, an X-ray examination of the urinary tract. It is performed by a radiologist or urologist, who instills a radio-opaque dye into a vein. The dye is then excreted by the kidneys and, in repeated films, gives excellent indication of the function and position of the various parts of the tract.

J

Jacksonian seizure: See EPILEPSY.

jaundice: a yellowish cast to the skin and whites of the eyes, also known medically as *icterus.* It is usually symptomatic of some problem involving the liver, gallbladder, or red blood cells; among the diseases and disorders that may (or may not) include jaundice are hepatitis, gallstones, yellow fever, and some types of anemia. If you believe your child has jaundice, you should take him to the doctor, who will probably want stool and urine specimens and will want to perform blood tests.

For an explanation of the mechanism of jaundice, see BILE. Also see, for a nonserious condition that shouldn't be confused with jaundice, CAROTENEMIA.

There is also a condition, called for lack of a better term "physiological jaundice," that is related to neither of the above; it occurs, specifically, in newborn babies — probably in at least half — starting about the third day after birth. The prenatal circulation contains more hemoglobin than is needed after birth. By about the third day, the destruction of those extra red blood cells begins, forming products that may make the baby appear jaundiced. Generally a bilirubin level is obtained to make sure the baby is all right, which is almost invariably the case. We add this reassurance for new parents, because young, inexperienced interns in hospitals tend to become unduly upset by this phenomenon.

jaw, broken: See FRACTURES.

jejunum: See INTESTINES.

jellyfish stings: See BITES AND STINGS.

"joint mouse": a loose fragment of bone or other calcified material within a joint, usually associated with some degree of inflammation; such a fragment can sometimes cause the joint to "lock."

joints: The body, you're doubtless aware, has a number of them. Some, such as the joining of the bones in the skull, are immovable, at least after infancy. Others, such as those in the spine, are slightly movable. Most are definitely movable, in a variety of ways: the knees, fingers, etc., are hinge joints, operating more or less like a door, as are the temperomandibular joints — TMJs, for short — at the sides of the lower jaw; the elbow joint has a pivotal action; the hips and shoulders are freely rotating ball-and-socket joints. All the movable ones have something in them to facilitate movement — disks of cartilage in the spine, connecting tissues and lubricants in the others.

Any pain or lack of mobility in a joint means that you should take the child to the doctor without delay; there are many situations in which continued use of the joint, without treatment, could cause the development of a much more serious condition.

For some of the disorders that can involve joints, see ARTHRITIS; BURSITIS; CLUBFOOT; DEFICIENCY DISEASES; DENGUE; DISLOCATION; EPIPHYSIS; FRACTURES; KNEE INJURIES; LEGG-PERTHES DISEASE; LUPUS; OSGOOD-SCHLATTER'S DISEASE; RUBELLA; SPRAINS; SYNOVITIS.

jugular: See BLOOD VESSELS.

K

Kafocin: a trade name for cephaloglycin; see ANTIBIOTICS.

kanamycin, Kantrex: See ANTIBIOTICS; the latter is a trade name for the former.

kaolin: a drug that acts on the inner surface of the intestines to absorb fluid and control diarrhea.

Kaopectate: a trade name for a product containing kaolin (preceding) and other ingredients. Do not give this or any similar product to your child without consulting your doctor.

karyotyping: the technical term for chromosomal analysis.

Keflex, Keflin, Kefzol: trade names for, respectively, cephalexin, cephalothin, and cefazolin; see ANTIBIOTICS.

keloids: See SCARS.

Kenacort: See CORTICOSTEROIDS.

keratitis: inflammation of the cornea as a result of injury, infection, overexposure to sun, etc.; the last, called *actinic keratitis,* is discussed under EYE INJURIES.

keratosis: an overgrowth and thickening of the outer, horny layer of the skin; it may look like a wart or a raised mole. A *seborrheic keratosis* is round and slightly elevated, and usually tends to get thicker and darker; it is, however, benign. A keratosis isn't serious, but it can resemble things that are, and you should leave the diagnosis to a dermatologist.

This type of growth can be removed and often is, chiefly for cosmetic reasons; removal is a relatively simple doctor's-office procedure.

Kesso-Pen: a trade name for penicillin G; see ANTIBIOTICS.

ketosis: a particular type of acidosis (a serious condition of overacidity in the bloodstream) involving a surplus of chemical compounds called ketone bodies; it signals a drastic disturbance in the normal chemical and water balance of the body, and the characteristic symptom is a vinegar-like smell to the breath. Ketosis may sometimes be a potential threat in diabetes, and if you have a diabetic child, you may be asked to check his urine periodically for excess ketones as well as for sugar.

kg: See KILOGRAM.

kidney infections: See NEPHRITIS; PYELITIS; PYELONEPHRITIS.

kidney stones: solid precipitations from the urine, formed in the kidney by the merging of tiny crystals of solid matter normally excreted; they may cause pain, and may also obstruct the flow of urine and damage the urinary passages by their roughness. Kidney stones may sometimes be small enough to be passed; in other instances, they must be removed surgically. It is believed that certain foods may precipitate the formation of kidney stones in susceptible individuals, and after the immediate problem has been dealt with, the doctor may recommend special dietary measures to help prevent future problems.

The condition is fairly rare in children.

kilogram: the unit of weight used in most of the rest of the world, and already employed in many U.S. hospitals that have switched to the metric system; it is equal to 2.204 pounds. To convert kilograms (abbreviated *kg*) to pounds, multiply by that number; to convert pounds to kilograms, divide by it.

Klebsiella: a genus of bacilli (see BACTERIA) often involved in urinary-tract infections — especially cystitis — as well as in pneumonia; it is among those bacteria normally found in the intestinal tract.

Klinefelter's syndrome: a congenital disorder in which a boy has received an extra X chromosome that somehow wandered away from its own egg or sperm cell at the time of fertilization and joined the developing embryo; the chromosomal pattern is thus XXY instead of the usual XY. It is probably the most common sex-chromosome abnormality, occurring at least once in every thousand — according to some estimates, once in every five hundred — male births.

Often, Klinefelter's becomes evident only at puberty, since the major effect is on sexual development: the testes are unusually small and fail to produce sperm, secondary sex characteristics — facial hair, etc. — may not emerge or do not develop fully, and body contours may not be typically male. (There may in some cases be personality disorders which lead to medical consultation earlier. And there are uncommon variants of Klinefelter's — XXXY and XXXXY — in which hypospadias is present at birth, a circumstance that may suggest the desirability of karyotyping at that time; see HYPOSPADIAS for further comment.)

At whatever age Klinefelter's syndrome is diagnosed, it is treated by administration of male hormones and, if necessary, psychiatric or psychological consultation.

Also see SEX CHROMOSOMES.

knee injuries: Any knee injury — a twist, sprain, or anything else — should be seen by a physician; it's not difficult to tear cartilage or ligaments in a severe twist of the knee, and if the youngster keeps walking on the leg, the tissues can be damaged further. A minor tear in cartilage can be corrected by surgery, and there is no permanent damage; so can torn ligaments, but both the surgery and recuperation from it are more complicated.

An unexplained pain in a knee also calls for a prompt visit to the doctor. Knees are subject to a number of inflammations and other ills — and a pain in the knee can also be the first signal of a problem elsewhere; see LEGG-PERTHES DISEASE.

If you suspect a child has a broken kneecap, see FRACTURES for first-aid measures.

knife wounds: What to do depends upon the nature and location of the wound. If the knife has made a slash, turn to CUTS. If the knife point has gone straight in, see PUNCTURE WOUNDS. If there is extensive hemorrhaging, see BLEEDING for first-aid measures. And if the wound is in the chest or abdomen, whatever its nature, rush the victim to the nearest hospital emergency room.

knock-knees: a condition in which the knees are bent inward, the toes usually turned out; it is typically a result of rickets (see DEFICIENCY DISEASES) but can also be caused, on occasion, by weak ligaments. If the problem is recognized early, it can generally be corrected by braces or special shoes; in an older youngster surgery may be needed. Your doctor will probably refer you to an orthopedist for consultation and treatment.

Koplik spots: See MEASLES.

Krebiozen: an alleged "cure" for cancer that has been found by experts to be totally worthless. Many cancers are now legitimately curable in early stages, and precious time (as well as money) can be lost by those who fall prey to the unscrupulous promoters of untested "miracle drugs."

kwashiorkor: a condition caused by severe lack of dietary protein; see DEFICIENCY DISEASES.

L

labial adhesions: a congenital condition involving inability of the labia minora (the inner folds or "lips" at the entrance of the vagina) to separate, because of bands of fibrous tissue between them. Usually, the bands break spontaneously during childhood, but if this hasn't occurred as puberty approaches, the separation must be done surgically in order to permit menstruation.

labyrinthitis: an inflammation of the inner ear, involving the intricate structures that are responsible for a normal sense of balance. There is usually some hearing loss, but the telltale symptoms are serious disturbances in balance and coordination; the youngster will be dizzy, will have difficulty in keeping physical perspective and judging distance, and may have the frightening impression that tall buildings are tilting toward him.

Treatment of the condition depends upon the cause, which can vary; among the possibilities are bacterial or viral infections, tumors, cysts, and allergic reactions.

laceration: a general term, used more in news reports and court cases than in doctors' offices, for a wound involving torn skin. See CUTS; SCRAPES AND SCRATCHES.

lactose: the disaccharide found in milk; this and other sugars are discussed under SWEETENERS.

Laetrile: an alleged cancer "cure" deemed by the Food and Drug Administration to be totally worthless, and outlawed in the United States and Canada since 1963. The drug, an extract of apricot pits, is still being produced and promoted, at this writing, in Mexico and some European countries; while it is not known to be specifically harmful, knowledgeable experts have warned of the danger of substituting such a useless nostrum for medically tested therapy.

laparotomy: a general term for any surgical procedure involving incision into the abdomen.

Larotid: a trade name for amoxicillin, a semisynthetic penicillin; see ANTIBIOTICS.

laryngitis: an inflammation of the larynx, or "voice box"; it usually, though not always, occurs in conjunction with a cold or sore throat — and sometimes signals a general throat infection. Symptoms are hoarseness (or even an inability to speak above a whisper), scratchiness, a dry cough, perhaps some discomfort in swallowing; there may or may not be fever, and the child may not even feel unwell. Nevertheless, you should consult a physician so that the infection can be diagnosed and treated.

There is a more serious form of laryngitis that can afflict very small children; see CROUP.

laryngologist: See SPECIALTIES, MEDICAL.

larynx: a more or less cylindrical structure in the neck, above the windpipe, defined by cartilage shields (one is the "Adam's apple"); it contains the vocal cords, two bands of tissue that vibrate to make the sounds used in talking, singing, etc. It is also referred to as the "voice box."

The larynx is sometimes subject to inflammation; see LARYNGITIS. Its growth can also cause minor difficulties for adolescent boys; see VOICE CHANGING.

lateral: toward the side, away from the midline of the body; the word is often used in differentiating similar structures succinctly (as, "upper left lateral incisor") or locating something precisely (as, "on the lateral surface of the right thigh").

lavage: You are likely to hear this term preceded by the word "gastric." It is commonly referred to as having one's stomach washed out, which just about says it.

laxative: See CATHARTIC.

lead poisoning: If your toddler has just gulped down a handful of paint chips or some other substance containing lead, turn to POISONING, HOUSEHOLD SUBSTANCES AND MEDICATIONS. What we shall discuss here is the chronic problem.

As you have doubtless heard, lead poisoning is a notorious killer and maimer of small children. The problem has been most prevalent in city slums where uncaring landlords have permitted rundown conditions that include flaking paint and plaster; the poisonous substance is white lead, present in much old paint and plaster as well as in some types of putty used around windowpanes. But these are not the *only* sources of lethal lead, as we shall shortly point out.

Lead poisoning — or as it is technically termed, plumbism — is a particularly insidious sort of poisoning. Its effects are usually cumulative rather than sudden, and symptoms — which may include fatigue, irritability, vomiting, fever, and/or convulsions — may appear only after a child has ingested the lead-containing material over a period of days, weeks, or even months. Once symptoms have appeared, more serious damage may already have occurred. The toxin strikes at brain cells, and causes both physical and mental impairment, including anemia, behavior disorders, and mental retardation.

If you do not live in a city slum, don't assume that this automatically precludes any possibility of lead poisoning from paint and other structural materials. A great many paints sold and used prior to 1960 were high in lead — meaning that underlayers of housepaint, as well as paint on secondhand furniture, may still have a high lead content; some paint still on store shelves may also be high in lead.

To be on the safe side, as far as paints go, we suggest the following:

• scrape down and repaint interiors if you come into possession of an old house, barn that you'll convert to living quarters, etc. — making sure that small children are not present during the scraping process, and that adults who are wear some sort of protection (lead poisoning will not cause grown-ups to become mentally retarded — not so far as is known, anyway — but it can make them very, very sick);

• scrape down and repaint any secondhand furniture or toys that will be used by a child young enough to nibble on things — of course including any infant furniture such as cribs or rockers;

• when purchasing paint for the aforementioned refinishing, see that it conforms to current federal standards (applying to any paints shipped by manufacturers in or after 1974), which mandate a maximum lead content of 0.06 percent in paint intended for indoor use (check the label — "lead-free" is even better);

• when purchasing either paints or painted toys for small children, make sure the label specifies that the paint is nontoxic;

• if you happen to be the tenant of an individual who has shown an unfeeling attitude about the dangers of the premises to your children, *agitate.*

There are also, as we noted earlier, a number of other sources of potential lead poisoning to which small children may be exposed, which may not require their active cooperation (as, nibbling something in their vicinity); some may affect adults, as well.

It has been pretty well established, at this point, that leaded gasoline can release enough of the substance into the atmosphere to create dangerous concentrations of lead — not especially for adults, or even for older children, but for those small children whose height brings them closer to the exhaust-discharge level. One report by the Federal Environmental Protection Administration calculated that a child swallowing ten teaspoonfuls of dust within a hundred feet of a "busy roadway" (turnpike? city street?) over an eight-month period would very likely become a victim of lead poisoning. It is certainly advisable to see that your small child does not play in such an atmosphere, and to support all efforts to diminish that particular source of atmospheric pollution.

Another source of lead poisoning of which you should be aware is earthenware (ceramics, pottery, other dinnerware). The hazard is not high in ordinary American-made, commercially sold ware; both the U.S. Potters Association and the National Ceramic Manufacturers Association maintain continuing programs to guard against it, including control of glaze content and assurance of proper manufacturing methods. The industry is federally monitored as well, and there is also a surveillance program covering imported dinnerware.

Nevertheless, some danger still exists — as a number of reports in recent years have testified. They have generally involved pottery purchased from small shops or roadside craftsmen, wares produced at home by hobbyists, or sometimes imported ware; a number of the latter cases have involved foreign-made wares (especially bowls) used for promotion by American food (especially cereal) manufacturers.

It's probably best to avoid buying such housewares. If you're a hobbyist, you should buy and use only glazes carrying labels verifying approval by the National Ceramic Manufacturers Association, and be sure, as well, that your application and firing procedures are correct (the NCMA's booklet on the subject should be available from craft dealers).

Should you have some of these objects on the premises, be aware that there is a truly serious danger of poisoning if they come in contact with any acidic food; toxic metals in glazes are not water soluble but are leached (dissolved) by acids. Acid substances include all fruit juices and soft drinks, wines, cider, vinegar, sauerkraut, and anything containing tomatoes. Although the Food and Drug Administration has officially stated that there is no danger in using such wares for quick serving, or in storing nonacidic foods in them, it seems preferable to avoid them altogether.

We've mentioned the building you live in, your child's toys, the air near ground level, and some of the contents of your kitchen cupboards. More? Yes, more.

The following items have also been implicated, over the last few years, as agents conveying excessive lead content to small children who have been inclined to nibble on them, as small children are wont to do upon almost anything: wrappers around confections from bakeries and frozen-food departments in supermarkets; color-printed sections of Sunday newspapers, notably magazine sections and comics; old pewterware (it doesn't matter what kind of food is kept in them — old pewter salt shakers, for example, are 80 percent lead); house dust in areas assaulted by high levels of lead pollution from traffic and other sources; some toothpaste tubes (a study reported in 1973); pencils (not the "lead," which isn't lead but graphite, but the paint on the outside); can-sealing materials for evaporated milk.

If you suspect that your child may be suffering from the effects of lead poisoning, lose no time in getting the child to your physician, a hospital, or your local health department for diagnosis. Treatment is speedy and simple: the child is given a medication that precipitates the lead out of the bloodstream, changing it to a harmless substance that is excreted. Be sure to take steps to remove the toxic substance from your home in order to prevent repetition.

Also see PICA, a condition that is sometimes a contributory factor in lead poisoning.

learning disability: a descriptive phrase for difficulty in, or lack of ability to keep up with, school work that is specifically not due to low intelligence, mental retardation, or emotional disorders (although it might create emotional problems); it is sometimes associated with detectable perceptual aberrations — e.g., the child, while passing standard vision and hearing tests, does not see, or does not hear, exactly the way other children do. It is essentially a facet of another "umbrella" entity; see MINIMAL BRAIN DYSFUNCTION.

LE cell: See LUPUS.

Ledercillin: a trade name for penicillin V; see ANTIBIOTICS.

lefthandedness: See DEVELOPMENT.

leg, broken: See FRACTURES.

Legg-Perthes disease: an aseptic

(noninfectious) necrosis (disintegration) of the upper end of the femur, or thigh bone, in which the head of the bone softens and yields to pressure; it is also known as Calvé-Legg-Perthes disease, or simply as Perthes disease (all three names are those of physicians who were among the first to describe the condition).

This disease is a mysterious one, even in medical circles. Its cause is completely unknown. It may strike, without warning, at any age between one and fourteen, although most of its victims are in the four-to-eight age group; some 85 percent of them are boys. In nine out of ten cases, the condition is unilateral.

There have been few studies of its incidence, but it is probably more widespread than is generally supposed. Based on reported cases only, the U.S. attack rate for the susceptible age group is estimated as at least one in 1200 (one in 740 for boys) — a figure that makes your youngster now some 640 times more likely to be a victim of Legg-Perthes than of polio. The figure may in fact be substantially higher; the important, and often elusive, factor is diagnosis of the condition, so that many — perhaps even most — cases are never discovered and reported.

Legg-Perthes generally begins with a slight limp. There may be a little pain in the hip joint itself, in the thigh, at the back of the knee, or even, rarely, in the foot. Unfortunately, the problem is often dismissed, by physicians who are unfamiliar with the disease, as simple muscle strain. Proper diagnosis requires X ray, and if you suspect that your child may have Legg-Perthes, you should insist on having X rays taken so that treatment, if necessary, can be started promptly.

It's true that the condition is never fatal, and that over a period of time it will spontaneously disappear; the usual pattern is a year (more or less) of degeneration of the bone, a similar period in which the condition stabilizes, and a third phase in which the bone is rebuilt and repaired and becomes normally hard again. There is, at this writing, no medication or treatment that can halt the first phase or hasten the third; surgery is possible but isn't generally recommended.

Treatment is important, however. It consists of removing weight from that leg, to prevent the softened bone from being pressed out of shape, and the child must use a brace, crutches, or similar device for a time. Treatment can be tedious and annoying to parent and child alike, but if these measures aren't taken, there is a strong possibility of malformation of the bone resulting in permanent deformity, as well as a chance of severe arthritis later in life. If the condition is recognized and treated, the youngster will recover with no ill effects whatever.

In the 10 percent of cases that involve both legs, surgery on at least one— generally involving bone graft — may be recommended in order to get the child on his feet (complete bed rest would be the only alternative), so that he won't miss months or years of schooling.

There are similar (and similarly mysterious) conditions affecting other bones, notably the upper end of the tibia; see OSGOOD-SCHLATTER'S DISEASE.

leishmaniasis: See PARASITES.

leprosy: See HANSEN'S DISEASE.

leptospirosis: an infection of animals — domestic ones in particular — caused by a type of bacterium called Leptospira. It is communicable to humans via the urine of infected animals, and typically produces a flulike illness but sometimes extremely critical inflammations of the kidneys, heart, or other organs. It is best avoided by seeing that dogs and farm animals are vaccinated against it, and by making sure your children never wade or swim in a pond that might be contaminated by susceptible animals.

Leritine: a trade name for anileridine, a morphinelike synthetic drug; see NARCOTICS.

lesion: broadly, any change in tissue or structure — some condition that shouldn't normally be present, whatever its cause. Thus a mosquito bite, a rash, a cut, or a break in a bone could all be called lesions. The word is most commonly used, however, to refer to skin conditions, and a physician will often use further descriptive terms to characterize the type of lesion; there are three of these you might encounter.

A *papule* is a circumscribed elevation, which may or may not be inflamed — such as a pimple or an ordinary insect bite.

A *vesicle,* which may develop from a papule, may be of any shape, and contains fluid of some sort; a lay person would most likely describe it as a blister. Vesicles are characteristic, for example, of poison ivy.

A *pustule* is the most serious of the three types, since it denotes an infection; it is a lesion filled with pus, and is usually yellowish and surrounded by inflammation. A boil is a familiar example of a pustule.

leucorrhea: See VAGINAL DISCHARGE.

leukemia: cancer of the blood-forming organs; it is the most frequent malignancy in children (though *not* a common illness in youngsters generally; see CANCER); leukemia accounts for about three out of ten malignancies in childhood. Although we shall use the singular here, there are in fact a number of distinct forms; in children, the major one is called *acute lymphocytic leukemia* (ALL).

There is a very strong suspicion of viral cause in leukemia, and it is already known that a particular virus can cause leukemia in cats (it's a different type, *not* communicable to humans) and that in some laboratory animals, vaccines can prevent the disease. It's believed that the cause of human leukemia will be pinpointed in the foreseeable future.

The onset of leukemia is insidious, the symptoms extremely vague; ALL has often been called the "great imitator," because its early symptoms can mimic almost anything — and, of course, vice versa. Typical manifestations might include one or more of these, all very common in a host of other conditions: unexplained fever, paleness, persistent respiratory infection, loss of appetite, fatigue, and irritability. And/or, less frequently: headache, joint pains, apparent bruises unexplained by injury, vomiting, swollen lymph nodes — all, again, much more commonly symptomatic of less serious conditions.

If leukemia is suspected on the basis of symptoms and examination of the child, the diagnosis must be confirmed by both blood counts and microscopic examination of bone marrow. These tests are necessary in order to exclude the many other ills that can simulate leukemia; the list includes mononucleosis (with which it has often been confused), anemia arising from other causes, tonsillitis, various rheumatic conditions, meningitis, mumps, other infections, and other malignancies.

Surgery is, of course, out of the question in leukemia, since it is by definition a disseminated disease; therapy now usually includes combinations of drugs and possibly irradiation as well. The prognosis is vastly better than it used to be — and parents of a child with leukemia who have read Dr. Ronald Glasser's novel, *Ward 402,* should be aware that the case of ALL described in that book is *not typical,* although it might have been in the 1950s or even the '60s. Most victims of the disease do *not,* like the young heroine of the book, succumb within months of diagnosis. In fact, it should not now be assumed that they must succumb at all. While recovery is by no means guaranteed, the odds have swung to favor young leukemia victims: in the '50s, the five-year survival rate (the statistical odds on at *least* that survival time) was estimated as no more than 25 percent, among even the most optimistic; the figure is now well over 60 percent and is improving steadily — to the extent that recent research reports are referring to *ten*-year survival rates and tentatively using the word "cured."

Parents of leukemia patients should be aware of another facet of the disease. The malignancy specifically involves the production of abnormal white cells. These tend to "take over" the bloodstream from the normal white cells, red cells, and platelets — the chief functions of which are, respectively, protection against infection, transport of oxygen, and normal blood clotting. A child with leukemia is thus unusually subject to — and should be guarded against — infections, malfunction of organs because of lack of oxygen (*any* unusual symptoms should be instantly reported to the doctor), and bleeding episodes (risky sports or crafts are unwise).

leukocytosis: an increase, demonstrated by a blood test, in the number of white blood cells, generally a sign of infection somewhere in the body; it may be one of several factors considered by the physician in making a diagnosis. It does *not* necessarily indicate leukemia (see preceding entry).

leukopenia: an abnormal reduction in the number of white blood cells, a condition that can occur in a number of situations, including some allergic reactions and certain — chiefly viral — infections.

leukorrhea: a variant spelling of *leucorrhea;* see VAGINAL DISCHARGE.

Levo-Dromoran, levorphanol: a morphinelike synthetic drug; the former is a trade name for the latter. See NARCOTICS.

Levoprome: a trade name for methotrimeprazine, a nonopiate but narcotic analgesic; see NARCOTICS.

levulose: another name for fructose, a primary sugar; see SWEETENERS.

Librium: a trade name for chlordiazepoxide, a tranquilizer and muscle relaxant; see SEDATIVES.

lice, body: We discuss two distinct types here. The kind generally referred to simply as "body lice" actually live not on the body, but in clothing; they emerge onto the body to feed (i.e., suck blood) every few hours. One bite may not be noticeable, but a series of bites will create a hives-like condition that's extremely itchy (but mustn't be scratched, since a secondary infection can easily be created). De-lousing with various insecticides or discarding the clothing are the only remedies. Be aware, too, if you've picked up such an infestation on travels through Europe, Africa, or Asia, that lice carry diseases, and a medical checkup is in order (see RELAPSING FEVER; TYPHUS FEVER).

Crab lice — so-called because that's what they resemble — are a different species. They infest coarse body hair; this may be eyebrows, armpit hair, or beards, but is usually pubic hair, and the lice are usually acquired by intimate contact. If there's an itch in that area, the presence of lice can be ascertained by checking with an ordinary magnifying glass; the lice themselves move about on and feed from the skin, the female attaching her eggs to the hairs. The condition is easily and quickly dealt with by any physician.

We feel obliged to add — because a number of readers apparently read this entry in our first edition quickly and, unfortunately, a bit carelessly — that "usually acquired by intimate contact" means just that. It *doesn't* mean *always.* Other documented modes of acquisition include borrowed clothing, bedding, sleeping bags, and ill-kept public restroom facilities. Someone consulting a physician for this problem is not, ipso facto, admitting to any socially (or parentally) condemned activity.

lice, head: They are a different variety of the body-louse species. The first symptom of their presence is severe itching; it's caused by a histaminic reaction to products released in the skin by the insect's bite. Nits (eggs) may be visible, attached to the hair.

Don't let the child scratch; that can create a secondary infection. If you know or suspect that your youngster has head lice, *do* consult the doctor promptly. There's no need to feel ashamed. The condition is common in schools, camps, and other places where children congregate; there's no implication of poor hygiene or neglect on your part. Your physician will be able to prescribe medication to get rid of the infestation fast.

It's wise, too, if you discover that a youngster has head lice, to examine all other members of the family as well as the child's regular playmates. And all combs and brushes in the family should be sterilized by boiling, or discarded.

life expectancy: It has increased by leaps and bounds in the past few decades. Your infant girl will probably live a minimum of 74 years (in 1900, the figure would have been less than 50), your baby boy a bit less, some 66 or 67 years. And the figure increases with each day of life. That is, each year's survival, assuming no fatal or severely debilitating ailment has been contracted, increases the overall expectancy by weeks or months. If a boy, for example, has lived 20 years, he can expect to live at least 50 more; a girl who has lived 20 years, 57 more; this increment continues throughout life.

ligaments: connective strands joining bones at the joints, and also serving to attach muscles to bones. They can sometimes be pulled, torn, or broken, conditions that can be diagnosed only by your physician. Depending upon the severity of the damage, an injured ligament may heal by itself or may require surgery.

limping: a symptom, not to be ignored, that something is wrong. If your child is limping, try to find out why. Ill-fitting shoes could be a cause; a stone or something else in a shoe could be another. If neither of these conditions exists, and there's no apparent injury, question the child closely as to when the limping started, whether or not there was a fall or other accident, precisely where the pain or discomfort is, etc. If there's no obvious explanation, take the child to the doctor; limping could signal a number of problems involving the feet, legs, and hip joints.

Lincocin, lincomycin: See ANTIBIOTICS; the former is a trade name for the latter.

lindane: See PESTICIDES.

lipids: substances that, when occurring in excessive quantities in the blood, tend to form fatty deposits in the arteries, occluding them and increasing the risk of coronary problems; cholesterol and triglyceride are just two of many such substances, also referred to generally as *lipoproteins.* Some terms that may be used to describe the presence of excess blood lipids are hyperlipemia, hyperlipidemia, hyperlipoproteinemia, and the more specific hypercholesterolemia.

For many years, it was believed that such conditions were (a) due solely to diet and (b) inclined to afflict only the elderly, or at least the reasonably advanced in years. It is now known that several of these disorders are familial (the patterns of inheritance vary, and some forms are more or less rare than others); some may even afflict small children — and, if left undetected and untreated, are likely to substantially reduce life expectancy. We strongly urge that, especially if any direct-line relative — parent, grandparent, aunt or uncle — experienced a heart attack before the age of forty, or yours are adopted children whose family histories are unknown to you, you have your children's lipid levels checked, and this should be started at the age of one year. Diabetes, longstanding obesity, and a family history of high blood lipids are also indications for annual checks.

If high lipid levels are found, there are two modes of treatment; one or both may be recommended in a particular instance.

One involves the administration of drugs designed to lower blood lipids. Among the leading medications in this group are cholestyramine (Questran), which is not generally used in children under six years but has been found effective in older children; clofibrate (Atromid-S), which is useful in some rare forms of the disorder, and is not advised for children; and dextrothyroxine (Choloxin), which has been found effective in the type of familial hyperlipoproteinemia that appears to be most common in early childhood (it is however, considered unacceptably risky in the presence of heart disease).

The drugs are typically used not alone, but in conjunction with dietary measures. Since they invariably have other metabolic effects in the body as well, your doctor may — depending upon the particular medication — want to check certain vitamin levels periodically and/or may give you special guidance concerning the taking of other medications.

Diet alone may be, and often is, the only therapy required (if the child is also obese, reduction to normal weight will be part of the goal, too). Basically, it will be a diet that avoids saturated fats — which promote lipid formation in the body — as well as foods that themselves contain cholesterol. The latter is not formed by plants, only by animals. All animal foods contain saturated fats (general clue: fats that are solid at room temperature), but some contain more than others; notably high are egg yolks and organ meats. Beef fat is about 50 percent the saturated kind, and beef generally is fairly high in fat content (four-fifths of the calories in a choice Porterhouse come from fat). Fish contains much less fat — cod, for example, only 3.5 percent — and one-third of the fat in most fish is polyunsaturated.

Being a vegetarian does not necessarily eliminate saturated fats from one's diet. Among substances high in it is coconut oil, which is a component of many nondairy coffee "creamers." Labels that state "hardened" or "partially hydrogenated" mean that unsaturated fat has been chemically converted to saturated fat in order to give it room-temperature stability. And we regret to report that peanut butter, alas, encourages high blood-lipid levels, too.

If, incidentally, you are wondering and worrying about milk — no need to. Skim milk is perfectly all right for children; only the fat has been removed, not any of the necessary nutrients. And it has, by the way, only 90 calories per eight-ounce glass, versus 160 for whole milk; there are also instant nonfat milks that come in dry form and are reconstituted with water, such as Alba, that have even fewer calories — and cost less, too. *None* of these comments apply to infants whose *only* source of calories is milk; skim milk is *not* adequate for their needs.

lipoma: a subcutaneous benign tumor composed of fatty material. A lipoma is basically harmless but is usually unsightly, tends to grow, and can sometimes become infected; hence, removal is usually recommended. The sooner the removal, the smaller the scar.

Liquiprin: a trade name for a liquid form of acetaminophen, an analgesic (it is *not* aspirin, despite its name). Although it is convenient to administer to small children and about as effective as aspirin in relieving pain and fever, it does not create the sense of well-being that aspirin does, nor is it effective against inflammation; many physicians prefer to recommend some form of aspirin instead.

Confusion about this product has been compounded by the fact that the trade name formerly signified neither aspirin nor acetaminophen, but salicylamide, still *another* analgesic.

Further, there is a *tablet* now made, carrying the very same trade name, which *is* aspirin — *not children's* aspirin, but an *adult* dosage.

We concur with the published comment of the American Pharmaceutical Association, the organization of professional pharmacists, that such doubly confusing use of a trade name is, and we quote, "irrational." The APhA has also pointed out that such substitution of medicinal agents by a pharmacist, in a prescription specifying a brand name, would be considered both unethical and illegal.

liquor: See DRINKING.

lisping: See SPEECH DISABILITIES.

liver: the largest gland in the body, and an organ essential to life; it's located in the upper abdomen, toward the right. The liver plays a number of major roles in circulation, digestion, and metabolism; among other things, it secretes bile for the digestion of fats, stores carbohydrates and some minerals and vitamins, synthesizes proteins, and helps in the formation of blood cells and antibodies.

A number of systemic illnesses can affect the liver to an extent, and the gland itself is liable to direct infection; see HEPATITIS.

lockjaw: See TETANUS.

Lomotil: an effective antidiarrheal medication, available only by prescription, that must be used with extreme care and should never be given to small children or kept where small children have access to it. For more details, see the discussion under DIARRHEA.

lordosis: See SWAYBACK.

Loridine: a trade name for cephaloridine; see ANTIBIOTICS.

Lotrimin: a trade name for clotrimazole, an antifungal agent; see ANTIBIOTICS.

L.P.N.: the abbreviation for Licensed Practical Nurse; see HEALTH PROFESSIONALS.

LSD: See PSYCHEDELICS.

lumbar puncture: See SPINAL TAP.

Luminal: a trade name for phenobarbital, a sedative and anticonvulsant; see SEDATIVES.

lungs: a pair of lobed organs in the chest, containing air sacs and many capillaries connected with blood vessels leading to and from the heart; breathing brings oxygen to the tiny air sacs, from which the oxygen is relayed to the blood — which is then returned to the heart through the pulmonary vein.

The lungs can become involved in any disorder of the rest of the respiratory tract (the nose, throat, windpipe, and bronchial tubes), and there are also a number of ills that can afflict the lungs more directly. See BRONCHIOLITIS; EMPHYSEMA; HISTOPLASMOSIS; HYALINE MEMBRANE DISEASE; PNEUMONIA; PSITTACOSIS; TUBERCULOSIS; VALLEY FEVER.

lupus: a chronic disorder, one of the collagen diseases in which that tissue, in the joints and/or elsewhere, suffers recurrent inflammation; the term is short for *lupus erythematosus,* which may be preceded by the word *discoid* (characterized by disc-shaped skin lesions, and affecting only the skin) or *systemic* (the two forms are sometimes referred to as DLE and SLE). Lupus afflicts perhaps a million Americans, two-thirds — and perhaps as many as five-sixths — of them female. Typically, it strikes during the twenties or thirties, but has been known, uncommonly, to start in the teen years; very rarely, it is diagnosed much earlier (the youngest patient on record was two years old).

The systemic form of the disease often starts with mild arthritic symptoms, which will occur sooner or later in nine out of ten patients. Other frequent early symptoms are fever — generally not the sole symptom — and a rash that often appears only on exposure to sunlight, classically in a "butterfly" conformation over the cheeks and nose.

Because the signs and symptoms of lupus are extremely variable, diagnosis can be difficult. If it is suspected, it must be confirmed by a number of tests, including biopsy of any skin lesions, urinalysis to check for certain proteins, blood testing for the presence of specific types of cells (called LE cells) and other factors.

The causes of lupus are not known; theories include viruses and other infectious agents, allergies, and — because of the sex ratio — hormones, as well as combinations of these. Treatment — which does not cure, but can relieve and control — generally includes avoidance of sunlight; safeguarding general health and avoiding emotional or physical stress, including infections; and medications which may vary from over-the-counter anti-inflammatory analgesics such as aspirin to more potent prescription drugs (see CORTICOSTEROIDS and IMMUNOSUPPRESSANTS).

lymph nodes: the things that are swollen in the condition called "swollen glands." Although the latter term is often used by physicians and patients alike, it's not really accurate.

There is, throughout the body, an interstitial circulation of lymph, a fluid that originates in blood vessels and contains infection-fighting agents; lymph nodes are simply clumpings of lymph channels and not by any definition "glands." They are located in the neck, armpits, and groin, at the back of the knees and the inner side of the elbows, and at various internal points in the body.

It is at the lymph nodes that some of the leukocytes (see BLOOD CELLS) are formed, and in the presence of certain kinds of infection, there is an increase in their production — hence, the swelling at these sites. The medical term for this swelling is *adenitis,* a word that is sometimes further qualified to specify the site of the swelling — as *cervical adenitis* (in the neck) or *mesenteric adenitis* (in the abdomen — where the swelling can sometimes cause pain, despite the fact that the illness or infection is in quite another part of the body).

Enlarged lymph nodes are a familiar accompaniment of ailments such as mononucleosis, rubella, and many infectious conditions both more and less serious; some youngsters tend to have swollen lymph nodes with every respiratory infection. They are, in any case, usually a symptom of *some* kind of infection *some*where in the body, and a signal that the child should see the doctor so that the problem can be pinpointed and treated.

lymphocyte: See BLOOD CELLS.

lymphogranuloma venereum: See VENEREAL DISEASES.

lymphoma: a term occasionally denoting a benign growth or polyp consisting of lymphoid tissue — and then normally preceded by the word "benign" — but usually denoting any of a number of malignant conditions involving lymph tissues and channels. Lymphomas account for one in ten cancers in children (see CANCER for general comment), but only one percent of malignancies at all ages. Half the total are a specific type called *Hodgkin's disease,* which is identified by a particular kind of malignant cell and is emphatically a disease of the young: fully half its victims are under the age of twenty-five.

In the lymphomas, perhaps more than in any other kind of cancer, suspicion of infectious organisms looms exceedingly large. There have been many observations of a phenomenon called "regional clustering" — unusual numbers of cases, beyond statistical expectations, in communities or among individuals who have been connected in some way (friendship, marriage, attending the same school, etc.). It has been established almost beyond doubt that a variety prevalent in certain parts of Africa, called Burkitt's lymphoma, is caused by a specific virus. (It is believed that the virus is transmitted by insect bite, not by person-to-person contact; there is no suspicion in any kind of cancer of direct transmission from one human being to another.) Some experimental studies employing transfusions or implants of infection-fighting tissues have reported gratifying responses, especially in Hodgkin's disease.

Animal experimentation has tended to support the theory — an exciting one, because it suggests the possibility of prevention. Marek's disease, for example, is a cancer of the lymph system that afflicts chickens; an effective vaccine has actually been in use for several years. Even more significant is the recent development of a workable vaccine against a type of lymphoma that occurs in monkeys — since they, like human beings, are primates.

Lymphomas typically begin with painless enlargement of lymph nodes — which of course can also mean anything from a simple cold to dozens of other common childhood infections (it's probably wise to become suspicious if lymph nodes remain enlarged, with no other clear sign of specific illness, for more than three weeks). There may also be other, rather vague symptoms including appetite loss, moderate fever, fatigue, and general "not feeling good."

Of course these symptoms may also be signs of something else, notably a systemic infection such as mononucleosis. Diagnosis of lymphoma can't be considered definite without a biopsy of lymph tissue in order to verify the presence of malignant cells and to identify them specifically. Following that, exploratory surgery may be recommended for the purpose of *staging* — determining exactly how far the disease has progressed and which parts of the lymph system have been affected; that, in turn, serves as a guide for therapy, which may consist of irradiation, chemotherapy (i.e., medications), or a combination of the two.

Over the last decade, multidrug treatment has been found especially effective in later stages of Hodgkin's and at various stages of some of the other lymphomas — particularly, a regimen that has come to be known by the acronym MOPP, combining the four drugs mechlorethamine, vincristine (Oncovin), procarbazine, and prednisone. MOPP has in fact been the major factor in reversing the previously dismal prognosis in advanced stages of Hodgkin's disease.

Thirty years ago, a diagnosis of lymphoma was truly equivalent to a death sentence, and exceptions made headlines. That is no longer true. Lymphomas in general, and Hodgkin's in particular (the odds now approach 90 percent for long-term survival), are now considered potentially *curable.* The shorter the interval between onset of symptoms and diagnosis and treatment, the greater the possibility of full recovery. But even if the disease is discovered only after it has had a chance to advance, the chances of survival are at *least* fifty-fifty.

M

Maalox: See ANTACIDS.

Madribon: a trade name for sulfadimethoxine; see SULFA DRUGS.

mafenide: See SULFA DRUGS.

magnesium carbonate: See ANTACIDS.

malaria: an infectious disease caused by a tiny parasite in the bloodstream and transmitted via the bite of a particular type of mosquito. Through concerted attacks on the insects and their breeding places — chiefly swamps and other bodies of stagnant water — malaria has been eliminated from many areas, including all of Europe and most of the United States. It is still a problem in a number of tropical and subtropical areas, however, including coastal Mexico, Central America, the northern part of South America, most of Africa (where it kills an estimated one million children yearly), and much of the Near and Far East; it has thus sometimes been contracted by travelers, including armed forces personnel.

The illness is an extremely unpleasant one and difficult to throw off. It begins, after an incubation period of five days to several weeks, with aching and nausea; this is followed by periodic attacks of violent chills and extremely high fevers, coming at intervals varying from one to three or four days (there are several types of malaria). There is treatment, with special antimalarial drugs, but they must be patiently administered over a long period of time to get rid of the infection completely. If your family is traveling to a place where malaria is endemic, discuss with your physician the possibility of protection in the form of certain drugs that are usually effective in preventing the disease (there is presently no vaccine against it).

Some persons have a natural resistance to malaria, associated with certain types of hereditary blood-cell defects; see ANEMIA.

malathion: See PESTICIDES.

malformation: an abnormally or incompletely formed or structured organ, limb, or other tissue; the word generally refers to a condition evident at birth — i.e., a congenital malformation. A malformation may be serious or inconsequential, depending upon the organ or part of the body involved.

malignant: describing a growth or condition that is not self-contained or self-limited and that, if untreated (or untreatable), will continue to spread; possibly cancerous; the opposite of *benign*. There are degrees of malignancy, based upon such factors as speed of growth and whether the condition tends to affect various types of tissue or only one.

malnutrition: lack of essential nutritional elements, either because they are missing from the diet or because the body is not assimilating or utilizing them properly. The definition involves quality, not quantity; a child suffering from starvation will certainly be afflicted with malnutrition as well, but the reverse is not necessarily true.

Also see DEFICIENCY DISEASES; NUTRITION.

malocclusion: a dental term meaning incorrect or abnormal "bite"; that is, the upper and lower teeth do not come together properly. The condition can usually be corrected by orthodontic measures.

Malta fever: See BRUCELLOSIS.

maltose: one of the disaccharides; this and other sugars, as well as synthetic substitutes, are discussed under SWEETENERS.

mandible: the anatomical term for the lower jaw.

mannitol: See SWEETENERS.

Mantoux test: a test for tuberculosis. See the comments under HEAF TEST.

MAO inhibitors: See ANTIDEPRESSANTS.

Maolate: a trade name for chlorphenesin, a muscle relaxant; this class of drugs is discussed under SEDATIVES.

Marezine: a trade name for cyclizine; see MOTION SICKNESS.

marijuana: See PSYCHEDELICS.

Marplan: a trade name for isocarboxazid; see ANTIDEPRESSANTS.

"master gland": the pituitary; see ENDOCRINE GLANDS.

mastitis: a very broad term meaning any inflammation involving breast tissue. Generally it is a bacterial infection, and not uncommonly occurs in nursing mothers; the initial symptom is fever, followed shortly by others including loss of appetite, and there are typically local symptoms as well. Treatment is with whatever antibiotic the physician judges appropriate; it is important to continue taking it as directed, even if symptoms have vanished in the meantime. Breast feeding may have to be discontinued while the infection lasts; your physician's advice should be followed.

mastoiditis: inflammation of the mastoid bone behind the ear, generally the result of a neglected and untreated middle-ear infection and considered quite serious because of the proximity of the site to the brain; prevention of this condition is one reason for prompt attention to any ear problem.

Symptoms of mastoiditis may include earache, a discharge from the ear, tenderness in the area behind the ear, fever, hearing loss, or a combination of these. Any one means the child should be seen by the doctor immediately. Treatment is with antibiotics and/or other drugs; surgery, once much used in the treatment of mastoiditis, is now rarely required.

masturbation: It is normal and natural for small children to masturbate, and a child shouldn't be made to feel otherwise; masturbation will not cause acne, insanity, or anything else. Bear in mind, too, that a young child's interest is not specifically sexual; he's exploring his body — all of it — and it's a major part of the learning process.

Nor should you be concerned if you discover that your teenage son or daughter masturbates; it's a normal sexual activity and, although it's not usually discussed socially, most people engage in it from time to time. If, on the other hand, you feel that it has become a constant preoccupation, then do discuss your concern with your physician.

maturation: See DEVELOPMENT; PUBERTY.

maxilla: the anatomical term for the upper jaw.

Maxipen: a trade name for phenethicillin, a semisynthetic penicillin; see ANTIBIOTICS.

mazindol: See DIET PILLS.

M.B.: in Great Britain, "Bachelor of Medicine"; equivalent to the American M.D. degree.

MBD: See MINIMAL BRAIN DYSFUNCTION.

McBurney's point: a term that is most likely to be mentioned by a young physician in an emergency room who would like to mystify you. What it is: a point on a straight line between the front edge of the right hipbone and the navel; poking it when a child is suffering from acute appendicitis will probably elicit a lot of screaming, because excruciating pain will result.

M.D.: the abbreviation for Doctor of Medicine, the degree that should, preferably, be held by the man or woman to whom you and your family turn for medical advice and treatment; also see OSTEOPATH for another kind of qualified practitioner. For the various specializations in subjects and services among M.D.s, see SPECIALTIES, MEDICAL.

measles: a highly contagious childhood disease, caused by a virus, formerly (prior to the introduction of a preventive vaccine in 1963) the most widespread of all the communicable diseases. Its medical name is *rubeola* (don't confuse this with German measles, or *rubella,* a completely different disease). The number of cases dropped markedly in the years that followed introduction of the vaccine; while some 600,000 cases a year was the norm a generation ago, only 7500 cases were reported to the Center for Disease Control for the epidemic year 1969–70 (October to October). But with that success came complacency, and the figures began to climb; 75,000 cases were reported in 1972–73. In 1973–74 New Jersey was hit by an epidemic; that state alone reported over 5000 cases.

Nonimmunization is definitely the reason for the rising rates; that was demonstrated by an event that couldn't have served better had it been purposely planned (which it wasn't). During the last six months of 1970, 633 cases of measles were diagnosed in Texarkana, a town that straddles the Arkansas-Texas border. Arkansas had previously initiated an immunization campaign, and 95 percent of children under ten in that part of town had been vaccinated; Texas had not. Only 27 of the town's cases were in Arkansas; 606 — 96 percent — were on the Texas side of the line.

Measles usually starts, after an incubation period of ten to fourteen days, with cold-like symptoms — runny nose, severe cough, general lethargy — plus fever and, on the third day, telltale white spots called Koplik spots in the child's mouth (you would likely not recognize them, but a physician would). On the fourth day the rash appears, beginning on the child's head and spreading downward over the face and body; the child feels sickest, and the fever is typically highest — up to 104° or 105° F. (40° or 40.5° C.) — at this time. By about the seventh day, the rash begins to fade, and there is — barring any secondary infection or other complication — fairly rapid improvement.

If a child does fall ill with measles, treatment consists only of measures to relieve discomfort: aspirin; calamine lotion for the rash; darkening the room if, as sometimes happens, there is sensitivity to light; cough medicine; and whatever else the doctor may recommend.

The physician's efforts will be, and yours should be, directed primarily toward guarding against complications. No one with a cold or any other contagious ailment should come near the child. An infant may, if the doctor judges it advisable, be given antibiotics to prevent secondary bacterial infection. Insofar as the child can be coaxed to eat, you should provide a well-balanced diet in order to keep resistance up. The child should be kept in bed while there is fever and for two full days thereafter.

Measles is, as we've previously noted, very contagious, via both contact and droplet infection, and for a ten-day period — from four days before, to five days after, the rash first appears. It's vital to be sure other youngsters in the household are protected. Any brother or sister who has neither been vaccinated nor had the disease (having it also gives permanent immunity) should promptly be given gamma globulin.

Although the disease itself is unpleasant enough, the major problem with measles lies in the possibility of serious complications, which can include bronchitis, pneumonia, and encephalitis; the last, which occurs once in every thousand cases, can cause permanent brain damage or death. Vaccination should take place at the age of one year (an older, unvaccinated child should of course be vaccinated immediately), and is generally given as part of a combination MMR (measles-mumps-rubella) shot; it is believed to give lifelong protection. A child who has, for some reason, been vaccinated earlier should be revaccinated at the age of one year; there isn't enough antibody-making ability to guarantee protection prior to that age.

Measurin: See PAIN RELIEVERS.

meatitis: an inflammation at the opening of the urethra. It occurs most commonly in boys — i.e., at the tip of the penis — and is often connected with diaper rash; the area becomes irritated when urine, which is normally acidic, passes over the rash. The meatitis will clear up when the diaper rash does. In the meantime, it's helpful to keep the child's diaper off as much as possible and leave the area exposed to the air.

Mebaral: a trade name for mephobarbital, a sedative and anticonvulsant; see SEDATIVES and EPILEPSY.

Meckel's diverticulitis: an inflammation in a little pouch in the wall of the small intestine; its symptoms are much like those of appendicitis, but generally include blood in the stool as well. Correction of the condition requires surgery.

meclizine: an antihistamine with antinausea properties; see MOTION SICKNESS.

meconium: the medical term for the material excreted in the very first bowel movements of a newborn baby; it is greenish-black in color and includes bile, mucus, and other waste materials accumulated in the intestines prior to birth.

medial: toward the midline of the body; the opposite of *lateral.*

Medic Alert: a concept and service that is, in the authors' opinion, a valuable aid to the parents of a child who may experience an away-from-home disability or emergency situation that could, with the wrong treatment or nonrecognition of a special condition, prove critical or even fatal. It is designed to provide crucial information to physicians, police, or similar individuals dealing with such an emergency.

The organization providing the service is the nonprofit Medic Alert Foundation, founded in 1956 by a California physician, Dr. Marion Collins, whose daughter had a potentially lethal allergy to horse-serum-based tetanus antitoxin. His design for a special identification bracelet for her to wear constantly led to the idea of offering a similar protective device for others, whatever the nature of their particular medical problems.

For a small (and tax-deductible) fee, a special necklace or bracelet is provided (for small children, the latter — enlarged as the child grows older — is recommended, since a necklace can easily twist around the child's neck or be yanked off). One side of the emblem bears the medical-identification

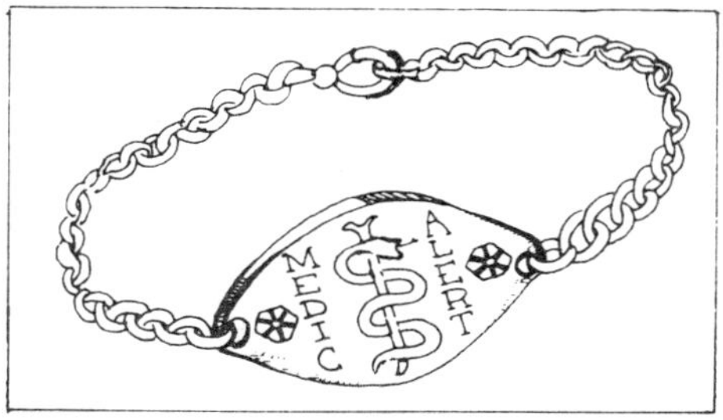

symbol and the words "Medic Alert" in red. On the other side is a special serial number assigned to the individual, a telephone number that may be called collect on a round-the-clock basis by medical or law-enforcement personnel, and whatever special emergency information is desired: "allergic to penicillin (or aspirin, or bee stings)" or "epilepsy," or "diabetes," or data regarding special medication the child takes, or the youngster's blood group. The telephone number is that of the foundation's central file, which keeps on record whatever additional medical information you care to provide, such as immunization and surgical histories, the name of the child's regular physician, and so on.

The foundation has advised us that there are affiliate organizations in a number of other countries, and that the emblem is registered in a total of some three dozen countries.

We would urge parents of a child with a serious and chronic medical problem to write Medic Alert Foundation, Turlock, California 95380, for further details about this service.

medicine chest: We find most families' stock of medical supplies is both something less and something more than it should be — on the one hand lacking in essentials, on the other containing a good many useless and even harmful items. You'll find, in various sections of this book, some comments on the latter, including a number of the ubiquitous decongestants, antacids, antiseptics, and pain relievers. Here, we'll offer a list of necessary — and sufficient — basics.

But first, some rules to follow on the keeping, giving, and taking of medications.

All swallowable medical supplies, whether pills or liquids, and including such ordinary things as aspirin as well as more exotic preparations, should be kept out of the reach of small children — which means under lock and key or some other device impossible for a tot to open; the only exception to this rule is syrup of ipecac, which is not harmful and should be handy for emergencies.

Any unlabeled and unknown medications should be discarded.

Each prescription medication should be labeled with the name of the drug, the person for whom it was prescribed, and the condition or illness for which it was prescribed (this in addition to the prescription number, physician's name, date, and dosage normally included by the pharmacy).

Never give a child (or take yourself) an old prescription for a new illness, unless the doctor specifically directs you to do so.

You needn't, no matter what you may have read elsewhere, discard a leftover medication automatically; instead, ask your doctor if it might be useful on another occasion, and keep it if it might be (fully labeled, as just noted).

Never grope for a medication in the dark; always turn on the light.

Always reread the label before giving a child any medicine, to make sure it is the right medicine and that you are giving it correctly. Do the same, of course, when you're taking medicine yourself.

YOUR HOME MEDICAL SUPPLIES

Now, here are the items you should have on hand, whether in the medicine chest per se, or elsewhere:

- this book, with the information in the back pages properly entered, and kept in a place known to the babysitter or anyone else caring for your children in your absence;
- an assortment of bandaging materials (see BANDAGES for a full list);
- absorbent cotton;
- a two-ounce bottle of syrup of ipecac *(syrup, not powder)* for emergency use as an emetic in case of accidental poisoning (but see POISONING before using it, since vomiting may be unhelpful and even harmful in the case of some poisons);
- cornstarch, for use as baby powder and also in a soothing bath for problems — such as poison ivy — involving extensive itching;
- petroleum jelly;
- rubbing alcohol — not for antiseptic use, but for soothing small itches such as insect bites, and for use (on your doctor's recommendation only) in sponge baths to reduce high fever;
- aspirin (plain aspirin, not "extra-strength" products or those with additional ingredients), both adult and children's types;

• an oral thermometer, and also a rectal type if you have an infant;

• an ice bag, or one of the recently introduced flexible cold packs (Cryogel) that is kept in the freezer until needed;

• a hot-water bottle or heating pad (a towel wrung out in hot water can also be used);

• calamine lotion (the plain type, not containing phenol);

• other medications your physician may recommend or suggest that you have on hand, including current prescriptions — which should be clearly labeled with all relevant data including the name of the drug and the person for whom prescribed (cover labels with transparent tape so they won't smear).

Also see FIRST-AID SUPPLIES for items to have in your garage or barn and to take on car, boat, and camping trips.

Mediterranean anemia: thalassemia; see ANEMIA.

Medrol: See CORTICOSTEROIDS.

megacolon: distension of the colon, the lower part of the large intestine; it may be congenital (see HIRSCHSPRUNG'S DISEASE), and may also result from a variety of causes later in life.

melanin: the brown-to-black pigment that normally occurs to some degree in skin and hair; its concentration in the skin is increased in response to the sun's rays.

melanoma: a pigmented skin cancer. A melanoma may stem from a mole that suddenly changes size and/or color, or may appear on normal skin as a small group of blue-black nodules. (The latter is statistically more likely; only one in about two million moles ever becomes malignant.) Either of these is a signal to take the child to the doctor without delay. Such a cancer can spread throughout the body, but if it is recognized and removed early enough, there will be complete recovery.

melanosis: abnormal darkening of the skin, from whatever cause.

melena: the medical term for dark, tarry-looking stools; melena is a signal of bleeding somewhere in the alimentary tract.

Mellaril: a trade name for thioridazine, a potent tranquilizer; see SEDATIVES.

menarche: the occurrence of a girl's first menstrual period.

Ménière's syndrome: a disorder of the inner ear, characterized by dizziness, nausea, and various hearing disturbances; it is extremely rare in children and teenagers.

meningitis: not the name of a particular disease, but a descriptive term for an inflammation — whatever its cause — of the membranes surrounding the brain and spinal cord; it tends to afflict children and adolescents more often than adults. It can result from primary infection by the meningococcus *Neisseria meningitidis* or certain other bacteria (see especially HEMOPHILUS INFLUENZAE), or it can be a secondary infection caused by the infectious agents of another illness, whether bacteria or viruses. Whatever the agent, it can be spread to and from others by droplet infection.

Incubation, depending upon the precise cause, can take from one day to seven. Symptoms vary not only with the type of infection, but with the age of the child as well; typically, they include fever, headache, vomiting, and a stiff neck. There may also be delirium or coma, muscular rigidity (especially a severe arching of the back), and, in one type of meningitis, a distinctive rash. If the doctor suspects this condition, the diagnosis must be confirmed by withdrawing and examining fluid from the spinal canal.

If *you* suspect meningitis, you should call the doctor immediately — and if you cannot reach your own physician, you should rush your youngster to the hospital. The condition is extremely serious, and the danger increases with the youth of the child. It must, in any case, be treated in the hospital. Generally sulfa drugs, antibiotics, and/or other medications will be used — again depending upon the exact nature of the infectious agent. Prior to the advent of these effective and fast-acting medications, meningitis was fatal for 90 percent of its victims; now, well over 90 percent recover.

If meningococcal meningitis is diagnosed in a child, the advisability of nose and throat cultures for the immediate family, and possibly prophylactic antibiotic therapy as well, should be discussed with the physician.

Although serious outbreaks have not occurred among civilians in the United States for quite some time, varieties of meningococcal meningitis — there are three types, A, B, and C — have caused epidemics in some other parts of the world (Brazil had epidemics in 1974 and 1975; two strains, Type A and Type C, were involved), and for some years posed a problem in U.S. military installations. A Type C vaccine developed by the armed forces proved extremely effective in that young-adult population. By 1973, it had been successfully tested in civilians, and the following year was licensed by the Food and Drug Administration (FDA licensing is not required for military-use-only drugs); large quantities were flown to Brazil to help meet that nation's emergency needs. A Type A vaccine had meanwhile been developed in Finland, where that strain has been epidemic, and by 1975 a combination vaccine was in use in Brazil. For the present, use of the vaccines — both are now fully licensed for manufacture and distribution here — is limited to such special situations involving actual or potential epidemic (the Type C vaccine is also available for travelers); they are not recommended for routine use in children or in pregnant women.

menstruation: the approximately monthly (the word comes from the Latin *mens,* meaning month) discarding of unneeded pregnancy-preparation material by the uterus. What happens, in sum, is that the ovary releases an egg — and meanwhile, the uterus manufactures a lining in preparation for the possible growth of an embryo. If the egg isn't fertilized, the lining is discarded, accompanied by some bleeding. This happens on an "average" of every 28 days, but hardly anyone is precisely average, and the cycle can vary from 21 to 35 days; teenagers in particular are typically irregular, and for the first couple of years after menarche, this is more or less expected and usually means nothing.

Regularity can also be *temporarily* upset by a number of things — including pregnancy, of course, but also including emotional upset or strain, and almost any illness (even a cold). Since glandular disease or malfunction — not necessarily of the ovaries themselves, but possibly of another of the endocrine glands — may be involved, it's best to discuss any question about your daughter's regularity or lack of it with your doctor.

The normal menstrual period lasts, depending upon the individual, anywhere from two to seven days (whatever its length, actual blood loss — again, normally — is minor, and won't cause anemia or any other ill effects). None of the old bugaboos are particularly valid, as far as activities and precautions go; it is perfectly all right for a girl to go right ahead with all her normal pursuits (unless, of course, she has been instructed otherwise by the doctor) — including swimming. And, it is perfectly all right for a teenager to use tampons if she finds them comfortable and feels that they permit her more freedom than sanitary napkins.

Menstruation is normally painless. Painful menstruation (the medical term is *dysmenorrhea),* which may involve abdominal cramps or pain in the thighs or back, is a sign that something is wrong, and a visit to the doctor is in order.

Amenorrhea is the medical term for absence of menstruation, whether it has failed to begin within the expected age range, or it has ceased at some later time.

mental retardation: a condition in which mental development is slow and is ultimately arrested at a point short of the normal range. It can result from a number of things, including certain congenital conditions, injury causing damage to the brain, some types of malnutrition, and certain kinds of poisoning, especially lead poisoning. In 75 to 80 percent of cases, the cause is unknown.

Mepergan, meperidine: see NARCOTICS; the latter is a morphinelike synthetic drug, the former the trade name for an analgesic combining meperidine and promethazine, an antiemetic.

mephenytoin: an antiseizure medication; see EPILEPSY.

mephobarbital: a sedative-anticonvulsant; see SEDATIVES and EPILEPSY.

meprobamate: a tranquilizer and muscle relaxant; see SEDATIVES.

Mercurochrome: See ANTISEPTICS.

Mesantoin: a trade name for mephenytoin, an antiseizure drug; see EPILEPSY.

mescaline: See PSYCHEDELICS.

mesenteric adenitis: See LYMPH NODES.

mesentery: a membrane connecting the intestine with the back of the abdominal wall; it contains blood vessels and lymph channels.

mesoridazine: a tranquilizer and antinauseant; see NAUSEA and SEDATIVES.

metabolism: the continuing activity of body cells — using oxygen and food, building tissues, breaking down and discarding waste materials; it involves all the body's organs, but especially the endocrine glands. Metabolism can be upset by almost any illness as well as by glandular malfunction; hypothyroidism and diabetes mellitus, for example, are metabolic disorders.

Basal metabolism, a term you may hear a physician use in connection with physical examinations or diagnostic testing, is a measure of the rate at which various basic processes take place in a particular individual under normal, at-rest conditions. Since that rate can change under various circumstances — including extreme emotional upsets, certain diseases, and other disorders — a measure of the rate at a given time can be a valuable diagnostic tool.

metacarpals: the five bones that connect the thumb and fingers to the wrist.

metastasis: the spread of disease from one part of the body to others, by way of the bloodstream or the lymph channels, or simply by proximity. The word is especially, and usually, used to mean the migration of cancer cells — but it can refer to other conditions, too.

metatarsals: the five bones that connect the toes to the ankle bones; the arch they form across the foot is the *metatarsal arch.*

metaxalone: a muscle relaxant; see SEDATIVES.

methacycline: one of the tetracyclines; see ANTIBIOTICS.

methadone: a morphinelike synthetic drug; see NARCOTICS.

methamphetamine, Methedrine: See AMPHETAMINES; the latter is a trade name for the former.

methaqualone: a nonbarbiturate prescription hypnotic; see SEDATIVES.

methicillin: a semisynthetic penicillin; see ANTIBIOTICS.

methocarbamol: a muscle relaxant; see SEDATIVES.

methohexital: a barbiturate used primarily in anesthesia; see SEDATIVES.

methotrexate: See IMMUNOSUPPRESSANTS.

methotrimeprazine: a potent analgesic; see NARCOTICS.

methsuximide: an antiseizure drug; see EPILEPSY.

methylphenidate: See HYPERKINESIS.

methylprednisolone: See CORTICOSTEROIDS.

methyprylon: a nonbarbiturate sleep-inducing drug; see SEDATIVES.

Meticorten: See CORTICOSTEROIDS.

MicaTin, miconazole: an antifungal agent (the first word is a trade name); see ANTIBIOTICS.

microcephaly: disproportionately small head size, symptomatic of a number of conditions.

midgets: See DWARFISM.

Midicel: a trade name for sulfamethoxypyridazine; see SULFA DRUGS.

Midol: See PAIN RELIEVERS.

migraine: a special and severe sort of chronic, recurrent headache, sometimes only on one side of the head, and often accompanied by nausea; the site of the ache and other symptoms are usually consistent in an individual.

There has been a good deal of speculation about the causes of migraine, and why some people are susceptible and others are not. The condition is generally familial, and leading neurologists now feel that there is a definite hereditary factor, although its pattern has not been established. There is a family history of migraine in almost two-thirds of cases, and frequently other members of the same generation — siblings or cousins — are also afflicted.

The word migraine can be traced back through French and Latin to the Greek *hemikrania,* "half-headed," and what is now known as *classic migraine* does indeed feature a headache that is strictly one-sided. It is also distinguished by a variety of neurological symptoms that appear during the period of half an hour or so prior to the headache and are called the *prodrome.* Sometimes these consist of numbness or tingling, weakness of an arm or leg, or speech disturbances — it varies from one individual to another — and occasionally include dramatic visual aberrations.

Most striking is the phenomenon called a *scintillating scotoma,* consisting of a dark patch in the visual field (one or both eyes may be affected), surrounded by bright zigzag lines that radiate outward to one or both sides. Visual prodromes may also take the form of clustered spots of bright color, pinwheel patterns, geometric shapes, images such as flowers or animals, or bizarre distortions in perception of the relative sizes of people or objects. Occasionally there is total darkening of all or part of the visual field, essentially a transitory blindness. When the prodromal symptoms are on one side, it is typically the side *opposite* to the headache; these symptoms disappear before the headache starts.

The headache itself is typically above or behind the eye or in the region of the temple; it can be, and usually is, quite severe. At the outset, the pain usually has a throbbing quality, gradually changing to a steady, intense ache. The headache is frequently accompanied by nausea and possibly vomiting; other symptoms may include sweating, weakness, nasal stuffiness, tearing and redness of tissues around the eyes, and acute sensitivity to noise and bright light. If no treatment is given, all this is likely to go on for four to six hours, or even longer.

Perhaps 10 percent of those with migraine have the classic type. The vast majority suffer from what is now known as *common migraine,* which is often bilateral (although in children, it is typically unilateral); prodromal symptoms may precede the headache by hours or even days, and are rather vague as compared with those of classic migraine — irritability, tension, mental "fogginess," occasionally gastrointestinal discomfort. The headache itself is similar to that of classic migraine — although accompanying symptoms (with the exception of the nasal ones) may be less severe and of shorter duration — and may last from several hours to several days.

There are also a few relatively rare types of migraine that have only in recent years been recognized *as* migraine. One of these occurs only in females, particularly adolescents and young adults, and is related to the menstrual cycle (it may be triggered, somehow, by hormonal events); prodromal symptoms may include dizziness, lack of coordination, speech difficulties, transitory blindness, prickling, and numbness, and the headache tends to be a throbbing one concentrated at the back of the head.

Classic and common migraine, too, seem to require "triggers" or provoking factors, which may vary considerably from one individual to another. They may include lack of food, certain kinds of weather, fatigue, loss of sleep, glaring or flickering light, alcohol, some foods (prominently chocolate, nuts, cheeses, and occasionally other dairy products), and emotional stress.

Migraine in a small child may be quite atypical. Even if you believe a youngster has migraine, it's important to let the doctor do the diagnosing and determine whether it is in fact migraine, or some other condition — such as an acute infection — requiring quite different treatment.

The home remedy for migraine headache is to make the youngster as comfortable as possible; have him lie in a quiet, darkened room, with the head still, and apply cold cloths or an ice bag if that seems to help. Aspirin is fine — but nothing stronger unless it's specifically prescribed by the doctor.

Prominent among the medications that have been found effective for migraine — but are *not* recommended, or normally prescribed, for very young children — is a derivative of a natural rye fungus called ergot, ergotamine tartrate (Ergomar, Gynergen). Ergotamine is also available in various combination drugs the physician may find desirable: Bellergal, for example, includes phenobarbital and belladonna alkaloids; Cafergot includes caffeine, and Cafergot P-B also pentobarbital and belladonna; Migral includes caffeine and cyclizine, an antinauseant; Wigraine includes caffeine, belladonna, and phenacetin. (Part of the doctor's decision may be dictated by the patient's ability to keep the medication down or to get it down in the first place. All these drugs are available orally. Gynergen can also be injected; Cafergot, Cafergot P-B, and Wigraine are also available in the form of rectal suppositories.) All of these have a legitimate place in the treatment of migraine. But they are very powerful drugs, and some are potentially habit-forming; the prescriptions must be followed *exactly.*

Migral: a preparation used in treating migraine; see the immediately preceding entry.

milk from baby's breast: See BREAST DEVELOPMENT.

milk of magnesia: See CATHARTIC.

Milontin: a trade name for phensuximide, an antiseizure medication; see EPILEPSY.

Milpath, Miltown: See SEDATIVES; the latter is a trade name for the tranquilizer meprobamate, the former a combination product containing meprobamate and an antispasm agent.

mineral oil: See CATHARTIC.

minerals: See DEFICIENCY DISEASES; NUTRITION.

minimal brain dysfunction: a broad term describing conditions in which there is a specific malfunction in the brain resulting in detectable physiological disabilities. There is no connection with intelligence, nor does this condition in any way relate to other neural disorders such as epilepsy, cerebral palsy, etc. Symptoms may range from minor reading difficulties, to problems with muscular coordination, to compulsive overactivity (hyperkinesis) and inability to concentrate.

Children with this problem, only recently recognized, used to be dismissed as either mentally retarded or emotionally disturbed. It is now estimated that at least 7.5 percent of U.S. youngsters — or a minimum of five million — are afflicted with MBD;

about 85 percent of them are boys (it is not yet known why).

If MBD is suspected in your child, your pediatrician or family physician may refer you to a neurologist for further examination and confirmation of the diagnosis. The condition typically does not persist past puberty. In the meantime, however, it is important that the youngster be able to cope and keep up with his schoolwork. Depending upon the precise nature of the problem, treatment may involve special reading instruction or tutoring, the administration of certain medications, and/or other measures.

Minocin, minocycline: one of the tetracyclines (the former is a trade name for the latter); see ANTIBIOTICS.

MMR vaccine: a recently developed triple vaccine that protects, with one injection, against measles, mumps, and rubella (German measles). For guidance on the scheduling of this and other vaccinations, see IMMUNIZATION.

moles: See BIRTHMARKS.

molluscum contagiosum: See WARTS.

mongolian spot: See BIRTHMARKS.

mongolism: See DOWN'S SYNDROME.

moniliasis: a form of candidiasis, sometimes called "vaginal thrush," which affects the vulvovaginal area. It's not at all uncommon in teenage girls and women (sexual maturity seems to be a prerequisite), and often appears during or following a course of antibiotic therapy. The organism causing it is typically *Candida albicans* (or, rarely, another member of the same genus), a fungus that is normally present but doesn't cause any trouble until sweeping antibiotic action depletes the number of harmless bacteria that normally keep the fungal population in line; oral contraceptives also seem to increase susceptibility in some women.

Typical symptoms are intense itching in the vulvovaginal area and visible evidence of the characteristic inflammation, combined sometimes with a vaginal discharge appearing much like soap residue on the vulva. If you suspect this condition, see the doctor; ointments, vaginal suppositories, and oral medications are available (by prescription only) which can take care of the problem within a few days — although susceptibility, under like circumstances at a later time, may persist.

Diaper rashes may also sometimes involve monilial organisms.

Monistat: a trade name for miconazole, an antimonilial fungicide; see ANTIBIOTICS.

mononucleosis: a contagious and stubborn, though not usually serious, disease that especially afflicts teenagers (although it can occur in children as young as four or five); it is also sometimes called "glandular fever" — a misnomer, since it rarely involves any glands, and there may or may not be fever. There have from time to time been epidemics in the high-school and college population, giving rise to its being nicknamed "kissing sickness"; such intimate contact isn't necessary, however, to communicate it. The exact cause has not been documented but is now believed to be the Epstein-Barr virus.

There is an incubation period of one to six weeks. Typically, the chief symptom is swelling of the lymph nodes ("swollen glands") in the neck, armpits, and groin; there are usually, though not always, a sore throat and headache as well. If there is fever, it generally hovers just above normal, rarely climbing higher than 101° or 102° F. (38.3°–38.9° C.). Rarely, there may be involvement of other organs such as the liver or spleen, or other symptoms such as jaundice or rash.

With such a vague set of symptoms, it would seem impossible to arrive at a diagnosis. For a lay person, that's true. But the disease is also characterized by certain aberrations in the number and type of white cells in the blood, and a special blood test can quickly tell the doctor whether or not your youngster has mononucleosis.

Treatment and recovery may take some time, and relapses — over a period of several weeks — are not uncommon; malaise, fatigue, and general weakness are often extraordinarily persistent. Antibiotics are of no avail, unless there is secondary bacterial infection. The main remedy is simply rest, although the doctor may also prescribe special dietary measures or certain medications, depending upon the individual situation.

monosaccharides: chemically elemental sugars; they include dextrose (glucose), fructose (levulose), and galactose. They are discussed, along with other sugars and synthetic substitutes, under SWEETENERS.

"mood elevators": See ANTIDEPRESSANTS.

MOPP: an acronym — employing the initial letters of four drugs — for a combination-chemotherapy regimen that has proved particularly successful in treating Hodgkin's disease; see LYMPHOMA.

Moro reflex: a generalized "startle response" by a newborn baby to certain sounds and other stimuli provided by the doctor. It is one of several neurological reflexes that are normal in the newborn and disappear as the child grows older.

morphine: an opium derivative; see NARCOTICS.

mosquito bites: See BITES AND STINGS.

motion sickness: Many children are subject to carsickness, bus-sickness, seasickness, etc., involving headache, dizziness, and especially nausea and vomiting while in or on a moving vehicle. It can come on suddenly and inconveniently and make the youngster miserable. But there are some effective preventives and remedies.

Whatever the vehicle, the condition is aggravated by lack of ventilation or unpleasant odors (car windows open to the breeze will help), and by loud noise. And of course, the more food in the stomach, the worse the situation — so don't let a child eat heavily just before a trip.

In a car, position the child so he can see out the window. Don't let him read or play with a toy; the constant refocusing of the eyes due to movement of the vehicle can precipitate the problem. Try to encourage the playing of games relating to the passing scene, if there's a whiling-away-time problem on a long drive.

On water, the question isn't likely to arise in small, open craft such as rowboats or outboards, but in larger boats. If you know the youngster is subject to the problem, or if symptoms of illness appear — don't send the child below to sleep it off; that will simply make it worse. Keep him on deck — preferably, if it's a motor cruiser and the sea isn't too rough, toward the bow of the boat — or on the flying bridge, if the boat has one. And have him nibble on something — a pretzel, a cracker, a piece of cold chicken, nothing complicated — slowly and cautiously; gets things going in the right direction, intestinally.

Finally, and most importantly — have antimotion-sickness pills with you. Your doctor can prescribe them. These are generally antihistamines with a strong antinausea effect. Most commonly used are cyclizine (Marezine), diphenhydramine (Benadryl), dimenhydrinate (Dramamine), hydroxyzine (Atarax, Vistaril), and meclizine (Antivert, Bonine). Some of these are available in liquid form, for children too young to swallow pills. Other drugs that may have been prescribed to curb nausea under other conditions should *not* be used for motion sickness; they won't work, and may have toxic side effects. The ones we've mentioned do work, and are perfectly safe — following prescribed dosages, of course.

motor: relating to muscle movement.

mouth-to-mouth resuscitation: See RESPIRATORY RESUSCITATION.

mouthwashes: By and large, these products are safe, even if accidentally swallowed. Three major brands, however, have been singled out by the American Pharmaceutical Association, the organization of professional pharmacists, as potentially toxic: Isodine, which contains iodine; Lavoris, the zinc chloride content of which can irritate the lining of the stomach; and Listerine, which contains boric acid and can poison a child who drinks eight ounces or more. It is well to check labels carefully; other, lesser known brands may also contain these possibly harmful ingredients.

MS: See MULTIPLE SCLEROSIS.

mucosa: the medical term for mucous membranes.

mucous membrane: the moist tissue lining the internal passages of the body — the respiratory tract, the gastrointestinal tract, etc.; it secretes mucus, a thick, clear fluid providing lubrication for passage through these areas.

multiple sclerosis: a crippling, but usually not fatal, disease of the central nervous system; its victims are rarely under the age of fifteen. In this ailment that affects some 250,000 Americans but remains a medical conundrum, the insulating sheath around the nerves degenerates and is replaced by scar tissue; the result is that nerve pathways are obstructed and both sensation and muscular control in various parts of the body are lost. The condition is not contagious.

Multiple sclerosis (MS) is generally not painful. Symptoms, which appear in varying order depending upon which nerves are attacked first, may include staggering gait, vision difficulties, tremors, partial paralysis, numbness, slurred speech, and problems involving elimination. There are no direct mental effects, although the victim can, understandably, become frightened and/or depressed as the disease progresses.

Expert diagnosis is vital, of course, since any one of the symptoms could conceivably signal some other condition. Treatment may, depending upon the patient's particular condition, include physical therapy, various drugs, and/or psychological counseling for the patient and possibly the family as well. Should your son or daughter have multiple sclerosis, we can give you no specific reassurance beyond the facts that it is not normally fatal, and that research is indeed going forward. There have been many remissions of varying duration — but at this writing, no complete recovery has been documented.

The precise cause of MS remains a tantalizing riddle, although there have been a number of provocative findings leading to a variety of theories. (Determining the exact cause is, of course, not merely an abstract scientific exercise but a prelude to effective treatment and, it is hoped, prevention. Without that knowledge, treatment must remain symptomatic.) Among the more intriguing facts: MS is far more prevalent in the North than in the South (almost forty times as common in Minnesota, for example, as in Mexico City); its onset is extremely rare before the age of fifteen or after the age of forty; familial "clusters" have been reported (families, of course, generally share environment as well as heredity); a number of investigations have revealed unusually high levels of immune factors, reacting to the measles virus and a few others, in the blood of MS victims; MS frequently assumes a relapse-and-remission, coming-and-going pattern, much like that of lupus and rheumatoid arthritis, and some therapeutic success with such drugs as immunosuppressants and corticosteroids has been reported.

Research into the etiology of MS has concentrated on the possibilities suggested by these facts. Among the hypotheses that are being explored: a "slow virus" process (see SSPE for further comment) involving a paramyxovirus, a poxvirus, or some similar organism; infection by a "defective" virus, possibly a mutant strain, that does not behave normally; a hypersensitive or "hyperimmune" reaction to a pathogen or other environmental factor; inherited or other congenital susceptibility or predisposition that causes a failure of, or defect in, the normal ability to resist infection; a combination of two or more of these, perhaps with some other, as yet unknown, factor or factors.

mumps: a contagious disease involving inflammation and painful swelling of the parotid (saliva-producing) glands, and sometimes other glands as well; it is medically termed *epidemic parotitis* and is caused by a specific virus (there are other conditions that can cause inflammation of the salivary glands, and *parotitis* describes any of them).

The swelling, appearing after an incubation period of two to three weeks, usually begins on one side, then may spread to the other; the glands involved are behind the jaw, just under the ears (they're *not* the things referred to in ordinary "swollen glands," which are not glands but lymph nodes). It lasts for a week or ten days and may be accompanied by fever or headache; because of the swelling, chewing and swallowing are often painful. The disease is contagious, by contact or droplet infection, from a full week before symptoms appear until they are completely gone.

Treatment of mumps consists simply of making the child as comfortable as possible; antibiotics and similar drugs are ineffective. Offer the child soft foods that will slide down easily and won't require a great deal of chewing. Gargling may help, as may hot or cold compresses (sometimes one makes a child feel better, sometimes the other). Aspirin, if your doctor approves, may be given during the painful period. Of course the youngster must be kept at home. Once a child has had mumps, there is lifelong immunity.

Most frequent victims of mumps are children between five and fifteen (it is quite rare under the age of three). Even prior to puberty, complications such as encephalitis, myocarditis, and permanent nerve deafness, though rare, can occur. In an adolescent, there is in addition a slight but nonetheless important chance of complications involving the sex glands, complications that can be especially destructive in boys.

For this last reason, immunization for all children is strongly recommended. The vaccine — which is believed to give lifelong protection — is usually given at the age of one year as part of the routine MMR (measles-mumps-rubella) shot, although some doctors prefer to wait until the child is approaching puberty. The earlier vaccination is preferable, chiefly because a youngster who contracts mumps can communicate the disease, with risk of complications, to susceptible older members of the household, including parents. Some cases of mumps may be so mild that they are not even diagnosed, although the infection may still be communicated to others. As of 1974, the Center for Disease Control warned that fewer than two out of five preschoolers had received mumps vaccine; we hope your children are in that minority.

muscarine: a toxin in certain wild mushrooms. See the "Mushroom Poisoning" section under FOOD POISONING.

muscles: There are three kinds: voluntary (striated) muscles, such as those controlling the arms and legs; involuntary (smooth) muscles, such as those of the intestines; and cardiac muscle — i.e., the heart — which is striated but involuntary, and is unique. Muscles make up about 40 percent of the average man's weight, about 30 percent of the average woman's, and less, of course, of a child's.

All muscles are elastic; they can stretch and contract, and have a property called *tonus,* meaning that they are always in a state of slight contraction and ready to contract further; even in sleep, muscles are not completely relaxed, although they're *more* relaxed then. Extreme cold can cause the voluntary muscles to contract involuntarily — which we call shivering.

Most of the muscles you'll hear mentioned by name are voluntary muscles. There are actually more than six hundred of these in the body, but only a few are likely to concern the average person or come up in nonmedical conversation. The anatomical names you're most likely to encounter are:

• *the biceps* — at the front of the upper arm and at the back of the thigh (yes, the name's the same for both), bends the arm or leg;

• *the deltoid* — at the shoulder, raises the arm away from the body;

• *the gastrocnemius* — the calf muscle that pulls the heel up in normal walking;

• *the gluteus maximus* — the buttocks muscle that pulls the leg into line with the torso, as when one stands up;

• *the pectorals* — in the upper chest, pull the arm across the body;

• *the quadriceps* — at the front of the thigh, straightens the leg (thus acting in opposition to the biceps);

• *the trapezius* — at the back and to the side of the neck, lifts the shoulder (it's the slanted one you can feel when you hunch your shoulder);

• *the triceps* — at the back of the upper arm, straightens the arm (in opposition to the biceps).

"Opposite-reaction" muscles, such as the arm's biceps and triceps, each contract to an extent when their opposite numbers are at work; this slows the action so that one bends or straightens one's arm smoothly, rather than with a sudden, violent snap. Muscles that straighten a limb when they contract, such as the triceps, are called *extensors;* those that bend a limb are *flexors.*

Muscles need fuel and oxygen to function, and their functioning produces certain chemical waste products; if, as a result of prolonged overwork, these products accumulate, the muscle is unable to contract — which is what we call fatigue, and is the most common cause of muscle soreness. It is remedied by a period of rest, which brings the chemical situation back to normal.

Another fairly common problem, caused not by fatigue but by a sudden strenuous effort, is a twisting or kinking of muscle fibers. This, too, corrects itself in time, chiefly with rest of the affected muscle; warmth (as, heating pads or hot baths) and massage can help, too.

See, for some of the problems — ranging from trivial to serious — that can afflict the voluntary muscles, BACK INJURIES; the section on spider bites under BITES AND STINGS; CEREBRAL PALSY; CHOREA; CONVULSIONS; CRAMPS, FEET AND LEGS; DEFICIENCY DISEASES; EPILEPSY; FACIAL PALSY; MULTIPLE SCLEROSIS; MUSCULAR DYSTROPHY; MYASTHENIA GRAVIS; RAT-BITE FEVER; TETANUS; TETANY; TRICHINOSIS.

muscular dystrophy: a wasting away, or atrophy, of the voluntary (striated) muscles, chiefly afflicting children. The cause of the condition has not yet been determined. It is known, however, that some forms of muscular dystrophy — there are several, and there is not complete agreement on their classification — are familial; i.e., there are hereditary factors involved.

One type, called *Duchenne's,* follows an X-linked recessive pattern of inheritance (see HEREDITY), thus affecting chiefly boys. It first attacks the hip and leg muscles, usually between the ages of two and four; the first symptom is generally difficulty in walking — the child falls easily and finds it hard to get up — and in climbing steps. The chest, shoulder, arm, and other muscles, too, grow progressively weaker, so that the child is almost completely helpless within six to twelve years. He is generally unusually susceptible to heart and respiratory ailments, as well. In this form of the disease, survival beyond the age of twenty is rare.

Other forms of muscular dystrophy, attacking girls as often as boys, strike in the late teens or even the early twenties. They may begin with other muscles — prominently, those of the arms, shoulders, and face — and tend to progress more slowly than the early-childhood type, so that, with orthopedic measures and physical therapy, the victim can look forward to productive years ahead.

Research is currently directed toward ascertaining just what causes the muscle deterioration in the various forms of muscular dystrophy, with hope of subsequently developing medications to halt or counteract it. There is at this writing strong suspicion of enzyme deficiency in the Duchenne's type, though not in the others.

mushroom poisoning: See FOOD POISONING.

mutation: a change in gene structure that occurs spontaneously or because of some outside influence (such as radiation), which can then be passed on to subsequent generations. Mutations take place frequently — perhaps, it has been estimated, affecting one in every five children conceived — but most are extremely minor. Only rarely do mutations result in major disorders or defects.

myasthenia gravis: a rare muscular affliction involving not atrophy, as in muscular dystrophy, but extreme fatigue and weakness of the muscles; as with muscular dystrophy, the cause is unknown (and is being intensively researched) — but here, the condition is known to be associated with a detectable decrease in certain chemical substances necessary for muscular contraction.

The onset of the disease — usually not before adolescence, although cases in infancy have been reported — is typically sudden, first affecting the muscles of the face, neck, and throat, later possibly other muscles such as those of the limbs as well; both speech and the ability to swallow may be among the first functions to suffer. Thereafter, the weakening is usually gradual.

There is no cure for myasthenia gravis, but the disease can be controlled to an extent by rest, physical therapy, and continuing treatment with certain drugs. Sometimes there have been spontaneous remissions, but they have proved to be temporary, and to date there have been no complete recoveries; therapy, however, is often highly effective.

A youngster suffering from this disease should carry identification in case of away-from-home disability; see MEDIC ALERT.

Mychel: a trade name for chloramphenicol; see ANTIBIOTICS.

Mycifradin, Myciguent: trade names for neomycin; see ANTIBIOTICS.

Mycitracin: a topical medication combining bacitracin, neomycin, and polymyxin; see ANTIBIOTICS for more about the three agents.

Mycoplasma pneumoniae: a little-known but extremely widespread infectious agent, often classified as a bacterium but technically neither bacterium nor virus. As its name implies, it can cause pneumonia. Usually, it doesn't; its repertoire appears to include a vast spectrum of conditions, all — appearing after an estimated incubation period of one to three weeks — involving the upper respiratory tract, and tending to affect different individuals in different ways (in many cases, the illness strongly resembles flu; it often involves fever, and can be quite severe). *Mycoplasma pneumoniae* epidemics are difficult to pinpoint, since symptoms are so variable, but they probably occur often among teens and young adults. The organism can be cultured, and is susceptible to treatment with erythromycin or tetracycline if necessary. A vaccine has long been sought, and it is hoped one will be available in the not too distant future.

Mycostatin: a trade name for nystatin; see ANTIBIOTICS.

myocarditis: See HEART DISEASE.

myopia: See NEARSIGHTEDNESS.

Mysoline: a trade name for primidone, an antiseizure medication; see EPILEPSY.

mytilotoxism: a type of shellfish poisoning; see FOOD POISONING.

myxedema: a severe condition of hypothyroidism involving swelling of subcutaneous tissues, dry skin, hair loss, lower than normal body temperature, weakness, and other symptoms; it is treated by administration of the missing hormonal substance.

myxoviruses: See VIRUSES.

N

nafcillin: a semisynthetic penicillin; see ANTIBIOTICS.

nail-biting: The cause of nail-biting varies from tension to boredom to emotional disturbances — and sometimes is just plain habit. Often, the more attention you pay to it, and the more you nag a child about nail-biting, the more he'll do it. Generally speaking, it's best to try and relieve any tension the child may be under, and to get him involved in more constructive or interesting activities requiring the use of his hands.

If the problem persists — and especially if it's associated with other signs of extreme tension or emotional disturbance — then discuss it with your pediatrician or family physician.

nail-cutting: Most infants are born with fully developed fingernails and, given the aimless groping activity of a tiny baby, they represent a danger. They should be cut right away; the best time is just after a feeding, when the baby has contentedly fallen asleep.

Children's fingernails, in general, should be kept quite short in order to prevent possible injury or infection when the child pokes curiously at genitals, ears, or eyes, or tries to scratch insect bites or rashes.

Toenails grow much more slowly than fingernails and usually need cutting infrequently, if at all, during a baby's first year or two. Cutting should be done straight across to prevent future problems (see TOENAIL, INGROWN).

An infant's toenails are very soft, and often curl at the ends due to pressure against a surface in crawling. This is no cause for concern; the nails will harden as the child grows.

nail injuries: A number of conditions can cause injury to the nails; they all require medical attention. Among them are a variety of skin conditions, including psoriasis; an infection at, or blow to, the nail bed, where the nail is produced; and violence done to the nail itself.

A blow to a nail usually means the area underneath the nail will turn a purplish color, and the nail may eventually drop off. A nail may also be ripped off, a mishap that's far from uncommon among youngsters (it frequently occurs when a bicycle's ridden too fast too close to a wall or other structure, and the hand gripping the handlebars comes into actual contact with the wall); it's a scary-looking injury but not really a serious one.

In either case, however, the youngster should be seen by a physician without delay in order to guard against possible infection and to have the wound properly dressed; if the nail has not been entirely lost, the doctor will generally try to keep it on as long as possible in order to protect the nail bed. New growth won't start until the nail bed heals.

narcolepsy: a condition characterized by a youngster's repeatedly falling asleep suddenly, at odd times, and not for reasons of fatigue (i.e., it happens when the child has had a normal amount of sleep); it is rare in very young children. It is sometimes erroneously referred to as "sleeping sickness"; true sleeping sickness, however, is a type of encephalitis.

Narcolepsy is not a disease but a symptom. The causes, which must be determined by a physician, may include emotional disturbances, brain injury or disease, tumors, and malfunction of certain endocrine glands; treatment, of course, depends upon what's at the root of the problem.

narcotics: powerful drugs with strong euphoric and/or analgesic (pain-relieving) effects. They are, by definition, potentially addictive and should never be used without prescription; if your doctor prescribes such a drug, however, you may be sure it is safe as long as the doctor's instructions are followed to the letter.

Addiction to any of them is a serious matter, and the problem is double-barreled since narcotics are (unlike amphetamines) addictive in *both* accepted senses of the word. There is heightened tolerance, meaning that larger and larger doses are required to achieve the sought-for effect; there is also a demonstrable physical dependence — that is, a change in the body's chemistry that makes withdrawal from or withholding of the drug a genuinely painful experience.

OPIATES

These drugs are all derived from opium.

Codeine is a legitimate ingredient of some cough medications — including, unfortunately, a few that have been available without prescription and have been a source of addiction problems among junior-high-school-age youngsters who have gone from drugstore to drugstore guzzling the stuff by the bottle (the actual codeine content per bottle is quite low).

Symptoms of addiction may include unaccustomed difficulty in rousing the child from sleep in the morning, increasing lateness coupled with falling grades in school, and possibly a drunklike gait; the eyes typically have an odd look, with narrowed pupils and redness in the whites of the eyes; there may be unexplained weight loss. In extreme cases, there may be convulsions.

Codeine is, of course, properly used in prescribed medications and is an effective cough suppressant in doctor-directed dosages; sometimes, however, it may be constipating. It may also be prescribed, in tablet form, to relieve severe pain; the doctor will undoubtedly caution you to administer it very sparingly, if possible keeping the frequency below the permitted maximum.

Heroin is not used for any legitimate medical purpose in the United States. Those addicted to it sniff the powder (the form in which it is sold) or melt it and inject it into the skin ("skin-popping") or into a vein ("mainlining") — thus risking the possibility of tetanus, septicemia, or serum hepatitis along with the addiction itself; other risks include those of a lethal overdose and the unknowable effects of adulterants that are commonly included when the drug is marketed.

The major effect of heroin is an extreme, euphoric lethargy; the pupils are typically unusually small; there may be constipation; there are generally needle marks somewhere on the addict's body. The effects last about four to six hours, when another "fix" or injection is needed. Without the drug, the addict will exhibit symptoms apparent both to himself and to others, among them general pain, nervousness and restlessness, profuse sweating, chills, sniffling, vomiting, and diarrhea.

Morphine is a very powerful antipain drug that *is* used by physicians; it is not normally prescribed for home use, but is administered by injection. Because it is so highly addictive, it is generally used only if the pain is extreme and must be relieved immediately, and the condition causing the pain can then be dealt with by other means (as, surgery); if the pain is of a chronic type, or of a longer lasting though limited nature (as, during recovery from a serious injury or from surgery), another medication is usually employed.

Symptoms of morphine addiction, much less widespread than heroin addiction, are much like those of addiction to heroin.

There are also a number of semisynthetic morphine derivatives, prominently hydromorphone (Dilaudid) and oxymorphone (Numorphan). These drugs, contrary to expectations when they were first introduced, are in a potency class with — and pose all the risks of — morphine.

Paregoric (tincture of opium) is an effective antidiarrhea drug and may sometimes be prescribed for that purpose. The dosage is always extremely small and must be followed exactly — and the drug must never be used for a *subsequent* occurrence of diarrhea unless the doctor has examined the child and explicitly directed you to do so. Never rub paregoric on a baby's gums as a teething remedy, no matter what old wives' tales you may hear advocating the practice; it can cause constipation, and it *is* a *narcotic.* Never use it for *any* purpose unless it is prescribed by your doctor.

NONOPIATES

There are three other groups of drugs that are not, strictly speaking, opiates, since they are not opium derivatives. What they are considered by the federal government is not particularly relevant, since federal drug classifications do not make a lot of pharmacological sense. (Cocaine, for example, is classified as a narcotic; it isn't. Alcohol and tobacco are not really looked upon as drugs at all; of course, they are.) Logically, they do belong in this class. Some are more risky, and have more potential for abuse, than others.

There is a fairly large group of synthetics that are quite like morphine, both chemically and in risk factors. They include alphaprodine (Nisentil), anileridine (Leritine), fentanyl (Sublimaze), levorphanol (Levo-Dromoran), meperidine (Demerol), methadone, and piminodine (Alvodine). They deserve to be treated with all the respect and caution that one would accord the opiates. They are subject to federal narcotics controls.

Not subject to those controls, and not even classed as narcotics, are ethoheptazine (Zactane), a chemical relative of meperidine, and propoxyphene (Darvon, Dolene, SK-65, et al.), which is chemically related to methadone; the latter is also marketed in such combinations as Darvon Compound (with APC) and Darvocet (with acetaminophen). In most published studies, neither drug has proved to be an especially effective pain reliever, being somewhat inferior to codeine and even, according to a Mayo Clinic study reported in 1972, to ordinary aspirin. Propoxyphene, however, can produce dependence similar to that of morphine, abuse has been widely reported, and there have been many overdose deaths; it appears probable, at this writing, that the drug will be placed under narcotics controls.

Finally, in an official limbo called "noncontrolled narcotics" are methotrimeprazine (Levoprome) and pentazocine (Talwin, also marketed in combination with aspirin as Talwin Compound). Theoretically, they have addiction potential; in practice, however, they have not caused that kind of problem (they must of course, like all these drugs, be used carefully and only according to prescribed directions). Both are effective pain relievers, though not in a class with morphine.

MIXTURES

The foregoing substances would seem the least wise of ingredients to toss in with others in combination medications, yet there are a number of products that do just that. Among those purveyed to physicians are Equagesic, combining ethoheptazine, meprobamate (an antianxiety agent with its own habit-forming potential), and aspirin; Mepergan, containing meperidine and the major tranquilizer promethazine; Percodan, which is oxycodone — a chemical analogue of codeine which is not used alone — combined with aspirin, phenacetin, and caffeine; Wygesic, combining propoxyphene and acetaminophen; and Zactirin, ethoheptazine plus aspirin.

Other mind-affecting drugs and substances that have posed social problems are discussed under AMPHETAMINES; DIET PILLS; DRINKING; GLUE-SNIFFING; PSYCHEDELICS; SEDATIVES (includes barbiturates and tranquilizers).

Nardil: a trade name for phenelzine; see ANTIDEPRESSANTS.

natal: relating or referring to birth. The adjective is rarely used alone; you'll usually encounter it with a prefix, as in the following terms:

antenatal — the same as prenatal (the latter is more common);

neonatal — immediately postnatal, relating to the first month of life (a newborn child, in this period, is a neonate);

perinatal — referring to the period surrounding birth, usually denoting the time from the beginning of labor until a day or two after the baby's birth;

prenatal — prior to birth, may refer to the entire period of gestation;

postnatal — after birth.

You may also hear such terms as *perinatology* and *prenatology*. They are fields of study centering on these periods and the events thereof.

naturopath: a practitioner who claims the ability to cure illness exclusively through the use of "natural" remedies such as foods and herbs; such a person is not a physician and is not qualified to treat you or your family. Don't confuse this word with OSTEOPATH; the latter *is* often qualified (see that entry).

nausea: a "queasy" feeling of wanting to vomit; it may be associated with dizziness, and may or may not be followed or accompanied by actual vomiting. It is a symptom of a multitude of conditions from infections to poisoning to motion sickness. Like any other symptom, persistent, unexplained nausea means the child should be seen by a doctor.

There are three main types of medications that have antinauseant properties, and which your physician may suggest under varying conditions. One is the group of antihistamines that are discussed under MOTION SICKNESS. Another, belladonna alkaloids such as atropine and scopolamine, which act as antispasmodics, relaxers of smooth muscle.

Third, there is a group of useful but potent drugs called phenothiazines that are structurally antihistamines — although they are not usually used for that purpose — and have heavy tranquilizing and antinauseant properties. They are more fully discussed under SEDATIVES. Among those that have especially useful antinauseant properties are chlorpromazine (Thorazine), fluphenazine (Prolixin), mesoridazine (Serentil), perphenazine (Trilafon), prochlorperazine (Compazine), promethazine (Phenergan), and triflupromazine (Vesprin). None of these should be used without medical consultation — and they should *not* be used for motion sickness.

There are also a number of medications combining sedatives or tranquilizers with specific antispasmodic agents. Among these are Combid, which includes prochlorperazine; Donnatal, which includes phenobarbital; Milpath and Pathibamate, which include the anti-anxiety drug meprobamate; and a number of medications used to counter such symptoms in migraine, which are listed under that topic.

navel in newborn baby: The stump of the umbilical cord, tied off or clamped and cut just after birth, will drop off after about a week or two. Until then, the baby should not be immersed in water. When the cord drops off, the child's navel may be rather messy-looking — moist, and possibly blood-tinged. Don't be alarmed; that's normal. Simply daub the area, once a day, with regular rubbing alcohol, which will help to dry it up. (The baby will generally squeal — not because it hurts or burns, but simply because it's unexpectedly cold). Any discharge, redness of the surrounding skin, or other unusual symptoms should, of course, be brought to your doctor's attention.

If your child's healed navel is the tucked-in kind, it requires some special attention. About once a week, either in the bath or while changing the baby, spread the puckers apart and cleanse the navel with soap and water, or with alcohol on a piece of cotton. If you omit this, secretions from the skin and urine from the diaper accumulate and eventually produce an odor; this material can also cause irritation, or even infection, in the surrounding area.

A not uncommon, and not serious, condition called umbilical hernia is discussed under HERNIA.

nearsightedness: the inability to see clearly at a distance because light rays are focused improperly and fall short of the retina; the medical term for the condition is *myopia.* It is usually hereditary.

A nearsighted youngster will tend to squint when focusing on distant objects; if you see this happening, you should promptly schedule an appointment with an ophthalmologist (if you don't know one, your family physician or pediatrician can recommend one). The condition can easily be corrected with proper glasses or contact lenses — and if it isn't corrected, it can hamper emotional and mental growth, narrowing the child's world both literally and figuratively.

Nebcin: a trade name for tobramycin; see ANTIBIOTICS.

neck problems: The muscles and tendons of the neck, like those of any other part of the body, are subject to stresses and strains, twists and tensions. If your youngster has any such pain or discomfort, though, it's best to have the doctor check it out to make sure it's nothing more serious than temporary muscle strain.

A special sort of neck problem that sometimes afflicts infants is called *wry neck* or, in medical terminology, *torticollis;* in this condition, the child's head is twisted to one side. It may be present at birth, disappearing with time. In an older child, it may appear suddenly; one possible cause could be a blow causing spasm of the muscles at that side of the neck, and there may be other causes as well, since it seems to occur at times without any apparent injury. It can, at any rate, be treated by application of heat and administration of various muscle-relaxing drugs; if you suspect your child has wry neck, call your doctor.

In an accident or fall, if you have any reason to think a child's neck may possibly be broken, turn immediately to BACK AND NECK INJURIES.

necrosis: the medical term for destruction or disintegration of tissues still in place and connected with healthy, living tissue; the condition may be caused by infection or not, may be extremely critical (as gangrene) or less critical and even temporary (as Legg-Perthes disease).

negative: a word used to describe the result of a test or examination; it means normal — that is, there is no evidence of the disease, condition, or problem for which the test or examination was made. A negative verdict on a VDRL test, for example, means that the patient does not have syphilis; a negative result of a test for pregnancy means that the patient is not pregnant; a negative physical examination has revealed no abnormal conditions.

Nembutal: a trade name for pentobarbital; see SEDATIVES.

Neobiotic, neomycin: See ANTIBIOT-

ICS; the former is a trade name for the latter.

neonatal, neonatology: See NATAL.

neoplasm: literally, "new growth," usually referring to a tumor; a neoplasm may be either benign or malignant.

Neo-Polycin, Neosporin: trade names for topical medications containing bacitracin, neomycin, and polymyxin; see ANTIBIOTICS.

Neo-Synephrine: See DECONGESTANTS, NASAL.

nephritis: an inflammation of the kidney; the term covers a group of disorders varying in cause but characterized by similar symptoms. Nephritis is a serious matter and prompt medical attention is crucial; there is complete recovery in well over 90 percent of cases, however, with early diagnosis and proper treatment. Untreated, it can cause other, even more serious, problems (see NEPHROSIS).

Symptoms of nephritis may include fatigue, poor appetite, headache, edema and fluid retention, increased blood pressure, and albuminuria; there may also be blood in the urine, a clear signal of something seriously amiss.

Bright's disease is a particular type of nephritis, medically termed *glomerulonephritis;* it is specifically an inflammation of the glomeruli, the small filtering units in the kidney. It is the most common kidney problem in children and frequently (though not always) is a complication of a prior respiratory infection. In addition to the symptoms previously noted, there may be high fever, vomiting, and — fairly typically — a great deal of blood in the urine. *Any* abnormality in your child's urine should be reported to the doctor immediately. The exact nature of the condition can be determined by urinalysis and other tests. Treatment of nephritis depends upon the cause of the problem and generally includes rest and dietary measures as well as medication.

nephrosis: a serious condition involving degeneration of certain tiny tubules within the kidney; it may be recurrent or chronic, and may result from nephritis that goes undiagnosed and untreated (see preceding entry). The chief noticeable symptom is edema — swelling due to fluid retention — in the abdomen, the chest, the area around the eyes, and sometimes the legs as well; albuminuria, not visible to the eye but easy to find by urinalysis, is also present.

Nephrosis is not itself an infection, but the child who has it is extremely susceptible to infection. Prompt diagnosis is vital, and hospitalization is usually needed; treatment generally includes various drugs, especially ACTH and cortisone, dietary measures, and precautions against infection, which may include preventive antibiotics. Most youngsters recover completely, although they may have one or more recurrences; the child's urine should be checked for albumin whenever he has any infection, particularly respiratory.

Nervine: an over-the-counter "tranquilizer"; see SEDATIVES.

nervous system: We define briefly, here, some terms you may hear and see referring to parts and functions of this intricate communications network.

Afferent and *efferent* are opposites

that can describe blood vessels too, but usually refer to nerves. The first means bringing toward the center, the second carrying outward. Thus, afferent nerves are those that bring messages — perceptions, sensations — from various parts of the body to the brain; efferent nerves are those that relay directions from the brain to muscles, etc.

The *central nervous system* (medically, often abbreviated to CNS) means the brain and spinal cord. Part of it is the *autonomic* nervous system, which is concerned with relaying impulses to those muscle tissues not under voluntary control: the heart, the muscles of the intestines, and so on. That, in turn, includes the *sympathetic* and *parasympathetic* divisions which send their messages from different parts of the CNS and — without getting overly technical — act more or less as a check on each other; it is the sympathetic network, for example, that speeds up the heart rate in response to excitement or alarm (and slows down intestinal contractions), while the functions of the parasympathetic system include slowing and steadying the heartbeat and getting digestion going.

Nerves outside the central system are called *peripheral.*

neuritis: an inflammation of nerves or nerve sheaths — a symptom, not a disease; the affected part of the body usually hurts, although there may sometimes be loss of sensation or even paralysis. It may be caused by, or associated with, a variety of conditions, including nutritional deficiencies, diabetes mellitus, certain types of poisoning, frostbite, and a number of infectious ailments. Once a diagnosis is made, the physician will give analgesics to relieve pain and will prescribe whatever treatment or drugs are necessary to deal with the basic cause of the problem.

neuroblastoma: a malignant growth (see CANCER for general comment) arising from embryonic sympathetic nerve cells that, for unknown reasons, develop in a deviant manner; it is the second most frequently seen solid tumor in children. Neuroblastoma occurs only in small children and generally appears quite early; almost a third of the cases are detected within the first year of life. It can occur anywhere in the body, but in two out of three cases, it arises somewhere in the abdomen.

Symptoms of neuroblastoma depend upon its location. Sometimes, a parent notices a mass or swelling. More often, there are other symptoms — among them listlessness, persistent diarrhea, or pain — that bring the condition to light; all of these, of course, can (and usually do) signal other problems, but they do call for medical evaluation. A diagnosis of neuroblastoma is based on X rays, blood tests, and other procedures that may vary depending upon the location; helpful in diagnosis is the fact that in about seven out of ten cases the tumor secretes a chemical that can be detected in the urine.

Early detection is very important, since that offers the best hope of surgical cure. If there has been little or no metastasis, especially if the child is under the age of two years, the chance of full recovery — with surgery, possibly backup irradiation and/or chemotherapy as well — is close to 90 percent.

neurologist: See SPECIALTIES, MEDICAL.

neurosis: an emotional illness often characterized by conflict between an individual's needs and desires and external pressures, which may produce feelings of anxiety or guilt; there is no essential disturbance in the perception of reality. For comparison, see PSYCHOSIS.

neurosurgeon: a specialist in surgery involving the brain and nervous system.

neurotoxic: particularly poisonous or harmful to components and circuits of the nervous system.

nevus: See BIRTHMARKS.

niacin: one of the B vitamins; see NUTRITION.

Niconyl: a trade name for isoniazid, an antituberculosis drug.

nicotinic acid: another name for niacin; see NIACIN.

Nidar: a combination of four barbiturates; see SEDATIVES.

Niemann-Pick disease: one of the relatively rare, hereditary lipid-metabolism diseases, like Gaucher's disease and Tay-Sachs disease transmitted by autosomal recessive inheritance (see HEREDITY) and — like these, Fabry's disease, and others — the result of an enzyme deficiency; the enzyme in this condition is one called sphingomyelinase. In Niemann-Pick disease, there are heavy accumulations of non-metabolized fatty materials in the liver and spleen, and possibly the bone marrow, lungs, and other sites as well. There is usually severe, progressive mental retardation, with death inevitable before the age of six years — although there are apparently some very rare forms in which life expectancy may be considerably extended or even normal.

No treatment is, at this writing, available for Niemann-Pick disease. It is, however, among those that can be diagnosed by fetal cell sampling (see AMNIOCENTESIS), and "carrier" parents can also be pinpointed. In future, it may be possible to replace the missing enzyme, treatment that is now at least theoretically possible in other similar disorders.

night blindness: a condition resulting from lack of vitamin A; see DEFICIENCY DISEASES. Also see RETINITIS PIGMENTOSA.

nightmares: Scary dreams can happen to anyone — to children more than to adults, because they're more impressionable and less experienced and can be seriously disturbed by stimuli ignored by adults. Late, heavy meals, late hours, and excessive excitement during the evening can be precipitating factors and should be avoided.

If a child does have a nightmare, he will be aware of the reason for waking up in a state of fright. You can help by reassuring him and bringing him quickly back to safe reality; have him recount the dream to you so he can get it off his chest and you can laugh at the obvious unreality of it together.

A child will generally not have a nightmare more than once in a single night, and the dream will often be triggered by a real event or experience of the previous evening; nightmares are different from night terrors (see following).

night terrors: This is something completely different from a nightmare (see the preceding entry). The youngster will wake up screaming and is indeed in genuine terror, although he has *not* had a bad dream that he can remember or recount. When you run to comfort him, you might find him totally disoriented; he may behave very strangely and may not even recognize you at first.

Don't panic. Be patient, and do whatever is necessary to comfort him. Do ask if anything hurts, in case there is really something physically wrong (generally there isn't). The situation will not go on all night; usually the child will eventually come to himself and go peacefully back to sleep — and may not even remember the incident the next day.

Night terrors are not uncommon and usually signal some emotional disturbance, but it's almost always of a temporary nature and will straighten itself out; you might try to find out, during the day, if something is bothering the child, or there is some insecurity. If night terrors recur frequently, or over a period of time, however, there may be a serious emotional problem for which professional help is needed; you should discuss the question with your pediatrician or family physician.

Nilstat: a trade name for nystatin; see ANTIBIOTICS.

Nisentil: a trade name for alphaprodine, a morphinelike synthetic drug; see NARCOTICS.

nit: the egg of an insect; see LICE for the only ones that are likely to pose a problem for people.

Nite Rest: an over-the-counter "sleep aid"; see SEDATIVES.

Nobese: a trade name for a combination-of-ingredients "diet pill"; see AMPHETAMINES.

Noctec: a trade name for chloral hydrate; see SEDATIVES.

NoDoz: a trade name for a "wake-up pill" sold without prescription; it contains caffeine. For comparison with more powerful substances, see AMPHETAMINES.

nolitetracycline: one of the tetracyclines; see ANTIBIOTICS.

Noludar: a trade name for the sleep-inducing drug methyprylon; see SEDATIVES.

Norflex: a trade name for orphenadrine, a muscle relaxant; this class of drugs is discussed under SEDATIVES.

Norgesic: a combination product containing aspirin, phenacetin, caffeine (see APC TABLETS), and the muscle relaxant orphenadrine (see SEDATIVES).

Norpramin: a trade name for desipramine; see ANTIDEPRESSANTS.

nortriptyline: See ANTIDEPRESSANTS.

nosebleed: A nosebleed may or may not be a symptom of something quite serious; generally it's nothing to worry about, except in the first two special instances mentioned in the second and third paragraphs following.

The first rule is: *don't panic.* Whatever the cause of the nosebleed, panic on your part is likely to arouse panic in the child — which tends, in turn, to make the nosebleed worse. Most nosebleeds appear to be more severe hemorrhages than they actually are; a teaspoonful of blood can easily cover a pillow. Stay calm and do what has to be done.

If the child has had a fall or other accident, nosebleed could be a symptom of skull fracture or internal injury. Don't stop for any first-aid measures whatever. Rush the child to the nearest hospital emergency room, keeping him flat on his back.

If the child's tonsils and/or adenoids were recently removed, keep the child lying down and quiet, and telephone the doctor who operated.

In other cases, nosebleed is generally due to hemorrhage from small blood vessels in the mucous membrane of the nose, which may have been irritated by a cold or an allergic condition or by the youngster's blowing his nose too hard or too often; or, the child may have actually scratched the membrane in picking the nose. In any case, the bleeding must be stopped. Forget the old wives' tales about cold keys on the back of the neck; they won't work. Nor should you pack the child's nose with anything.

Have the child sit up, and keep him sitting up. Pinch the nostrils (or the one nostril, if bleeding is from one side only) closed and hold them that way for three to five minutes. Then gradually release the pressure. If bleeding is continuing, or immediately begins again, repeat the nostril-pinching procedure. If it still doesn't work, take the child to the nearest hospital emergency room; there may be a circulatory problem that requires immediate medical attention.

If you have managed to stop the bleeding, dip a cotton swab in some ordinary nose drops and gently daub it on the mucous membrane of the septum (you'll probably be able to see,

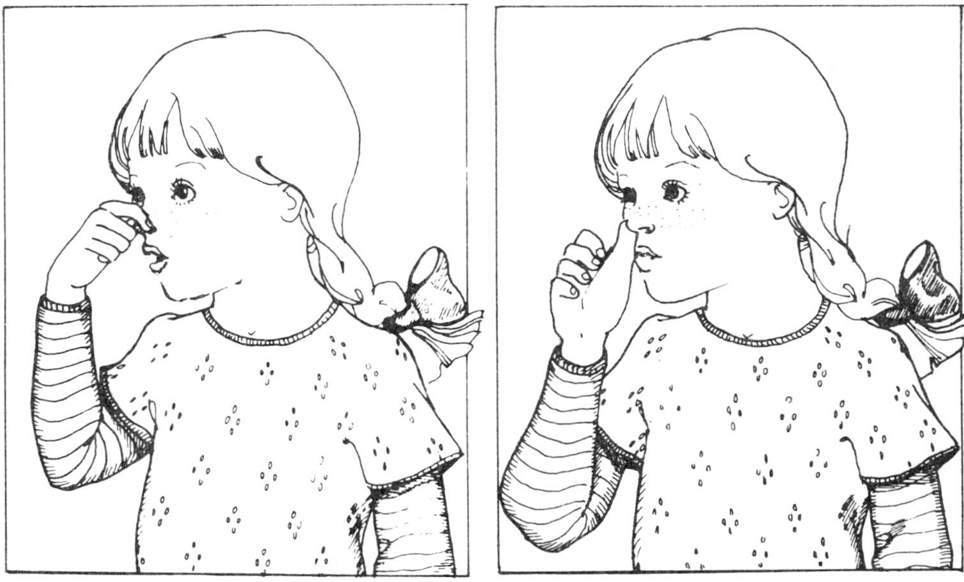

Stopping an Ordinary Nosebleed

The affected nostril or nostrils should be held closed for three to five minutes — by the child if old enough, by an older person if the child is too small to exert pressure; see text for further measures.

at this point, where the bleeding came from; if not, daub it as far up as you can); this will help to constrict the capillaries. Apply a little petroleum jelly at bedtime for the next few nights to soothe the area.

nose-blowing: a feat that is rarely mastered at the age of a year, uncommonly by two, often not until much later. At whatever age your youngster seems ready to tackle it, it's important that it be done properly — which means one nostril at a time, and not holding the tissue too tightly. Children are quite susceptible to middle-ear infections because of their relatively short eustachian tubes. Holding both nostrils tightly when blowing tends to force infectious material from the nose-throat area into those tubes.

nose, broken: See FRACTURES.

nose drops: See DECONGESTANTS, NASAL.

nose, object in: The child may be able to eject the object himself if you can induce sneezing; try having him sniff some pepper. If that doesn't work, don't make any attempts to remove the object yourself; take the child to the doctor.

nose shape, change in: See PLASTIC SURGERY.

nose sprays: See DECONGESTANTS, NASAL.

Novahistine: See ANTIHISTAMINES.

numbness: a deprivation, total or partial, of feeling and/or motion. Severe cold, for one thing, can cause it. Also, following a cut, even a small one, a child may complain of numbness or a "funny feeling" around the area; this means that some of the tiny nerves have been severed, and it will take a long time before normal sensation is restored, if ever (these nerves may slowly regenerate, but sometimes they will not).

If there is no apparent cause for numbness, the child should be seen by a physician.

Numorphan: a trade name for oxymorphone, a semisynthetic morphine derivative; see NARCOTICS.

nurse, nurse-midwife, nurse's aide: See HEALTH PROFESSIONALS.

nursing: See BREAST FEEDING.

nutrition: More than forty distinct elements, nutritionists have found, are necessary for maintenance of your children's normal growth and continued good health — but you need not be concerned with most of them. There are just a handful of basic constituents, vitamins, and minerals whose absence can cause serious problems (see DEFICIENCY DISEASES); if your children get enough of those, they'll be getting the minor elements too.

Nor need you do your shopping armed with sets of nutritional charts; if you see that your family gets a good assortment of various *kinds* of foods — breads and cereals, meats and dairy products, fruits and vegetables, and so on — then their diet is bound to be nutritionally balanced, too.

Weight problems needn't and shouldn't interfere with this effort. It's perfectly possible to avoid fattening foods and maintain nutritional balance; see CALORIES.

In most parts of the United States today, there is no need to supplement your children's diet with vitamins or other food supplements; everything they need can be obtained from readily available foods. There are exceptions, of course; your doctor may at times recommend vitamin and/or mineral supplements for a very young infant whose all-milk diet may be inadequate, for a child with a definite deficiency of some sort, or for one whose nutritional needs are greater; you should then, of course, follow your physician's instructions.

Here are some facts about the functions and sources of the major nutritional elements, both for your general information, and for your guidance if the doctor should advise your increasing or decreasing a particular element in your child's diet.

BASIC ORGANIC CONSTITUENTS

These are the elements of which our bodies are actually made — the elements, in fact, of which all living matter is made. Protein is the most important of them, by far; there's little sugar, and even less spice, involved, despite the old rhyme about the alleged components of little girls. (The snails and puppy dogs' tails attributed to small boys were meant to sound unappetizing, but perhaps came closer; at least they were proteins.)

Protein constitutes at least half the dry matter in the human body (the body is some 70 percent water); something over one-third of the protein is in muscles. Protein is needed daily to build, repair, and renew body tissues, since the body cannot store a great deal of it. The protein we eat is broken down, in the process of digestion, into components called amino acids; these, in turn, become the "building blocks" of the new proteins in our bodies.

Animal life provides by far the best source of protein; that includes meats, poultry, fish, eggs, milk, and milk products such as butter and cheese. There are some reasonably good vegetable sources, too — soybeans, nuts, dry beans and peas — that can occasionally substitute for more expensive things in the first group. And there's some protein, too, in whole-grain cereals, breads, fruits, and vegetables; but these relatively inferior sources become more beneficial if they're eaten with high-protein foods — vegetables with meat, for example, and cereal with milk.

Fats provide heat and energy, and some contain vitamins A and D or help in their utilization. They're stored in the body, so they're not needed daily, and in fact you needn't make any special effort to include them in your family menu; many foods contain fats, though not always obviously — among them meats, eggs, butter, whole milk and milk products, and all fried foods.

Carbohydrates include starches and sugars, and these too provide heat and energy; in the latter function, they're somewhat faster-acting than fats, and they do have a place in the diet of the active youngster who uses up energy fast. Refined-sugar foods such as candy, though, tend to have destructive effects on the teeth, and it's better for children to get this element from foods that have other nutritional benefits, such as ice cream; fruits are excellent natural-sugar sources, too. See SWEETENERS for more about this class of nutrients and substitutes for them.

VITAMINS

There are some forty vitamins (that's how many are known; there may be more), but only a few that you even have to think about. If your youngster gets these, he'll be getting the others as well, since there are no unique food sources for the latter.

The word "vitamin" was coined from the Latin *vita,* "life"; a vitamin is, you might say, a "life-chemical," a substance presumably necessary for existence, or at least reasonably healthy existence. Over the years, as these substances known or believed to be essential to human health have been discovered, they have been named and given alphabetical designations (some with sub-numerical designations as well), all the way from A to such little-known ones as T and U. (There are also others that have been found vital to the lives of fish, chickens, and other creatures, but not to human beings or to our fellow mammals.)

Their discoveries have usually occurred under dire circumstances, involving the diagnosis of a disorder that is found to respond to the chemical together with the finding that it has been missing from the diet (or is in the diet but is for some reason not being utilized). Probably the earliest and most famous example was the eighteenth-century realization that sailors who were at sea for long periods of time suffered from the severe ailment called scurvy. An observation that the one element missing from their diets was citrus fruit led to the remedy; by 1795, British sailors were being issued a daily ration of lime juice, and shipboard scurvy faded into memory. Not until 1928, however, was the essential element identified as vitamin C.

It has become clear, as vitamins have been isolated, that they are indeed essential, and that their absence or marked deficiency causes serious illness. It is clear only to certain pill manufacturers and to ill-informed promoters of nutritional nonsense that taking it upon yourself to dose your children with extra quantities of these chemicals is in the least desirable. In fact, it is increasingly apparent to physicians and to respected nutritionists that popping these pills into your family's mouths is distinctly *un*desirable — not merely unnecessary, but potentially harmful. There are several reasons.

One is that the *third of a billion dollars* annually funneled out of the American family budget for these products is cash that could more wisely be spent for better quality diet, increased medical insurance, healthful recreation, and things similarly beneficial to the American family's health. In short, it's wasted money. We like the way Dr. Philip White, Director of the American Medical Association's Department of Foods and Nutrition and a leading authority on the subject, puts it: "Ingesting unneeded quantities of vitamin supplements is about as logical as assuming one can sweep more efficiently with two brooms than with one."

Only small quantities of the vitamins are needed for continued health, and only when there is marked deficiency or a special situation is replacement or addition needed. A deficiency might result from inadequate nutrition, from an inability of the body to use the vitamin even though it's available in the diet (in both these cases, there would be detectable signs and symptoms), or — temporarily — from disinclination to eat during a serious illness; prolonged high fever, extreme fluid loss, or extensive burns might also pose a threat of temporary deficiency.

Certain other circumstances might also suggest a need for supplements. They may be prescribed in pregnancy, since the developing child's nutritional needs must be taken into account. They may be advised, at times, for a nursing mother. They are generally added (in liquid form) to an infant's diet to fill needs not met by milk or formula alone. Additional supplements may be needed for a premature infant whose ability to utilize nutrients in milk may not be fully developed at birth. And they may be suggested for a child who is allergic to an entire group of foods containing a particular vitamin.

All of the foregoing, importantly, are situations in which the need is determined, and the remedy advised, by a physician. The purpose is therapeutic, to remedy or to prevent a particular problem. None of this applies to the average child or adult.

A second reason not to succumb to the pleas of the pill-pushers is that dispensing vitamin supplements to your children can lead to a false sense of security on your part, with resulting carelessness in seeing that their diet is well balanced. Bear in mind that other nutritional elements, besides vitamins, are needed; no number of pills can guarantee your child an adequate intake of protein, or of carbohydrates. Further, vitamin pills often do not include minerals — which are essential too — or, if they do, it is not necessarily the full range in the required amounts. And they typically do *not* contain any of those dozens of minor vitamins that are needed in very tiny amounts and *are* present in the food sources of the major vitamins.

There is a third very good reason to eschew unprescribed vitamin supplements: certain of these substances can actually be *toxic* in sufficient quantities — yes, poisonous — and in smaller but still excessive quantities can create a good deal of havoc in the body; in the cases of others, the effects of extra, unneeded amounts are unknown and *may* be distinctly harmful. Infants and children are most susceptible to the adverse effects of vitamin overdosage (but teenagers and adults are by no means immune to them).

The federal government has, at this writing, taken two small steps to protect the gullible public from itself; they do not make it impossible for people to poison themselves with vitamin pills, just a little more tedious. RDAs — which stands for recommended daily allowances — have been established by the Food and Nutrition Board of the National Research Council for the major vitamins, denoting those amounts that will maintain good health (they are well above amounts needed to prevent deficiency diseases). And dosages of vitamins A and D (which have proved especially hazardous in large quantities) exceeding certain levels are sold only by prescription.

We shall detail functions, sources,

and overdose hazards of the major vitamins, in alphabetical order. First, a brief mention of one of the minor vitamins, one of the few minor ones for which both function and deficit have been pinpointed: vitamin K.

Vitamin K is not included in over-the-counter products, and no RDA has in fact been established for it; the necessary quantities are infinitesimal, the sources the same as those for several of the major vitamins. It acts to maintain normal blood levels of prothrombin, a factor needed for blood clotting (it is sometimes called the "antihemorrhage vitamin"). Deficiency is extremely rare and, as you may imagine, is usually discovered rather quickly. It is administered therapeutically to a woman shortly before delivery or to an infant right after birth in order to prevent hemorrhage in the newborn, and also in instances of overdose of anticoagulant drugs.

Now to vitamins A through E, the major "life-chemicals."

Vitamin A, most widely known as a preventer of "night blindness" (actually subnormal vision under dusk or dimly lit conditions), is also vital to overall vision, to growth and bone development, and to the health of the skin and mucous membranes. Its utilization by the body requires protein, so the diet must include an adequate amount of that substance. Deficiency can thus result from lack of protein; it can also occur in disorders, including cystic fibrosis, that interfere with the digestion of fats.

Eggs, butter, cheese, and fortified milk all contain lots of vitamin A (there is enough in human milk for a breast-fed infant; a bottle-fed baby needs either a fortified formula or prescribed supplements). Meats, liver in particular, are also good sources. Deep-yellow and dark-green vegetables — carrots, spinach, squash, etc. — contain carotenes, substances that are converted to vitamin A by the body. Most margarines are fortified with either carotene or the vitamin itself (check labels).

Vitamin A is one of the three fat-soluble vitamins; it is stored by the body, and deficiencies are therefore — except in cases of long-term deprivation, invariably involving multiple deficiencies — extremely rare. (That is also the reason for its high potential toxicity: large doses over a period of time can create perilous buildup.) Dosage is measured in international units; the RDA is 2500 to 5000 I.U. — a bit less for children under five, a bit more for pregnant women and nursing mothers (that's true for all vitamins). Which means that one cup of canned sweet potatoes (17,000 I.U.) will more than adequately supply the vitamin A needs of three to six people for a day. Some other interesting examples of vitamin A content: half a cantaloupe, 6540 I.U.; three raw apricots, 2980 I.U.; a cup of cooked spinach, 14,580 I.U.; two ounces of beef liver, 30,000 I.U.; a cup of collard greens, 10,260 I.U.; a ten-ounce package of frozen chopped broccoli, 6500 I.U.; one raw carrot, 5500 I.U.

It should be clear that the average person does not need supplements. The medical literature abounds with case reports of vitamin A's toxic effects from prolonged excessive use, and we are not going to recount them all here. Suffice it to say that among the documented results of overdosage are bald spots, mouth ulcers, anemia, severe liver damage, hypertension, neurological problems, physical stunting in children, and an alarming condition called pseudotumor cerebri — a buildup of pressure within the head that mimics brain tumor.

The B vitamins ("B complex") include a variety of substances, which appear to work together to an extent, of which more shortly. Six of them have been clearly pegged as essential and have been assigned RDAs, although you need really be concerned only about the first three we shall list, since the others are needed in truly minuscule quantities; actually, few foods contain massive quantities of B vitamins, but most, as it happens, contain some (and a balanced diet will provide enough). As a group, they are important to the body's overall functioning, especially in the areas of the nervous system, the circulatory system, digestion, and metabolism. The six major B vitamins:

• Thiamine (B_1) plays a major role in the health of the nervous system and in carbohydrate metabolism; severe deficiency, as is well known, causes the debilitating disease called beriberi. Deficiencies (of thiamine and usually of other B vitamins too) have also been known to occur occasionally in certain intestinal disorders that interfere with digestion and absorption of food sources. Primary sources are whole-grain and enriched breads and cereals; most meats contain significant amounts, too. The RDA is 0.75 to 2.25 milligrams; there have been no reports, to date, of toxic overdoses.

• Riboflavin (B_2, G) performs primarily in metabolism at the cellular level. Deficiency hardly ever occurs alone, but accompanies pellagra (niacin deficiency) and/or other B-complex deficiencies. It's found in milk (the major source), meats, eggs, nuts; the RDA is similar to that for thiamine and can be entirely supplied by one pint of milk (whole or skim). No adverse effects of overdosage have been documented.

• Niacin (nicotinic acid) is especially important in sugar metabolism; deficiency causes the degenerative disease called pellagra (which, again, rarely occurs without other B-complex deficiencies as well). The body actually manufactures a good deal of the niacin it needs from an amino acid called tryptophan, which is present in practically all foods (prime sources are milk, meat, eggs, nuts, and legumes). The RDA is ten to thirty milligrams — but because of that tryptophan factor, don't try to figure it out; again, a balanced diet will provide what's needed. There have been reports of adverse effects of overdosage via unneeded supplements; they include liver dysfunction and jaundice, gastrointestinal irritation and aggravation of peptic ulcer, increased levels of uric acid (which can lead to kidney stones in some people), distortion of laboratory tests, and increased histamine release (which could be inimical to children with asthma or other allergic disorders).

• Pyridoxine (B_6) is one word covering three slightly different chemical substances — pyridoxine itself, derived from plants, and pyridoxal and pyridoxamine, from animal foods. It plays a part in protein metabolism and, to a lesser degree, in some other bodily processes. The RDA is only one to three milligrams, and deficiency (except as part of overall B-complex deficiency) is practically unheard of. You run virtually no risk of it, whatever your family eats; there is a vast list of sources, including bananas, cereals, poultry, meat, fish, shellfish, eggs, green vegetables, nuts, prunes, potatoes, raisins, and we could go on for another page. Liver damage has been reported from excessive amounts.

• Folic acid (folicin, M) acts in collaboration with cyanocobalamin (following) in assuring healthy blood function. Its therapeutic use is limited to a particular type of anemia (certain drugs can sometimes deplete folic-acid levels, and supplements are of course given when such depletion is diagnosed). The RDA is really tiny, less than half a milligram; major sources are liver, dark-green vegetables, nuts, and lentils.

• Cyanocobalamin (B_{12}) works, as we've mentioned, in conjunction with folic acid. Deficiency causes a specific kind of anemia, sometimes due to abnormal absorption of the vitamin; despite what you may have heard about people receiving B_{12} shots for "pep-up" purposes, cyanocobalamin is properly given only to correct such an anemia (if there is a chronic, inherent absorption problem, replacement therapy continues indefinitely), and unneeded supplementation is a waste of money (no specific adverse effects have been reported). The RDA is a mere three to nine *micro*grams (a microgram is a millionth of a gram); sources are foods of animal origin only, including eggs, meats (especially organ meats such as liver and kidney), cheeses, fish, and shellfish.

Because the B-complex vitamins work, as we said, in concert, they need one another. Many authorities believe that a possible hazard of taking extra, unneeded quantities of some of them may thus lead to what could be, in effect, a "created deficiency" of others.

A second perilous aspect of B-vitamin overdosage as a group is that certain of them are known to interact with other drugs (and there may also be other, as yet unknown, interactions) — which could lead to quite serious trouble. Riboflavin, for example, can counteract the benefits of tetracycline taken for an infection; excess folic acid can lower blood levels of the anticonvulsant drug phenytoin (Dilantin); overdosage of the complex as a whole can increase blood-clotting time, thus posing a critical threat of hemorrhage to anyone with even a slight bleeding problem.

Vitamin C (ascorbic acid) plays a part in many bodily processes essential to health maintenance and resistance to infection; a severe deficiency causes the tissue-degeneration disease called scurvy. The supply must be refreshed daily, because human beings — unlike most other mammals — can neither synthesize nor store the vitamin. Therapeutically, it's administered beyond normal levels to treat diagnosed deficiency (mild deficiency can cause gum problems, degeneration of connective tissue, and delayed wound healing), in severe injuries when abnormally low blood levels of the vitamin have been found, and frequently in cases of severe and extensive burns.

A mere ten milligrams a day of vitamin C (one ounce of orange juice contains over 15 mg) is sufficient to prevent scurvy; the RDA is 30 to 90 mg. You undoubtedly know that citrus fruits (grapefruit, lemons, limes, oranges, tangerines) and their juices are prime sources. But so are many other fruits and vegetables; here are some other examples of vitamin C content: an average raw tomato, 42 mg; a cup of strawberries, 88 mg; half a cantaloupe, 63 mg; a ten-ounce package of frozen chopped broccoli, 143 mg; a cup of cooked cauliflower, 66 mg; a cup of cooked mustard greens or turnip greens, 68 mg.

Does processing destroy vitamin C? Yes — some kinds, under some conditions. Not canning; canned orange juice, for example, retains 98 percent of its original vitamin C content. Cooking, though, can deplete the food value — not because the vitamin dissipates, but because it dissolves readily in water. The answer is simply to use as little liquid as possible when cooking a vitamin C-rich vegetable (and to reuse the liquid later for such things as rice) — and to avoid water entirely if you can (e.g., by baking potatoes and sweet potatoes instead of boiling them).

What about the recurrent question of whether or not extra vitamin C can prevent colds? Since the theory was first proposed, via a best-selling book, in 1970, there have been several studies — which have admittedly been difficult to carry out because of the subjective nature of cold symptoms. It has been pretty clearly established that it would not cause a person to have significantly fewer colds; results *have* suggested, however, that colds *may,* as a result, be milder and perhaps shorter (demonstrated by fewer days missed from school or work).

Should you, on that basis, provide your children with 100- (or 250- or 500- or 1000-) mg supplements? We don't think so. For one thing, the study results cited are not considered conclusive, and have not been consistent from one investigation to another among the few that have been conducted. For another, long-term results of massive vitamin C doses (including possible effects on an unborn child) are not yet known — and some adverse short-term effects *are* known.

It has been observed that high doses of the vitamin can cause diarrhea, can shorten coagulation time (subjecting some people to heightened hazards of blood-clot formation), and can dangerously deplete blood levels of the B vitamin folic acid. They may also increase the chance of kidney stones in some people, produce adverse effects on growing bone, and interfere with testing for diabetes mellitus (as well as with urine testing in diagnosed diabetes).

Vitamin D, the so-called "sunshine vitamin," is actually formed within the body (as well as occurring in, or added to, foods), so some scientists think it should be called a hormone. Sunshine does play a part in the process.

Human skin contains a substance called 7-dehydrocholesterol, located just beneath the stratum corneum, the outermost layer of the skin. That substance, under the influence of the sun's rays, undergoes a series of chemical conversions, the end result of which — while not in fact a single substance — can, for all practical purposes, be called vitamin D, and is the substance in foods and in vitamin products.

Nature obviously intended young children to receive more of this substance: infants' skin contains twice the adult concentration of it and, regardless of race, the skin of infants is thinner and more lightly pigmented than that of adults of similar coloring; the decrease in concentration and increase in pigmentation occur gradually over the years. The reason: vitamin D is essential for assimilation of calcium and other minerals for proper bone development.

Tiny amounts are needed, too, for those whose skeletal growth is completed, but the need decreases radically. While the RDA for infants, pregnant women, and nursing mothers is 200 to 400 I.U. (like vitamin A, vitamin D is measured in international units), there has been no RDA established for others; the best estimate is about 70 I.U. — a little less for those with lighter than average skin, a little more for those who are darker.

Vitamin D deficiency in infants and toddlers can cause rickets, maldevelopment in growing bones; in adults, deficiency may result in blood-calcium imbalance, creating a muscle disorder called tetany. Deficiency can stem from dietary lack, from difficulty in absorbing the vitamin from food sources, or — in small children — lack of sunshine (another count in the case against smog). The leading food sources of vitamin D are fortified milk, margarine, and cereals; butter; eggs; liver; and salt-water fish such as tuna, salmon, and sardines. Deficiencies are rare except where there has been an extreme lack of sun plus a seriously unbalanced diet.

Like vitamin A, vitamin D is fat soluble, is stored by the body, and can be highly toxic in large, unneeded doses (products containing more than 400 I.U. in a single dose are now available only by prescription); highly individual reactions to overdoses have been documented, and there is often a very narrow margin between helpful and harmful amounts. Nausea, vomiting, headaches, appetite loss, and weakness — which do not sound truly critical — have been known to occur. And so have a number of clearly serious conditions, including kidney stones, increases in blood-lipid levels, bone fragility, calcification of vital organs, and increased blood pressure. There is concern at this writing that excessive doses during pregnancy may cause congenital blood-vessel malformation — in particular, stenosis of the aorta. And some recent studies have raised the possibility that overdose over a period of time may substantially raise the risk of heart attack.

Vitamin E, like C, has been heavily promoted as a panacea, to the sole benefit of its exploiters. Its purveyors have claimed, variously, that it will combat angina, prevent heart attacks, soothe tired feet, avert miscarriage, relieve constipation, stabilize blood pressure, strengthen muscles, reverse mental retardation, improve vision, heal wounds, smooth wrinkles, banish body odor, relieve arthritis, and boost sexual prowess — among other things. Not a single one of these claims is true.

"Vitamin E" refers to a group of substances called alpha-, beta-, gamma-, and delta-tocopherol; often only the first, alpha-tocopherol, is mentioned, since it is the most active and constitutes 90 percent of the total. The vitamin's function is still not completely understood. It appears, in part, to play a protective role in relation to vitamin A; it may also play a role — at the cellular level — in helping to prevent the premature development of disorders of aging that have been known to occur in response to environmental stresses. This is at normal levels, not via massive supplements. The RDA, 15 to 45 I.U., is easily obtained from common foods that are also sources of other major vitamins: vegetable oils, margarine, green leafy vegetables, whole-grain cereals.

The only known deficiency disorder involving vitamin E is one that occurs — rarely — in premature infants; it is believed due to an absorption disability related to prematurity. (There is no connection with the still-unsolved mystery called "crib death.") There have been a number of reports of cumulative overdose effects, not unexpected since E, like A and D, is a fat-soluble vitamin and is stored by the body; among them are headaches, nausea, dizziness, blurred vision, gastrointestinal problems, and weakness. There may well be others.

MINERALS

As is the case with vitamins, there are a host of minerals the body needs, but only a handful that need to be considered in menu planning; if these are present, the minor minerals will be obtained as well. Minerals may perform their good works singly, in combination with one another, or in collaboration with certain of the vitamins.

Calcium is one we've already mentioned in connection with vitamin D; it works together with phosphorus and with that vitamin, and it's truly crucial to the health of a growing youngster. Calcium is stored by the body, about 99 percent of it used for building bones and teeth. The remaining one percent is small but nonetheless vital in a number of areas, especially as a "binding" element in holding cells in place within the tissues of the body; it is also essential for normal muscle contraction and is a minor factor in blood clotting.

Milk and milk products are the prime sources of calcium; greens, especially turnip greens and mustard greens, are good secondary sources, as are a few other vegetables — among them, broccoli, cabbage, cauliflower, celery, onions, asparagus, and green beans. Whole-grain foods and eggs also contain small amounts.

Iron is a major factor both in the manufacture of red blood cells and in transporting oxygen to the various parts of the body. Meats — liver, in particular — and poultry are the prime sources of it; leafy vegetables like spinach and lettuce are good secondary sources, as are a number of other foods, including eggs, dried fruits, molasses, whole-grain breads and cereals, clams and oysters, peas, beans, nuts, raisins, dates, prunes, cooked greens, beets, and brown sugar.

Iodine is a must for proper thyroid function (see ENDOCRINE GLANDS for more about that). The source is sea water. If you live in a coastal area, there's not likely to be a problem; there's some iodine in your drinking water, as well as in the soil — so there are traces in all locally grown foods. Inland, you should be sure that your family uses iodized salt, and it's wise to also serve them saltwater fish or shellfish occasionally.

Other minerals include copper, which works with iron; phosphorus, which, as we've already mentioned, works with calcium and with vitamin D; magnesium; sodium; potassium; etc. You don't have to worry about specific food sources for these; they'll be present in the necessary amounts (which are quite small) in a well-balanced diet.

Also see "HEALTH FOODS"; VEGETARIANISM.

Nydrazid: a trade name for isoniazid, an antituberculosis drug.

nystatin: See ANTIBIOTICS.

Nytol: an over-the-counter "sleeping aid"; see SEDATIVES.

O

obesity: See OVERWEIGHT.

Obetrol: the trade name for a combination-of-ingredients "diet pill"; see AMPHETAMINES.

obstetrician: See SPECIALTIES, MEDICAL.

occipital: referring to the back of the head; the bone at the back of the skull is called the occiput.

occlusion: See HEART DISEASE. In terms of dentistry, the word means "bite"; see MALOCCLUSION.

occult: describing a condition or disease process that remains hidden because symptoms are absent or not readily evident. Occult *blood* (or *bleeding*) specifically denotes blood (from somewhere in the gastrointestinal tract) that appears in the stool in amounts too small to be visible but that can be detected by chemical analysis.

oculist: a now obsolete term for ophthalmologist; see SPECIALTIES, MEDICAL.

O.D.: the abbreviation for Doctor of Optometry (see OPTOMETRIST). Don't confuse this with D.O. (see OSTEOPATH). Both *O.D.* and *o.d.* are also used in medication instructions; see PRESCRIPTIONS.

olfactory: referring or relating to the sense of smell.

omentum: a membrane at the front of the abdomen, functioning chiefly as a storage area for fat; it is part of the peritoneum, the membrane lining the whole abdominal cavity. The omentum can sometimes be involved in umbilical hernia (see HERNIA).

Omnipen: a trade name for ampicillin, a semisynthetic penicillin; see ANTIBIOTICS.

oncologist: See SPECIALTIES, MEDICAL.

Oncovin: a trade name for vincristine, an anticancer agent; see LYMPHOMA.

oophoroma: an ovarian growth, not necessarily a malignant one.

ophthalmologist: See SPECIALTIES, MEDICAL.

opiates: See NARCOTICS.

optician: a manufacturer of, and dealer in, lenses for eyeglasses. An optician is qualified to fill prescriptions for glasses but is *not* qualified to examine, test, or treat eyes, or to write prescriptions.

Optimil: a trade name for methaqualone, a prescription hypnotic; see SEDATIVES.

optometrist: a professional who is qualified to test and measure vision and to prescribe corrective eyeglasses in case of visual defects; some optometrists are also opticians or associated in business with opticians (see the earlier entry), but for obvious reasons, it's best to patronize one who isn't. An optometrist is not a physician and is not qualified to treat diseases of, or injuries to, the eyes, or to prescribe medications; an optometrist who notes or recognizes a medical problem in the course of examination is obliged to refer you to an ophthalmologist.

OPV: the abbreviation for oral polio vaccine; see IMMUNIZATION.

oral hygienist: See HEALTH PROFESSIONALS.

oral surgeon: See SPECIALTIES, DENTAL.

orbit: the bony structure surrounding the eye.

orchitis: inflammation of the testis caused by disease or injury.

organic foods: See "HEALTH FOODS."

organophosphates: See PESTICIDES.

Oricillin: a trade name for propicillin, a semisynthetic penicillin; see ANTIBIOTICS.

orphenadrine: a muscle relaxant; this class of drugs is discussed under SEDATIVES.

orthodontist: See SPECIALTIES, DENTAL.

orthopedist: See SPECIALTIES, MEDICAL.

orthostatic: relating to, or caused by, standing erect; for two examples, see ALBUMINURIA and BLOOD PRESSURE.

O.S.: See PRESCRIPTIONS.

Osgood-Schlatter's disease: an aseptic necrosis of the upper end of the tibia or shinbone. It is somewhat different from the other major aseptic necrosis, LEGG-PERTHES DISEASE (see that entry). Osgood-Schlatter's tends to occur around the age of puberty, and its most frequent victims are boys; the condition may take several years to heal completely. Treatment does not require complete rest, but activities that may cause pain in the knee — such as jumping for rebounds in basketball — should be avoided.

osteochondroma: a benign tumor, but see the comment under SARCOMA.

osteochondrosis: degeneration of the growing portion of a bone, the characteristic symptom of a number of conditions affecting, usually, children and adolescents (see, for example, LEGG-PERTHES DISEASE and OSGOOD-SCHLATTER'S DISEASE). Osteochondrosis is an aseptic necrosis — that is, it is not demonstrably caused by a bacterium or other invading organism — and is not contagious; it is invariably temporary and self-limited but does require medical diagnosis; treatment depends upon the site involved.

osteomyelitis: an inflammation of bone and bone marrow; it is an infection, usually secondary to an injury or to an infection elsewhere in the body. Symptoms include pain at the affected site and fever which may range from low to high; there may also be visible swelling in the area. The condition can usually be treated with antibiotics, but occasionally surgery is necessary.

osteopath: a physician of a sort, not the holder of an M.D. degree, but that of D.O. or Doctor of Osteopathy. Originally, osteopathy was a system of medicine placing major, if not sole, emphasis on the presumed ability of the body mechanism (bones, joints, etc.) to maintain health and fight diseases by itself, assuming adequate nutrition and a healthful environment.

In recent years, osteopathy has been much modified and modernized, and no longer shuns the use of drugs and other medications and measures in the treatment of illnesses; the training and methods of a D.O. are now quite close to those of an M.D., and there are even some physicians who have both degrees. Your first choice in seeking someone to treat your child should be an M.D. In a situation requiring immediate medical attention, however, if an M.D. is not available, don't hesitate to turn to a *young* — i.e., recently trained — osteopath.

Don't confuse this qualified professional with others who are *not* qualified to treat the ills of your family. See CHIROPRACTOR; HOMEOPATH; NATUROPATH.

osteosarcoma: See SARCOMA.

o-t-c: See OVER-THE-COUNTER.

otitis: inflammation of the ear, especially the middle ear; the full medical name for the latter condition is *otitis media.* It usually occurs as a complication of an infection — such as measles, scarlet fever, or inflamed adenoids — in the nose and throat that travels to the ear via the eustachian tube; children are especially susceptible to such secondary infection because their eustachian tubes are shorter and straighter than those of adults.

Otitis media usually begins with pain in the affected ear, and there is fever that can vary from low to 105° F. (40.5° C.) or even higher; often a telling sign will be a sudden rise in temperature after the primary infection seems to have subsided. There may also be a discharge from the ear. An infant, of course, will not be able to tell you about an earache, but there will generally be changes in behavior that suggest pain, such as inability to sleep well and/or awakening screaming; the screams often subside when the baby is picked up and held in a vertical position (the pain of otitis media is invariably worse when the child is horizontal). Sometimes a baby will rub an ear or turn the head from side to side.

Otitis externa is an inflammation of the outer ear — that is, the passage outside the eardrum; it can be caused by swimming in contaminated water, or by infection from an injury, such as the child's poking something into the ear. Symptoms may include visible redness and itching, and there is definite pain when the ear is pulled at; here, too, there may be a discharge.

Either type of otitis requires prompt medical attention; if you suspect either condition, have the doctor see the child without delay. A continuation of the condition could cause both generalized infection and possible hearing loss. Treatment usually requires sulfa drugs or antibiotics and possibly, in the case of otitis media, drainage of infectious material from the ear. If the latter is necessary, it will usually be performed by a specialist.

otolaryngologist, otologist: See SPECIALTIES, MEDICAL.

otoscope: an instrument that permits the physician to examine the interior of the ear.

O.U.: See PRESCRIPTIONS.

out-patient: a patient receiving treatment from hospital personnel or facilities, and visiting the hospital periodically for that purpose, but not staying in the hospital.

ovaries: See ENDOCRINE GLANDS; SEX ORGANS.

overdose of drugs: See POISONING, HOUSEHOLD SUBSTANCES AND MEDICATIONS.

over-the-counter: the term for medications legally sold without prescription, often abbreviated *o-t-c*.

overweight: Generally speaking — there are exceptions, but they're rare — excess weight is the result of excess food; the child is eating more than is used up in terms of growth, ongoing body functions, energy for activities, and so on (see CALORIES). Sometimes there are emotional factors that lead to the overeating. Sometimes it's an environmental problem; a child whose parents constantly overeat and are overweight can't be expected to forgo the goodies his elders devour.

Don't nag an overweight child; sometimes the more you harp on the subject, the more the youngster will overeat. Don't ever put a child — or permit a teenager to put himself or herself — on a so-called "crash" diet of any type, whether it involves avoiding certain food categories, eating one food exclusively, or any other gimmick. Nor should reducing pills or candies be used; they're either worthless or dangerous (see DIET PILLS).

The calorie-measured canned liquids that are designed to substitute for certain meals and are often pleasantly flavored are nutritionally well-balanced and, usually, safe — but should be used *only* if they are approved by your doctor. In some instances, there can be gastrointestinal side effects; in a child with any chronic condition, digestive or not, no such deviation from normal eating should be undertaken without medical consultation.

By and large, the best thing you can do is simply see that the child gets a balanced diet (see NUTRITION) that emphasizes low-calorie sources of the nutritional elements. Bear in mind that *you set the example.* You can't heap your own plate with mashed potatoes and then deny a child a second helping. (If you're one of those rail-thin types who can eat and eat and never gain an ounce, do your extra nibbling when the child's not around.) And don't tempt the child; don't have forbidden cakes and candies in the house.

If none of this seems to work, do discuss the problem with your physician; there may be other factors involved. In the case of a *teenager,* however, let the *youngster* talk with the doctor — *privately.*

So far as teenagers go, there is one other possibility. You may know of the organization called Weight Watchers, specifically designed for those with a continuing, chronic weight problem. The group uses no gimmicks, simply special dietary regimens (which are medically sound, nutritionally balanced, and quite safe) plus the attendant sympathy and encouragement of others with similar problems; they have also devised a great many recipes to safely satisfy the fat youngster's yen for rich-looking, rich-tasting treats. Weight Watchers has special diet plans for teenagers and has branches in many communities; international headquarters of the organization is 175 East Shore Road, Great Neck, New York.

ovulation: the periodic release of an egg cell from an ovary; it occurs approximately midway between menstrual periods.

oxacillin: a semisynthetic form of penicillin; see ANTIBIOTICS.

Oxalid: a trade name for oxyphenbutazone; see ANTI-INFLAMMATORIES.

oxazepam: a muscle relaxant and tranquilizer; see SEDATIVES.

oxycodone: a codeine analogue that is not employed separately, but is incorporated in some combination products; see NARCOTICS.

oxymorphone: a semisynthetic morphine derivative; see NARCOTICS.

oxyphenbutazone: See ANTI-INFLAMMATORIES.

oxytetracycline: one of the tetracyclines; see ANTIBIOTICS.

P

PABA, Pabafilm, Pabanol: See SUNSCREENS.

pacifiers: These are little "nipples" without holes, attached to plastic or rubber disks to prevent a baby from swallowing the whole thing. Once they were somewhat controversial, thought by many to betray laziness or some similar sin on the parents' part; now just about all pediatricians agree that they're fine, useful devices, and can make life more peaceful for parent and baby alike.

Some babies need to suck more than is needed to get the amount of milk they require (not all babies have this instinctive urge). If the baby is being bottle fed, sucking can be prolonged by switching to nipples with smaller holes. A nursing mother might offer just one breast at a feeding (it may provide enough sustenance for that feeding, and can be emptied in five to seven minutes) and let the baby have a few minutes of nonproductive sucking. Neither of these ideas may work — in which case, a pacifier is an excellent answer (if it is not provided, chances are that thumb, fingers, fist, or anything else available will probably be used).

Essentially, sucking functions as a tension reliever, relaxing the infant and promoting sleep. Sometimes parents find it difficult to determine whether, when a baby wakes up crying — and they have determined that he is not wet, fevered, or in pain — he wants a milk-dispensing nipple or the pacifier. The answer is to offer one or the other; there is a fifty-fifty chance of being right. If he spits it out after a few minutes and screams with annoyance, then give the other.

It occurs to most parents that it might be helpful to have the pacifier handy in the baby's crib so if that's what's wanted it can be found quickly and easily, the rest of the household need not be aroused, and the aforementioned guessing game can be avoided. There are a number of ways to do this. (One way *not* to do it is to tie the pacifier around the baby's neck, which could lead to strangulation.) Some parents have tried scattering several pacifiers around the crib, on the theory that the child is bound to bump into one of them; maybe yes, maybe no (on occasion, eight pacifiers can mysteriously find their way to one end of the crib while the baby gropes in vain at the other). Tying the pacifier to a wrist might work — except that if it slips around to the other side, there is no way a small baby can figure out how to reposition it. For a baby who tends to stay in one position while sleeping (many don't), a good solution is to run a rolled-up diaper through the ring on the pacifier, place the pacifier in convenient position for the baby, then pin the diaper firmly to the sheet (with pins close to the pacifier, so it won't slide). None of these methods is guaranteed.

It should be emphasized that a pacifier is *not* meant to serve as a round-the-clock tranquilizer, but simply as something to help the baby fall asleep contentedly. Crankiness during normal daytime waking hours should be dealt with by offering a new stimulus: moving the baby about, playing with him, talking to him.

As soon as your baby has any teeth, check the pacifier frequently; if there are signs of disintegration, replace it. When a pacifier is old and falling apart, there is always the possibility that small pieces could break off and choke the child.

Most children — assuming the foregoing advice has been followed — will, by the age of two or three, completely relegate the pacifier to bedtime, and would not think of appearing in public with it. If nothing else, peer pressure not to "act like a baby" will generally do the job. It's not harmful for the pacifier to be used at bedtime, even at three or four — but if it continues much after that, there is some cause for concern; permanent teeth may begin arriving as early as age five, and if pacifier use continues after that, the teeth could be pushed out of line. If you are still having trouble persuading your child to give up the pacifier at that point, it's best to discuss the question with your dentist.

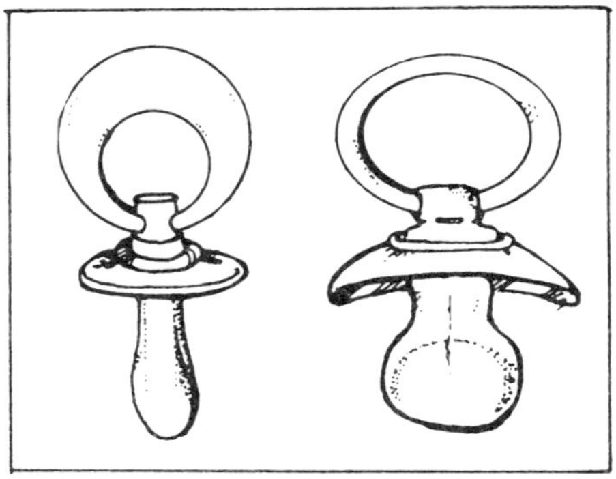

Pacifiers
At left, the usual type; at right, the Nuk pacifier, with differently structured "nipple," believed by many orthodontists less liable to cause possible distortion of bite.

A special note: Early in 1975, the American Academy of Pediatrics issued a warning, and requested federal action, regarding imported "pacifiers" designed to resemble actual pacifiers but made of hard candy; the "nipple" can easily break, posing a serious choking hazard for infants and small children (the packages have been labeled, "not for infants," but few infants can read labels). Subsequently, the Food and Drug Administration ordered the recall of the products. We hope that, by the time you read this, the candy "pacifiers" will all have been withdrawn; if they have not, and you have an infant or small child, see that these items do not find their way into your house.

Such are the dangers to which parents of small children must be constantly alert.

padimate: See SUNSCREENS.

pain: a sensation produced by irritation of sensory nerve endings in the affected part of the body. It's a protective mechanism, and has, generally, a threefold purpose: it prevents injury or recurrence of injury (as, the pain of extreme heat when touching something that could cause a burn); it signals something amiss that might otherwise be unnoticed (most internal pains are in this category); it enforces the rest necessary to healing (as, the pain of attempting to use a pulled muscle).

An infant who can't yet talk will nevertheless react to pain in some way. The baby will certainly cry and will often also do things that are clues to the location of the pain. Abdominal pain may be signaled by legs drawn up tightly, or stretched out stiffly, for example; pain in the ear, by turning the head from side to side or groping toward the ear; pain in a leg or foot (in a child old enough to walk), by limping or favoring that leg.

If the child is old enough to talk, it's important to find out the exact location and nature of the pain. Have the child point to the precise place it hurts, if there is a precise spot — and if there isn't, find that out too. Try to discover how bad the pain is; you might do this by comparing it with other hurts or ills the child has had (i.e., is the pain "worse than" or "like" or "not as bad as" others?). Try to find out, too, whether the pain is sharp or dull, whether it throbs, whether it is continuous or intermittent (coming and going), whether it is present when the child is at rest or only on movement, whether it is relieved by assuming a particular position.

Then, when you have as much information as you can get about an unexplained pain, call the doctor.

Also see, if the pain is in that area, ABDOMINAL PAIN; CHEST PAIN; EARACHE; HEADACHE.

pain relievers: No one who possesses a television set need be told of the dozens of pain relievers promoted to the public. Without exception, they are designed only to combat mild pain (we'll come, in a moment, to how well they do that); really severe pain needs stronger stuff, available only by prescription or by a doctor's administration (see NARCOTICS).

Now, what's in those over-the-counter products? As you may have guessed, almost all the major brands contain aspirin, the mysterious "ingredient doctors recommend most" referred to coyly by one advertised brand (Anacin's *other* ingredient — and there are only two — is simply caffeine, the waker-upper in coffee). Yes, aspirin *is* what doctors recommend most, because it is by far the most effective pain reliever available without prescription. But doctors *don't* generally recommend that the aspirin be combined with something *else.* Just plain aspirin is fine, and it *is* something that you should have in your medicine chest; see ASPIRIN for a full discussion of keeping it and using it, and how and when.

Other ingredients commonly appearing in those "extra-strength" or "fast-acting" or "combination-of-ingredients" products include: other analgesics similar to, but not as effective as, aspirin, such as acetaminophen (it doesn't work against inflammation, which aspirin does), phenacetin (the infamous "P" in APC tablets, which has been implicated in kidney disorders), salicylamide (the most similar to aspirin, but with an occasional tendency to cause depression), and antacids, which have nothing to do, obviously, with relieving a headache. Acetaminophen may, however, be recommended by your physician if there's a sensitivity to aspirin and inflammation is not the problem; it is available generically as well as under a number of trade names, most prominently, Datril, Tempra, Tylenol, and Valadol.

And the others? We cannot list them all; there follow some examples.

Measurin is simply aspirin, formulated for release over a period of time; Ecotrin is also aspirin, coated in an effort to protect the gastrointestinal tract of those sensitive to it. They are useful products, but consult your physician before you use them or give them to your children. Cama is another time-release aspirin that also includes antacids (the aspirin dosage is at the adult level) and should be used only on a doctor's advice. Enderin is acetaminophen (each tablet contains ten grains rather than the usual five) plus caffeine.

A number of products combine aspirin with antacids such as sodium bicarbonate, magnesium carbonate, magnesium hydroxide, aluminum hydroxide, or calcium carbonate. The theory underlying the inclusion of these substances is that they will speed the action of aspirin and will also exert a protective effect against the stomach irritation aspirin may sometimes cause in some people. In fact, much depends both on the quantity of antacid and on the form of the medication. Taking aspirin in effervescent solution, as is the case with Alka-Seltzer, for example, does result in faster absorption (although taking aspirin with hot water speeds it even more), and some studies have concluded that the antacid content of this particular product does act in a protective capacity. In other instances, the combination has been less successful. The Food and Drug Administration has, for example, termed two advertised claims for Bufferin — that it acts "twice as fast" as plain aspirin and that it "helps prevent" stomach upsets caused by aspirin — misleading. ("Most of the published studies," said the FDA statement, "indicate there is little difference in the incidence of stomach upsets after ingestion of Bufferin or plain aspirin.")

Other aspirin products that include antacids in their formulations are Congesprin, a highly promoted product for children (which indeed contains only the aspirin in a standard children's tablet but also tosses in the decongestant phenylephrine in addition to the antacid); Cope, which also includes caffeine and an antihistamine; and Vanquish, which also incorporates caffeine and acetaminophen.

The other heavily touted products (an exception is Liquiprin, which is discussed separately under its own entry) are combinations of analgesics, with or without other ingredients. They vary almost to the extent that we might conclude — if we were not charitably inclined — that manufacturers might simply have looked around for a formulation that was "different" (never mind *better*). Empirin Compound is an APC drug. Excedrin offers A and C, plus acetaminophen and salicylamide — except tha

Excedrin-PM drops the C (remember that's caffeine) and includes an antihistamine (which is likely to have some minor sedative effect). Trigesic's name suggests that it has three analgesics; in fact, it consists of only two — aspirin and acetaminophen — plus caffeine. Comeback offers acetaminophen and salicylamide combined with caffeine. Bromo-Seltzer contains no aspirin; its active ingredients are phenacetin and acetaminophen, and it also contains caffeine and antacids (the potentially toxic bromide compound that gave the product its name has apparently been quietly dropped since our earlier edition).

Finally, what of the products that claim some special property that will relieve that vague condition, "menstrual tension and discomfort"? Well, judge for yourself. Femicin is a combination of salicylamide and acetaminophen with caffeine, an antihistamine, and a bromide compound that might in larger quantities relieve stomach upset (but will not do so in the quantity included in this product). Midol combines aspirin and caffeine with an ephedrine salt that is claimed to act specifically against uterine spasms or cramps, a claim that has been seriously questioned. And Pamprin, despite its name, contains no aspirin but is a combination of phenacetin, salicylamide, an antihistamine, and a diuretic, another ingredient that seems highly questionable to many experts.

palate: Anatomically speaking, it consists of two parts. The *hard palate* is just another term for the roof of the mouth. The *soft palate* is a group of muscles, just behind the hard palate, that play a part in speech and in swallowing; the *uvula,* that wobbly little thing dangling at the back of the mouth, is part of the soft palate. For discussion of one congenital problem, see CLEFT PALATE.

palliative: a medication or treatment given to relieve symptoms of pain or discomfort (as opposed to treating the basic cause of the problem), e.g., aspirin to relieve a headache, calamine lotion for the itching of a rash, compresses to dull the pain of a bruise.

Palocillin: a trade name for penicillin G; see ANTIBIOTICS.

palsy: entire or partial paralysis or absence of muscle control. See BELL'S PALSY; BRACHIAL PARALYSIS; CEREBRAL PALSY.

Pamprin: See PAIN RELIEVERS.

pancreas: See DIGESTION; ENDOCRINE GLANDS. For comment on some ailments and disorders involving the gland, see CYSTIC FIBROSIS; DIABETES MELLITUS; PANCREATITIS, following.

pancreatitis: an inflammation of the pancreas, generally considered quite serious; it may be caused by a back-up of bile from the liver or gallbladder, or by bacterial or viral infection. (In children, it is not uncommonly connected with mumps and in this instance is considered a little less serious.)

Treatment — which usually takes place in a hospital — may include, depending upon the specific circumstances, blood transfusion, drugs to relieve pain, antibiotics (if the infection is bacterial), drawing off of secretions (if a duct is blocked), and dietary measures; in rare instances, surgery is required.

pandemic: a very widespread epidemic

(the *pan* part comes from the Greek word for "all"), reaching across an entire country, or even around the whole world; flu, for example, was pandemic in 1918 and again in 1968.

Panmycin: a trade name for tetracycline; see ANTIBIOTICS.

panniculitis: See BLOTCHES.

papilla: a small elevation on the surface of the skin or mucous membrane — as, a taste bud on the tongue; also, a special structure at the bottom of a follicle that conveys nourishment to the hair root.

Pap test: the popular term for a diagnostic procedure, also called a "Pap smear," in which a sample of secretions is taken from the cervix of the uterus for analysis. The procedure — performed quickly and painlessly in the doctor's office — is used to detect cervical cancer and other pathological conditions in this area; it is named for Dr. George Papanicolaou, its originator.

It is now felt that this procedure is advisable as part of routine physicals for teenagers as well as adults, since a high correlation has been established between cervical cancer — as well as precancerous cell changes — and sexual intercourse. The precipitator, it is believed, may be an otherwise innocuous transmittable virus. Cervical cancer is virtually 100 percent curable if it is detected early.

papule: See LESION.

Paracort: See CORTICOSTEROIDS.

Paradione: a trade name for paramethadione, an antiseizure medication; see EPILEPSY.

Paraflex: a trade name for chlorzoxazone, a muscle-relaxant agent; see SEDATIVES.

parainfluenza viruses: See VIRUSES.

paralysis: the inability to move a muscle or muscles; it may be temporary or permanent. Paralysis is a symptom, not a disease, and can mean many things — infection, poisoning, tumor, physical injury — that might somehow have affected the nerves involved. Following a fall, it may mean a serious injury to the spinal cord — and the child *must not be moved* (see BACK AND NECK INJURIES).

In any case, you should call your physician immediately, reporting the extent of the paralysis, the circumstances under which it appeared, and any other symptoms accompanying or preceding it.

paramethadione: an antiseizure medication; see EPILEPSY.

paramyxoviruses: See VIRUSES.

paranasal sinuses: See SINUSES.

paranoia: a mental disorder characterized by a specific set of delusions, usually of persecution, in a person who is otherwise rational.

paraphimosis: a condition that can afflict an uncircumcised boy, involving inflammation of the foreskin, with constriction below the head of the penis; symptoms include swelling around the foreskin and pain on urination. It requires immediate treatment, since it can interfere with the functioning of the entire urinary tract.

It can usually be avoided by making sure that the foreskin is fully retracted at least once daily. The parent should do this until the boy is old enough to do it properly himself. If there is any question about complete retractability of the foreskin, have your doctor check it.

parasites: There are many, many microscopic primitive life forms, and some larger and less primitive, that are known to live on or in, and feed off, humans, usually to the detriment of the latter. Broadly speaking, the term can include fungi, lice, and — to the extent that they feed on the material of living cells — viruses; but the terms "parasitic disease" and "parasitic infection" generally refer to ills not caused by any of those organisms. A number of the parasitic diseases, with whose names the reader is probably familiar, are discussed under their own entries: DYSENTERY, one form of which is caused by an ameba; MALARIA; TOXOPLASMOSIS; TRICHINOSIS; and WORMS, which entry includes the three major types found in the United States.

Many such parasites afflict natives of various other parts of the world, and physicians here are in fact unfamiliar with most of them, because in the past they have rarely been seen in this country. We single out, here, several that have been posing an increasing problem in recent years as more and more travelers have returned carrying unsuspected "souvenirs." All can be diagnosed and treated. With care, they can be avoided.

Filariasis is caused by several species of parasites that use people (and in some areas, monkeys as well) as hosts; it is endemic in Southeast Asia and some other parts of the Orient, and in most tropical areas. It is transmitted from host to host by the bites of mosquitoes, which serve as intermediate hosts in which the larvae develop; mature larvae are then deposited in the bloodstream of the next human host by another bite. The adult parasites cause severe pain and swelling in the lymph nodes, particularly in the groin.

Giardiasis, a condition involving intestinal troubles, is caused by a protozoan called *Giardia lamblia,* which enters the body via sewage-contaminated food or water. Formerly believed limited to tropical and subtropical areas, the problem is now known to occur all over the world, and there may even be sizable incidence as far north as Scandinavia; in 1974, several hundred visitors to the Soviet Union were reported to have contracted it from ordinary tap water. Food eaten in foreign climes should be thoroughly cooked, and any doubt about local sanitation suggests that water should be boiled or otherwise disinfected. Outbreaks in a number of U.S. locations have also been documented; a number of these have resulted from drinking untreated water from apparently clean mountain streams in the West.

Symptoms of giardiasis, appearing after an incubation period of one to three weeks (occasionally longer), include diarrhea and, frequently, severe abdominal cramps; diagnosis is established by stool analysis. A number of effective drugs may be used in treatment, prominently one called quinacrine (Atabrine).

Leishmaniasis is caused by two species of another protozoan, each endemic to different areas and causing inflammation of different parts of the body; both are carried among the many mammals — including humans — that serve as their hosts by the bites of sandflies. Visceral leishmaniasis, also known as "dumdum fever," involves inflammation of the spleen and liver, generally fever and swelling of the lymph nodes, and possibly anemia due to invasion of the bone marrow; the parasite is found in China, the Indian subcontinent, parts of the U.S.S.R. and northern Africa, and parts of South America (Brazil in particular). Cutaneous leishmaniasis involves inflammation and ulceration of the skin and/or mucous membrane and is known locally by a number of different names ("Baghdad boil," "Turkestan ulcer," etc.); it is endemic in various parts of northern Africa, the Middle East, the southern U.S.S.R., and the Indian subcontinent.

Schistosomiasis or "snail fever" is an extremely serious and debilitating condition caused by three separate species of blood flukes called *Schistosoma;* they are distributed through South America, Puerto Rico and other Caribbean islands, Africa, the Middle East, and the Orient, and may attack either the gastrointestinal or urinary tract. The fluke has a couple of unusual characteristics. One is the unique life cycle that gives the condition its popular name: the eggs, released from untreated human sewage, can develop only within the bodies of certain fresh-water snails; the organisms leave the snails as free-swimming larvae to seek the next necessary host, a human body. The second is that the larvae can enter the body through unbroken skin; having done so, they proceed to internal organs via the bloodstream. The snail hosts thrive in relatively still waters, and thus construction of dams and irrigation canals in "developing" nations has helped ensure the flukes' development as well (above the Aswan High Dam, schistosomiasis was reported by the end of 1974 to afflict an astounding 76 percent of the local population). When traveling in such areas, it is well to avoid immersion in fresh-water streams, no matter how clean they may appear to be — and to be very sure of the source of water used for drinking and bathing.

Trypanosomiasis occurs in two different parts of the world and is caused by various protozoans of the genus *Trypanosoma;* in both instances, the condition is an extremely critical one, involving high fever, liver and spleen dysfunction, myocarditis and/or pericarditis, meningitis, and encephalitis. In South America, it is also known as Chagas' disease; the parasite uses both humans and a variety of animals (both wild and domestic) as hosts, and is transmitted from one to another by the bite of various local sucking insects, including the "kissing bug" and "assassin bug." In Africa — where it is found between the latitudes of 15° N and 20° S — it is known generally as African sleeping sickness (untreated, it proceeds to extreme lethargy and terminal coma), specifically by locale names (West African sleeping sickness, Rhodesian sleeping sickness, etc., caused by slightly different varieties of the parasite); the parasite is carried among hosts, which include game and domestic animals as well as humans, by the bite of the tsetse fly.

parasympathetic nerves: See NERVOUS SYSTEM.

parathion: See PESTICIDES.

parathyroids: See ENDOCRINE GLANDS.

paratyphoid fever: a bacterial infection that tends to be endemic in the same areas, and under the same conditions, in which typhoid is found; it is caused by a related but slightly different *salmonella* organism (there are tests — of blood, urine, and stool — to determine exactly what the agent is). It may be spread by contaminated food — especially eggs and poultry — and also by human contact, whether the person is ill with the disease or is simply a carrier.

The disease is similar to, but milder than, typhoid fever; it was once thought to be simply a mild version of the latter. Aside from fever, generally the only symptom, which appears after an incubation period varying from one to ten days, is an attack of diarrhea, which can sometimes be so mild that its appearance goes unnoticed (it will, however, persist as long as the infection is there); or, it may be acute. Treatment, once the condition is diagnosed, involves rest, antibiotics to combat the infection, and dietary measures. Having paratyphoid fever gives long-lasting immunity — but only to this particular bacterium, not to other *salmonella* infections (such as typhoid fever and some kinds of food poisoning).

There is a combination vaccine against both typhoid and paratyphoid, and your youngsters should be vaccinated if they are traveling to an area where poor sanitation facilities and/or polluted water are likely (the destination should be discussed with your physician). Vaccination is also recommended in the event of flood or other disaster that may lead to contamination of a community water supply.

paregoric: camphorated tincture of opium. For discussion of its uses and nonuses, see NARCOTICS.

parenteral: not involving the intestines. The word is occasionally used to describe a condition, but more often in *parenteral nutrition,* meaning intravenous feeding. A *parenteral diarrhea* is not related to illness in the intestines but is a secondary concomitant of another condition.

Parest: a trade name for methaqualone, a sleep-inducing drug; see SEDATIVES.

Parnate: a trade name for tranylcypromine; see ANTIDEPRESSANTS.

paronychia: an infection around a fingernail or toenail, involving inflammation, swelling, and sometimes abscess. Occasionally, it can be caused by a fungus infection; more often, the infection is bacterial and follows an injury to the area, an improperly treated ingrown toenail, or a carelessly handled condition such as a hangnail. Treatment consists of hot soaks and such medications as antibiotics or sulfa drugs, topically and possibly internally as well.

parotid glands: saliva-producing glands at the sides and to the back of the mouth; they are located just under the ears. These are the glands that become swollen in mumps; such swelling can sometimes be caused by other conditions as well, including certain allergic reactions.

parotitis: an inflammation of the parotid glands. For discussion of *epidemic parotitis,* see MUMPS.

paroxon: See PESTICIDES.

parrot fever: See PSITTACOSIS.

patch test: See ALLERGY TEST.

patella: the anatomical term for the kneecap.

Pathibamate: a combination product containing the tranquilizer meprobamate and an antispasm agent; see SEDATIVES.

Pathocil: a trade name for dicloxacillin, a semisynthetic penicillin; see ANTIBIOTICS.

pathogen: any disease-causing organism or substance.

pathognomonic: literally, "naming the disease"; describing a sign or symptom that is unique or so characteristic that, if it is present, the disorder is clearly identified.

pathologist: See SPECIALTIES, MEDICAL.

"patterning": a widely publicized but unproved and medically unaccepted method of handling retarded children by training them to creep and crawl. Its benefits have never been demonstrated by qualified physicians.

P.B.I.: a test for thyroid function (see ENDOCRINE GLANDS); the letters stand for protein-bound iodine.

P.C.: an abbreviation with two meanings. Appearing after a physician's name and degree, the letters signify "professional corporation." For the other meaning, see PRESCRIPTIONS.

"PCP": a street term for phencyclidine, a potent animal tranquilizer; see PSYCHEDELICS.

pectin: a polysaccharide; see SWEETENERS.

pectorals: See MUSCLES.

Pedacillin: a trade name for penicillin G; see ANTIBIOTICS.

Pediamycin: a trade name for erythromycin; see ANTIBIOTICS.

pediatrician: See SPECIALTIES, MEDICAL.

pediculosis: the medical term for lice infestation; you will find it discussed under LICE, BODY and LICE, HEAD.

pedodontist: See SPECIALTIES, DENTAL.

peeling skin: There are three conditions under which peeling skin is perfectly normal and isn't a matter for concern on your part or your physician's.

A newborn baby's skin peels for the same reason yours might if you'd been washing a lot of dishes; the infant has just emerged from nine months in a liquid medium.

Sunburned skin will peel off as new skin develops underneath the burned layer.

Diseases involving a rash often end with a certain amount of peeling skin; in scarlet fever, for example, there is typically peeling of the palms and soles.

In all these cases, just be sure to let the peeling proceed at its own pace; don't rip off shreds of skin. You can apply some lubrication, such as simple petroleum jelly, if you like.

Other causes of peeling skin include various allergies and nutritional deficiencies; both diagnosis and treatment require medical expertise. If there's no apparent reason for your child's peeling skin, consult your physician.

pellagra: a disease resulting from a severe lack of niacin, one of the B vitamins; see DEFICIENCY DISEASES.

pelvis: an anatomical term that may, depending upon the context in which it's used, denote three different things. The word can refer to the bones of the hip area, sometimes also called the "pelvic girdle" — a basin-shaped arrangement that supports the abdominal organs and to which the legs are connected. Or, it can mean the whole area, including the lower abdominal organs such as the lower intestines, bladder, internal sex organs, etc. And, it can refer to a similarly shaped part of a particular organ — such as the pelvis of the kidney, which is the part from which the ureter leads to the bladder.

pemoline: a medication used in the treatment of hyperactivity; see HYPERKINESIS.

pemphigus: a rare skin disease that can afflict persons of any age, even newborn infants; its cause is completely unknown. It involves blistering, itching, and burning, and can occur on mucous membrane as well as on skin itself; the blisters, which may be pea-sized or larger, contain clear serum.

The condition is considered serious, since there can be substantial serum loss, and in some instances there may be disconnection of the layers of the skin. Pemphigus is curable; it's generally treated with ACTH, cortisone, and other drugs.

Penapar: a trade name for penicillin V; see ANTIBIOTICS.

Penbritin: a trade name for ampicillin, a semisynthetic penicillin; see ANTIBIOTICS.

penicillamine: a penicillin derivative used in the treatment of lead poisoning; it is also used in Great Britain for the treatment of severe rheumatoid arthritis, but there are a number of serious side effects in such usage and it has not been approved in this country.

penicillin: see ANTIBIOTICS.

penis: the male genito-urinary organ that acts as a conduit for both copulation and the excretion of urine. Also see CIRCUMCISION; MEATITIS; PARAPHIMOSIS.

Pensyn: a trade name for ampicillin, a semisynthetic penicillin; see ANTIBIOTICS.

pentazocine: a potent analgesic; see NARCOTICS.

Pentids: a trade name for penicillin G; see ANTIBIOTICS.

pentobarbital, Pentothal: See SEDATIVES; the former is a sleep-inducing drug, the latter a trade name for thiopental, a barbiturate used primarily in anesthesia.

Pen-Vee: a trade name for penicillin V; see ANTIBIOTICS.

"pep pills": See AMPHETAMINES.

peptic ulcer: an ulcer in the upper part of the gastrointestinal tract; the term can imply either a gastric ulcer (in the stomach itself) or a duodenal ulcer (in the first segment of the small intestine), usually the latter because it's more common. An ulcer in this area is an erosion of the mucous membrane lining the tract. The immediate physical cause is excess acid production, but what causes *that* isn't completely clear; there could be hereditary tendencies and the precipitating factor often seems to be of emotional origin.

"Classic" symptoms of peptic ulcer include pain in the upper abdomen that's relieved by eating, possible constipation, and possible nausea; there may also be indications of blood in the stool (not bright red blood, but a tarry, near-black color to the stool itself) — and if that's so, it indicates that the condition is quite serious. Symptoms in young children, however (yes, children *can* have ulcers), tend to be atypical, so these aren't necessarily good guidelines — and they are, in any case, possible symptoms of other conditions as well. The wisest course is to have your physician check out *any* unusual situation, whether it involves pain or stool peculiarities; if an ulcer is suspected, X ray will confirm the diagnosis.

Rest, special dietary measures, and medications are the usual remedies for peptic ulcer; surgery is needed only in extreme instances.

Pepto-Bismol: a widely advertised over-the-counter product suggested for relief of "upset stomach." It contains bismuth subsalicylate, salol, and zinc phenolsulfonate, none of which are particularly effective medications. If your youngster has gastrointestinal symptoms, consult your doctor rather than using doubtful medications that may not be helpful.

Percodan: a combination-product analgesic that contains oxycodone plus aspirin, phenacetin, and caffeine (APC); oxycodone is a chemical analogue of codeine (see NARCOTICS) that has a fairly high dependence-creating potential and is not used alone.

percussion: a diagnostic procedure in which the physician taps the chest, back, or other part; the sound elicited gives various information about the organs and structures within.

Periactin: a trade name for the antipruritic agent cyproheptadine; see ANTIHISTAMINES.

pericarditis: See HEART DISEASE.

perinatal: See NATAL.

periodontist: See SPECIALTIES, DENTAL.

peripheral nerves: See NERVOUS SYSTEM.

peristalsis: See INTESTINES.

peritonitis: a general inflammation of the peritoneum, the membrane lining the entire abdominal cavity; it is typically caused by the rupture of an inflamed and infected appendix or other organ within the abdomen. There is invariably pain, either localized or general, usually accompanied by a rising temperature, a generally sick feeling, and rigidity and tenderness of the abdomen; there may also be vomiting.

Peritonitis, actual or suspected, is considered a medical emergency, and if you suspect it, the child must be rushed to the nearest hospital without delay. Treatment will include antibiotics for the infection, probably surgical removal of the appendix, and possibly transfusions and other measures, depending upon the circumstances. Peritonitis was once inevitably fatal; it need not be so now, if treatment is prompt.

Permapen: a trade name for penicillin G; see ANTIBIOTICS.

pernicious anemia: See ANEMIA.

peroxide: See HYDROGEN PEROXIDE.

perphenazine: a potent tranquilizer that is also employed for its antispasm action. See NAUSEA; SEDATIVES.

Perthes disease: See LEGG-PERTHES DISEASE.

Pertofrane: a trade name for desipramine; see ANTIDEPRESSANTS.

Pertussin: See COUGHS.

pertussis: See WHOOPING COUGH.

pesticides: They have been, as you doubtless know, a continuing source of controversy. We must necessarily restrict ourselves, here, to comment on safety for your family in general and your children in particular (rather than long-term ecological considerations). The danger, at this writing, does not appear to lie primarily in food residues (no ills in human beings have thus far been traced to such residues), but in encounters with the substances themselves, whether through accident or carelessness.

The major pesticides in use on farms and in homes and gardens over the past few years belong to one of two chemical groups, chlorinated hydrocarbons (DDT, DDE, aldrin, dieldrin, endrin, lindane, chlordane, heptachlor, and others) and organophosphates (parathion, malathion, paroxon, DFP, chlorthion, soman, EPN, phosdrin, TEPP, and others). Main difference between the two: their persistence after use.

The chlorinated hydrocarbons aroused concern quite a few years ago when it was found that they could and did linger (in the atmosphere) and build up (in animal and human tissues). Long-term effects — on unborn children, on nursing infants, on everyone should the chemicals prove carcinogenic (which some had, in laboratory animals) — led some states to take early action. New York, for example, at the end of 1970 enacted legislation completely banning DDT, DDE, endrin, and several others and requiring special permits for highly restricted use of aldrin, chlordane, dieldrin, heptachlor, and lindane; at the same time, several dozen others — including parathion, EPN, phosdrin, and TEPP as well as such substances as cyanides and strychnine — were removed from retail sale and restricted to use by those holding professional permits.

In 1972, the federal government acted to ban DDT except for a handful of highly specialized purposes; aldrin and dieldrin met the same fate in 1974. Production of chlordane and heptachlor was suspended in mid-1975 pending further investigation. Meanwhile, in early 1973, the American Academy of Pediatrics warned its members to "be on the lookout for a sharp increase in poisoning from toxic pesticides which have replaced DDT . . . parathion and other potential replacements are highly toxic by the oral, dermal and respiratory routes. Exposure can result in fatalities in a matter of a few hours." And that is precisely the problem. While the organophosphates are not as persistent in the atmosphere as the chlorinated hydrocarbons (although they *can* persist in *soil* for months or even years), they are much more toxic. As the quoted warning points out, the poison need not be breathed or eaten; even its contact with the skin can cause systemic toxic effects. And most of the victims have been children.

If you can completely avoid the use of pesticides in and around your home, we urge you to do so. If you cannot, we hope you will take the following minimal precautions in order to protect yourself, your children, and your pets.

Store such substances far from the kitchen, and locked away from any possible access by children or pets.

Read labels very carefully; follow all instructions and specified precautions.

Never transfer a pesticide from its original, labeled container to another, unlabeled one.

When spraying a pesticide outdoors, be sure there is no wind that could carry the lethal material elsewhere. Wear head-to-toe protective clothing, including natural-rubber gloves (neither synthetics nor ordinary cloth gloves offer protection) and one of the special respirators that has been tested and approved for this purpose.

After using any pesticide, wash your hands and face thoroughly with soap and water.

After spraying an organophosphate, see that the clothes you were wearing are washed — immediately, and separately from other laundry: children playing with boots or gloves worn during pesticide application and tossed carelessly in a corner have been known to go into convulsions within minutes.

When a pesticide container is empty, get rid of it — completely. Such containers left in backyards have figured prominently in reported cases of child poisonings.

petit mal: See EPILEPSY.

pets: Many aspects of choosing and caring for pets are of course outside the purview of this book. Strictly from the health and safety viewpoint, however, there are a few rules that you should keep in mind.

When you buy a dog or cat, make sure that the animal is free of disease; have it examined by a veterinarian before you bring it into your home.

If you have very small children, don't buy a grown animal raised in a childless home; older animals unused to the quick movements and careless romping of youngsters can become nervous, irritable, and unpredictable.

Never let a child keep a stray animal of any kind; such an animal is, more often than not, ill. A lost or stray animal should be turned over to the ASPCA; or if you live in a rural area, it should be isolated until you have had a veterinarian pronounce the animal a healthy one.

Don't purchase a baby wild animal as a pet believing that it will grow up to be as gentle as a dog or pussycat. It's true that the animal's relationship to its owners will generally be friendly, and perhaps even affectionate — but its *reflexes* will remain purely instinctive; one swat of a half-grown lion's paw could be lethal to a child — whether or not the beast *intended* harm.

Keep your pet in good health and free of parasites and other things that could carry disease. Keep it clean. See that it has all necessary vaccinations, including rabies shots. Have it regularly examined for ticks and fleas that could transmit diseases to your children. Be aware that troublemaking substances can be carried innocently by a dog or cat; the oils of poison ivy, for example, can cling to fur — causing no discomfort to the animal, but quite a bit to humans who come in contact with it. Also see RINGWORM, to which both pets *and* children are susceptible. Animals' internal worms, however, do *not* normally infect children — unless the child actually gets the animal's feces in his mouth.

Assuming you've taken all the above precautions, don't worry if your puppy or kitten gets very chummy with your baby and even licks him; there is no recorded case of friendly licking causing any harm.

Don't, on the other hand, *ever* leave an infant or very small child *alone* with a dog or cat. Most pets are very good with babies, and as long as an adult is present, nothing is likely to go wrong. But remember that a small child is unaware of potential dangers. If a tot innocently and ignorantly attacks the pet — perhaps not meaning any harm, but actually hurting the animal — the animal will, in all likelihood, behave logically; it will retaliate.

Animals, like humans, have been known to suffer emotional aberrations, although it's fairly rare. Most pets will not harm a human being unless the person strikes first. But if a pet *does* attack even one person for no apparent reason — get rid of it.

If you're thinking of acquiring a pet turtle, think again. They have frequently been a source of salmonella infections, to the tune of an estimated 280,000 cases a year (not because of pet-shop carelessness, but due to contamination carried from the breeding locations). Federal regulations banning importation of pet turtles and regulating their interstate shipment went into effect in 1973, but the Food and Drug Administration determined that these controls were inadequate, and that the turtles were highly susceptible to recontamination from bacteria in water and in their food — with the result that huge numbers of disease-carrying animals were still reaching the retail market. In mid-1975, the FDA announced a complete ban on commercial distribution and sale of baby turtles (those with a shell length of less than four inches) and fertile turtle eggs, except for scientific and educational purposes. The ban will probably be healthful for the turtles, too: the Animal Welfare Institute, in a statement applauding the ban, noted that with proper care, the type of turtles generally sold in pet shops can grow to eleven inches and live for forty years — but 90 percent of those purchased as pets have survived only a few months.

Snakes are not very good pets unless the child is a teenager and is familiar with the care and feeding of the animal. To be sure that the snake is not poisonous, buy it from a reputable reptile dealer — not from discount merchandisers, variety stores, or mail-order firms, which have been known to occasionally purvey potentially lethal baby rattlers.

How about small unusual mammals — monkeys, gerbils, hamsters, guinea pigs? The last three are fine, frequently educational pets for youngsters old enough to care for them — and they're laboratory bred, so won't carry rabies (assuming they're kept indoors and have no contact with wild creatures). We advise against monkeys. Aside from the fact that they are messy and inclined to bite, they are prey to many of the viral ills that afflict human beings — which is like having another source of childhood contagion in your home (except that pediatricians and family physicians don't treat monkeys, and most veterinarians don't either).

For some other precautions relating to pets, see ASTHMA; PSITTACOSIS; TOXOPLASMOSIS.

Pfizerpen: a trade name for penicillin G; see ANTIBIOTICS.

pH: You may sometimes see this combination of letters, followed by a number, on various preparations — such as soaps and shampoos — designed for use on skin or scalp. It is a statement of acidity versus alkalinity; the letters stand for *percentage of hydrogen,* a chemical measurement that's significant in determining this quality. The values are represented on a scale that ranges from 0 to 14, with 7 the neutral point; values below 7 are acid, those above 7 alkaline. On the average, the pH of human skin is between 4.5 and 6, i.e., slightly acidic (most soaps, detergents, etc., are alkaline, although some are more so than others); thus a neutral or low-pH preparation may be more soothing to the skin.

phagocytes: "scavenger cells" that make it their business to ingest unwanted or unneeded substances in the body. There are two types: one, a certain subclass of leukocytes, ingests chiefly bacteria and foreign (i.e., invading) material; the other, another subclass with a different structure, functions largely at the microscopic level, taking care of cells that have died (which goes on all the time in our bodies; new cells are constantly produced to replace the old ones). The process of ingesting these particles is called *phagocytosis.*

phalanges: the bones of the fingers and toes; the singular is phalanx, from the Greek for "a line of soldiers." The joints between them, including the knuckles, are called *interphalangeal* joints.

pharmacist: a graduate of a school of pharmacy, who has special training in chemistry and the compounding of medications and is qualified to follow your physician's directions in filling prescriptions. Whether or not your neighbors address such an individual as "Doc," a pharmacist is *not* a Doctor of Medicine and is emphatically *not* qualified to diagnose, or suggest remedies for, your family's ills.

pharmacologist: a specialist in the study of drugs and their actions and reactions in the body. A pharmacologist may or may not be a Doctor of Medicine.

pharyngitis: See SORE THROAT.

phenacetin: See APC TABLETS; PAIN RELIEVERS.

phenaglycodol: an anti-anxiety medication; see SEDATIVES.

Phenaphen: a combination-product analgesic that contains aspirin, phenacetin, belladonna derivatives, and phenobarbital (see SEDATIVES).

phendimetrazine: See DIET PILLS.

phenelzine: See ANTIDEPRESSANTS.

Phenergan: a trade name for promethazine, a tranquilizer and antispasmodic. See NAUSEA; SEDATIVES.

phenethicillin: a semisynthetic penicillin; see ANTIBIOTICS.

phenmetrazine: See DIET PILLS.

phenobarbital: a sedative and anticonvulsant. See EPILEPSY; SEDATIVES.

phenothiazines: a class of drugs that have been found useful in two distinct areas, based upon their propensity for calming. See NAUSEA; SEDATIVES.

phensuximide: an antiseizure medication; see EPILEPSY.

phentermine: See DIET PILLS.

phenylbutazone: See ANTI-INFLAMMATORIES.

phenylephrine: See DECONGESTANTS, NASAL.

phenylketonuria: a hereditary deficiency in an enzyme involved in the breakdown of a particular amino acid; the name of the condition (often abbreviated to PKU) stems from the fact that its victims' urine contains a detectable chemical substance called a phenylketone, and this was the basis of the first diagnoses. There is now a blood test, required by law in most states for all newborn babies, which should be performed on or after the sixth day after birth (there is a significant incidence of false-negative results before that); if the test is positive, it is then confirmed by urinalysis.

Hereditarily, the defect is unqualifiedly recessive (see HEREDITY for an explanation). It occurs in approximately one in ten thousand births, and afflicts boys and girls equally; all races and peoples, too, are affected, although the incidence is proportionately higher in Europeans and people descended from Europeans. It is estimated that one person in every fifty is genetically a PKU "carrier" — but the chance of marrying another carrier, thus creating the only conditions under which a child may be afflicted, is only about one in 2500 (in such a marriage, there is one chance in four that a child will have the condition).

If PKU is undiagnosed and untreated, there will be inevitable mental retardation, and it will usually be evident by the time the child is three or four months old (treatment can still be started at this point, or in fact even later). By the age of two or three years, a below-50 I.Q. will be obvious in some 90 percent of PKU victims (about 10 percent, exceptions to the rule, show only mild retardation). The child will not walk or talk until much later than normal, if at all, and is likely to be irritable and destructive as well; he may also have chronic convulsions and other problems. About 80 percent of PKU victims have lighter hair than their parents and normal siblings, since the action of the missing enzyme also plays a part in pigment formation.

All this can, however, be avoided. Phenylketonuria can be treated by providing the child with a special diet; if the regimen is started early, it will be fully effective. Even if the condition is not discovered until later, if the child is still under the age of three years, treatment should be attempted. Whether the diet will help an as-yet-untreated older child is up to the doctor's judgment of the individual case.

The diet keeps a substance called phenylalanine — which constitutes about five percent of the protein in normal food — to a very low level. It is based chiefly on special synthetic formulas that provide amino acids but are unusually low in phenylalanine; among such formulas are Ketonil and Lofenalac in the United States, Cymogram and Minafen in Great Britain.

This basic regimen, taking the place of mother's milk or ordinary formula, is supplemented by vitamins, iron, and very small amounts of milk, and, after a time, by low-protein fruits and vegetables. Later, carbohydrates are introduced, and still later, other variations including special-recipe deserts (usually there is no restriction on sweets per se). What must be avoided are all the normal protein sources — meat, poultry, fish, eggs, and normal amounts of ordinary milk. The diet is continued until adolescence or sometimes may be terminated sooner (medical opinion varies).

These restrictions can be a trial to both child and parents — but they're worth it, since they'll insure that the child will live a normal life thereafter, without the tragic handicap of retardation. He or she should, of course, take precautions against producing a child with either a PKU victim or a carrier. And it is important for *you,* if PKU has been discovered in your baby, to have other children in the family checked immediately — and to inform your *own* brothers and sisters (and your spouse's), who may also carry the trait, so they may be alert to the possibility of PKU in *their* children (although the odds, as we've noted, are against it).

It is not, at this writing, possible to detect PKU in an unborn child, although it probably will be; it *is* possible to detect the "carrier" state in a prospective parent.

phenylpropanolamine: See DECONGESTANTS, NASAL.

phenytoin: a major anticonvulsant. See DILANTIN; EPILEPSY.

Ph.G.: the abbreviation for Graduate in Pharmacy.

phimosis: a condition in which the foreskin of a baby boy is unusually adherent; it is a definite indication that circumcision should be performed. Phimosis does not mean that a problem exists (the problem is a potential one; see PARAPHIMOSIS). It should also be noted that the foreskins of all newborn boys are to some degree adherent; the physician is in the best position to judge whether or not there is cause for concern.

pHisoHex: See HEXACHLOROPHENE.

phlebitis: inflammation of a vein; it may or may not be due to the presence of a thrombus, or clot, and can sometimes occur as an aftermath of prolonged bed rest, fracture, or surgery. Treatment depends upon the location and precise nature of the problem and may involve anticoagulants, external treatment to reduce swelling, and sometimes surgery.

phlegm: the abnormally thick mucus coughed or spit up from the throat, bronchial tubes, or lungs in instances of infection or congestion.

phobia: an unfounded, irrational fear. Words have been coined to characterize many phobias; for the pleasure of those who delight in collecting esoteric terms, herewith a sampling. Some are rather common; others are decidedly rare. (The first word is the thing feared.)

air: aerophobia
animals: zoophobia
being stared at: scopophobia
blushing: ereuthophobia
books: bibliophobia
change: neophobia
colors: chromatophobia
crowds: ochlophobia
dawn: eosophobia
dirt: mysophobia
eating: phagophobia
empty rooms: cenophobia
enclosures: claustrophobia
everything: panophobia
fear: phobophobia
flowers: anthophobia
glass: crystallophobia
hair: trichophobia
heights: acrophobia
machinery: mechanophobia
marriage: gamophobia
meteors: meteorophobia
money: chrematophobia
names: nomatophobia
oneself: autophobia
open space: agoraphobia
people: anthrophobia
pleasure: hedonophobia
rain: ombrophobia

rust: iophobia
spirits: demonophobia
thinking: phronemophobia
thirteen at table: triskaidekaphobia
time: chronophobia
walking: basiphobia
winter weather: cheimaphobia
work: ergasiophobia

phosdrin: See PESTICIDES.

photosensitivity: unusual reaction to sunlight, or to light in general; often, it suggests some sort of eye or skin reaction. Such a situation may exist temporarily as a result of injury (see the section on sunburn under EYE INJURIES) or particular therapy, as with tetracyclines (see ANTIBIOTICS); chronically in some conditions (see, for example, LUPUS); or sometimes, congenitally (see ALBINO).

phrenic nerves: neural connections with the diaphragm; for a common problem connected with them, see HICCOUGH.

physiatrist: a physician specializing in the practice of physical medicine and rehabilitation.

physical examinations: Your baby's first complete physical should — and normally does — take place right after birth; it is then that many congenital problems can be discovered and dealt with immediately. Thereafter, to assure continued good health, your child should be examined by your pediatrician or family physician once a month until the age of a year; every three or four months during the second year; at six-month intervals until the age of six; after that, once a year.

These regular visits are also an excellent time to discuss with your doctor any general questions you may have as well as aspects of your child's psychological and emotional development.

physical therapist: See HEALTH PROFESSIONALS.

physician: a person who, having been regularly admitted to a medical school duly recognized in the country in which it is located, has successfully completed the prescribed course of studies in medicine and has acquired the requisite qualifications to be legally licensed to practice medicine (comprising prevention, diagnosis, treatment and rehabilitation), using independent judgment to promote community and individual health.

And that's official — the definition issued by the World Health Organization in 1972.

pica: the medical term for a habit of eating substances that are generally considered inedible — paint, plaster, dust, paper, fabrics. It is often highly selective: one child may seek out paint chips, another strands of wool from a blanket, still another house-plant soil. The reason is unknown. Sometimes, it is believed, the child may be seeking to compensate for some diet deficiency; in other cases, there may be some emotional disturbance; there may well be additional causes.

Pica seems to be self-limited; it generally does not persist beyond the age of five or so. But in the meantime, whatever the child has chosen to nibble upon may well cause serious damage — in particular, paint or plaster, which are prominent causes of lead poisoning; about 30 percent of children who exhibit pica have been found to suffer from lead poisoning. If you believe your child has this habit, prompt examination — by your physician, a hospital, or your local health department — is called for.

pigeon breast: a congenital deformity of the sternum, or breastbone, so that it projects much like the breast of a pigeon. There's no functional interference with the child's health, and the condition tends to be less noticeable as the child grows; thus it is usually simply ignored unless it's so very unattractive that it becomes a matter of concern to the youngster — in which case it can be diminished surgically.

pigeon toes: a way of walking with the toes turned in (which pigeons, incidentally, don't do). There are a number of different problems that can cause a child to walk this way, ranging from difficulties at the hip joint to deformities of the knee to a variety of foot troubles; if you observe this condition in your youngster, a visit to your physician is in order.

piles: See HEMORRHOIDS.

piminodine: a morphinelike synthetic drug; see NARCOTICS.

pimple: a small infection originating in a clogged oil gland at the base of a hair shaft; see ACNE for a full discussion of causes and remedies.

pink eye: See CONJUNCTIVITIS.

pinworms: See WORMS.

pituitary: See DIABETES INSIPIDUS; ENDOCRINE GLANDS: GROWTH HORMONE.

pityriasis: a not-uncommon skin disease characterized initially by the appearance of a patch of red, generally somewhere on the torso, often on the chest; this "herald patch," as it is medically termed, develops pinkish-gray scales and proceeds, within a week or so, to spread — usually to the rest of the trunk, seldom to the arms and legs, almost never to the face.

There may be some itching accompanying the lesions, or there may not. After a period of time, varying from six weeks to three months, the whole business disappears spontaneously.

Pityriasis is not contagious, and no one has the slightest idea what causes it. Aside from its unsightly appearance and the possibility of itching (for which calamine lotion seems to give some relief), it isn't considered serious. There's no particular treatment for it, except that early exposure to sunlight can sometimes cut it short a bit.

If you suspect that your child has pityriasis, though, consult your doctor. The condition can be confused — by a lay person, not by a physician — with other problems, including psoriasis, that *do* require treatment.

PKU: See PHENYLKETONURIA.

placebo: a "control" medication often used in research — not a true drug, but an inert substance devised, for purposes of a study, to resemble (in appearance, taste, and/or other appropriate facets) the actual drug under study. Frequently, codes are used so that physicians administering the substances are also ignorant of which substance each patient receives (see DOUBLE-BLIND). The purpose is to measure true effects of the real substance against results that may occur spontaneously or by suggestion.

placenta: an organ formed within the uterus — partly from the outermost layer of the embryo, partly from the uterine lining — which serves as a "way-station," during pregnancy, between mother and child; it is via the placenta — although there is not a direct mixing of fetal and maternal blood circulations — that oxygen and nutrients are conveyed to the developing child, and waste materials are excreted. After it has fulfilled its purpose, the placenta becomes the "afterbirth."

Placidyl: a trade name for ethchlorvynol, a sleep-inducing drug; see SEDATIVES.

plague: This highly contagious scourge, caused by the bacillus *Yersinia pestis,* is not merely of historical interest; contrary to popular supposition, it is still endemic — and *can* become *epidemic* — in some parts of the world. It is no longer widespread in Europe, where perhaps 25,000,000 died of plague in the 1300s and raging epidemics occurred as late as the latter part of the seventeenth century. But it *is* endemic in parts of Africa and South America, and it represents a real problem in Southeast Asia; about half the world's cases are believed to be in Vietnam, where at least several hundred, and perhaps several thousand, persons are struck each year. And it's not unknown in the United States.

Plague is a zoonosis; that is, it infects certain animals — in this case, chiefly rodents — as well as people and can be carried to humans (usually by fleas) from infected animals (although it can be transmitted person-to-person, by droplet infection, as well). The great plague epidemics of history were spread primarily by rats, which carried the infection from one port to another as unlisted passengers aboard ships. Once people became aware of this, rodent control eliminated much of the danger; but where pest control breaks down or is nonexistent, the infection can persist in the rodent population.

This situation is true even in part of the United States. Although it's not now generally known, there was a plague epidemic in San Francisco in 1900; it was stopped, by an intensive rat-control effort, before it spread across the country — but not before the infection had been transmitted to ground squirrels in the surrounding countryside. Once that became known, the squirrels too were destroyed in huge numbers. Some of their descendants, however, have kept the infection alive and transmitted it to other wild rodents such as rats, mice and prairie dogs, and plague is considered endemic in some sparsely populated areas of the western — particularly southwestern — United States. The last major outbreak in this country occurred in 1924, when there were 38 cases, 34 of them fatal. But scattered cases have continued over the years. There were thirteen (with one death) reported in 1970, two in 1971, one in 1972, at least two in 1973. In mid-1974, after reports of several cases and one death, a serious outbreak was avoided by the evacuation and temporary closing of a national park camping ground in New Mexico; reported cases for the year totalled eight (one victim died), and the Center for Disease Control believes there were at least three others. In 1975, 22 cases (with four deaths) were reported, the highest number in the last half-century.

It is believed that the foregoing figures may be deceptively low because of misdiagnosis. Physicians unfamiliar with plague can easily confuse it with a number of other conditions, especially tularemia — many presumed cases of which may actually have been plague; if plague is suspected, however, blood tests can reveal the presence of the specific bacteria.

Throughout history, plague has been a subject of dread — and rightly so. Its onset, after a brief (two-to eight-day) incubation period, is abrupt and debilitating, with high fever, severe chills, intense headache, and often delirium. If it progresses, there is typically capillary breakdown in the skin and mucous membranes, resulting in internal bleeding and vomiting of blood and in small subcutaneous hemorrhages; it was the latter, causing visible dark patches, that gave plague its familiar nickname of "black plague" or "black death." Its other name, bubonic plague, derives from the other characteristic symptom — swelling, and possible ulceration, of the lymph nodes; such swellings were called buboes.

In the past, plague was often fatal within days. Now — assuming medical help is available — it can be cured, since sulfa drugs and several of the antibiotics are effective against the bacterium; such drugs can also prevent illness if given quickly after exposure. The disease is, however, obviously best avoided entirely. Vaccination (consisting of three injections, the first two thirty days apart and the third four to twelve weeks later) is essential for travel to Southeast Asia. Your doctor may also consider vaccination advisable if your family plans a camping trip in Arizona, New Mexico, or adjacent parts of California, Utah, Colorado, or Texas — the area of reported cases in recent years. The vaccine is effective for four to six months.

plantar warts: See WARTS.

plaque: an invisible build-up on a tooth consisting of mucin (a protein constituent of saliva), food and cellular debris, and bacteria, for which plaque provides an excellent growth medium; depending upon its content and location, plaque may be either cariogenic (causing caries, or tooth decay) or periogenic (causing disease of the gums and soft tissues). The problem can be prevented by thorough brushing.

plasma: the fluid, constituting about 50 percent of the blood, in which the blood cells are suspended; it can be obtained from whole blood by removing the cells, usually by centrifuge. Whole blood is preferable for transfusion purposes, but under special circumstances, plasma may be used to treat such conditions as shock; it is stored and transported more easily than whole blood, so that it may be more readily available in certain situations — as in a battle or disaster area.

plastic surgery: a term covering a variety of surgical techniques employed to restructure skin and/or bone or other tissues, in order to correct an undesirable or unwanted appearance; the condition being corrected may be congenital or may be caused by scarring, injury, etc.

Plastic surgery undertaken specifically to change a congenital feature that may be unattractive but is not actually deformed is called *cosmetic surgery.* It should never be undertaken lightly — both because it is quite expensive, and because it must be ascertained that the approach of the patient (and of the parents, if a child is involved) is a clear-eyed one and that surgery is not expected to magically banish unrelated personality problems. A physician specializing in this type of surgery must be consulted, and in many cases the plastic surgeon may advise psychological consultation as well, prior to performing the operation, in order to explore the patient's motives and to make sure that hopes regarding the outcome are realistic.

The shape of a nose may be changed by an operation called *rhinoplasty,* performed from inside the nose; i.e., there are no scars. It generally involves two or three days in the hospital and ten days or so for at-home recuperation; some swelling around the nose and beneath the eyes usually continues for several weeks, and the patient must follow certain precautions regarding nose blowing as well as overall physical activity.

A receding chin can be recontoured by the insertion of a small piece of cartilage. This operation is sometimes performed from inside the mouth, in which case there is no scar at all, and sometimes from beneath the jaw, leaving a hairline scar under the chin. There are, again, two or three days of hospitalization; convalescence usually takes about two weeks.

Protruding ears can be repositioned closer to the head by plastic surgery; here, there must be in-depth discussion because ears can grow at different rates, and sometimes the operation must be repeated at a later date (each case is different, and a qualified physician will be able to advise on the prospects for a particular child). The small scars resulting from this type of surgery are behind and underneath the ear, thus unnoticeable. Generally the operation requires two days in the hospital; healing is complete in a week to ten days.

For methods of dealing with scarred skin, see CHEMOSURGERY; DERMABRASION.

platelets: See BLOOD CELLS.

Plegine: a trade name for phendimetrazine; see DIET PILLS.

pleurisy: an inflammation of the pleura, the membrane lining the chest cavity. It can occur alone, but it is most commonly associated with pneumonia, tuberculosis, or some other infection involving the respiratory tract and especially the lungs; it is then treated simultaneously with the primary infection.

Pleurisy is characterized chiefly by pain in the chest (and/or the sides or back), especially on breathing; there may also be a dry cough, as well as fever. Treatment, in addition to medications to combat infection, may include analgesics to relieve pain; in some instances there is also fluid accumulation in the chest and drainage may be needed.

plumbism: See LEAD POISONING.

pneumonia: an inflammation of the lungs; it may be caused by a variety of infectious agents. The word without further qualification usually means *lobar pneumonia* (affecting one or more lobes of the lungs), caused by a bacterium called the pneumococcus; if both lungs are involved, it may be referred to as *double pneumonia.* If the condition begins in the bronchial tubes and involves only small patches of the lungs, it is called *bronchopneumonia.* If the causative agent is a virus rather than a bacterium, the illness is described as *viral pneumonia.*

Either pneumonia or bronchopneumonia, but particularly the latter, can occur not only as a primary infection, but also as a complication of other conditions such as measles, bronchitis, flu, a strep infection, etc. The time involved for the condition to develop varies with the precise cause: the pneumococcal type generally takes only two to five days, while the incubation period for the viral type (as a primary infection) may be a week or two, depending upon the virus involved. (This may be the right place to further confuse you by noting that the term viral pneumonia is usually synonymous with the phrase *primary atypical pneumonia* — except when the same sort of illness is caused by a specific virus with another name; psittacosis or parrot fever, for example, also causes a viral pneumonia or bronchopneumonia.)

Pneumonia, whatever the cause, is characterized by fever, chills, cough, and general weakness. Fever may be moderate to high, and the degree of it isn't necessarily indicative of the severity of the illness; a child may be in critical condition with a temperature of 100° F. (37.8° C.), in a less serious state with a temperature of 105° F. (40.5° C.) If there is also pleurisy, or inflammation of the chest-cavity lining (as there often is in double pneumonia), there will also be pain when breathing and coughing.

All kinds of pneumonia are contagious (though not highly so) and serious, posing a special threat in infancy; immediate medical attention is, of course, a must. Treatment depends upon the cause. The bacterial type, which in the old days was some 25 or 30 percent fatal, can now usually be knocked out in a day or two with antibiotics or sulfa drugs (which *must be continued as long as instructed,* even if symptoms are gone and the child no longer feels ill). The viral kind is a little less serious but may be more difficult to deal with, and relief of symptoms — rest, aspirin, etc. — may be the only remedy possible; sometimes, however, antibiotics, especially the tetracyclines, are effective in combating the infection.

A vaccine against the pneumococcal type of pneumonia has been developed and findings from international field trials, announced in 1976, are heartening: the vaccine appears to be 80 percent effective in preventing this type of infection. Approval for general use by physicians is expected within a year or two.

There is, however, little or no prospect for vaccines against viral and other bacterial pneumonias. The only preventives are keeping up your child's general resistance by good nutrition, adequate rest, and so on, and making sure that less serious conditions — flu, sore throats, other respiratory-tract infections — are promptly diagnosed and treated.

Pneumonialike symptoms may also be caused by some parasites; see WORMS.

podiatrist: an individual with special training in the care of minor foot problems such as corns and bunions and who may also, under a physician's direction, care for chronic foot problems that may develop as a concomitant of certain ills later in life. (Such individuals originally dealt with both hands and feet and were known as *chiropodists; chiro* stems from the Greek word for "hand.") A podiatrist is not a physician. The individual you should consult about your youngster's foot problems should be your physician or a specialist — such as an orthopedist — whom your physician may recommend.

poisoning, food: See FOOD POISONING.

poisoning, household substances and medications: This entry deals with first-aid measures; see the following entry for advice about *preventing* poisoning accidents in your home.

WHEN IN DOUBT, ASSUME THE WORST

If you *see* a child eat or drink a poisonous or possibly poisonous substance, of course there is no doubt; similarly, if you find the child ill or unconscious next to an empty container. But there may be instances when there is some question.

If you find a substance gone unexpectedly, and there was an opportunity for the child to eat or drink it, immediately try to find out. If the child can talk, ask. If not, and the circumstances suggest that he *might* have consumed the stuff, assume he *did.*

If a youngster walks up to you, smiles sweetly, and announces brightly, "I ate the rat poison!" — do *not* dismiss the announcement as a joke. Have the child show you, immediately, what is claimed to have been eaten or drunk (and if it's on a high shelf, don't automatically assume it was inaccessible; children are ingenious climbers). If the substance is gone, demand to know whether it was actually eaten or flushed down the toilet (or whatever). If you are still in doubt, *believe;* in most such situations, children tell the truth.

None of the emergency procedures will harm the child who has *not* swallowed anything poisonous; *failing* to act if the child *has* could cause a *great deal* of harm.

WHAT TO DO

Do not panic. Remain calm, and take the following steps, *in order.*

1. See if the child is breathing. If not, turn to RESPIRATORY RESUSCITATION and follow the instructions there. Have someone phone for an ambulance, and continue resuscitative measures until medical aid arrives. Don't attempt any other treatment.

2. If the child is unconscious but is breathing (or has resumed normal breathing), do not attempt any treatment whatever, and do *not* give the child *anything* by mouth, even water. Simply rush the child to the nearest hospital for emergency treatment. Take along the container from which the poison came, if it is available.

3. If the child is conscious, proceed as follows:

First, check the bottle, can, or other container for emergency instructions; if you find any, follow them.

If there are no such instructions but you know what the substance is, look for it (or its major ingredient) on the alphabetical list that follows.*

If you find it on the list, note the letter

*If the substance is a medication and you have no idea in what category it belongs, check the overall encyclopedia entries. Many common over-the-counter medications, as well as many widely used prescription drugs, have been included in the poisonous-substances list; hundreds of others are entered — by both generic and trade names — in the appropriate alphabetical locations throughout the book.

EMERGENCY PROCEDURES

Reminder: Be sure you have reviewed the basic steps preceding the list of poisonous substances. Do not attempt to get *anything* out of, or put *anything* into, a child who is not fully conscious.

(A) Induce vomiting; see EMETIC for methods. Have a pan or other container ready to catch and retain the vomited material. If the child has not vomited in fifteen minutes, repeat the emetic. If the child has still not vomited after ten minutes more, rush him to the nearest hospital emergency room; take the pan with you in case he vomits on the way, and also take the container from which the poisonous substance came.

If the child does vomit within the allotted time, keep the vomited material in the pan. Call your doctor; report what and how much you think the child consumed, and the appearance and odor of the vomited material. If you cannot reach your doctor, report this information to the nearest poison control center (see APPENDIX E if the number has been entered there, or find it in APPENDIX D).

(B) Induce vomiting; see EMETIC for methods. Have a pan or other container ready to catch and retain the vomited material. If the child does not vomit immediately, rush him to the nearest hospital emergency room; take the pan with you in case he vomits on the way, and also take the container from which the poisonous substance came.

If the child does vomit immediately, follow the last paragraph of (A), above.

(C) Do *NOT* induce vomiting, or give the child anything whatever by mouth. Check in and around the mouth for evidence of burns or other injury; if you find any, apply ice or a cold pack to dull the pain. Then rush the child to the nearest hospital emergency room. Take the poison container with you if it's available.

(D) Do *NOT* induce vomiting. If you have transportation immediately available, and can get the child to the hospital within fifteen minutes, do so. If you don't have transportation available, call for an ambulance. While you're waiting for the ambulance — or before you leave, if it will take more than fifteen minutes to get to the hospital — give the child some milk to drink.

Before you leave for the hospital, check the child's mouth for evidence of burns or other injury; if you find any, apply ice or a cold pack to dull the pain. Take the poison container with you to the hospital.

(E) Do *NOT* induce vomiting. If you have transportation immediately available, and can get the child to the hospital within fifteen minutes, do so. If you don't have transportation available, call for an ambulance. While you're waiting for the ambulance — or before you leave, if it will take more than fifteen minutes to get to the hospital — give the child some acid substance to drink (orange, lemon, lime, or grapefruit juice — or, if you have none of these, diluted vinegar).

Before you leave for the hospital, check the child's mouth for evidence of burns or other injury; if you find any, apply ice or a cold pack to dull the pain. Take the poison container with you to the hospital.

(F) If the label or container carries any drug name whatever — whether a brand name or a chemical name — call the nearest poison control center (see APPENDIX E or APPENDIX D for the number), reporting what the label says and how much you believe the child consumed. If for any reason you cannot reach the poison control center, induce vomiting (see EMETIC for methods), keeping a pan or other container ready to catch and retain the vomited material. If the child vomits immediately, take him *and* the vomited material to the nearest hospital emergency room; if he does not, take him to the hospital and take the pan with you in case he vomits on the way; in either case, be sure to take along the bottle or other container from which the medication came.

If the substance is a prescription medication identified only by a number, call the pharmacy whose name is on the label, explain the problem, and get the name of the medication; try to get brand name, chemical name, and general class of drug. Then see if any of those words or terms appear on the list or among the encyclopedic entries (which may lead to a word on the list). If so, follow whatever procedure is indicated. If not, do as indicated in the preceding paragraph.

If there is no drug name on the label or container and you cannot reach the pharmacy, then try to contact the prescribing physician. If you cannot do so, again proceed as in the first paragraph of (F).

following it; find that letter on the page facing the list (it is repeated throughout the list section) and follow the instructions indicated.

If you do not find it on the list, telephone the nearest poison control center for advice (see APPENDIX E if the number has been entered there; if not, find it in APPENDIX D).

If you do not know what the poisonous substance is, follow procedure (C) on the facing page.

POISONOUS SUBSTANCES

Follow the emergency procedure indicated by the letter following the substance — *exactly.* Be sure you have reviewed the basic steps preceding this list.

Acetaminophen (A)
Acetone (B)
Acids (D)
After-shave lotion (A)
Alcohol, ethyl (liquor) (B)
Alcohol, isopropyl (rubbing) (A)
Alcohol, methyl (wood) (B)
Alkalies (E)
Ammonia (E)
Amphetamines (A)
Anacin (A)
Analgesics (A)
Antacids (A)
Antibiotics — not poisonous, but call doctor and ask advice
Anticoagulants (C)
Antidepressants (A)
Antifreeze (B)
Antihistamines — not usually toxic, but consult doctor promptly
Antiperspirant (A)
Antiseptics (B)
Ant poison (B)
APC tablets (A)
Appetite suppressants (B)
Arsenic (B)
Arthritis medication (F), unless otherwise specified under type
Aspirin (A)
Asthma medication (F)
Atropine (B), and also wrap the child in cold wet cloths if there is fever
Auto polish (C)
Azalea (B)

Barbiturates (B)
Battery acid (D)
Belladonna — see Atropine
Benzedrine (A)
Benzene (C)
Bilberries (A)
Birth control pills (A)
Bleach (D)
Bluing (D)
Boric acid (B)
Bromides (A)
Brush cleaner (D)
Bufferin (A)
Butazolidin (B)

Calamine — not poisonous, but call doctor and ask advice
Campho-Phenique (A)
Camphor (A)
Candle wax (A)
Carbolic acid (D)
Cascara (A)
Castor oil (A)
Cathartics (A)

EMERGENCY PROCEDURES

Reminder: Be sure you have reviewed the basic steps preceding the list of poisonous substances. Do not attempt to get *anything* out of, or put *anything* into, a child who is not fully conscious.

(A) Induce vomiting; see EMETIC for methods. Have a pan or other container ready to catch and retain the vomited material. If the child has not vomited in fifteen minutes, repeat the emetic. If the child has still not vomited after ten minutes more, rush him to the nearest hospital emergency room; take the pan with you in case he vomits on the way, and also take the container from which the poisonous substance came.

If the child does vomit within the allotted time, keep the vomited material in the pan. Call your doctor; report what and how much you think the child consumed, and the appearance and odor of the vomited material. If you cannot reach your doctor, report this information to the nearest poison control center (see APPENDIX E if the number has been entered there, or find it in APPENDIX D).

(B) Induce vomiting; see EMETIC for methods. Have a pan or other container ready to catch and retain the vomited material. If the child does not vomit immediately, rush him to the nearest hospital emergency room; take the pan with you in case he vomits on the way, and also take the container from which the poisonous substance came.

If the child does vomit immediately, follow the last paragraph of (A), above.

(C) Do *NOT* induce vomiting, or give the child anything whatever by mouth. Check in and around the mouth for evidence of burns or other injury; if you find any, apply ice or a cold pack to dull the pain. Then rush the child to the nearest hospital emergency room. Take the poison container with you if it's available.

(D) Do *NOT* induce vomiting. If you have transportation immediately available, and can get the child to the hospital within fifteen minutes, do so. If you don't have transportation available, call for an ambulance. While you're waiting for the ambulance — or before you leave, if it will take more than fifteen minutes to get to the hospital — give the child some milk to drink.

Before you leave for the hospital, check the child's mouth for evidence of burns or other injury; if you find any, apply ice or a cold pack to dull the pain. Take the poison container with you to the hospital.

(E) Do *NOT* induce vomiting. If you have transportation immediately available, and can get the child to the hospital within fifteen minutes, do so. If you don't have transportation available, call for an ambulance. While you're waiting for the ambulance — or before you leave, if it will take more than fifteen minutes to get to the hospital — give the child some acid substance to drink (orange, lemon, lime, or grapefruit juice — or, if you have none of these, diluted vinegar).

Before you leave for the hospital, check the child's mouth for evidence of burns or other injury; if you find any, apply ice or a cold pack to dull the pain. Take the poison container with you to the hospital.

(F) If the label or container carries any drug name whatever — whether a brand name or a chemical name — call the nearest poison control center (see APPENDIX E or APPENDIX D for the number), reporting what the label says and how much you believe the child consumed. If for any reason you cannot reach the poison control center, induce vomiting (see EMETIC for methods), keeping a pan or other container ready to catch and retain the vomited material. If the child vomits immediately, take him *and* the vomited material to the nearest hospital emergency room; if he does not, take him to the hospital and take the pan with you in case he vomits on the way; in either case, be sure to take along the bottle or other container from which the medication came.

If the substance is a prescription medication identified only by a number, call the pharmacy whose name is on the label, explain the problem, and get the name of the medication; try to get brand name, chemical name, and general class of drug. Then see if any of those words or terms appear on the list or among the encyclopedic entries (which may lead to a word on the list). If so, follow whatever procedure is indicated. If not, do as indicated in the preceding paragraph.

If there is no drug name on the label or container and you cannot reach the pharmacy, then try to contact the prescribing physician. If you cannot do so, again proceed as in the first paragraph of (F).

Caustic lime (E)
Caustic soda (E)
Chloral hydrate (B)
Cleaning fluid (C)
Clinitest (D)
Clorox (D)
Cocaine (B)
Codeine (B)
Coffee (A), applying only to very large amounts and very small children
Colchicine (B)
Cold pills (A), unless otherwise specified under brand name
Cologne (A)
Compazine (B)
Compoz (A)
Contac — see Atropine
Contraceptive pills (A)
Cope (A)
Copper cleaner (C)
Coricidin (A)
Corn remover (C)
Cortisone (B)
Cough medicine (A)
Coumarin (C)
Crayons (C)
Cuticle remover (A)
Cyanide (C)

Daffodil bulbs (B)
Dalmane (B)
Darvon (B)
DBI (C)
Decongestants (A)
Demerol (B)
Denatured alcohol (B)
Denture cleaner (C)
Deodorant (A)
Depilatories (A)
Detergent (C)
Dexedrine (A)
Diabetes medication (C)
Diabetes urine test pills (D)
Dieffenbachia (dumb cane) (C)
Diet pills (B)
Digitalis (B)
Dilantin (B)
Dishwasher detergent (C)
Dishwashing liquid (A)
Diuretics — not toxic, but call doctor and ask advice
Donnatal (B)
Douching solution (A)
Drain cleaner (E)
Dramamine (B)
Dristan (A)
Drug, unknown (F)
Dumb cane (Dieffenbachia) (C)
Dye (A)
Dymelor (C)

Empirin (A)
Ephedrine (A)
Epilepsy medication (B)
Epinephrine (B)
Epsom salts (A)
Equanil (B)
Ergotamine (A)
Eskatrol (B)
Estrogen (A)
Eucalyptus oil (A)
Excedrin (A)
Eye drops — see Atropine

Fabric dye (A)
Fabric softener (A)
Fiorinal (B)
Fireworks (B)
Floor cleaner (E)
Floor wax (C)
Flowers (A), unless otherwise specified under plant name
Flypaper (A)
Furniture polish (C)

Gasoline (C)
Glue (A)

EMERGENCY PROCEDURES

Reminder: Be sure you have reviewed the basic steps preceding the list of poisonous substances. Do not attempt to get *anything* out of, or put *anything* into, a child who is not fully conscious.

(A) Induce vomiting; see EMETIC for methods. Have a pan or other container ready to catch and retain the vomited material. If the child has not vomited in fifteen minutes, repeat the emetic. If the child has still not vomited after ten minutes more, rush him to the nearest hospital emergency room; take the pan with you in case he vomits on the way, and also take the container from which the poisonous substance came.

If the child does vomit within the allotted time, keep the vomited material in the pan. Call your doctor; report what and how much you think the child consumed, and the appearance and odor of the vomited material. If you cannot reach your doctor, report this information to the nearest poison control center (see APPENDIX E if the number has been entered there, or find it in APPENDIX D).

(B) Induce vomiting; see EMETIC for methods. Have a pan or other container ready to catch and retain the vomited material. If the child does not vomit immediately, rush him to the nearest hospital emergency room; take the pan with you in case he vomits on the way, and also take the container from which the poisonous substance came.

If the child does vomit immediately, follow the last paragraph of (A), above.

(C) Do *NOT* induce vomiting, or give the child anything whatever by mouth. Check in and around the mouth for evidence of burns or other injury; if you find any, apply ice or a cold pack to dull the pain. Then rush the child to the nearest hospital emergency room. Take the poison container with you if it's available.

(D) Do *NOT* induce vomiting. If you have transportation immediately available, and can get the child to the hospital within fifteen minutes, do so. If you don't have transportation available, call for an ambulance. While you're waiting for the ambulance — or before you leave, if it will take more than fifteen minutes to get to the hospital — give the child some milk to drink.

Before you leave for the hospital, check the child's mouth for evidence of burns or other injury; if you find any, apply ice or a cold pack to dull the pain. Take the poison container with you to the hospital.

(E) Do *NOT* induce vomiting. If you have transportation immediately available, and can get the child to the hospital within fifteen minutes, do so. If you don't have transportation available, call for an ambulance. While you're waiting for the ambulance — or before you leave, if it will take more than fifteen minutes to get to the hospital — give the child some acid substance to drink (orange, lemon, lime, or grapefruit juice — or, if you have none of these, diluted vinegar).

Before you leave for the hospital, check the child's mouth for evidence of burns or other injury; if you find any, apply ice or a cold pack to dull the pain. Take the poison container with you to the hospital.

(F) If the label or container carries any drug name whatever — whether a brand name or a chemical name — call the nearest poison control center (see APPENDIX E or APPENDIX D for the number), reporting what the label says and how much you believe the child consumed. If for any reason you cannot reach the poison control center, induce vomiting (see EMETIC for methods), keeping a pan or other container ready to catch and retain the vomited material. If the child vomits immediately, take him *and* the vomited material to the nearest hospital emergency room; if he does not, take him to the hospital and take the pan with you in case he vomits on the way; in either case, be sure to take along the bottle or other container from which the medication came.

If the substance is a prescription medication identified only by a number, call the pharmacy whose name is on the label, explain the problem, and get the name of the medication; try to get brand name, chemical name, and general class of drug. Then see if any of those words or terms appear on the list or among the encyclopedic entries (which may lead to a word on the list). If so, follow whatever procedure is indicated. If not, do as indicated in the preceding paragraph.

If there is no drug name on the label or container and you cannot reach the pharmacy, then try to contact the prescribing physician. If you cannot do so, again proceed as in the first paragraph of (F).

Grease remover (C)
Gun cleaner (C)

Hair dye (A)
Hair remover (A)
Hair-setting lotion (A)
Headache remedies (A), unless otherwise specified under brand
Heart medication (F), unless otherwise specified under type
Herbicide (B)
Heroin (B)
Hydrochloric acid (D)
Hydrofluoric acid (D)
Hydrogen peroxide (C)

Indocin (B)
Ink (A)
Insecticide — see Pesticides
Insect repellant (A)
Iodine, tincture of (B)
Iron pills (B), and also give sodium bicarbonate to neutralize
Isoniazid (B)

Jequirity beans (B)
Jimsonweed — see Atropine

Kerosene (C)

Lactic acid (C)
Larkspur (B)
Laurel (B)
Laxatives (A)
Lead in paint: if just eaten, (B); cumulative, see LEAD POISONING
Leather polish (B)
Leaves (B), unless otherwise specified under plant name
Lemon oil (A)
Librium (B)
Lighter fluid (C)
Lily of the valley (B)
Lime, caustic (E)
Linseed oil (A)
Liquor (B)
Lomotil (A), and watch for delayed symptoms, including respiratory depression
LSD (A)
Lubricant (C)
Luminal (B)
Lye (E)

Matches, safety (A)
Matches, sulfur or "strike anywhere" type (C)
Medication, content unknown or not listed here (F)
Meperidine (B)
Meprobamate (B)
Mercurochrome (B)
Mercury compounds (A)
Mercury from thermometer — not toxic, but rush child to hospital if glass may have been swallowed
Mescaline (A)
Metal cleaner, polish (C)
Methadone (B)
Methedrine (A)
Methyl (wood) alcohol (B)
Migral (A)
Milk of magnesia (A)
Milkweed (A)
Milpath, Miltown (B)
Mineral oil (A)
Mistletoe (B)
Moth repellent (B)
Motion sickness medication (B)
Motor oil (C)
Mouthwash (B)
Mushrooms — see FOOD POISONING

Nail polish, polish remover (B)
Naphtha (C)
Naphthalene (B)
Narcotics (B)
Nembutal (B)

EMERGENCY PROCEDURES

Reminder: Be sure you have reviewed the basic steps preceding the list of poisonous substances. Do not attempt to get *anything* out of, or put *anything* into, a child who is not fully conscious.

(A) Induce vomiting; see EMETIC for methods. Have a pan or other container ready to catch and retain the vomited material. If the child has not vomited in fifteen minutes, repeat the emetic. If the child has still not vomited after ten minutes more, rush him to the nearest hospital emergency room; take the pan with you in case he vomits on the way, and also take the container from which the poisonous substance came.

If the child does vomit within the allotted time, keep the vomited material in the pan. Call your doctor; report what and how much you think the child consumed, and the appearance and odor of the vomited material. If you cannot reach your doctor, report this information to the nearest poison control center (see APPENDIX E if the number has been entered there, or find it in APPENDIX D).

(B) Induce vomiting; see EMETIC for methods. Have a pan or other container ready to catch and retain the vomited material. If the child does not vomit immediately, rush him to the nearest hospital emergency room; take the pan with you in case he vomits on the way, and also take the container from which the poisonous substance came.

If the child does vomit immediately, follow the last paragraph of (A), above.

(C) Do *NOT* induce vomiting, or give the child anything whatever by mouth. Check in and around the mouth for evidence of burns or other injury; if you find any, apply ice or a cold pack to dull the pain. Then rush the child to the nearest hospital emergency room. Take the poison container with you if it's available.

(D) Do *NOT* induce vomiting. If you have transportation immediately available, and can get the child to the hospital within fifteen minutes, do so. If you don't have transportation available, call for an ambulance. While you're waiting for the ambulance — or before you leave, if it will take more than fifteen minutes to get to the hospital — give the child some milk to drink.

Before you leave for the hospital, check the child's mouth for evidence of burns or other injury; if you find any, apply ice or a cold pack to dull the pain. Take the poison container with you to the hospital.

(E) Do *NOT* induce vomiting. If you have transportation immediately available, and can get the child to the hospital within fifteen minutes, do so. If you don't have transportation available, call for an ambulance. While you're waiting for the ambulance — or before you leave, if it will take more than fifteen minutes to get to the hospital — give the child some acid substance to drink (orange, lemon, lime, or grapefruit juice — or, if you have none of these, diluted vinegar).

Before you leave for the hospital, check the child's mouth for evidence of burns or other injury; if you find any, apply ice or a cold pack to dull the pain. Take the poison container with you to the hospital.

(F) If the label or container carries any drug name whatever — whether a brand name or a chemical name — call the nearest poison control center (see APPENDIX E or APPENDIX D for the number), reporting what the label says and how much you believe the child consumed. If for any reason you cannot reach the poison control center, induce vomiting (see EMETIC for methods), keeping a pan or other container ready to catch and retain the vomited material. If the child vomits immediately, take him *and* the vomited material to the nearest hospital emergency room; if he does not, take him to the hospital and take the pan with you in case he vomits on the way; in either case, be sure to take along the bottle or other container from which the medication came.

If the substance is a prescription medication identified only by a number, call the pharmacy whose name is on the label, explain the problem, and get the name of the medication; try to get brand name, chemical name, and general class of drug. Then see if any of those words or terms appear on the list or among the encyclopedic entries (which may lead to a word on the list). If so, follow whatever procedure is indicated. If not, do as indicated in the preceding paragraph.

If there is no drug name on the label or container and you cannot reach the pharmacy, then try to contact the prescribing physician. If you cannot do so, again proceed as in the first paragraph of (F).

Nitric acid (D)
Noctec (B)
Noludar (B)
Norgesic (B)
Nose drops (B)
Nytol (A)

Oil, lubricating (C)
Oleander (C)
Opiates (B)
Orinase (C)
Oven cleaner (E)
Oxalic acid (C)

Pain reliever, over-the-counter (A)
Pain reliever, prescription (B)
Paint, liquid (C)
Paint thinner (D)
Paint from wall — see Lead
Paregoric (B)
Paris green (B)
Paste (A)
"Pep pills" (A)
Perfume (A)
Permanent-wave solution (A)
Peroxide (C)
Pesticides

Chlorinated hydrocarbons such as aldrin, dieldrin, endrin, DDT, DDE, chlordane, heptachlor, lindane, toxaphene (B).

Organophosphates such as parathion, malathion, paroxon, DFP, chlorthion, soman, EPN, phosdrin, TEPP — systemic poisoning may occur through skin or by inhalation as well as by mouth. Symptoms include salivation, sweating, blurred vision, headache, nausea, difficulty in breathing; if large dose, may lead to convulsions and respiratory failure. Without treatment, death may follow quickly. Rush child to hospital for immediate administration of atropine plus specific antidote, pralidoxime chloride. Do not attempt any first-aid measures.

Phenacetin (A)
Phenobarbital (B)
Philodendron leaves (C) — rarely systematically toxic, but may cause severe throat inflammation and swelling, with threat to respiration
Plants (B), unless otherwise specified under plant name
Plaster — see Lead
Plaster of paris (C) — not toxic, but may harden and require surgical removal
Pokeweed (A)
Polish remover (B)
Potato leaves, stems, berries (B)
Prednisolone, prednisone (B)
Putty — see Lead

Quaalude (B)
Quicklime (E)
Quinine (B)

Rat poison, arsenic (B)
Rat poison, strychnine, warfarin, or type unknown (C)
Reducing pills (B)
Relaxants (B)
Reserpine (B)
Rhododendron (B)
Ritalin (A)
Roach killer (B) usually, but see Pesticides
Rubber cement (A)
Rubbing alcohol (A)
Rug cleaner (C)
Rust remover (D)

Saccharin (A)
Saddle soap (A)

EMERGENCY PROCEDURES

Reminder: Be sure you have reviewed the basic steps preceding the list of poisonous substances. Do not attempt to get *anything* out of, or put *anything* into, a child who is not fully conscious.

(A) Induce vomiting; see EMETIC for methods. Have a pan or other container ready to catch and retain the vomited material. If the child has not vomited in fifteen minutes, repeat the emetic. If the child has still not vomited after ten minutes more, rush him to the nearest hospital emergency room; take the pan with you in case he vomits on the way, and also take the container from which the poisonous substance came.

If the child does vomit within the allotted time, keep the vomited material in the pan. Call your doctor; report what and how much you think the child consumed, and the appearance and odor of the vomited material. If you cannot reach your doctor, report this information to the nearest poison control center (see APPENDIX E if the number has been entered there, or find it in APPENDIX D).

(B) Induce vomiting; see EMETIC for methods. Have a pan or other container ready to catch and retain the vomited material. If the child does not vomit immediately, rush him to the nearest hospital emergency room; take the pan with you in case he vomits on the way, and also take the container from which the poisonous substance came.

If the child does vomit immediately, follow the last paragraph of (A), above.

(C) Do *NOT* induce vomiting, or give the child anything whatever by mouth. Check in and around the mouth for evidence of burns or other injury; if you find any, apply ice or a cold pack to dull the pain. Then rush the child to the nearest hospital emergency room. Take the poison container with you if it's available.

(D) Do *NOT* induce vomiting. If you have transportation immediately available, and can get the child to the hospital within fifteen minutes, do so. If you don't have transportation available, call for an ambulance. While you're waiting for the ambulance — or before you leave, if it will take more than fifteen minutes to get to the hospital — give the child some milk to drink.

Before you leave for the hospital, check the child's mouth for evidence of burns or other injury; if you find any, apply ice or a cold pack to dull the pain. Take the poison container with you to the hospital.

(E) Do *NOT* induce vomiting. If you have transportation immediately available, and can get the child to the hospital within fifteen minutes, do so. If you don't have transportation available, call for an ambulance. While you're waiting for the ambulance — or before you leave, if it will take more than fifteen minutes to get to the hospital — give the child some acid substance to drink (orange, lemon, lime, or grapefruit juice — or, if you have none of these, diluted vinegar).

Before you leave for the hospital, check the child's mouth for evidence of burns or other injury; if you find any, apply ice or a cold pack to dull the pain. Take the poison container with you to the hospital.

(F) If the label or container carries any drug name whatever — whether a brand name or a chemical name — call the nearest poison control center (see APPENDIX E or APPENDIX D for the number), reporting what the label says and how much you believe the child consumed. If for any reason you cannot reach the poison control center, induce vomiting (see EMETIC for methods), keeping a pan or other container ready to catch and retain the vomited material. If the child vomits immediately, take him *and* the vomited material to the nearest hospital emergency room; if he does not, take him to the hospital and take the pan with you in case he vomits on the way; in either case, be sure to take along the bottle or other container from which the medication came.

If the substance is a prescription medication identified only by a number, call the pharmacy whose name is on the label, explain the problem, and get the name of the medication; try to get brand name, chemical name, and general class of drug. Then see if any of those words or terms appear on the list or among the encyclopedic entries (which may lead to a word on the list). If so, follow whatever procedure is indicated. If not, do as indicated in the preceding paragraph.

If there is no drug name on the label or container and you cannot reach the pharmacy, then try to contact the prescribing physician. If you cannot do so, again proceed as in the first paragraph of (F).

Salicylates (A)
Scopolamine — see Atropine
Seconal (B)
Sedatives (B)
Shampoo (A)
Shellac (B)
Shoe polish (B)
Silver nitrate (B)
Sleep-Eze — see Atropine
Sleeping pills, over-the-counter — see brand name
Sleeping pills, prescription (B)
Soap (A)
Soda, caustic (E)
Soma (B)
Sominex — see Atropine
Spot remover (C)
Strychnine (C)
Styptic pencil (C)
Sulfa drugs (A)
Sulfuric acid (D)
Suntan lotion (B)

Talcum powder (B)
Talwin (B)
Tar (C)
Terpin hydrate (D)
Thiazides — see Diuretics
Thorazine (B)
Tobacco (B)
Tofranil (A)
Toilet cleaner (D)
Tolinase (C)
Toluene (C)
Tranquilizers (B)
Triavil (B)
Tuinal (B)
Tulip bulbs (B)
Turpentine (D)
Tylenol (A)
Typewriter cleaner (C)

Upholstery cleaner (C)

Valadol (A)
Valium (B)
Varnish (C)
Vick's VapoRub (A)
Vitamin-and-mineral pills (B)
Vitamin pills (A)

Warfarin (C)
Washing soda (C)
Wax (C)
Wax remover (E)
Weed killer (B)
White lead — see Lead
Wintergreen, oil of (A)
Wood alcohol (B)
Wood preservative (C)

Zactane, Zactirin (B)

poisoning, prevention of: If you have a child under the age of five in your home, it is vital that you take precautions. The peril is, we assure you, a very real one. Children in this age group account for two-thirds of all poisonings, 90 percent of which occur in the home. There are hundreds, if not thousands, of commonly available household items that can poison; the National Safety Council has estimated that the average American home probably contains at least forty of them.

Of course that fact does not pose much of a problem for adults, teenagers, or even older children — who are unlikely to deliberately drink insecticide or floor cleaner, nibble on mothballs, or down an entire bottle of aspirin. But amazing as it may seem, small children have been known to do so;

studies have shown that their sense of taste and smell just doesn't work the same way, and they are often attracted to things older folks would find repellent. Couple this proclivity with curiosity, lack of knowledge and experience, and inability to read labels; you can, we trust, see why small children must be protected from themselves.

We urge you to observe the following bare-minimum safeguards, for your child's sake.

Keep detergents, disinfectants, insecticides, and all other potential troublemakers under lock and key; for the full list, see the entry immediately preceding this one — everything there is listed because it *has* been known to cause trouble. Tucking things on high shelves isn't enough; small children can climb amazingly well.

Keep all medicines — except for syrup of ipecac, which isn't poisonous and should be handy for emergencies — locked away, in a locked suitcase for instance. Or get a special hook-and-eye spring lock, too hard for a tot to open (e.g., the Kindergard latch) for your medicine chest. This precaution applies not only to habit-forming drugs, sleeping pills, and that sort of thing, but also — in fact, particularly — to such everyday items as aspirin (the leading child poisoner; two out of three cases involve children's aspirin), vitamins (number two on the list), and minerals; iron pills pose a special danger, because they are sugar coated, taste good, and generally come in bright, attractive colors. *Don't* depend on safety caps: they are not yet mandated for all medications — and even when they're there, adults frequently forget or neglect to close them properly.

Reread the label, and do so in good light, each time you give anyone medicine. Don't ever characterize a medication as "candy" or something similarly appealing; medicine is medicine, to be taken only when given by you or some other adult authority.

When you take medications yourself or give them to an older youngster, do so, if you can, out of the sight of toddlers; small children are strongly inclined to ape the actions of their elders.

Watch for hazards that may be *brought into* your home inadvertently by guests — pills in purses, for example, and medications in coat or jacket pockets that a child can reach even when the coat's hung up; children *have* been poisoned in both those ways. Similarly, keep an eye on your child when *you're* visiting *others* — especially homes with no small children, where your hosts may not be conscious of the problem. And accompany your youngster on any visits to the bathroom in other people's homes; there's no telling what might be readily accessible.

Be aware that there are at least seven hundred species of poisonous plants in the United States, and many children have died or become severely ill after nibbling on them; they include many common plants found in and around the home. Among them are many trees, vines, and shrubs that are poisonous to some degree or in some part (including English ivy, privet, wisteria, oleander, mountain laurel, and black locust), a number of familiar bulbs, and many garden flowers —

plus many wild-growing plants including the evening primrose and the ordinary buttercup. (Even parts of some food plants are toxic; the leaves of peach trees, potatoes, rhubarb, and tomatoes are among them.) And the leaves of quite a few popular house plants contain toxins. We suggest that you make it your business to learn the names of all plants growing in and around your home, and then consult your local library, extension service, or horticultural society for information on their toxicity.

Also see FOOD POISONING, PREVENTION OF; LEAD POISONING; PESTICIDES.

poison ivy, poison oak, poison sumac: These three infamous plants are actually all the same, botanically speaking — all varieties of the species called *Rhus toxicodendron,* and all causing the same sort of trouble for *Homo sapiens.*

Poison ivy, with its red-stemmed leaves in groups of three, is the most widespread; it thrives as a vine or shrub throughout the United States except for the Southwest. Poison oak, with a similar leaf arrangement, grows chiefly as a bush, and is limited to the West Coast. Poison sumac, found only in the eastern part of the country —

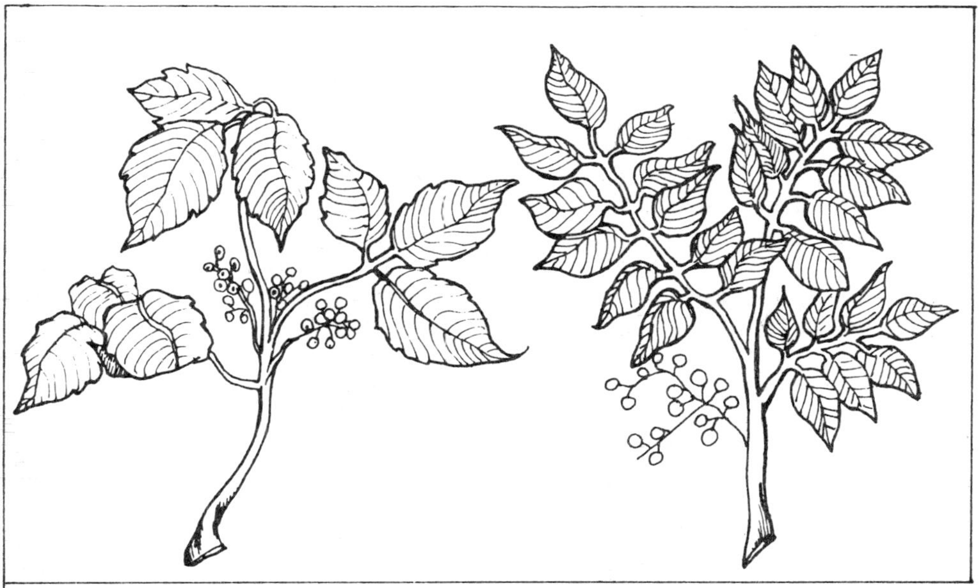

Poison Ivy and Kin

RHUS TOXICODENDRON *(the species name translates literally as "poison tree") is found in three forms and displays two leaf formations.* LEFT: *Red-stemmed leaves in groups of three mark poison ivy, thriving throughout most of the United States as a climbing vine or ground cover; poison oak, the bush or shrub form found only on the West Coast, has similar leaves.* RIGHT: *Poison sumac, confined to the East (chiefly boggy areas), is a shrub or small tree; its leaves are mostly paired, with three to seven pairs on each stem or twig and a single leaf at the end. All three forms bear clusters of loosely hanging small, yellowish-white berries in season.*

chiefly in boggy areas — takes the form of a low-growing tree; its leaves are paired, with three to seven pairs on each stem or twig and a single leaf at the end of the stem. We'll refer simply to poison ivy from here on, but what is said here applies to all three.

The "poison" isn't really a poison in the strict sense of the word, but an allergen — a chemical called urushiol, contained in the oils secreted by the plant, to which three out of four people are allergic. Urushiol is found in every part of the plant — leaves, flowers, berries, twigs, stems, roots — and is not destroyed by winter cold, water, drying, or burning. Burning is, in fact, especially dangerous because it disperses the chemical in the air, where it can affect the eyes and also be inhaled.

(The way to destroy poison ivy found growing on or near your property, recommended by the National Audubon Society because it is effective, safe, and not harmful to other plant or animal life: Cover yourself completely, by wearing long sleeves, long pants, and gloves. Cut the stems of the individual plants, very close to the ground. Apply Ammate to the cut stems.)

The best course is to avoid poison ivy entirely. Heavy clothes aren't especially helpful, since the oils get on the clothes, which have to be handled in the course of removing them. It is well to teach your children to identify these plants and to give them a wide berth. Also be aware that animals, who are not allergic to urushiol, can pick up the plant's oils on hair or fur and thus convey it to human beings.

If you know or believe exposure has occurred, but no problem has yet arisen, the allergic reaction can sometimes be prevented by fast action; if the chemical hasn't penetrated the underlayers of the skin, there's a chance of removing the oils before they cause trouble. The child should be washed all over with strong soap, thoroughly dried, and then given a brisk alcohol rub. Clothing and pets that may have picked up the oils should also be thoroughly washed with strong soap.

The characteristic blistery rash may erupt at any time from six hours to several days after exposure; it's usually of a linear nature — that is, following the path of the child's brush with the plant. There will typically be intense itching, and possibly some swelling as well.

With the exceptions noted in the next paragraph, poison ivy doesn't need medical attention. Don't let the child scratch, because that can cause infection. Nails should be cut short. Do everything you can to relieve the itching. Calamine lotion, or the spray version incorporating an antihistamine (Caladryl), is fine. As is a cornstarch or baking-soda bath (put enough of either in the tub to definitely cloud the water). Aspirin or a similar mild pain reliever may also be helpful.

That's all you should do without medical advice. A systemic antihistamine may be useful, but check with your doctor first. Also consult your physician if a very extensive area is involved, if any signs of infection appear (pus, a great deal of redness, increased swelling, fever), or if the itching and discomfort don't respond to the remedies we've suggested. The doctor must also be seen if the child's face or eyes are involved.

Uncomplicated poison ivy is not contagious. It can be "caught" only if some of the oils are still on the skin and are touched by another allergic person; the blisters and their contents do not contain the allergen.

Families in which urushiol allergy has been manifested should be aware that the chemical can also be found in a number of other plants and plant products. Among them: cashews and pistachios, which come from the same botanical family (and indeed allergies have been known to coincide — although it's not necessarily consistent); some india inks used for laundry marking; cashew oil, which is used in some glues and other products; and certain oils of various Oriental trees, used primarily in lacquers — and rather ubiquitously, as travelers have found, on toilet seats in that part of the world.

polio: a viral infection of the central nervous system; the word is short for *poliomyelitis*. Polio has also been known as "infantile paralysis," but that's a double misnomer; the infection rarely causes paralysis and, although it's true that over 50 percent of its victims have been under ten, about 25 percent have been over twenty. The disease, highly contagious and often epidemic among children in the summer months, was rightly dreaded; although half its victims recovered completely, one in twenty died, and some 15 percent were permanently crippled (President Franklin D. Roosevelt, who developed the disease as an adult, was one of those).

With the introduction of vaccine, the incidence dropped — from a peak of 58,000 cases in 1952 to a mere nineteen, with no deaths, in 1969. Since then, however, the Center for Disease Control has repeatedly warned that complacency could easily renew the threat of widespread epidemic. By 1974, the Center estimated that some 40 percent of American children had not been immunized, and that proportions were even higher in some parts of the country. A 1972 "mini-epidemic" in a Connecticut private school left seven children partially or severely paralyzed. With increased international travel, the danger is multiplied. Polio incidence has been rising in many African, Asian, and Latin American countries, especially the last; within the past decade there have been epidemics or major outbreaks in Argentina, Ecuador, Mexico, Nicaragua, Peru, and Trinidad.

In fact, children may now be at higher risk than they would have been a generation ago. Before the advent of vaccine, many youngsters contracted subclinical infections — not serious enough to make them sick, but sufficient to give them immunity. Today's children have never encountered the wild, natural virus; without immunization, they are completely unprotected. We urge you to see that *your* children *do* receive protection.

The original, injected vaccine is no longer in use. Your child should receive TOPV (trivalent oral polio vaccine, which covers all three forms of the virus) at the approximate ages of two months, four months, six months, a year and a half, and five years; boosters are given every three or four years thereafter, possibly indefinitely (follow your own physician's advice) — and should certainly precede travel to any locale where polio has been prevalent.

Polycillin: a trade name for ampicillin, a semisynthetic penicillin; see ANTIBIOTICS.

polymyositis: See DERMATOMYOSITIS.

polymyxin: See ANTIBIOTICS.

polyp: a mushroom-shaped (that is, having a "stalk") growth arising from mucous membrane; polyps can occur in the nose, throat, sinuses, intestines, and other sites. Rarely, polyps may be a precancerous condition; usually, however, they are harmless and are not removed unless their size or position is such that they are causing obstruction of the particular passageway. They're easily removed, especially if they're in a conveniently accessible site such as the nose, throat, or rectum.

Polyposis describes the presence of a number of polyps. *Familial polyposis* is a rare inherited condition (it is autosomal dominant; see HEREDITY) characterized by chronic formation of polyps in the colon only, typically beginning in late childhood.

polysaccharides: a category of chemically bonded sugars, the most familiar of which is starch. See NUTRITION for general discussion of carbohydrates; sugars and their synthetic substitutes are discussed under SWEETENERS.

Polysporin: a topical medication combining bacitracin and polymyxin; see ANTIBIOTICS.

porphyria: an uncommon — though not as rare as once supposed — hereditary disorder of metabolism in which there is faulty handling of a pigment called porphyrin, presumably because of deficiency of one or more enzymes. The disorder is in fact common in a few areas, notably in South Africa, where it has been traced back to a single early Dutch settler. It occurs in two or possibly three forms, the mildest of which follows a recessive pattern of inheritance, the most severe a dominant one (see HEREDITY for explanation of the terms).

The severe form — from which England's King George III, as well as a number of his forebears (including Mary, Queen of Scots) and five of his children, is now believed to have suffered — is called acute intermittent porphyria (AIP), which describes it well. It is characterized by acute attacks that may begin in the late teens or the twenties; the attacks begin with physical symptoms — generally acute abdominal pain, weakness, sweating, and a typical wine-red color to the urine (imparted by porphyrin) — followed by a variety of neurological and mental symptoms that may include severe headache, insomnia, visual disturbances, difficulty in swallowing, convulsions, irrational behavior, and delirium. Before the cause was known, the physical symptoms were often ignored or dismissed and the condition viewed as insanity (subsequently a "psychogenic" disorder) — which was what happened to George III, long thought to be "mad." Months or years may intervene between attacks.

Only in recent years was it discovered that certain drugs, among them some that were sometimes given to porphyrics to relieve pain in an acute attack, can make such attacks worse and even actually initiate them. There is now a blood test that can detect AIP even if no attacks have yet occurred; since there is a 50–50 chance of inheriting the disorder, anyone in whose family AIP has been diagnosed should be tested. Those who have inherited the gene, whether or not they have had any symptoms, should avoid alcohol, sulfa drugs, estrogens (including birth-control pills), chloroquines (drugs used to treat malaria and some other conditions), and sedatives in general and barbiturates in particular (barbiturate anesthetics, such as methohexital and thiopental, must not be used in surgery — and those affected should carry a warning to that effect).

A second form — it may be a milder version of AIP, and is sometimes called erythropoietic protoporphyria — appears earlier, often in late childhood, and is characterized chiefly by severe photosensitivity of the skin, which upon minimal exposure to sunlight burns, itches, swells, and reddens, with possible blistering and scarring. (Some of those with the condition are susceptible to the reaction only in warm weather.) Sunscreens do not appear to help, but recent studies suggest that the reaction can be lessened considerably by administration of a substance called beta-carotene, a vitamin A precursor; although it creates a change in skin color (see CAROTENEMIA), serious adverse effects such as hypervitaminosis A have not been reported.

A third form of the disorder is congenital and becomes evident as soon as the child has teeth, which appear somewhat pinkish; there may be some photosensitivity as well, but this mild form of porphyria is believed to be distinct and transmitted by recessive inheritance.

Diagnosis of any form of porphyria can be confirmed by fecal sampling; because of porphyrin traces, a fecal solution will appear red when examined under ultraviolet light (normal solution will be green).

port wine stain: See BIRTHMARKS.

positive: a result of a test or examination, meaning the condition for which the physician is testing or looking has been found. A positive result of a blood test for syphilis, for example, means that the patient *does* have syphilis; a positive result of a test for sugar in the urine means that sugar is present; a positive pregnancy test means that the patient is pregnant.

postnasal drip: drainage of mucus from the back of the nose into the throat; whatever the cause — a cold, sinusitis, adenoidal infection, or allergic reaction — it's usually worse during the night and gives rise to a good deal of coughing in the morning. If you believe your youngster has a postnasal drip, consult your physician so that the underlying cause can be diagnosed and corrected; don't try to treat it yourself with patent medicines.

postnatal: See NATAL.

postpartum: relating to, or occurring during, the period (in the mother's life) following childbirth; for her baby, the period is *postnatal.*

postprandial test: a type of diagnostic test conducted after the consumption of food — usually food specified by the physician — in order to determine the body's reaction to, or handling of, the food. It may involve taking specimens of urine and/or blood samples, either a particular time after eating, or several times at certain intervals.

potassium: a minor but essential mineral, also a key blood chemical (see ELECTROLYTES). Potassium replacement may be administered or advised if there has been inordinate fluid loss, which may occur because of illness, injury, diuretic drugs, and some types of poisoning.

potentiate: to increase the effects of (a drug), beyond those normally expected — usually (although there are exceptions) something to be avoided. Potentiation often occurs when a patient, unknown to the physician, has added another drug (e.g., alcohol) to an already prescribed one (e.g., a sedative).

Pott's disease: tuberculosis of the spine.

poxviruses: See VIRUSES.

practical nurse: See HEALTH PROFESSIONALS.

precancerous: describing a lesion, or cellular changes detectable on microscopic analysis, not indicative of present malignancy but known — through past experience — to precede the development of a malignancy. Removal (as of a skin lesion) or other treatment (sometimes consisting simply of close observation) is generally advised in order to prevent the occurrence of cancer or to treat it early if it appears.

prednisolone, prednisone: See CORTICOSTEROIDS.

pregnancy: For several years after menarche, the presence or absence of a period isn't necessarily indicative of anything: menstrual irregularity, with missed or late periods, is fairly common during the teen years — and on the other hand, it's possible (though unusual) to have a period or two after becoming pregnant.

It's important in our view, for parents to establish an atmosphere that will encourage a daughter to seek *your* counsel, without fear of violent recriminations, if she believes she may be "in trouble." (Both you and she should know, too, that "the pill" and other measures are designed to prevent *pregnancy only,* and *aren't* safeguards against *infection;* see VENEREAL DISEASES.)

We are neither moralizing nor suggesting what your attitudes should be regarding premarital sexual relations; your attitudes, and the standards you set for your children, are your business. What *is* our concern is your daughter's health; it's vital that, if there is any possibility of pregnancy, she feels free to come to *you — without delay* — rather than resort to some doubtful action that could cause her permanent injury.

New and faster laboratory tests, using samples of the patient's urine, have replaced the older, tedious methods — injecting material into mice, rabbits, frogs, etc. — of detecting pregnancy; they are also both more reliable and less expensive. They can give a dependably accurate answer in a matter of hours, providing more than two weeks have passed since the missed menstrual period (a blood test has been developed, and may soon be generally available, that can detect pregnancy a week after conception, even before a missed period). False-positive results (i.e., indicating pregnancy erroneously) are extremely rare and generally due to technical error; false-negative results can occasionally occur in early pregnancy (repeating the test a week later, to make sure, is usually advised).

For related discussion, see ABORTION.

Preludin: a trade name for phenmetrazine; see DIET PILLS.

prematurity: By arbitrary medical definition, a baby is termed premature if born before the 37th week of pregnancy; birth weight, formerly the criterion, no longer applies (see SMALL FOR DATE). About 10 percent of babies are born prematurely; in the majority, the reason is unknown. Known causes include various disorders in the mother and premature separation of the placenta.

Whether a premature baby needs special care, and what that special care should consist of, are decisions made by the physician who examines the baby after birth; they will be based both on the length of pregnancy and whether or not the doctor feels there are any other problems.

If it is judged necessary, the baby is placed in an incubator that provides proper levels of warmth and humidity, controls the amount of oxygen the baby receives, and also lets medical personnel monitor the child's heart and respiratory rates. The physician may also sometimes direct that the baby be transferred to another hospital with special facilities (you might hear the terms "preemie unit," or "intensive care nursery"); this is no reason for alarm on your part — it's just extra insurance.

The baby is kept in an incubator or special unit until — again, in the physician's judgment — he is strong enough for regular nursery care. If a premature baby is properly cared for, there are usually no permanent ill effects, either mental or physical.

prenatal: See NATAL.

Presamine: a trade name for imipramine; see ANTIDEPRESSANTS.

Pre-Sate: a trade name for chlorphentermine; see DIET PILLS.

prescriptions: directions written by a physician or dentist to a pharmacist for medication, including the total amount, exact dosage, and directions for administering it. (Directions to an optician for the formulation of corrective eyeglasses are also prescriptions.)

The pharmacist fills the order, assigns the prescription a number, and labels the medication with date, number, physician's name, and instructions for use. That information is a basic legal requirement. The label should also carry the patient's name, so that look-alike medications do not get confused. More and more physicians feel that the label should also bear the name of the drug: the generic name, plus the trade name, if applicable. We entirely agree. For several reasons:

• the information in this and other books will make a lot more sense, and you will be able to use it intelligently;

• discussions with your physician are greatly facilitated ("I've been giving Johnny those little yellow pills" may not be very helpful information);

• because there are potentially hazardous interactions among various drugs, it is important to be able to tell one physician what another has prescribed (different doctors may be consulted for different conditions);

• precious moments can be saved, when a drug is taken by accident, if you can immediately name it when you phone your physician or a poison control center.

Ask your physician to specify such labeling on the prescription form, and do *not* accept a pharmacist's laziness — or protest that such information cannot be put on the label. That's not true. The pharmacist must include on the label whatever the physician directs.

You will often find mysterious abbreviations included in prescriptions the doctor writes. They are abbreviations for Latin phrases, used not to mystify you but to save time and space and because — like many scientific terms, including generic names of animals, plants, bacteria, etc. — they cut across language lines and are understood everywhere. Among the common ones:

ad lib — freely, generally pertaining to refill instructions
a.c. — before meals
b.i.d. — twice a day
co., comp. — compound
d. — per day
dur. dol. — while the pain lasts
e.m.p. — as prescribed
gr. — grain, grains (a grain equals roughly 65 milligrams)
gtt. — drops
h.s. — at bedtime
mg — milligrams
o.d. — every day
O.D. — in right eye
O.S. — in left eye
O.U. — in each eye
p.c. — after meals
p.r.n. — as needed
pro us. ext. — for external use
q.h., q. 2 h., etc. — every hour, every two hours, etc.
q.i.d. — four times a day
q.n.s. — as much as necessary
sig. — label
s.o.s. — if necessary
stat. — immediately
t.i.d. — three times a day
ut dict. — as directed

Of course the physician's instructions for administering medication must be followed to the letter. And (admonitions you will see in a number of other places in this book) be sure that (1) the medication — pertaining especially to treatment of infection — is taken for as many days as the doctor specified, even if symptoms have disappeared before that; (2) the physician is promptly advised of any adverse reaction to any medication (if you are not sure it is a reaction to the drug, report it anyway and let the doctor judge).

For some other important guidelines on the keeping and giving of medications, see MEDICINE CHEST; POISONING, PREVENTION OF.

PreSun: See SUNSCREENS.

prickly heat: See HEAT RASH.

primaquine sensitivity: See FAVISM.

primidone: an antiseizure medication; see EPILEPSY.

Principen: a trade name for ampicillin, a semisynthetic penicillin; see ANTIBIOTICS.

p.r.n.: See PRESCRIPTIONS.

probarbital: See SEDATIVES.

procaine: See ANESTHETIC.

prochlorperazine: one of the phenothiazines, a tranquilizer and antinauseant. See NAUSEA; SEDATIVES.

proctologist: a gastroenterologist (see SPECIALTIES, MEDICAL) specializing in problems of the anus and rectum, particularly in surgical treatment thereof.

proctoscopy: visual examination of the rectum.

prodrome: See MIGRAINE.

prognosis: literally, "knowing before" (from the Greek) — of course an impossibility. In everyday use, the word means outlook or educated guess as to the probable course of a disease and the outcome for the patient, based both on medical statistics and physician's judgment of the condition of the individual patient. (The statistical prognosis in a disease, and the prognosis for a particular patient who has that disease, may be quite different.)

projectile vomiting: See PYLORIC STENOSIS; VOMITING.

Prolixin: a trade name for fluphenazine, an antinauseant and tranquilizer. See NAUSEA; SEDATIVES.

promazine, promethazine: two of a group of potent tranquilizers; the latter is also used as an antinauseant. See NAUSEA; SEDATIVES.

prophylaxis: a procedure designed to prevent illness, disease, or other problems; the word might refer to preventive medicine or dentistry, or to measures taken by the ordinary person. Examples of prophylaxis include immunization against infectious disease, professional cleaning of the teeth by a dentist or oral hygienist, washing one's hands after going to the bathroom, taking steps to prevent pregnancy.

propicillin: a semisynthetic penicillin; see ANTIBIOTICS.

propoxyphene: an analgesic chemically related to narcotics and discussed under that entry.

proprietary hospital: See the discussion of hospitals in APPENDIX A.

proprietary name: brand, or trade, name.

prostaglandins: You have probably heard something of these substances, and you will doubtless hear more in future; they represent one of the most active and promising frontiers of current biomedical research.

Most medical terms, while complex, make a certain amount of logical sense. This one doesn't, although it seemed to when the word was coined. The substances were first discovered in the early 1930s in fluid from the prostate gland, and it was assumed at the time that their sole location had been established and that they played some role in the male reproductive process — hence the coinage, which appeared entirely appropriate.

It is now known that these substances — at least fifteen distinct ones have been identified at this writing — are in fact continuously produced in all kinds of tissues throughout the body and play an active part in many physiological processes. They are synthesized within the cells through the action of certain enzymes, and their activities appear to depend upon interaction with other cellular enzymes and the renowned "second messenger" (see CYCLIC AMP); some investigators have in fact postulated that prostaglandins may play an early role in the hormonal-message relay, perhaps acting as the second messenger while cyclic AMP may be not the second but the third. The prostaglandins do, at any rate, modulate the actions of many hormones and appear generally to play roles in metabolism as well. Once released, they do not seem to live long, so it is assumed that their actions and effects are strictly local, taking place in or near the cells where they are produced.

What is especially intriguing about the prostaglandins thus far identified is that the actions of some seem to contradict the actions of others. It is thus possible that a number of ills and disorders may represent an imbalance — i.e., too much or too little of one of them — which might be rectified by remedying a deficiency or administering an "antidote" for an excess.

Based on elements of their chemical structure, the identified prostaglandins fall into four groups, designated A, B, E, and F, further differentiated by subscripted numbers and sometimes by Greek-letter suffixes. The Es and Fs appear most prevalent and active. Following, to give you just a small idea of the therapeutic potential, are some of the actions of various prostaglandins that have been documented.

Both PGE_2 and PGF_2-alpha stimulate uterine contractions and have been approved for clinical use for that purpose (the only two that have been synthesized and are available commercially thus far, they are marketed as Prostin E_2 and Prostin F_2-alpha); they are employed to induce labor as well as to initiate abortion in the second trimester. PGF_2-alpha is also known to reduce secretion of a hormone necessary for implantation of a fertilized egg, which suggests that it, or some variation of it, might have a role to play in contraception; as available now, it is not so used nor is such use contemplated, because of side effects.

PGE_1 is a bronchodilator, stimulating the release of cyclic AMP which in turn relieves bronchial spasm. PGE_2, on the other hand, decreases cyclic AMP release, and the PGFs also promote bronchial constriction (at least one study has found abnormally high serum levels in asthma patients). The use of PGE_2 or PGF_2-alpha to induce abortion or labor is thus not advised in a woman with either a personal or family history of asthma.

PGE_1 inhibits blood clotting, while PGE_2, which is the main prostaglandin synthesized in human skin, promotes clotting and is formed markedly faster following a wound or burn. But PGE_2 also encourages sickling in the blood of those with the sickle-cell trait, although it has no such effect in others.

The PGAs and PGEs reduce blood pressure; the PGFs lower pressure in cats and rabbits but raise it in dogs, rats, and humans.

PGE_2 can significantly reduce gastric secretion and acid production, both of which play a part in creating and exacerbating peptic ulcer; preliminary clinical trials suggest it may be useful in treatment.

The PGEs dilate blood vessels (and can thus produce severe headache); PGF_2-alpha constricts them.

PGE_1 has been found in laboratory animals to reduce the inflammation of experimentally induced arthritis. PGE_2 and PGF_2-alpha, on the other hand, apparently play active roles in creating inflammation; aspirin and other anti-inflammatory agents act, at least in part, by attacking a precursor substance and preventing formation of these prostaglandins.

Prostaphlin: a trade name for oxacillin, a semisynthetic penicillin; see ANTIBIOTICS.

prosthesis: an artificial — i.e., manufactured — substitute for a missing or lost part of the body; prostheses include false teeth as well as replacements for hands, legs, etc.

prosthodontist: See SPECIALTIES, DENTAL.

protein: See NUTRITION.

proteinuria: the presence of certain proteins in the urine in excess of normal quantities, a finding that may, together with other test results, have diagnostic significance. Also see ALBUMINURIA.

protriptyline: See ANTIDEPRESSANTS.

"proud flesh": overgrown tissue sometimes seen on an unhealed wound before new skin has formed; it consists of blood vessels and connective tissue and usually subsides by itself in the course of healing.

pro us. ext.: See PRESCRIPTIONS.

proximal: nearer to, or in the direction of, the trunk; the opposite of *distal.*

pruritus: itching.

pseudohermaphroditism: See HERMAPHRODITISM.

psilocybin: See PSYCHEDELICS.

psittacosis: a type of viral infection, also known as parrot fever; it afflicts both people and birds — not only parrots, but also parakeets, pigeons, canaries and others often kept as pets. It tends to start with a bird — who may not, incidentally, appear noticeably ill — and is transmitted to a person via contact with the bird itself, its cage, its droppings, etc. Thereafter, the human who has been infected can communicate the virus to other people by droplet infection.

Symptoms of psittacosis, which appear after an incubation period of four to fifteen days (the average is ten), include chills, high fever, constipation and loss of appetite, followed by coughing and general debilitation. As with many other ills, such symptoms are typical of other conditions as well, but a diagnosis of psittacosis can be confirmed by a special blood test. Unlike most viral infections, this one responds to some antibiotics; the tetracyclines and erythromycin are most effective. Remember that psittacosis is contagious; the child who has it should be kept away from others for the course of the illness — usually about two weeks.

There is no vaccine or other immunization against psittacosis. Simply make very sure any pet birds are completely healthy (have them checked periodically by a veterinarian), and teach your children to avoid wild birds (pigeons in particular) and their droppings.

psoriasis: a skin condition manifested by silver-scaled red patches, appearing most commonly on the arms and legs (especially elbows and knees) and scalp, but sometimes on other parts of the body — chest, back, and so on. There is usually no itching, and there is no particular effect on the general health. About 10 or 15 percent of cases include arthritis.

It is more widespread than most people think; estimates are that two to five percent of the U.S. population has psoriasis at one time or other. Nor is it true, as some articles in popular periodicals have said, that psoriasis never appears in children; it can afflict even infants — although it's rare under the age of three years and still uncommon under ten.

Psoriasis is a medical mystery, as far as its cause is concerned. Theories have included metabolic disturbance, an unknown infectious agent (although it is *not* contagious), allergy, and emotional factors — or some combination of these. Whatever the immediate cause, heredity does seem to be a predisposing factor; the condition often occurs repeatedly in the same family (too often for mere coincidence), even when family members are not living together (thus excluding environmental elements).

If you suspect that your youngster has psoriasis, don't attempt to diagnose or treat it yourself, no matter what the ads say. In the first place, it may not be psoriasis at all. In the second place, if it *is* psoriasis, there are a number of effective methods of treatment, some of which work better with some individuals, some with others. None are advertised on television.

Exposure to sunlight seems to do some good with most victims. Dietary measures — in some a low-protein diet, in others a low-cholesterol regimen — have an effect sometimes. And there are a number of medications that have often been found beneficial, including both topically applied ointments and substances given internally; some of these are employed in combination with carefully controlled exposure to ultraviolet light. A new treatment known by the acronym PUVA, combining a photosensitizing oral drug called a psoralen with long-wave ultraviolet-A irradiation, appears in clinical trials to be quite promising; careful testing is necessary, however, to determine dosages that will have optimum therapeutic results and minimize the risk of burns and other side effects.

All these can control or relieve the condition in varying degrees, but there is no single cure. Psoriasis may last for weeks, months, or even years; it may depart as mysteriously as it arrived.

PSS: See SCLERODERMA.

psychedelics: substances that effect varying degrees of change in perception and/or sensation on the part of the individual using them; the effects may range, depending upon the substance, from a mild shift of mood to actual hallucination ("seeing things"), and may involve physical changes as well.

The psychedelics are not addictive: they do not require higher and higher dosages in order to achieve the sought-for effect, nor do they create a physical dependence. They may create a psychological dependence, but such dependence is far weaker than that upon amphetamines and probably not as strong as a long-time reliance on ordinary cigarettes. The chief danger in uncontrolled use of the more powerful types is the trouble they can cause while the effects last, trouble that's sometimes of a permanent nature.

Marijuana is a familiar example of the mildest type of psychedelic. Most powerful are the chemical concentrates such as LSD — which, it is estimated, is about a thousand times as powerful as marijuana.

These substances have found widespread use among young people in recent years. It is necessary and important that you, as a parent, have some basic facts about the drugs and their effects.

MARIJUANA

Marijuana is composed of the dried leaves, stalks, and flowers of the *Cannabis sativa* plant, which grows just about anywhere (hashish, widely used and abused in the Near East and some other parts of the world, is a far more powerful substance that comes from another part of the plant). It has a vocabulary all its own, and has been variously known as "boo," "charge," "grass," "hemp," "pot," "weed," "tea," and, most recently at this writing, "dope," a term formerly reserved exclusively for narcotics. It is generally smoked — either in a pipe (of the ordinary variety, or a hookah) or rolled as a cigarette (termed, past and present, a "reefer," "stick," or "joint") — or, occasionally, incorporated in foods.

There is, frankly, no medical proof that marijuana is seriously harmful (except for its use by injection, which has severely toxic effects). So far as is known at this writing, its effects are less dangerous than those of liquor or of ordinary (tobacco) cigarettes. A recent two-year study of marijuana smoking in Jamaica — where it is widely used and is known as *ganja* — found no ill effects in chronic smokers; it should also be noted that the Jamaican ganja smoker uses ten to twenty times as much of the substance as the average American user, and that the Jamaican product is far stronger than the Mexican or South American marijuana typically used in this country.

At this point — we of course reserve the privilege of second thoughts, should new evidence of serious adverse effects of marijuana come to light — we are inclined to side with those who have recommended the removal of criminal penalties for marijuana use. They include such distinguished groups and individuals as Drs. Joel Fort, Lester Grinspoon, Benjamin Spock, and Dorothy V. Whipple; the National Commission on Marihuana and Drug Abuse; Consumers Union; the American Bar Association; the National Education Association; many state and local investigatory groups; and an increasing number of prominent legislators at the federal, state, and local levels. It seems to us incongruous for a society to jail young people for the use of a substance that has not caused demonstrable harm to themselves or to others (1974 arrests for the possession of marijuana numbered over four hundred thousand) — while looking with forbearance upon the use by those same young people of such things as alcohol, which is well known not only to damage the drinker but to trigger antisocial and sometimes violent behavior. Not to mention permitting their use of such potentially lethal weapons as the automobile, which kills some fifty thousand Americans each year.

As of mid-1976, eight states — Alaska, California, Colorado, Maine, Minnesota, Ohio, Oregon, and South Dakota — had reclassified possession of small amounts of marijuana as a misdemeanor or civil violation. But with these exceptions, marijuana use is still classed as a criminal activity. There are three possible results.

First, it means that its users of whatever age (and marijuana smoking has been reported among children as young as ten or twelve) are breaking the law, thus running the risk of police records that can pursue them all their adult lives. Second, it means that importation, distribution, and wholesale purveying of the drug are often in the hands of professional criminals — who can and sometimes do make intensive efforts to "trade up" their customers to more profitable, and far more dangerous, merchandise such as amphetamines and narcotics. Third, since there are no brand names and no controls of quality or content, marijuana can be, and occasionally is, adulterated with those addictive drugs or with far more potent psychedelics.

The effects of smoking marijuana, unlike those of drinking, may be almost unnoticeable to the observer. There is no staggering or thickness of speech; neither physical nor mental efficiency is markedly impaired (but continued concentration may be difficult); although the eyes may be slightly bloodshot, the pupils are not necessarily dilated. The smoker may, sometimes, appear unusually talkative. Beyond this, the effects are essentially subjective, including a mild elevation of mood, decreased awareness of time, slight increase in pulse rate, increased appetite, and some loss of peripheral vision. Recent experiments suggest that driving performance is affected substantially less by marijuana than by alcohol — although it *is affected;* no one under the influence of *any* psychotropic drug should drive.

There have been, we should note, some tentative suggestions that marijuana (or its active ingredient) might have therapeutic potential, including acting as a mild analgesic and tranquilizer, lowering blood pressure, countering nausea, relieving asthma, and controlling glaucoma.

One continuing source of controversy concerning the use of this drug by young people has been an alleged relationship with heroin. It is estimated that perhaps 85 percent of heroin addicts have used marijuana — but that an even higher percentage have used alcohol. Obviously, most users of alcohol do not go on to become heroin addicts. Nor do most marijuana smokers; 99 percent, in fact, do not. Which should come as a relief to parents, since it is now estimated that one-quarter to two-thirds of all U.S. high-school and college students (the studies have varied) have used marijuana.

LSD

LSD — short for lysergic acid diethylamide, and sometimes known simply as "acid" — is quite another kettle of fish. It is a semisynthetic chemical compound, first discovered in the 1940s, derived from ergot, a fungus that grows on rye. It was soon found that this chemical, injected into the bloodstream in minute, controlled amounts, could temporarily conjure up all the symptoms of a full-blown psychosis — an effect that offered great hope for progress in the study and treatment of mental illness.

Unfortunately, a few misguided researchers began advocating its use — by injection or by mouth (as a liquid, it is tasteless and odorless) — as a so-called "mind expander." Students, ignorant of its dangerous nature, began to experiment with it; during the 1960s other groups of young people, despite increased publicizing of LSD's lethal effects, joined what has been ironically dignified by some of its leaders as a "movement" or even a "religion." It is a movement in the direction of suicide, for in uncontrolled, nonmedical use, LSD is totally unpredictable; one leading physician has referred to "turning on" with it as "chemical Russian roulette."

What can LSD do? It can, as already mentioned, create what is for all practical purposes a psychosis — which can be something different for each individual. It changes perceptions, thoughts, and moods — often violently — and has physical effects as well, altering heart rhythm and constricting blood vessels. Among the results that may occur singly or in combination are extreme panic, terror, bizarre behavior (not excluding suicide or homicide), and — in an estimated 25 percent of users — "flashback" hallucinations that may appear up to several weeks, or even months, after the drug is taken.

Like some other illicit drugs, LSD can be — and often is — adulterated in one direction or another. Sometimes, "LSD" sold on the street is actually a far weaker chemical, not much stronger than marijuana. More often, it is LSD-*plus* — plus amphetamines or other mind-affecting substances; plus phencyclidine (on which further comment will follow); frequently plus such lethal stuff as strychnine.

These warnings are not, as some advocates of LSD use have suggested, either guesswork or jittery ramblings of an overly rigid political or medical "establishment." They are quite serious, and they are factual; it's advisable for the young and curious, and their parents, to take them to heart.

COCAINE

Cocaine has assumed increasing importance in the drug-abuse picture over the past few years; it is a chemical derived from the leaves of the coca plant, a South American shrub that has provided a fairly useful mind-affecting substance for deprived and depressed natives of the Andes for several thousand years. If the name of the plant rings loud bells, yes, it was in fact a major ingredient of a popular soft drink introduced in the United States in the 1880s; that beverage, as of 1903, contains nothing stronger than caffeine.

Part of its current popularity undoubtedly derives from two concurrent phenomena. One is the fact that Sigmund Freud, the deservedly famed Viennese neurologist and psychoanalyst, espoused it as a "wonder drug" (for a time; he later backtracked) and a possible aid in the treatment of morphine addicts; the other, the revelation that Sir Arthur Conan Doyle, creator of the superlogician Sherlock Holmes (described as a cocaine devotee in the stories), was apparently himself fond of taking a bit now and then.

Cocaine is still a legitimate part of the pharmacopaeia, although its use is very strictly controlled. Penalties for its illegitimate use (the only legitimate use is in very limited kinds of surgery) parallel those for trafficking in narcotics — although cocaine does not in fact fit into that category.

Cocaine has a number of properties in common with amphetamines, others that are quite different. Sniffed — the usual method of taking it — it is a powerful nasal decongestant (and was in fact the first drug employed for that purpose; it has of course since been replaced by far safer agents). It is hardly, however, the ideal sinus clearer. It is rapidly absorbed by the mucous membranes; ensuing systemic effects include stimulation of the central nervous system, euphoria, depression of appetite, a deceptive feeling of unbounded energy and great acumen, and what might be termed an "internal acceleration" that results in rapid heartbeat, increased blood pressure, and rising temperature. (Injected, a route that a few devotees have used, cocaine can be lethal even in small doses — and death occurs too quickly for any treatment to be of help.)

Cocaine is not addictive in the sense that a narcotic is: tolerance (the need for increased amounts to achieve the same effect) does not develop, nor are there usually physical withdrawal symptoms if use of the drug is stopped (though some exceptions have been reported). There is, however, a marked psychological dependence, and repeated use tends to become compulsive. With chronic use, there are additional effects, both physical and mental. There is destruction of the mucous membrane of the nose, ultimately of the bone as well. Because of appetite depression, severe malnutrition may result. Insomnia and convulsions are likely. Marked depression when effects wear off leads to more frequent use of larger doses, which, in turn, lead inevitably to full-blown psychosis, with paranoia and a variety of unpleasant hallucinations involving a number of the senses, notably the sensation of insects — occasionally, snakes — crawling on or under one's skin.

Needless to say, some users' efforts to prevent or counter these effects by combining or following cocaine with depressants such as heroin or barbiturates are not helpful.

OTHER DRUGS

From time to time misguided youngsters in search of new kicks have also turned to other substances, both natural and concocted in the laboratory. Among the former are *mescaline,* derived from the peyote cactus, and *psilocybin,* which comes from a particular species of wild mushroom.

Chemicals have included, in addition to LSD and THC (short for tetrahydracannabinol, the concentrated active ingredient in marijuana and hashish): "STP," with effects similar to those of mescaline; "DMT," similar in action to psilocybin; phencyclidine, an animal tranquilizer; and assorted results of amateur laboratory experimentation. All of these are frequently adulterated with one another, as well as with LSD. They are in a potency class with LSD and should be viewed as posing similar risks.

One of the foregoing — phencyclidine, known popularly by various nicknames, most prominently "angel dust" and "PCP" — merits additional comment. Phencyclidine is produced commercially for use as an animal tranquilizer, but most of it purveyed on the street (alone, in combination with one or more of the other psychedelics, or masquerading as one of the latter) is concocted illicitly. In humans, its effects are extremely unpredictable, and there have in recent years been an increasing number of reports of serious poisonings. Low doses, depending upon the amount and route (it may be smoked, injected, or taken orally), may result in blurred vision, amnesia, anxiety, nausea and vomiting, increase in blood pressure, loss of muscle control, and, paradoxically, either profound depression or central nervous system stimulation. At higher doses, phencyclidine's documented effects include psychosis, critically low blood pressure, cardiac arrhythmia, uncontrollable convulsions, coma, respiratory arrest, and death.

The possible inclusion of this potent and potentially lethal substance in — or substitution of it for — other drugs illustrates the danger of uncontrolled drug distribution we mentioned earlier. Two reported studies of randomly purchased drugs purporting to be other substances found that 50 percent to 77 percent of the samples analyzed contained phencyclidine.

For a discussion of some other dangerous thrill-seeking pursuits, see: AEROSOL-SNIFFING; AMPHETAMINES; DIET PILLS; DRINKING; GLUE-SNIFFING; NARCOTICS; SEDATIVES.

psychiatrist: See SPECIALTIES, MEDICAL.

psychogenic: of emotional origin or cause. Also see PSYCHOSOMATIC, which is different and describes illness in which emotional factors play a precipitating role but are not the basis for the condition. A psychogenic problem generally requires psychotherapy.

psychologist: a professional who is not an M.D. but usually has at least an M.S. or M.A. degree and often a Ph.D. as well; such a person is qualified to do intelligence and personality testing and is also trained to treat certain emotional problems. A psychologist may be qualified, and may be recommended, to deal with a youngster's emotional problems, although in certain instances a psychiatrist may be considered preferable because of medical background, understanding of physiological as well as psychological processes, and ability to prescribe medications. In making a recommendation, your pediatrician or family physician will consider both the nature of the problem and the personalities of both patient and consultant.

psychomotor epilepsy: See EPILEPSY.

psychosis: mental illness which may result from either functional or organic factors and is essentially characterized by disturbance in the perception and/or interpretation of reality. (For comparison, see NEUROSIS.)

Psychosis in childhood (i.e., before the teen years) is typically characterized by inability to form a special relationship — whether of love *or* hate — with parents or others who take major responsibility for child care; rebellion is not a symptom of psychosis, but withdrawal may be. For two kinds of childhood psychosis, see AUTISM; SCHIZOPHRENIA.

psychosomatic: describing illness triggered by emotional factors; the term is a combination of the words *psyche* (mind, from the Greek word for soul or the intangible part of the self) and *soma* (body).

Such an illness is in no sense unreal or imaginary; rather, it is a combination of a physical weakness, allergy, or similar condition and an emotional experience or situation that sparks or intensifies the problem, in a sense breaking down the body's ability to resist or withstand the illness. Respiratory allergies (such as asthma) and intestinal sensitivities are highly susceptible to this kind of mechanism, but any involuntary organs of the body can be similarly affected — including the heart and circulatory system, urinary tract, endocrine glands, and skin.

Only a physician can separate the factors and make the diagnosis, though; don't try to do it yourself. A child's sudden bed-wetting, for example, could be of psychosomatic origin; but it could also signal an infection of the urinary tract or other condition needing prompt medical attention.

psychotherapy: counseling or treatment, using various techniques appropriate to the patient's age, comprehension, and problems, based primarily upon communication and interaction between patient and therapist (as opposed to chemotherapy or other techniques, which may of course be employed as adjuncts in psychotherapy if deemed desirable). Psychotherapy may be administered by various specially trained individuals, including psychiatrists, psychologists, and psychiatric social workers.

psychotropic: describing drugs or other substances that have a mood-altering or consciousness-changing effect.

"ptomaine poisoning": See FOOD POISONING.

ptosis: drooping of the upper eyelid; it may be due to muscular, neurological, or other causes.

puberty: by medical definition, the point at which reproduction becomes physically possible — the beginning of menstruation and ovulation in girls, and sperm production and enlargement of the testes in boys. The age at which puberty takes place varies considerably. Menarche, for example, might take place anywhere between the ages of nine and sixteen (or even a little earlier or a little later); the present U.S. average is twelve and a half years and has gradually become a little lower over the past several generations (there is some disagreement as to whether that trend will continue or not). Boys generally reach puberty, on the average, a little later than girls. And there is a definite hereditary factor; parents who reached puberty appreciably earlier or later than average are likely to see similar patterns in their children.

Also see, for related discussion, ADOLESCENCE; BREAST DEVELOPMENT; MENSTRUATION; SEX ORGANS.

pulmonary: relating to and affecting the lungs, though not necessarily referring to the lungs themselves; the pulmonary artery, for example, is not within the lungs, but carries blood from the heart to be oxygenated by the lungs.

pulmonary stenosis: congenital narrowing of the pulmonary artery (see the preceding entry); it may vary from mild to serious, depending upon the degree of obstruction. Symptoms, too, may vary — there is usually diminished exercise tolerance, but there may be other symptoms as well (and sometimes none at all). The condition may be noted any time from infancy to adolescence. In a severe case of pulmonary stenosis, surgery may be required; in a very mild case, there may be no treatment needed at all.

pulse: the heartbeat rate per minute, detectable by listening to the child's chest as well as by placing your fingertips on the inner surface of the wrist, just inside the outer bone of the forearm when the hand is held palm upward (don't use your thumb to take a pulse; it has a pulse of its own).

In an emergency, if you have no thermometer but do have an accurate watch with a second hand, the pulse rate can give an indication of a child's condition, since it tends to rise with fever; therefore, it's good to know your child's normal, at-rest pulse rate (the rate can also be raised by excitement or exercise). An increase of ten beats per minute in the pulse rate generally means a one degree Fahrenheit (about half a degree Celsius) rise in temperature. There are, however, some exceptions to this rule: in typhoid fever, and in meningitis and inflammations involving the brain, the pulse rate may be normal, or even lower than normal, despite a high fever; in some heart problems, a higher-than-normal pulse may be detected even when the temperature is normal.

As we've implied, normal pulse rate varies considerably from one individual to another. It also varies with age and with sex: the pulse rate of females, at any age, is typically higher than that of males. "Average" pulse rates at birth may range from 120 to 140; during the first year, from 100 to 130; during the second, from 95 to 115; during the third, from 85 to 105; from the fourth to about the fifteenth year, from 75 to 90. Thereafter, the rate tends not to vary much, staying usually within the 60-to-90 range.

The wrist is not the only point at which the pulse can be felt; that one is called the *radial* pulse, because it is near the radius, one of the two forearm bones. Other major pulse points are the *carotid*, in the neck just beside the adam's apple; the *temporal*, at the temple, in front of the ear; and the *femoral*, at the top front of the thigh, toward the groin.

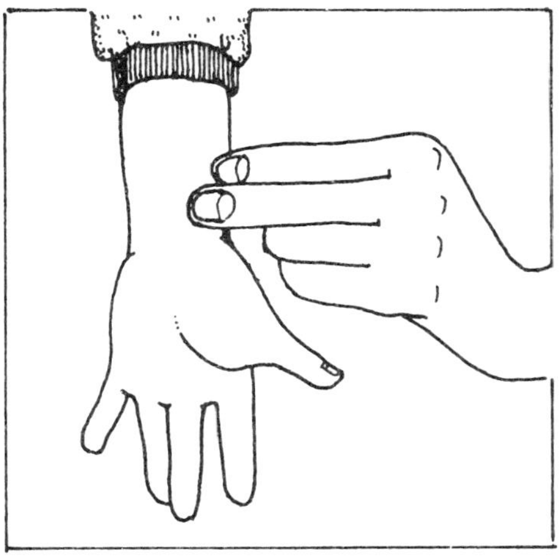

Taking a Pulse
The radial pulse, at the inside of the wrist, is the best known, but there are several other sites where the pulse can also be felt; see text.

puncture wounds: those made by objects that have a small entry point and penetrate to a marked extent, leaving a deep, narrow wound. Such a wound can be created by any long, sharp instrument — nail, needle, knife, fishhook, ice pick, animal fang, etc. — or by a missile such as a bullet or arrow. They are especially critical because they pose the risk of tetanus; the deeper and narrower the wound, the greater the danger. *All* puncture wounds require that the child be taken to the nearest hospital emergency room as quickly as possible, pausing only for minimal first-aid measures.

If the wound is in the chest, the prime concern is respiration. If the object is still there and is protruding from the wound, leave it there; it will act as an effective plug. If it is not, the wound must be securely covered to prevent air from being sucked into the chest cavity and compressing the lungs, and it should be done in a particular way: watch the child's breathing carefully — then move quickly to place something over the wound just at the end of an exhalation, which will minimize the amount of trapped air in the chest cavity; if a bullet or other object went completely through the chest, also cover the exit wound. For the covering, use sterile gauze if you have it; if you don't, use anything available, the cleaner the better. Don't give the child any food, drink, or medication.

On the way to the hospital, be alert for breathing difficulty, and give the child aid if necessary (see RESPIRATORY RESUSCITATION).

If the wound is in the abdomen, it must be considered a matter of life and death; there are many essential organs in this area. A gunshot wound is most critical of all, because a bullet rips through tissues with high momentum (the organs sometimes slide away from a knife or other object that enters more slowly). If the object is still in the wound, make no effort to remove it; if the wound is open, simply cover it with whatever clean cloth is available, and rush the child to the hospital. Don't give the child anything to eat or drink, or any medication.

If the wound is elsewhere — again, don't give the child anything whatever by mouth, and don't apply any antiseptic or other medication to the wound itself. *Do* take the following steps:

1. Remove the puncturing object if it is still in, and protruding from, the wound — *unless* you don't have the necessary equipment to do so without causing additional damage, as from the barbs of a fishhook (see illustration for how to remove a fishhook safely).
2. If or when the object is not protruding from the wound, wash the wound and the immediately surrounding area with soap and water.
3. Cover the wound with sterile gauze or with a clean handkerchief or any other available clean cloth, and get the victim to the hospital.

purpura: purplish patches on the skin and/or mucous membrane, caused by bleeding under the skin — a symptom rather than a disease; the condition may or may not be serious, depending upon the cause and whether or not the cause is readily apparent.

The term describes multiple patches rather than a single one, as in an ordinary bruise; purpura might,

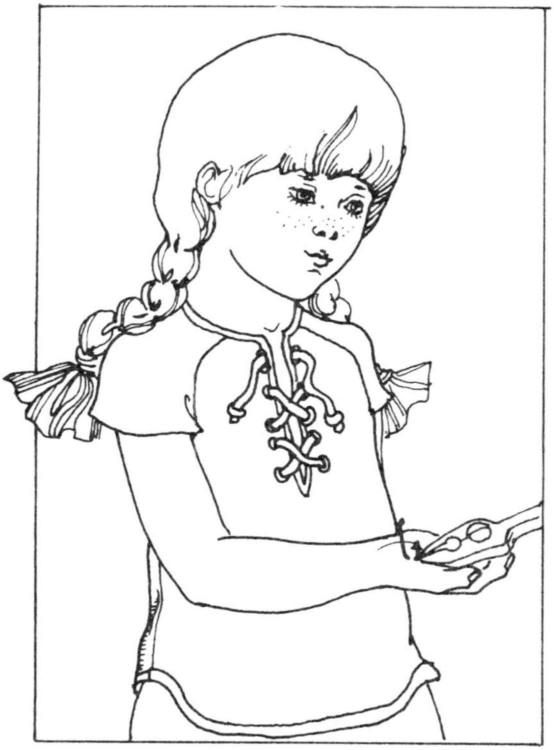

Removing a Fishhook

First, clip off the barb with wirecutters; this step is essential, since attempting to pull the barb back through the flesh would cause extensive tissue destruction, not to mention excruciating pain. (If the barb is not projecting, push the hook through in the direction in which it entered, until the barb does emerge.) Then carefully remove the shaft by pulling it back through the flesh in the direction of the arrows.

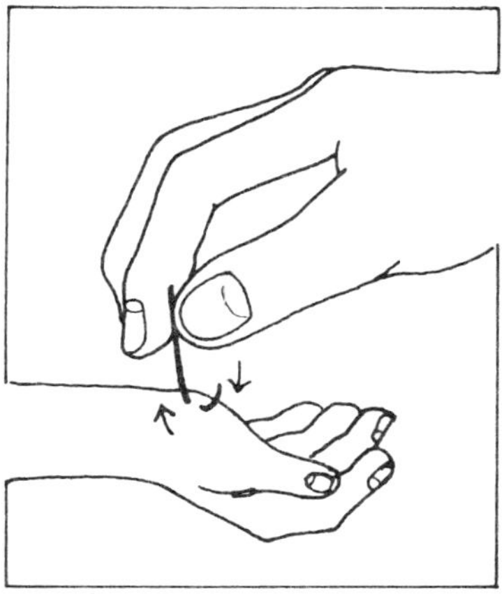

though, also be caused by some types of trauma (violent injury), and if such a cause is obvious — or determined by questioning the child — then there's no cause for worry.

Purpura can also occur in a number of other situations; all require prompt medical diagnosis. Among the things that can cause purpura are certain blood-cell imbalances, liver problems, extreme allergic reactions, and some types of poisoning; the fact that there is subcutaneous bleeding, in the absence of specific external injury, indicates only that there is *some* interference with normal blood coagulation. Treatment will of course depend upon the physician's determination of the underlying cause and may include medications, transfusions, or other measures.

purulent: a medical term that simply means *containing pus.*

pus discharge: Pus is a thick, yellowish fluid containing bacteria plus white blood cells, which congregate in such a manner only in the presence of infection. If you notice a discharge of pus from a wound or from any body opening (such as an ear), consult your physician without delay.

pustule: See LESION.

pyelitis: a type of kidney inflammation specifically involving the pelvis of the kidney, the outlet area from which the ureter leads to the bladder; symptoms may include back pain, frequent urination, pus or blood in the urine, and sometimes fever.

Pyelitis is usually caused by blockage either at the junction of the kidney and ureter, or between the bladder and urethra; it may also follow a bout of cystitis, a bladder infection. If you suspect this condition — or, for that matter, *any* condition involving the urinary tract — prompt medical attention is vital; an infection can spread and cause very serious trouble. Treatment will depend upon the doctor's diagnosis of the cause of the problem; it is likely to involve rest and antibiotics or sulfa drugs.

pyelogram: See IVP.

pyelonephritis: an inflammation involving both the pelvis of the kidney and other areas as well. See NEPHRITIS; PYELITIS.

pyloric stenosis: a constriction of the pylorus, the junction of the lower end of the stomach and the beginning of the small intestine. The cause of this condition is not known, but the medical consensus is that it seems to be familial and may be hereditary; it doesn't seem to cause any problems, however, until the second week of life, and possibly not until the tenth week. And it seems to affect more boys than girls — so that if it is hereditary, it is likely to be a sex-linked trait.

The chief symptom of pyloric stenosis is projectile vomiting — spurting of vomit with great force — soon after feeding. Other, less obvious, symptoms may include visible stomach spasms, weight loss or absence of expected gain, constipation, dry skin, and dehydration.

Rarely, a case of pyloric stenosis occurs because of an allergic reaction. Usually, though, it's the mysterious constriction we've mentioned, and the child must usually have surgery as quickly as possible; the operation takes care of the problem, and the infant is generally fine within two or three weeks.

Pyopen: a trade name for carbenicillin, a semisynthetic penicillin; see ANTIBIOTICS.

pyrexia: the medical term for fever.

pyrilamine: See ANTIHISTAMINES.

pyuria: the medical word for pus in the urine; it is a symptom, not a disease. Pyuria indicates infection in the urinary tract — in the bladder (see CYSTITIS), the kidney (see NEPHRITIS; PYELITIS), or elsewhere; it is more common in girls than in boys, because the tract is shorter and more subject to contamination. The causative organism is identified by urine culture; the physician will prescribe appropriate antibiotics or other medications.

Q

Q fever: a rickettsial infection (for other such infections, see RICKETTSIALPOX; TICK FEVER; TYPHUS FEVER) found primarily in Australia, Central America, the Mediterranean area, and parts of the U.S. Southwest and West.

Q fever is contracted by contact with infected cattle, sheep, or goats (or products thereof) or by the bite of a tick that infests such animals and can thus transmit the disease to humans. Symptoms, which appear after an incubation period of two weeks to 26 days, are similar to those of flu — fever, chills, headache, general weakness — plus, sometimes, a rash similar to that of typhus fever, consisting of flat, dark red spots.

Unlike flu, Q fever responds to antibiotics, especially tetracyclines; with proper diagnosis, the infection can be banished within a week or so (to be sure the infection's gone, medication must be continued for several days after temperature is normal). There is no means of immunization.

q.h., q.i.d., q.n.s.: See PRESCRIPTIONS.

Quaalude: a trade name for methaqualone, a sleep-inducing agent; see SEDATIVES.

quadrant: a quarter of a circle, used for anatomical description (as, in locating a pain) of areas that can be conveniently divided vertically and horizontally. Most commonly — and always, when the word is used without further qualification — it refers to the abdomen, imaginary lines through the navel demarcating the four quadrants; thus, a symptom below and to the right of the navel would be located in the right lower quadrant.

quadriceps: See MUSCLES.

quarantine: detention or restriction limiting entry to and/or departure from premises, or a country, in cases of communicable disease or the suspicion of communicable disease. Several decades ago, it was much used in the United States for the common childhood diseases; that has changed with the advent of widespread immunization and the public's awareness of precautionary measures. Quarantine is sometimes still applied to international travelers coming from an area where a particular disease is widespread.

Questran: a trade name for cholestyramine, a blood-lipid-lowering agent; see LIPIDS.

quinsy: See TONSILLITIS.

R

rabbit fever: See TULAREMIA.

rabies: a viral infection of the brain and nervous system to which all mammals, including human beings, are susceptible. It may be acquired by the bite of an infected animal, or by licking of broken skin or mucous membrane by an infected animal — and very possibly by exposure to the dust of caves inhabited by rabid bats.

There is a vaccine for domestic animals, and you should be sure that your dog has been vaccinated (cat-carried rabies is almost unknown). But the major danger lies in contact with wild-animal carriers. The chief carriers in North America are now believed to be the skunk in the United States and the fox in Canada; other major carriers are now raccoons and the aforementioned bats. Bites by squirrels, rabbits, and other rodents such as rats and mice have not been proved to cause rabies in humans — although it is theoretically possible — and generally speaking, city dwellers bitten by rats need not fear rabies, since urban rats apparently have no contact with the wild virus reservoir; no known case of rabies following a rat bite has ever occurred in New York City, where there are several hundred rat bites reported each year. (These pests do present other perils, however; see RAT-BITE FEVER.) Laboratory-raised animals — such as gerbils, white mice, hamsters, and guinea pigs — are not sources of rabies, assuming they have not been let loose to encounter wildlife.

The incubation period of the disease in an animal is three to five days; it can transmit the infection during this period as well as after it has become ill. Symptoms typically begin with restlessness and difficulty in swallowing; the animal's mouth will hang open, and it will drool. This is followed by howling, snapping, and moving about in a bizarre fashion, followed by paralysis, convulsions, and inevitable death.

Symptoms in humans are roughly similar; there is the same tightening of throat muscles and inability to swallow, with eventual panic at the sight of water, and at the end complete delirium — and there is no cure. (In early 1971, a single — and, if correctly diagnosed, the first — case of apparent "cure" was reported in a young boy who had been bitten by a bat that had been caught, killed, and demonstrated to be rabid. It must be assumed, however, that rabies is *not* curable, since there have been no claimed cures before or since.)

The incubation period in humans,

however, is longer than that in animals — generally ten days to six weeks, sometimes several months. If the animal is under observation, it is an easy matter to discover whether or not it was harboring the infection at the time of a particular bite; if so, it is obviously ill, or will become obviously ill within a few days. You can forget about rabies if the animal is alive and healthy a full week after it has bitten someone.

If the animal is ill, or becomes ill during that period, it can then be killed and autopsied to confirm or rule out the presence of the virus. In any instance in which rabies is confirmed — or the animal is not available for observation or examination (including cases involving a wild animal that has escaped) — the person bitten must receive rabies-immune serum plus a fairly lengthy series of vaccinations.

Don't forget that a child who has been bitten by an animal may require a tetanus injection, whether or not there is danger of rabies.

radiation: a general word for the phenomenon of X-ray generation, whether from space or from sources on our planet. A slightly different word is usually used to denote the deliberate use of such rays for beneficial purposes in medicine; see IRRADIATION.

radiodontist: See SPECIALTIES, DENTAL.

radiologist: See SPECIALTIES, MEDICAL.

radius: one of the two bones in the forearm, the one attached to the thumb side of the wrist; it is positioned in such a way that the lower end crosses over the other bone (the ulna) when the wrist is turned inward.

"rainbows": a slang term, among some drug abusers, for a combination of two barbiturates, amobarbital and secobarbital; see SEDATIVES.

rales: one of the sounds that may be heard through a stethoscope as the patient breathes; it is an indication of some problem involving the lungs or bronchial tubes and can provide an additional clue for the physician in diagnosing such ills as bronchitis, tuberculosis, and pneumonia.

rashes: eruptive manifestations on the skin; they may be reddish or pinkish, smooth or scaly, blotchy, pimply or blistery. Rashes may be symptoms of innumerable things ranging from allergy to insect bites, from localized skin conditions to a host of infectious diseases. Don't try to describe a rash over the telephone if you can help it; the best description in the world is no substitute for the physician's actually *seeing* the rash. And be sure, if you *are* phoning, to tell the doctor about other symptoms such as fever, cough, sneezing, or a feeling of general illness.

Here, as a quick checklist, are some of the most common problems typified by a rash, together with brief characterizations of the rashes' distinguishing features and accompanying symptoms of the conditions. You'll find more details about each condition under its own entry. This list is not intended, of course, for diagnosis — which must be performed by your physician — but only to alert you to the possibilities. Most rashes itch, but that's not necessarily so in children under the age of two or three.

Cellulitis — diffuse redness and swelling, possibly with fever.

Chickenpox — tiny raised pimples, appearing possibly a day or two after initial symptoms of fever and headache. The rash begins on the back, chest, or scalp and spreads to the rest of the body, ending with the palms and soles, and is usually very itchy; the pimples turn into small blisters and eventually form crusts.

Dengue — pale pink, appearing on the third or fourth day, possibly during remission of a previously high fever; follows initial symptoms that include nausea, vomiting, and severe pain in bones and joints. The rash begins on the knees, ankles, and elbows and spreads from there to the rest of the body.

Diaper rash — pimply, affecting the area covered by diapers.

Erysipelas — red, shiny, accompanied by swelling and high fever.

Erythema infectiosum — bright red, on the cheeks, subsiding after a few days and followed a day or two later by a spotty rash on arms and legs, possibly on the torso as well. The rash comes and goes for two or three weeks.

Heat rash — red pinpoints on a generally flushed area, often the back of the neck, underarms, or groin. It is usually itchy or prickly.

Hives — itchy welts, possibly accompanied by swelling of hands, feet, and/or the area around the eyes.

Impetigo — red, spotty, typically appearing on face, arms, legs, buttocks, or scalp; the spots gradually change to blisters, rupture, and form light brown crusts. Atypically, impetigo can appear to be a cluster of insect bites or a severe abrasion.

Measles — pinkish spots appearing on the fourth day, following coldlike symptoms and fever. The rash begins on the head and spreads downward, usually accompanied by a rise in temperature.

Pemphigus — suddenly appearing blisters, pea-size or larger, with an itching, burning sensation.

Pityriasis — a red patch on the torso, usually on the chest; within a week, gray scales form and the rash spreads to the rest of the torso. It usually does not progress to the arms, legs, or face.

Poison ivy — blistery, itchy, possibly with slight swelling; appears at the site of contact with the plant (or its oils) six hours or more after exposure.

Psoriasis — silver-scaled red patches, appearing anywhere, but typically on arms, legs, or scalp.

Q fever — flat, dark red spots accompanied by flulike symptoms.

Rat-bite fever — pink or purplish, appearing within three weeks of the bite; accompanied by fever and by various other respiratory, gastrointestinal, or muscular symptoms, depending upon the type of infection.

Rickettsialpox — similar in character to the rash of chickenpox, appearing on the third or fourth day following initial symptoms of fever, headache, and sensitivity to light.

Roseola — light rosy-red, similar in character to the measles rash, usually appearing only on the torso. It always follows four days of fairly high fever, and is accompanied by a drop in temperature. Roseola affects only children under the age of three years.

Rubella (German measles) — splotchy, appearing on the second or third day following initial headache and possibly other symptoms; spreads steadily from the face downward.

Scarlet fever — scarlet, appearing one to three days after initial symptoms of sore throat and fever. It usually starts on the chest and under the arms, spreading from those areas to the rest of the body; it may or may not involve the face.

Shingles — small blisters on a reddened area, roughly in single file, on one side of the body only; it may be preceded by fever. It appears usually on the chest, sometimes on neck, face, or back. It is painful, not itchy.

Tick fever (Rocky Mountain spotted fever) — slightly raised pink spots, appearing first on the wrists and ankles and progressing to the palms and soles, then to the rest of the body. It is accompanied by flulike symptoms, sometimes also by sensitivity to light.

Typhoid fever — splotchy, accompanied by a group of severe symptoms that include high fever, diarrhea, headache, and abdominal pain.

Typhus fever — flat, dark red spots; follows initial symptoms of high fever, headache, severe gastrointestinal distress, and blood in the stool and urine.

Certain *bites* may *appear* to be rashes. See BITES AND STINGS; LICE, BODY; SCABIES.

rasping: See COUGHS; CROUP; HOARSENESS.

rat bite: For first-aid procedure, see BITES AND STINGS; also see RAT-BITE FEVER, following, for discussion of possible complications.

rat-bite fever: a term covering two different diseases (there may also be others) transmitted by the bite of an infected rat. They are caused by two different types of bacteria.

The type most commonly found in the United States (it is often carried by the ubiquitous Norway rat) is caused by a bacillus, and is also known as Haverhill fever; the incubation period is variable but generally shorter than that of the second kind of rat-bite fever (following). The illness is flulike, with sore throat, fever, some general aching; there is usually also nausea and vomiting, and often a mild rash. This type may also be contracted by eating food that has been contaminated by rat urine or droppings.

The second type, caused by a spirochete, is more serious, chiefly attacking the nervous system. Symptoms, which appear after an incubation period of one to four weeks, usually include fever and severe chills, swollen lymph nodes, and increasing rigidity in the muscles; there may also be a purplish rash. If the condition is untreated, the child is likely to become delirious and lapse into coma.

In both types, there is often discoloration at the site of the bite, which may appear to have healed during the incubation period.

Rat-bite fever should be suspected if a child develops any of these symptoms within three weeks or so of being bitten by a rat, or if there is any possibility of food contamination by rats. If you do suspect it, get the child to a physician, or to a hospital, quickly. Antibiotics — especially chlortetracycline and pencillin — are effective against either type of infection.

RDS: See RESPIRATORY DISTRESS SYNDROME.

recessive: See HEREDITY.

rectum: the lower part of the large intestine, terminating in the anus; this part of the intestinal tract can be easily examined, tactilely and visually, by a physician.

"red devils": a slang term, among drug abusers, for the barbiturate drug secobarbital; see SEDATIVES.

reducing pills: See DIET PILLS.

reduction: a medical term that applies to two different procedures, depending upon the condition to which the physician is referring. In the fracture of a bone, reduction means the setting of the fracture, the aligning of the broken parts; in hernia, it means correction of the condition, placing the tissue back in its proper position.

reflex: an involuntary response to a stimulus; examples include laughing when tickled (if the subject is "ticklish"), jumping upon hearing a loud noise, blinking the eyes when a strong light is flashed into them, and the familiar knee-jerk reflex in which a specific tendon is struck, normally resulting in a particular muscular contraction. The absence of an expected reflex may indicate, to the physician, some problem involving the nervous system.

refractory: a word that may have one of two meanings, depending upon the context. In the general sense, it means "obstinate" — that is, describing a condition or problem that seems to be resisting treatment. In a more specific sense, it is the same as "refractive" and may be used to describe a visual problem; in that case, it refers to some problem involving the resolution of light rays through the lens of the eye, and such a problem can generally be remedied by corrective lenses.

registered nurse: See HEALTH PROFESSIONALS.

rejection: the response to a transplanted organ or tissue that apparently declares it "foreign matter" and prevents it from "taking"; rejection is believed to be related to the body's system of defense against foreign bodies in general.

Rela: a trade name for carisoprodol, a muscle relaxant; see SEDATIVES.

relapse: the recurrence of an illness, or the reappearance of symptoms, after progress has been made toward recovery or definite improvement has been noted.

relapsing fever: a term covering a group of similar infections, caused by spirochetes, that infect rodents as well as human beings and are transmitted by lice or ticks. Relapsing fever is found in the United States only in parts of the Southwest, where it is tick-borne; it is endemic in large areas of the rest of the world, however, including southern Europe (where it tends to be lice-borne), northern and western Africa, the Near East, and parts of the Far East.

The illness is characterized by headache, general weakness, and especially chills and high fever tending, as the name implies, to follow a recurrent pattern: the patient will be sick for a few days (usually five to seven), will apparently recover, then after another few days will have a relapse; the pattern continues, if the infection is untreated, for up to six or eight weeks. It can be cut short, however, by antibiotics, especially tetracyclines and penicillin.

relaxant: See SEDATIVES. This term usually applies to an anxiety-relieving agent that acts either primarily or secondarily by relaxing skeletal-muscle tension.

remission: the disappearance of signs or symptoms of an illness — not necessarily the basic condition or ailment itself, and not necessarily permanently; *spontaneous* remission means this has happened without specific treatment.

REM sleep: short for rapid-eye-movement sleep, so called because such movements have been detected at this particular level of slumber. It is a period of dreaming and is apparently necessary for continued well-being; deprivation of REM sleep, whether by abrupt waking or via hypnotics that have a depressive effect on this activity, has been found to be emotionally and mentally injurious.

renal: pertaining to the kidney(s).

reoviruses: See VIRUSES.

resect: to remove or rectify by surgery; a *resectable* condition is thus one that can be dealt with by surgical means.

resident: a hospital physician who is a medical-school graduate, has served an internship, and is now gaining further experience — under the direction of experts — in a particular specialty. The *chief* resident in a hospital department has nearly completed the residency, and will soon go on to become an attending physician at the hospital or a specialist in private practice.

respiratory distress syndrome: a general term covering various conditions, occurring congenitally or shortly after birth, that cause breathing difficulty in a newborn infant (hyaline membrane disease is one example, but there are a number of others); treatment will of course depend upon the precise nature and cause of the condition, and it is best handled in an intensive-care nursery.

respiratory resuscitation: We detail here the most effective means of "artificial respiration" — direct, person-to-person breathing, also called expired-air ventilation, since it uses the rescuer's own exhaled air to ventilate the victim's lungs. It may be done either directly mouth-to-mouth or by using an oral airway — a plastic device that is widely available and that is good to have on hand. (If you are reading this ahead of time: it is wise to practice respiratory resuscitation — and have older children and teenagers do so as well — long before it is needed.)

EMERGENCY PROCEDURE

1. Lay the child on his back, turn the head to one side, and quickly remove any vomit, mucus, or foreign matter that may be in the mouth; use whatever is available — gauze, a clean handkerchief, your fingers if necessary. Then turn the head back in line with the body.
2. *(see illustration)* Put something under the child's shoulders — a towel, a piece of rolled-up clothing, anything — if it's available (if not, don't waste time looking). Tilt the head back as far as you can, so the chin is pointing upward — that's to keep the airway clear — and pull the jaw

slightly forward to keep the tongue out of the way.

3. *Mouth-to-mouth:* Approaching from the child's side *(see illustration),* take a deep breath, open your mouth wide and place it over the victim's mouth, at the same time pinching the nostrils closed. (If it's a baby or very small child, and you can cover both the nose and mouth with your mouth, do so.) Exhale into the child's mouth.

Using an airway (use this method for an infant or very small child only if you have a special junior-size airway): Position yourself behind the child's head. Hold the tongue forward against the lower teeth with one hand, and insert the S-shaped airway *(see illustration)* with the other. Insert the shorter end for a child, the longer end for a teenager; in either case, one end of the S should be pointing toward the child's feet, the other end curving up and toward you. The flange at the middle of the tube should rest against the child's lips. Place your

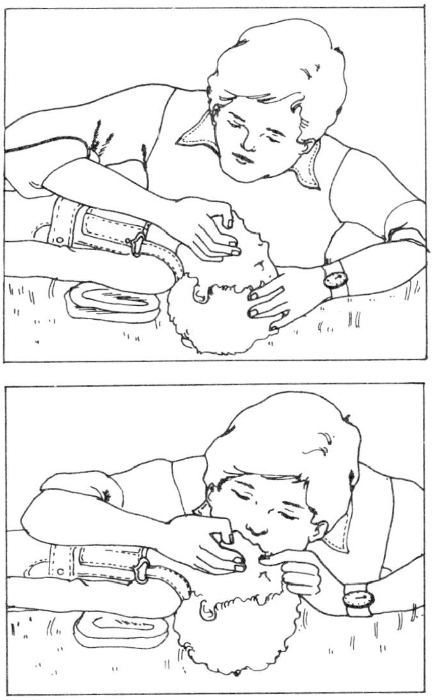

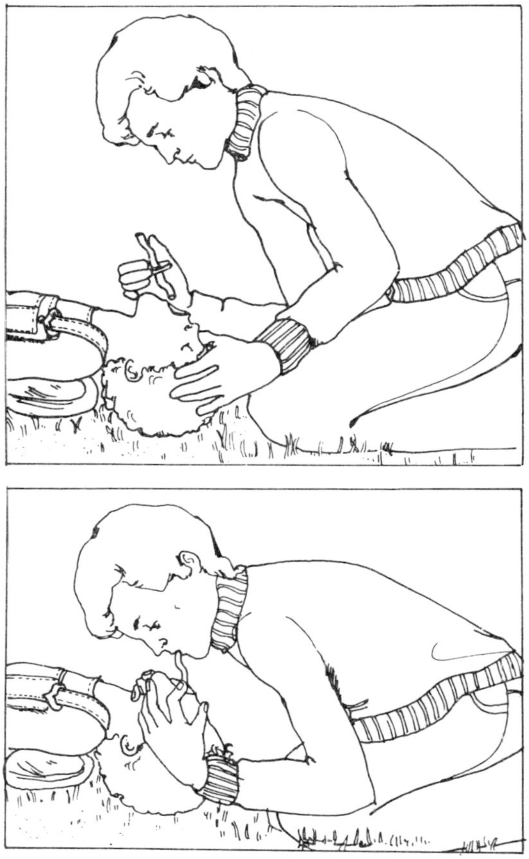

Respiratory Resuscitation
Shown are the correct approaches and positions for direct, mouth-to-mouth breathing and for resuscitation using a plastic oral airway; see text for step-by-step details.

hands at each side of the child's mouth *(again, see illustration)*: thumbs pinching the nostrils closed, index fingers pressing the flange tightly against the lips, the other fingers curling under the jawbone to hold it up and toward you. Take a deep breath, and exhale into the airway.

With either method, exhale forcefully if the victim is a teenager or older child, more gently if he is a small child (whose lung capacity is smaller).

4. Remove your mouth and watch and listen for a return of air. If it occurs, go directly to step 6. If there is no return of air, double-check the child's head and tongue positions — and if you're using an airway, be sure there's no air leak around the flange. Press gently on the child's abdomen to release any air that may be there. (If that makes the child vomit, quickly turn his head to the side — remove the airway, if you're using one — and go back to step 1.)
5. Repeat steps 2 and 3. Again watch and listen for a return of air; if there is one, go directly to step 6. If not, quickly turn the child on his side — again, remove the airway if you're using one — and slap him smartly between the shoulder blades to dislodge any foreign matter that may be blocking the respiratory tract; exploration of the back of the mouth with your fingers may detect the object, if there is one. Then repeat steps 2 and 3.
6. Continue, at a regular rate of about twelve breaths a minute — one every five seconds, approximately — for an older child or teenager; if the victim is an infant or very small child, use about twenty shallower breaths a minute, one every three seconds.
7. If the child begins to breathe weakly but more or less regularly, continue the resuscitation, but time your breaths to coincide with his: blow when he inhales, then take your mouth away quickly (and release his nostrils) to let him exhale.
8. Continue until the child is breathing normally or medical help arrives. Even if the child *is* breathing normally, stand by and watch carefully, and be ready to resume resuscitation if necessary.

retching: an unsuccessful attempt to vomit, usually accompanied by nausea. It means that the child has nothing in the stomach to bring up — but if he *had,* he *would.* If a child retches, something is wrong and you should call the doctor.

retina: the back of the eyeball, on which images are focused and thence transmitted, by particular nerves, to the brain. *Detached* retina is a condition in which small areas of the retina have separated from the underlying tissue; it may be caused by injury, infection, or tumor, and is very rare in children.

retinitis pigmentosa: chronic, progressive inflammation of the retina, with pigmentary infiltration and, usually but not inevitably, blindness; it appears to be a familial affliction of predominantly recessive or modified-recessive inheritance (see HEREDITY). The first symptom may be "night blindness," diminished dusk vision, followed by "tunnel vision," narrowing of the visual field. There is not, at this writing, realistic hope of reversing the damage; with increased interest and research, it is hoped that ways of improving the vision of afflicted children may be found. No way has yet been found of identifying "carriers" of the RP gene or of discovering afflicted children before birth.

retrolental fibroplasia: a condition involving injury to the blood vessels of the retina, resulting in partial or total blindness; it may be caused by an overdose of oxygen in the newborn period and, before the cause was discovered, was the basis of many tragic cases of blindness in premature infants and others who spent time in atmosphere-controlled situations.

All physicians are now aware of this danger, and you may be sure that if oxygen must be given your baby, the concentration will be well within safe limits. Potentially dangerous levels of oxygen are now used only in life-threatening conditions in which there is no other alternative.

Reye's syndrome: a critical — and, as we write this, still mysterious — phenomenon that is rare but occurs in sufficient numbers to be of concern; it attacks children following some viral infections. It most probably has existed for some time, but the syndrome was first described as a distinct entity by the Australian pathologist Ralph D. K. Reye and his associates in 1963. Although the exact cause is unknown and the question of treatment still unresolved, one fairly consistent fact has emerged: early diagnosis is distinctly helpful, and *may* in fact insure survival. (Too little is presently known to promise that it *will.*)

We shall, at any rate, summarize current knowledge, in order to alert parents — and, we hope, help to save some young lives.

The syndrome typically follows a viral illness — but the reverse is far from true; it befalls perhaps one in two thousand children (ages have ranged from mere months to mid-teens) who are struck by the virus in question. It is highly selective: rarely have there been two children in a family who were both struck by Reye's, although they may have had the same illness. The most likely viral diseases to precede Reye's syndrome are, in order of prevalence: influenza B strains; chickenpox; and assorted upper-respiratory-infection viruses that have been associated with scattered cases.

As with almost all reportable conditions, official statistics are probably absolutely low but proportionately accurate. They indicate that there is an extremely high correlation between incidence of the B-strain influenza viruses (the strains are discussed under INFLUENZA) and Reye's. During the epidemic year 1970–71, when there was fairly significant influenza-B activity, 83 cases of Reye's were reported in this country, almost half in the New York–New England area. The following year — the connection with the flu virus was not yet evident, and physicians around the country were presumably on the alert — only 12 cases were reported; that year's prevalent flu virus was an A strain. In 1973–74, the B flu strain that had been previously isolated in New England surfaced again, with much more widespread incidence. The B strains tend to cause milder illness. But there were, that season, 356 reported cases of Reye's syndrome — and seven out of twenty of the affected children, 35 percent, died.

Reye's syndrome has never been diagnosed in anyone over the age of seventeen; it is not known why. The median age of those struck by it is — statistically — eleven (but bear in mind the age range we mentioned earlier): following B-strain flu infection, a little older, twelve to fifteen; following chickenpox, much younger, averaging about six. It shows no special preference for either sex.

Symptoms tend to appear about a week after onset of the viral infection, which is usually mild and from which the youngster is apparently recovering. The first symptom is, almost invariably, persistent vomiting — sometimes dismissed as a secondary effect of the flu or other viral infection. This can indeed occur — but if it is just a concomitant annoyance with flu, it tends to appear earlier. At any rate, the vomiting in Reye's is extremely persistent and, if the child has had little to eat, there is dry retching. The ensuing symptoms are likely to be behavioral. The child may act "hyperactive" or "manic." Delirium is possible, and seizures may ensue, but apathy and dullness are more likely. Sooner or later, the child falls into a coma, from which there may or may not be recovery. The condition is not contagious.

It is strongly suspected that sudden liver malfunction is at the root of the problem. Why it occurs is not known, and viruses have not been clearly identified in the livers of children having the illness (although a number of researchers have reported the presence of microscopic particles described as "myxoviruslike" or "paramyxoviruslike" and have suggested that perhaps Reye's represents a simultaneous attack by two or more viruses acting synergistically). But liver malfunction has been documented by finding excessive amounts of ammonia in the bloodstream (ammonia, a metabolic by-product, is normally converted to urea and excreted) as well as fatty degeneration, which may also involve other internal organs. The major symptoms we've mentioned are caused by ammonia, which damages brain cells.

Profound coma is a discouraging sign; it indicates that extensive brain damage has probably occurred (we use the word "probably" advisedly; that's usually, but not always, the case). One extremely frustrating fact is that there is no predicting how fast this will occur: children have been known to go into coma within hours or to go through a variety of preceding symptoms for days.

Obviously, if your child has just recovered from flu, chickenpox, or any other relatively mild upper respiratory infection, you should keep an eye on that child, and should report to your doctor any symptoms that seem the least bit strange. If you cannot reach your own doctor and the foregoing description leads you to believe your child may be developing Reye's syndrome, you should immediately take the child to the nearest hospital.

There is nothing you can do at home for Reye's syndrome, and don't try. No single treatment has been found universally effective, but a number of therapies have been found helpful in a significant percentage of cases. They include dialysis, intravenous administration of glucose, transfusion, and others that may be indicated, depending upon the condition of the individual child. If Reye's syndrome is suspected, the child *must* be *hospitalized.*

rhabdomyosarcoma: See SARCOMA.

rheumatic fever: a condition medically considered a hypersensitive reaction to a recent streptococcus infection or to the chemical products of strep infection. It is now uncommon, since it is largely preventable by proper and successful treatment of the original infection.

Children between the ages of five and ten who live in cool climates appear most susceptible to rheumatic fever; it may occur as a result of a variety of untreated, or improperly treated, strep-caused illnesses, including certain ear infections, erysipelas, scarlet fever, strep sore throat, and tonsillitis (but despite the fact that these are contagious, rheumatic fever isn't).

Symptoms may vary from one victim to another, but typically include migratory joint pains (that is, they travel from one joint to another), fever (sometimes low, sometimes high), recurring nosebleeds, weight loss, general weakness, and fatigue. The diagnosis can be confirmed by blood tests and other procedures.

Rheumatic fever can, without prompt treatment, result in involvement of the heart (it has been responsible for most of the noncongenital heart problems in children); if the condition is suspected, you should see that the child gets expert medical attention without delay. If you do so, chances of full recovery, without any lasting ill effects, are good.

Bed rest, possibly for several weeks, is generally advised, and the child is also given various drugs — among the possibilities: analgesics, hormones such as ACTH and cortisone, antibiotics, and sulfa drugs — depending upon the physician's assessment of the child's condition.

rheumatic heart disease: See HEART DISEASE.

rheumatoid arthritis: See ARTHRITIS.

rheumatologist: See SPECIALTIES, MEDICAL.

Rh factor: a factor found in most people's blood, which can sometimes cause special problems in transfusion and in the neonate; its name comes from the *Rhesus* monkey — the factor having been discovered via experiments with this particular primate.

Those with the factor, who are termed *Rh positive,* constitute some 85 percent of all Caucasians, and even higher percentages of other races. The problems arise with those few who are *Rh negative* — whose blood doesn't have the factor.

Those who are Rh negative possess a "rejection mechanism" that goes into action against the factor and actually destroys the "alien" red blood cells. Thus, in event of a transfusion, someone who is Rh negative *must* receive negative blood. When we said in our earlier discussion of transfusion (see BLOOD GROUPS) that persons with type AB blood are "universal recipients" because their blood will not reject those of other types, that was not quite true; AB-*negative* blood *will* reject any Rh-*positive* blood — so that it is those whose blood is type AB and also Rh positive who are really the "universal recipients." Similarly, type O individuals are truly "universal donors" only if their blood is also Rh negative.

Like the blood groups themselves, the presence or absence of the Rh factor is a hereditary matter. Genetically, the Rh-negative quality is recessive (see HEREDITY for an explanation), so that if both parents are negative their children will be negative too; if both are positive and carrying no recessive Rh-negative genes, all their children will be Rh positive; if both are of mixed heredity, one in four children will be negative. But it is none of these situations that cause a possible problem of mother-baby incompatibility.

That problem can occur only if the *mother* is Rh *negative,* and the *father* is Rh *positive.* In such a case, it is possible (in fact certain, if the father is *not* of mixed heredity; otherwise, there is a fifty-fifty chance) that children will be Rh positive. If all these possibilities coincide, there is still no problem with the first child.

But *if* some of that Rh-positive baby's blood reached the mother's through the placenta, then, shortly after pregnancy, she *may* begin manufacturing anti-Rh-factor antibodies. If she should carry a second Rh-positive child, those antibodies, if present, *may* seek out and destroy the baby's red blood cells, producing a condition called *erythroblastosis fetalis,* a hemolytic anemia; the result may be miscarriage or stillbirth, or the baby may be born alive but critically ill, requiring one or more immediate or delayed exchange transfusions to replace all his blood with the Rh-negative type. Until 1968, thousands of infants were lost each year because of erythroblastosis fetalis. (Such children often exhibit jaundice, which has led to the term "yellow babies.")

In that year, however, a new preparation called RhoGAM, an "Rh-immune globulin," was introduced. If RhoGAM is administered (by injection) to an Rh-negative mother *within 72 hours* after she has given birth to her first Rh-positive child, development of antibodies is prevented, and her next baby is protected; this must be done, of course, after the birth of each Rh-positive child. And to be on the safe side, all Rh-negative women should receive RhoGAM after each abortion, spontaneous or deliberate.

rhinitis: the medical term for an inflammation in the nose — due to allergy, a cold, or some other factor.

rhinoplasty: See PLASTIC SURGERY.

rhinoviruses: See VIRUSES.

RhoGAM: a preparation introduced in 1968 to combat a major incompatibility problem in pregnancy; see RH FACTOR for details of the problem and what the product does.

rhythm method: See CONTRACEPTION.

rib, broken: See FRACTURES.

riboflavin: one of the B vitamins; see NUTRITION.

rickets: a condition resulting from severe lack of vitamin D and/or calcium; see DEFICIENCY DISEASES.

rickettsia: a type of disease-causing organism. Although sometimes classed as bacteria, rickettsiae are smaller than the usual bacteria, albeit larger than viruses. Unlike bacteria, and like viruses, they require living tissue for survival; all members of this class of microorganisms are parasitic, living chiefly on certain arthropods, especially lice, ticks, and mites. The diseases caused by rickettsial organisms, as far as is known, are all transmitted mainly by these arthropod carriers, by biting or by excretion on human skin (resulting in itching, then scratching, then broken skin that provides an entryway for the organism); they are not contagious by person-to-person contact. The rickettsiae were named for Howard Ricketts, the pathologist who discovered them; there is no connection with the deficiency disease called rickets.

The diseases caused by rickettsiae tend to be somewhat similar — usually involving fever and chills, some sort of rash, general malaise — and are usually quite debilitating; some are considered serious, others less so. Such diseases tend to be endemic in particular areas frequented by the arthropod vectors. They are all effectively treated by antibiotics, especially tetracyclines.

For discussion of major rickettsial infections, see Q FEVER; RICKETTSIALPOX; TICK FEVER; TYPHUS FEVER.

rickettsialpox: a rickettsial infection (see preceding entry), generally considered the least serious of the group, and the only one that has occurred in U.S. urban areas; it appears to have been endemic in parts of Queens, a borough of New York City, in the 1950s.

Rickettsialpox is carried to humans by mites (smaller relatives of ticks) from house mice, possibly from rats as well. Symptoms, appearing after a seven- to ten-day incubation period, typically include fever; headache; severe general malaise; sensitivity to light; and a rash, somewhat similar to that of chickenpox, that appears on the third or fourth day (often the rash is especially prominent at the site of the bite).

As with the other rickettsial infections, tetracyclines — Aureomycin and Terramycin in particular — are effective; medication must be continued for 24 hours after the fever is gone. There is no immunization for rickettsialpox; the only preventive measure is rodent control.

Rifadin, rifampin, Rimactane: See ANTIBIOTICS; the first and third words are trade names for the second.

ringworm: a fungus infection (there are no worms involved) that tends to start in a small spot and spread in a widening ring; it can occur anywhere on the body, although two sites are more commonly affected than others. The medical term for it is *tinea* — *tinea pedis* if it occurs on the feet (this form is discussed separately; see ATHLETE'S FOOT), *tinea capitis* on the scalp (the second common site; here the condition is also known as *favus*), and *tinea corporis* elsewhere on the body.

Ringworm of the scalp is highly contagious and can easily be epidemic among youngsters in a school, camp, or neighborhood — by direct contact, by borrowing combs and brushes, via unsterilized barber-shop implements, even by the children's leaning against things like the backs of seats in movie theaters.

The infection is in the hair follicles, and the first symptom is likely to be a patchy, "moth-eaten" look at the back of the head, accompanied by itching.

As dead skin scales off, yellowish crusts form. The condition can go on spreading for months if it's untreated.

If you suspect your child may have ringworm, consult the doctor without delay; other things can cause similar symptoms, but the doctor can pinpoint the problem by examining the child's head with a special light that reveals the presence of the fungus. It's easily and quickly curable with fungidical antibiotics — usually applied topically, sometimes given internally as well.

Don't let the child scratch his head. Scratching could cause a secondary scalp infection; ringworm can also attack fingernails, and the damage there could be quite serious. Wrap the child's head up with something, if necessary.

Cats and dogs are also subject to ringworm and can transmit it to people by direct contact — and dogs have been known to contract it via infected clippers used by professional groomers, just as children can get it from barbers; the same sort of treatment (by a veterinarian) is effective for animals. Young animals are especially susceptible to ringworm, as are young humans, apparently because their skin is thinner.

Ritalin: a trade name for methylphenidate hydrochloride, a stimulant which, like certain amphetamines, has been found effective in calming overactive children; see HYPERKINESIS.

R.N.: the abbreviation for Registered Nurse; see HEALTH PROFESSIONALS.

RNA: the abbreviation for ribonucleic acid, part of the material in cells. It is active in the synthesis of proteins and, like the better-known DNA, plays a part in the hereditary mechanism; while DNA is the material of which genes are made, RNA is the substance that carries genetic information to other parts of the cell. Like DNA, RNA is composed of phosphates and sugars, but its chemical makeup is different.

See HEREDITY for more about the kinds of information RNA carries.

Robaxin: a trade name for methocarbamol, a muscle-relaxant agent; see SEDATIVES.

Robicillin: a trade name for penicillin V; see ANTIBIOTICS.

Robitet: a trade name for tetracycline; see ANTIBIOTICS.

Robitussin: See COUGHS.

Rocky Mountain spotted fever: See TICK FEVER.

roentgenologist: radiologist; see SPECIALTIES, MEDICAL.

Romilar: See COUGHS.

Rondomycin: a trade name for methacycline, one of the tetracyclines; see ANTIBIOTICS.

rose fever: See HAY FEVER.

roseola: a condition affecting very small children; its name is short for *roseola infantum,* and it is also known medically as *exanthem subitum* (which is simply Latin for "sudden eruption"). Don't confuse this with two totally different ailments that have similar-looking names, rubeola (measles) and rubella (German measles).

The susceptible age range for roseola is generally six months to two years; it's very rare after the age of three. It starts with fever that may be fairly high — up to 104° or 105°F. (40° or 40.5°C.) — and is sometimes accompanied by convulsions. Fever persists for four days, then — *after* the child's temperature has returned to normal — a light rosy-red rash, something like that of measles, appears, usually on the chest, abdomen, and back. (This late-appearing rash is the distinctive feature of the illness — although your doctor may pinpoint the problem earlier via a blood count.) The rash may last a day or two, or it may exist for only a few hours — and may thus go unnoticed, particularly if it happens to come and go during the night.

Fever and rash are the only two consistent symptoms. Occasionally there may be puffiness around the eyebrows, enlarged lymph nodes, or sore throat; but often, the child doesn't really feel ill or uncomfortable.

Roseola is not considered serious. Antibiotics are ineffective, and treatment generally consists of aspirin, sponging, and other measures to reduce fever. Follow your own doctor's advice.

No one knows exactly what causes roseola; it's believed to be a virus. It *is* known that once a child has had it, he cannot get it again. And it is contagious. Usually, because of the child's age, it's not communicated directly to other infants; it can, however, be carried by adults and older children who are not susceptible themselves, but isolation of the infant's contacts is not necessary. Once the rash appears, it is no longer contagious.

roughage: If your doctor mentions this category of food (sometimes called "fiber"), as something to be either increased or avoided, the reference is to high-residue foods, those containing a high proportion of elements not readily absorbed in the intestinal tract; examples are the skins of fruit, celery, lettuce, other fresh salad greens, and bran.

roundworms: See WORMS.

rubbing alcohol: See ALCOHOL.

rubella: a highly contagious viral infection also known variously as "German measles" or "three-day measles," though it has no relation to measles itself (rubeola), which is caused by a different virus. Tending in the past to recur in epidemics at six- to nine-year intervals, rubella is usually quite a mild disease in children, a bit less so in adults.

Typically, rubella begins — after a two- to three-week incubation period — with a slight headache; from this point on, symptoms may vary considerably. There may or may not be slight cold symptoms, such as a runny nose, and there may or may not also be slight fever, generally no higher than 101° to 102° F. (38.3° to 38.9° C.). There may or may not be swollen lymph nodes, especially in the back of the neck and in the groin. A splotchy rash usually appears, spreading from the face downward, a day or two after the first symptoms; a confusing aspect is that sometimes, though rarely, there's no rash at all. In teenagers and adults, but seldom in youngsters, the rash is sometimes accompanied by noticeable redness of the gums and the mucous membranes around the eyes, and also by joint pains, which can persist for days or even weeks. Rubella is contagious, via droplet infection, from a week before the rash appears until the rash is gone.

There's no specific treatment for rubella, other than keeping the child home and away from others, especially susceptible women who are, or who might become, pregnant — including the child's mother — for reasons we'll get to in a moment. Once an individual has had rubella, immunity lasts for life.

We've said that contagion is possible only until the rash is gone; there's one exception to that rule. It is possible, although it happens very rarely, for a baby to be born with the disease, if the child's mother has had it at the very end of her pregnancy. Rubella is quite serious in a newborn child, but some 80 percent of such children do recover without complications; they are, however, contagious for approximately *nine months.*

By far the most tragic aspect of rubella has been its effect on the unborn children of women who contracted the disease early in pregnancy; somehow, the virus strikes the embryo during crucial stages of development, causing unpredictable congenital deformities, blindness, deafness, circulatory and heart defects, mental retardation, and even death. It is estimated that in the United States, as a result of the rubella epidemic of 1964, there were a minimum of thirty thousand damaged babies, with another possible thirty thousand miscarried or stillborn; in New York City alone, probably one in every hundred pregnancies during that year was a rubella casualty.

This fact about rubella has been known for years, and it was long felt that the best solution was to deliberately expose young girls to the disease whenever possible, so as to avoid their contracting it later. That wasn't always convenient, of course. Thus many girls did grow up without immunity — and at this writing, it is estimated that some 10 to 30 percent of all women of childbearing age are still susceptible.

In 1969, a vaccine was introduced with a great deal of imaginative fanfare (was there a youngster who didn't demand a "rubella umbrella"?) It worked. The next epidemic peak would have occurred in 1970, '71, '72, or '73 — and that peak never came. (Not all cases, of course, occur in epidemic cycle years.)

Since then, as with a number of preventable childhood diseases, the Center for Disease Control has found it necessary to issue repeated warnings; still, by early 1975, three out of eight children had not been immunized and reported cases for the first half of 1975 were 60 percent higher than 1974. It must be emphasized that whether or not a woman personally plans to have future children is beside the point; her rubella, or her child's, can be communicated to her pregnant neighbor (who should herself have been previously vaccinated — and if you want to spread the word, that's fine with us).

As we mentioned earlier, symptoms of rubella can vary considerably, and mild cases of other viral infections can also mimic rubella — so a history of having had the disease is not dependable proof of immunity. There is, however, a blood test, which your doctor can perform, that will reveal antibodies to the infection if they are present, thus avoiding unnecessary vaccination. (The vaccination will not actually harm someone who has already had the disease — but it can sometimes be followed by the same sort of arthritic discomfort as the illness itself, and there's no point in inviting that unnecessarily.) Every susceptible person in your family over the age of one year (that's the age for routine childhood vaccination, generally as part of the MMR shot; see IMMUNIZATION) should be vaccinated, with two — possibly three — exceptions.

One exception is any condition or drug regimen that produces lowered resistance to infection, including use of corticosteroids or immunosuppressants. If a child is suffering from some other infection that involves fever, the doctor will also likely suggest postponing a rubella (or MMR) shot.

Another, and there's some difference of opinion here: many rheumatologists feel that in a child who has juvenile rheumatoid arthritis — whether or not any of the drugs we've mentioned are being employed — the vaccination should wait until the condition has entered a remission (inactive) period. The reason is that the vaccine, since it can itself cause arthritic manifestations, may aggravate a preexisting arthritic condition. As we said, there is not complete agreement here; follow your own physician's advice.

Finally — there is no controversy on this point — the vaccine's effect on an unborn child is uncertain and potentially damaging. A pregnant woman, or one who might become pregnant within three months, should not be vaccinated. A nonimmune woman who receives the vaccination should then take care not to conceive a child within three months. (We are being conservative; many physicians feel a period of two months is sufficient.)

If you are now pregnant, and are reasonably sure you did not have rubella during the early months of your pregnancy (if you think you *did,* discuss the question with your obstetrician), you should have the blood test for immunity immediately following childbirth. Results can be made available within 24 hours; you can then, if necessary, be vaccinated — an excellent time, since most women are unlikely to become pregnant within three months of giving birth.

There is a rubella gamma globulin, but it is not considered dependable; while it typically prevents active illness in a pregnant woman who has been exposed to rubella, there is no guarantee whatever that it can keep the virus from damaging the developing embryo. It is recommended only if there is exposure to rubella in early pregnancy and the mother cannot accept the idea of abortion in case of infection.

rubeola: See MEASLES.

runny nose: See COLDS.

rupture: See HERNIA; PERITONITIS.

S

Sabin vaccine: formerly, a term used to differentiate this polio vaccine, given orally, from Dr. Jonas Salk's vaccine, given by injection. The oral vaccine is now *the* vaccine, referred to usually as TOPV (trivalent oral polio vaccine) or simply OPV; see POLIO.

saccharides, saccharin: See SWEETENERS.

sacroiliac: relating to the sacrum, the next-to-last segment of the spine (the last is the coccyx, the "tailbone"), and the ileum, the largest of the bones that form the pelvic girdle — and also to various connectives, especially ligaments, between them.

safety: See ACCIDENTS, PREVENTION OF; FIRE EXTINGUISHERS; FIRE-RETARDANT CLOTHING; FOOD POISONING, PREVENTION OF; MEDICINE CHEST; PESTICIDES; PETS; POISONING, PREVENTION OF; TOYS; TRAVEL PRECAUTIONS.

"Saint Vitus' dance": See CHOREA.

salicylamide, salicylates: The second word is a class of mild analgesics, or pain relievers; for the most effective and most widely used, see ASPIRIN. Salicylamide is a minor member of the group; see PAIN RELIEVERS.

saliva: the secretion of the salivary glands; it keeps the mouth moist and also contains enzymes helpful in the digestion of starches. It can carry bacteria and other organisms, too, which is the reason that spitting in public is not only unesthetic, but possibly dangerous. Human bites that penetrate the skin — rabies aside — are infinitely more serious than similar dog bites.

There are few troubles with the salivary glands, but for a discussion of one of them, see MUMPS.

Salk vaccine: See the comment under SABIN VACCINE.

Salmonella: a genus of bacilli that can cause a variety of problems. See FOOD POISONING; PARATYPHOID FEVER; PETS; TYPHOID FEVER.

"salting out": See ABORTION.

San Joaquin Valley fever: See VALLEY FEVER.

San-Man: an over-the-counter "sleep aid"; see SEDATIVES.

Sanorex: a trade name for mazindol, an appetite depressant; see DIET PILLS.

sarcoidosis: a systemic condition, often referred to simply as "sarcoid," characterized by formation of granular nodules (of a type usually suggesting an inflammatory reaction) in the lungs and frequently also other sites including the skin, lymph nodes, liver, spleen, salivary glands, finger or toe bones, and/or eyes. It rarely appears before the age of twenty. The cause is unknown. Some feel that it may be a specific disease caused by an as yet unidentified virus or other organism; others feel that it represents a hypersensitive sort of response to certain pollens, common bacteria, or the like. Sarcoid may range from mild to severe, depending upon the tissues involved, and sometimes disappears spontaneously; it is generally treated, if necessary, with corticosteroids.

sarcoma: a cancer of structural tissue. Sarcomas account for only three percent of all malignancies but for more than a quarter of all cancers in children and young teenagers. They include bone tumors, relatively rare cartilage tumors (chondrosarcomas), and a condition called rhabdomyosarcoma, almost entirely limited to children.

The most prominent type of bone tumor arises in the bone ends and is called osteogenic sarcoma (what we say about it here applies to chondrosarcoma as well). Since it generally occurs in arm or leg bones, there is theoretically a good chance of complete cure by amputation. But diagnosis may be delayed, since the tumor can mimic, and be confused with, other conditions having similar symptoms (pain and/or swelling in a limb): local infections, aftereffects of injury, glandular malfunctions, certain nutritional deficiencies, several forms of arthritis, cysts, and *benign* tumors. (The last are not uncommon in young people. One in particular, called osteochondroma, usually occurs in the typical osteogenic sarcoma site; there is about a one-in-five chance that it may *become* malignant, so it must of course be removed.)

Once the diagnosis is established, amputation is usually performed as close to the torso as possible, to catch any tumor spread that may not be detectable. Peculiar to these tumors is the possibility of "micrometastases" — tiny clumps of malignant cells that cannot be seen on X ray and may migrate slowly to distant parts of the body, eventually starting new tumors. Surgery is thus usually followed by a fairly lengthy — perhaps two years — course of chemotherapy to prevent future problems. The prognosis is directly related to promptness of diagnosis, and for that reason has statistically not been rosy — but is not unfavorable in an individual case that *has* been caught and treated early. There are also new drugs that show promise of improving the outlook even in more advanced cases.

Ewing's sarcoma is a less common type that develops in the main shaft of the bone. Because there may be systemic as well as localized symptoms, including such vague ones as fever and malaise, diagnosis is difficult; this tumor also metastasizes unusually fast. For those reasons, the outlook has been poor in the past; but it has been improving recently, with emphasis on earlier detection and increasing use of combination therapy.

Rhabdomyosarcoma, more prevalent in children than other sarcomas, arises from embryonic precursors of skeletal muscle cells and can occur anywhere in the body where there is muscle tissue — but in fact, the vast majority occur in the head and neck area, and about one in five in an arm or leg. Peak occurrence of rhabdomyosarcoma is between the ages of two and six, although it has been known to appear as late as the early teens; it is very rarely found before the age of one year. It is often first found by a parent, since in well over nine-tenths of cases the major sign is a noticeable lump or swelling. Other symptoms depend upon the location; there may be a vision problem, for instance, if the growth is near the eye, or hoarseness or difficulty in swallowing if it is in the neck.

That early observation often means earlier diagnosis than is usual in some other cancers — which, of course, means a higher likelihood of the tumor's confinement to a single area and a better prospect for full recovery; statistics also suggest that the younger the child, the brighter the outlook, in general. Treatment is usually by surgery and irradiation; since 1970, long-term postsurgery chemotherapy — generally with a combination of drugs — has usually followed and has been found to increase the chance of full recovery, even when the tumor has not been strictly localized. Survival rates have, in fact, improved to the extent that rhabdomyosarcoma is now spoken of by oncologists as "potentially curable."

scabies: a skin condition caused by the burrowing of a tiny arthropod, *Sarcoptes scabiei,* popularly called the "itch mite." The female of the species is the troublemaker. Picked up by a child from soil — or from a playmate — the mite tunnels under the top layer of the skin, releasing a substance that causes intense itching (except in very small tots of a year or two, who sometimes don't itch).

Scabies is found worldwide, although the incidence in our country was quite low until the 1970s. There has been a vast increase in this decade, sufficient to be termed "epidemic" by some concerned observers. One source may be adoptions of small children from foreign nations, particularly from Southeast Asia; significant numbers of the latter have been found to be carrying the infection. (Increased travel abroad by our own citizens has also doubtless played a part.) Scabies may also be, and often is, transmitted venereally. And a variety of the same genus of mite, primarily infesting dogs — as with humans, young ones in particular — is transmittable to humans as well.

Usually, the mite picks sites where the skin is tender and easiest to penetrate — the inside surfaces of fingers and toes, ankles, backs of knees, wrists; but it can attack other areas as well. The visible evidence is a tiny linear elevation something like a slight scratch, with a little bump at one end (that's the mite's entry point); once established, the mite lays eggs and the larvae proceed to excavate their own tunnels.

If you suspect your youngster has scabies — and it's often difficult for a lay person to spot — consult your doctor; the mite can be eliminated by application of various topical medications. And don't let the child scratch; that can lead to secondary infections such as impetigo. Cut the child's fingernails very short and do everything you can to relieve itching.

Remember, too, that scabies is contagious. If it's been diagnosed, the child's clothes and bedding should be sterilized by boiling — and other members of the family should be examined by the doctor to make sure they haven't picked up the condition; some physicians advocate prophylactic treatment of the entire family, even if no symptoms are evident.

scaling skin: See PEELING SKIN. Or, if scaling is accompanied by redness or other manifestations, see RASHES.

scalp: the skin covering the head. It has many, many small blood vessels, and can bleed copiously as the result of a very small wound. If your child does suffer a scalp wound, don't be panicked by the sight of a great deal of blood. Simply stop the bleeding by applying pressure with a clean, dry handkerchief, and then take a good look; often, you'll find a quarter-inch cut.

For some other problems that can beset the scalp, see BALDNESS; CRADLE CAP; DANDRUFF; LICE, HEAD; PSORIASIS; RINGWORM; SEBORRHEA. The scalp is usually prominently involved in rashes accompanying certain childhood diseases, too — especially chickenpox and measles. And of course it's possible for the scalp to be affected by a number of generalized skin conditions.

scan: in general, any diagnostic procedure utilizing a series of discrete images that are subsequently combined to form an overall image. The term is now often used to denote a particular technique; see COMPUTERIZED AXIAL TOMOGRAPHY.

scapula: the anatomical term for the shoulder blade.

scarlatina: See SCARLET FEVER, following.

scarlet fever: an infectious disease caused by streptococcal bacteria, the same group that cause erysipelas, strep sore throat, and other problems; it is also known as scarlatina — a term that has sometimes been used erroneously, by physicians as well as others, to mean a mild, or less serious, case. The severity of scarlet fever does vary; but it must always be viewed as a serious matter because of the organism involved and the many possible avenues of critical complications.

Children between six and twelve are the most frequent victims of scarlet fever, and the illness strikes most commonly in late winter and spring. The infection needn't be picked up from someone who actually has the disease; it can be caught from someone with a sore throat or other strep infection — or from someone carrying the bacteria, who isn't sick at all. Symptoms, appearing after a two- to five-day incubation period, usually include sore throat, chills and fever — which may go up to 104° F. (40° C.) — headache, and possibly vomiting; fever may, rarely, cause convulsions in a very young child.

Typically, a scarlet rash erupts one to three days after the first symptoms appear. It generally starts on the chest and underarm areas, proceeding from there to the rest of the body; the face is little involved, if at all. The rash begins to fade in two or three days and is gone within a week. At the conclusion of the illness, in some 80 percent, there is peeling of the skin, especially on the palms and soles.

None of this is terribly serious in itself, and the child may feel little discomfort if the throat is not very sore and the fever not very high. The two potential problems are complications and, as far as the rest of the family is concerned, contagion.

The second problem is easily and quickly solved: if scarlet fever has been diagnosed, all other members of the family, *including adults,* should receive antibiotics — preferably penicillin or erythromycin — for *three days.* You should also notify anyone outside the family who has been in contact with the child from the day the first symptoms appeared (it's not contagious prior to that).

The sick child must also receive antibiotics — again, preferably penicillin or erythromycin — and *treatment must begin promptly* (which means you must lose no time in calling the doctor, if you even *suspect* scarlet fever). Each day's delay doubles the possibility of complications, so that by the fourth day, if treatment hasn't started, there is a one-in-three probability of complications — which may range from rheumatic fever to involvements of the eyes, ears, kidneys, or lymph nodes. The child must also be kept at home for 48 hours after antibiotic treatment has begun; after that, it's no longer contagious.

It is vital, however, that the youngster continue receiving the antibiotic for *ten full days,* even if recovery is apparently complete, in order to assure prevention of rheumatic fever and other problems. With treatment, the sore throat will probably be gone quickly, the fever within three days; there will probably be no effect on the duration of the rash. But stopping the medication before the end of the ten-day period has frequently been found to result in relapse and to substantially increase the risk of complications.

Additionally, the child should be watched carefully for at least *three weeks* from the onset of the illness. Any symptom of possible complication — a reappearance of fever, earache, urinary peculiarities, swollen lymph nodes, etc. — either during the actual illness or after the child has apparently recovered, should be reported to the doctor immediately.

It's rare to have scarlet fever per se more than once, but, contrary to prior thinking, it is now known to be possible. Because of the many and potentially serious problems posed by streptococci, there has been and continues to be intensive search for an effective vaccine that might offer long-term protection.

scars: If scars are extensive and seriously disfiguring — as, from burns, serious injury, or extensive acne — you should discuss with your physician, or with a dermatologist or plastic surgeon, the possibility of correction of the problem; there are a number of effective procedures.

Keloids are unusually large, thickened scars. The word is properly used only in reference to a scar that remains oddly thickened even when the redness is gone and the scar has lightened as scars normally do; a temporary thickening that subsides spontaneously is not truly a keloid.

Keloids are actually benign tumors of fibrous tissue; why they occur — and it's not predictable — is unknown. They may occur after healing of any kind of break in the skin from a pimple or insect bite to major surgery. They are more common in dark-skinned people — and we mean individuals, not races; actual skin color seems to be an operative factor.

Sometimes, they can be diminished by special techniques; again, the question should be discussed with your physician.

Schick test: See DIPHTHERIA.

schistosomiasis: See PARASITES.

schizophrenia: a broad term referring to a group of mental disorders characterized by illogical reactions, limited range of emotional response, a degree of detachment from reality, and possibly delusions, hallucinations, or other symptoms, combining to an incapacitating extent. (The so-called "split personality" phenomenon is not necessarily present.)

The definition of *childhood schizophrenia* (i.e., prior to the teen years) is a little more specific. It is characterized by a regression or arrest in ego development and a distinct lag in the process of maturation, with disturbed behavior encompassing all areas of central-nervous-system function: motor control, perception, intellect, emotions, and social relationships. Whether childhood schizophrenia is a distinct illness limited to children, or a precursor of adult illness, is still an open question.

No one has yet pinpointed the precise cause(s) of schizophrenia (in child or adult), but current theory postulates a congenital predisposition, or susceptibility. Some who are inclined toward this hypothesis believe the predisposition may be inherited, and that one or more biochemical factors will ultimately prove to be implicated (some studies have suggested that reactions to certain food elements, especially particular proteins in wheat and other cereal grains, may be involved); others have suggested that there may be some correlation with gestational factors such as season of conception, prenatal diet, or maternal infections.

Schizophrenia requires treatment by a specialist — generally including both psychotherapy and chemotherapy — and, when a child is affected, loving support and cooperation on the part of parents and other members of the family.

sclera: the medical term for the translucent membrane covering the eyeball — the white of the eye.

scleroderma: a rare condition (especially so in children) classed, along with lupus and dermatomyositis, as a collagen disease; it is also less commonly, but more accurately, known as *progressive systemic sclerosis* (PSS). It generally begins with fever and diffuse aches. As the word "scleroderma" suggests, there may be skin involvement; if so, the affected area may become shiny and waxy-looking and later harden (the Greek *skleros* means "hard"), shrivel, and lighten. The joints are often involved, with swelling and discomfort similar to that of rheumatoid arthritis, though milder. Other manifestations may include muscular weakness, localized edema, and/or gastrointestinal difficulties.

Despite the broad assortment of symptoms, the diagnosis of PSS can be established by biopsies and other laboratory tests, and such tests will be performed, if it is suspected, in order to rule out the many other conditions that might cause similar symptoms. There is no specific therapy for PSS, since the cause is completely unknown (based on a high incidence of abnormal lymphocytes in PSS patients, current theory postulates an infectious agent, perhaps a virus); treatment is generally symptomatic, including analgesics, anti-inflammatory medications, and, rarely, corticosteroids.

sclerosis: an abnormal hardening of tissues; the most common kind, arteriosclerosis, involves the walls of arteries and does not affect children. For the types that (uncommonly) do, see MULTIPLE SCLEROSIS; SCLERODERMA.

scoliosis: a sideward curvature of the spine. Causes may vary and include disorders and diseases of the hip, spine, and back muscles, as well as inequality in length of the legs. Sometimes the precise cause is not known, as in a type — generally termed *idiopathic scoliosis* — that afflicts young teenagers, mainly girls, and appears to be to a degree familial (i.e., it is known to occur in relatives, and not infrequently upon diagnosis a slight, nearly undetectable curvature will be observed in a sibling or parent).

If idiopathic scoliosis is untreated, the curvature progresses until the completion of skeletal growth, requiring extensive surgery to correct the marked deformity. Treatment is carried out by an orthopedic specialist and involves, usually, a brace or other device to hold the spine in correct position; it may include physiotherapy designed to promote proper posture and strengthen the back muscles. These measures are continued until full growth is reached (a point determined by X ray — which is also used periodically to check the effectiveness of therapy). Sometimes, a certain amount of surgery is still needed when the growth period is completed (or even before, if the brace fails to halt or reverse the curvature), but in many cases, the long-term therapeutic program may eliminate that need.

The affected youngster must understand that it is vital to follow the physician's directions, however cumbersome the brace may be — not only to prevent deformity of the spine itself, but to protect internal organs that can be thrown out of line by postural distortion.

scopolamine: a belladonna alkaloid that has little therapeutic use; although it is effective against motion sickness, it has been abandoned in favor of drugs unlikely to have scopolamine's fairly lengthy list of adverse effects both physical and mental. (The drugs now used are listed under MOTION SICKNESS.) It is, however, incorporated in some over-the-counter "sleep aids"; see SEDATIVES.

scorpion sting: See the section on this subject under BITES AND STINGS.

scotoma: See MIGRAINE.

scrapes and scratches: By and large, these minor injuries heal quickly and without problems, and don't need medical attention. The only thing you should do is clean the area and protect the wound from infection. Cleansing is especially important with knees and elbows, where dirt's often imbedded in the skin.

First (and only)-aid procedure is to wash the area vigorously with soap and water; if it's one of those grimy scrapes, "wash" means *scrub,* with a washcloth — which will be temporarily painful for the child, but necessary if infection is to be prevented.

Once the wound is clean, don't put iodine, Mercurochrome, or anything else on it. Just leave it open to the air to heal, unless it's in an exposed area where outdoor play is likely to result in dirt and further injury; do, then, cover it with an adhesive strip bandage or square of gauze held with adhesive tape — but remove the bandage when the child's through playing outside for the day.

When a scab has formed, don't let the child scratch or pick at it. Tearing off the scab before healing underneath is completed could cause infection or permanent scarring.

Do take the youngster to the doctor if any sign of infection appears — pus, or extensive reddening or swelling, or red streaks on the skin from the wound toward the center of the body.

Also see CAT-SCRATCH FEVER. Occasionally, what seems to be a scraped-raw area could actually be another condition; see IMPETIGO.

scratch test: See ALLERGY TEST.

screening: denoting a program designed to detect disease (or other inimical condition) that may not be evident without special testing procedures, within a given population. The population is generally one at high risk or one in which the particular condition could prove extremely hazardous, as: breast cancer in women; the gene for Tay-Sachs disease in persons of eastern European Jewish descent; venereal disease in pregnant women; lead poisoning in children exposed to heavy automotive pollution or to old, dilapidated housing; hypertension in people in general.

scrotum: See SEX ORGANS.

scurvy: a condition resulting from severe deficiency of vitamin C; see DEFICIENCY DISEASES.

seafood poisoning: See FOOD POISONING.

seasickness: See MOTION SICKNESS.

sebaceous cyst: See CYST.

seborrhea: a condition of overactivity of the sebaceous (oil) glands in the skin. Normally, these glands excrete a substance called sebum; its function is to soften and lubricate the skin (and hair) and also to carry off waste materials such as dead, sloughed-off cells. Overactivity of the glands is often related to such problems as acne and dandruff. In a more serious form, however, it can cause seborrheic dermatitis, involving extensive crusting and scaling of the scalp, ears, chest, and other areas; such a situation needs medical care.

sebum: See SEBORRHEA, preceding.

secobarbital, Seconal: See SEDATIVES; the latter is a trade name for the former.

secretion: the process by which certain organs (as, glands) produce particular substances (as, hormones) physically and chemically different from the producing organ (the word comes from the Latin word for "separate"); the substance produced by such a process. Such substances are designed for use within the body — which is the difference between this word and *excretion*, the elimination of waste materials that are *not* usable.

Sedacaps: an over-the-counter "sleeping aid"; see SEDATIVES.

Sedaphen: a combination product containing phenobarbital plus several bromides; see SEDATIVES for comment on individual ingredients.

sedatives: Dictionaries, both medical and general, characterize these drugs as substances that "quiet" or "calm."

That, it is obvious, can mean anything from making one feel less anxious to putting someone into a deep (perhaps even permanent) sleep. In fact, many medications, having a broad range of properties, do indeed fall into this category; some are referred to as sedatives, while others are characterized as sleeping pills (or "aids"), tranquilizers, and a number of other things. A few of them can perform at either extreme of the range, depending upon dosage.

Before we list chemicals, we should perhaps define some terms that are used to describe the actions of these drugs. Anything that has a *sedative* effect acts, broadly speaking, to decrease excitement or anxiety and may, in sufficient dosage, act as a hypnotic. A *tranquilizer* is generally understood to be a sedative that enables one to enjoy decreased anxiety (or other psychic disturbance) without being sedated to the point of falling asleep. A *relaxant* is a tranquilizer that acts particularly in the area of muscle relaxation, relieving "uptightness" both literally and figuratively. *Hypnotic* drugs are designed primarily to induce sleep. There are, as you will see, a number of cross-categories among the relevant drugs as they are usually classed.

The phrase "under sedation" may imply the use of any of the drugs in this category, whether used to slightly calm or to place in deep sleep. Which, as we've said, may or may not be the same drug.

None of the medications we are about to describe should be given to a child — or, for that matter, taken by anyone in your family — without a physician's advice. None should ever be combined with alcohol (that particular combination can in fact be *fatal*) or with any other medication containing a sedative, tranquilizer, narcotic, or antihistamine. And of course recommended dosage should never be exceeded. These warnings apply not only to those products that require prescriptions, but to over-the-counter products as well.

RX: "MINOR" TRANQUILIZERS AND RELAXANTS

These mildly sedative agents are, as a group, used in three ways: to relieve anxiety and tension associated with neurotic conditions, to relieve anxiety that might arise in reaction to situations of temporary stress, and to relax painful muscle spasm that can accompany injury or a flare-up in some types of arthritis. These combined properties make them sometimes useful as sleep-inducers as well.

Among those that are basically anti-anxiety agents are, prominently: chlormezanone (Trancopal); hydroxyzine (Atarax, Vistaril), which also has some antinauseant effect; meprobamate (Equanil, Miltown); phenaglycodol (Ultran); tybamate (Solacen, Tybatran); and a group of chemically similar drugs called benzodiazepines, which include chlordiazepoxide (Librium), clorazepate (Tranxene), diazepam (Valium), and oxazepam (Serax). Meprobamate and the benzodiazepines also have significant muscle-relaxant properties. Clorazepate and diazepam have also proved useful, in some cases, in controlling convulsive seizures. Meprobamate is also a component of some multi-ingredient products, notably in combination with an antispasm agent (Milpath, Pathibamate) and with aspirin and ethoheptazine (an analgesic of questionable value; see NARCOTICS) in Equagesic.

Those drugs employed primarily as relaxers of skeletal muscles include carisoprodol (Rela, Soma; Soma Compound also includes phenacetin — see PAIN RELIEVERS — and caffeine), chlorphenesin (Maolate), chlorzoxazone (Paraflex), metaxalone (Skelaxin), methocarbamol (Robaxin), and orphenadrine (Norflex).

Responses to these medications may vary tremendously with the individual, and if one does not work, another might; similarly, if one causes unwanted drowsiness, another might not. All drugs in this group, the primary anti-anxiety agents in particular, have potential for creating physical dependence — addiction — and must not be overused.

RX: "MAJOR" TRANQUILIZERS

These drugs are quite potent, and are generally reserved (with some exceptions) for treatment of acute emotional and mental problems involving such symptoms as extreme panic, withdrawal, and hostility, whether associated with schizophrenia or with toxic or other conditions; they are not prescribed or administered to allay everyday anxiety.

The major ones, including all those we shall list, belong to a class of agents called phenothiazines; they include acetophenazine (Tindal), chlorpromazine (Thorazine), fluphenazine (Prolixin), mesoridazine (Serentil), perphenazine (Trilafon), prochlorperazine (Compazine), promazine (Sparine), promethazine (Phenergan), thioridazine (Mellaril), trifluoperazine (Stelazine), and triflupromazine (Vesprin). Side effects, particularly of the neuromuscular variety, are not uncommon; any untoward reaction of any kind should be reported promptly to the prescribing physician.

Several of these drugs are also effective against nausea and vomiting, but are — because of their potency — not used lightly for that purpose. The ones so used (usually in smaller dosage) are chlorpromazine, fluphenazine, perphenazine, prochlorperazine (which is combined with isopropamide, an antispasmodic, in Combid), promazine, triflupromazine, and promethazine; the last is employed chiefly for this purpose and is also an effective antihistamine (but, because of its other actions, far from first choice for that purpose). Mepergan is a product combining promethazine with meperidine (see NARCOTICS).

RX: BARBITURATES AND OTHER HYPNOTICS

All these drugs, barbiturates and nonbarbiturates, should be handled with cautious respect. All are capable of producing addiction — both physical and psychological dependence — and, in sufficient dosage, toxicity and death; they should if possible be employed in smaller-than-prescribed doses, certainly never in larger ones. (The single exception: if a barbiturate is prescribed for control of epileptic seizures, the dosage directed by the physician should be followed exactly; apparent ineffectiveness or adverse effects should be discussed with the doctor, who may direct that the dosage be increased or reduced appropriately.) They are employed primarily as sleep-inducers, occasionally for daytime sedation (less commonly since the anti-anxiety agents have become available), some as anesthetics or adjuncts thereto.

The major barbiturates used as sedative-hypnotics are amobarbital (Amytal), aprobarbital (Alurate), butabarbital (Bubartal, Butisol), mephobarbital (Mebaral), pentobarbital (Nembutal), phenobarbital (Eskabarb, Luminal, Stental), probarbital (Ipral), and secobarbital (Seconal); mephobarbital and phenobarbital are also anticonvulsants and are used in epilepsy. Two others — methohexital (Brevital) and thiopental (Pentothal) — have an extremely short period of action, thus are not useful for treating insomnia, but are widely used in anesthesia; some of the others are employed for presurgery sedation.

There are also a number of products that combine barbiturates with one another and/or bromides (or bromidelike drugs). Such a combination poses a risk of cumulative toxicity and makes dosages very difficult to control; the products are not considered useful, and we mention a few of the major ones here only for purposes of information. Carbrital is pentobarbital plus carbromal; Ethobral is a mixture of butabarbital, phenobarbital, and secobarbital; Nidar contains those three barbiturates plus a fourth, pentobarbital; Sedaphen is phenobarbital and three bromides; Tuinal combines amobarbital and secobarbital.

Prominent nonbarbiturate sedatives, which are used exclusively to induce sleep, include chloral betaine (Beta-Chlor), chloral hydrate (Noctec, Somnos), ethchlorynol (Placidyl), ethinamate (Valmid), flurazepam (Dalmane), glutethimide (Doriden), methaqualone (Optimil, Parest, Quaalude, Somnafac, Sopor), and methyprylon (Noludar). Flurazepam, which is — like some of the tranquilizers — a benzodiazepine, appears the least likely of these to interfere with REM (dream) sleep.

Parents of teenagers should be aware that extensive abuse has been reported with methaqualone, as well as barbiturates.

Finally, a number of prescription sedative-hypnotics have been incorporated in a variety of medications with other types of drugs — some rationally, some not. Donnatal and a number of other products combine phenobarbital with belladonna alkaloids — probably a useful type of product in dealing with spasmodic intestinal upset. Several "diet pills" combine barbiturates and stimulants; see our comment under AMPHETAMINES. Cafergot P-B includes pentobarbital and belladonna alkaloids in its basic ergotamine-plus-caffeine formulation; this is intended for use in migraine, with its pain and concomitant intense nausea. The rationale for two other drugs promoted for mild analgesic use is doubtful; these are Fiorinal (butalbital — a barbiturate not employed separately — plus aspirin, phenacetin, and caffeine) and Phenaphen (phenobarbital, aspirin, phenacetin, and a belladonna derivative).

OVER-THE-COUNTER: "SLEEP AIDS" AND "TENSION RELIEVERS"

These products do not contain any of the foregoing powerful, potentially habit-forming drugs. Some do, however, contain ingredients that many physicians would not prescribe because they are considered too risky. It is helpful to know, if you are stirred by soothing voices pushing "little blue pills" and promising "safe, restful sleep," just what you are being urged to ingest.

The main ingredient in most of these products is methapyrilene, an antihistamine, which has a minor sedative action; some also include pyrilamine, which is similar. They are probably reasonably safe, although the sedative effect is not dependable — and tends to disappear altogether if the product is used continually over a period of time.

Some also — or instead — contain bromides or scopolamine. Both do act effectively as sedatives; the trouble is that they have other effects as well. Bromides have been largely abandoned in medicine because of the risk of bromism, a condition of chronic toxicity with continued use; because bromides are excreted very slowly, their effects are cumulative, and a toxic level can be reached by gradual buildup in the body. Symptoms include an acnelike rash, verbal and muscle-coordination disturbances, dizziness, and gastrointestinal dysfunction.

Scopolamine (also known as hyoscine) is an alkaloid derived from belladonna; it acts quickly, even in small doses, as a depressant of the central nervous system. Beyond that, it is more than a little unpredictable. In some people, drowsiness is preceded by a period of disorientation, possibly including hallucinations. It can be dangerous for anyone with glaucoma. "Side effects" may include cycloplegia, paralysis of the eye muscle that is responsible for focal accommodation. In high enough doses, it has been known to set off a full-blown psychosis.

A number of brands include salicylamide or another minor analgesic, which may be helpful if aches and pains are preventing sleep (salicylamide has a depressant side effect, but not at the doses in the pills — although that's apparently the rationalization for including it rather than a more effective pain reliever such as aspirin). A few products contain thiamine and niacin, which are two of the B vitamins; turn to NUTRITION to see how much sense *that* makes. And a handful (not including any that we are about to mention) add a soupçon of passion-flower extract, which is apparently a hand-me-down from the old patent-medicine heyday and just about as useful as the "snake oil" and similar nostrums peddled then.

Dormin, Sedacaps, and Somnicaps are among those products that consist solely of methapyrilene, probably the best bet for occasional use (remember that effectiveness diminishes after continuous use) if your doctor feels such a product may be helpful. Probably equally harmless are such products as Nytol, which is simply methapyrilene and salicylamide (the capsule form contains more of both drugs than the tablet). Quite a number of products combine methapyrilene and scopolamine, including Compoz (which, though promoted for daytime use, contains more scopolamine than some products designed to induce sleep, and also includes a second antihistamine), Nite Rest, San-Man, Seedate, and Sleep-Eze. Sominex, Sure-Sleep and others add salicylamide to their methapyrilene and scopolamine. Alva-Tranquil offers methapyrilene, a bromide, a salicylate, and those B vitamins. And Nervine has none of the antihistamine, just the vitamins along with three bromides.

sed rate: the commonly used, short form for erythrocyte sedimentation rate, sometimes abbreviated to ESR; a measure of the sinking velocity of red cells within a quantity of drawn blood. Elevation of the sed rate is a nonspecific indication of infection or inflammation somewhere in the body; it may occur in conditions as disparate as rheumatoid arthritis and the common cold.

Seedate: an over-the-counter "sleep aid"; see SEDATIVES.

seizure: See CONVULSION; EPILEPSY.

seltzer medications: See ANTACIDS; PAIN RELIEVERS.

semen: the ejaculate of the penis; it is a thick fluid containing sperm plus fluid secretions of various associated glands.

septic: infectious; containing, or caused by, infectious organisms; the opposite of *aseptic.*

septicemia: a bacterial infection of the bloodstream itself, sometimes called "blood poisoning"; it is now uncommon. Septicemia is not a primary infection, except when it stems from the use of infected needles (as, by drug addicts); it typically results from an infected wound or other condition that has been untreated or improperly treated, thus permitting the infectious agent to invade other parts of the body. Symptoms are general malaise and very high fever, possibly accompanied by jaundice. It is treated, depending upon the exact nature of the infection, by antibiotics, transfusion, or other measures, and is best managed in the hospital.

septum: any thin dividing wall in the body; the word usually refers, however, to the dividing cartilage between the nostrils. If it is twisted or bent — a condition called *deviated septum* that may be congenital, or may occur as a result of nose fracture — it sometimes interferes with proper drainage in the nose, thus aggravating such problems as colds or sinus infections. It can be corrected surgically, but the operation is generally not recommended unless the deviation and the difficulty it causes are quite severe.

For advice on coping with bleeding from the septum, see NOSEBLEED.

sequelae: the medical term for residual aftereffects, as of an illness or injury.

Serax: a trade name for the tranquilizer oxazepam; see SEDATIVES.

Serentil: a trade name for mesoridazine, a major tranquilizer; see SEDATIVES.

serum: the liquid part of the blood containing disease-fighting antibodies — i.e., plasma minus the clotting elements. There are various serums for treating specific ailments; they are made by immunizing an animal or person, then extracting the antibody-containing serum from the blood; injection of antiserum thus gives prompt passive immunity.

Serum sickness is an allergic reaction to such a serum, especially one derived from animals. Allergy to tetanus antitoxin, until recently available only in horse serum, is not uncommon; now there is a human serum available — but vaccination is still preferable, so that the necessity for administering antitoxin can be avoided altogether.

serum hepatitis: See HEPATITIS.

sex chromosomes: Each of us normally receives two of them, one from each parent: a girl, one X chromosome from each; a boy, an X chromosome from his mother and a Y from his father. (Under HEREDITY, we discuss some of the disorders that can be transmitted via the X chromosome. That discussion presumes the usual number of sex chromosomes per person.)

Occasionally, through some accident at or about the time of conception, a child receives a different number. (Whatever the number, the child is a boy if they include at least one Y chromosome.) Two such situations, which have been given names, are discussed separately: KLINEFELTER'S SYNDROME, the XXY boy; and TURNER'S SYNDROME, the XO (having a single X chromosome) girl.

A third, unnamed situation, because it has received quite a bit of publicity — much of it inaccurate and distorted — deserves comment. That is the one in which a boy has received an extra Y chromosome — i.e., is XYY instead of the usual XY.

A few years back, newspaper headlines announced excitedly that a mass murderer whose deed had horrified the public had been found to be XYY. Subsequently, the newspapers duly reported that the story had been in error; these reports ran, as they are wont to do, in small paragraphs tucked in the back pages, and we have no doubt that many of our readers did not know until this very moment that Richard Speck was not XYY after all.

The reports — the original ones, that is — spurred many researchers to speculate about the possible connection between this chromosome aberration and the inclination to commit crimes. They hastened to analyze the chromosomes and personalities of a number of prison populations—and lo, their findings tended to bear out the theory. While the incidence of the XYY configuration has been variously estimated as occurring once in every three hundred to one thousand male births (0.1 to 0.3 percent), figures far exceeding those emerged from the prison populations — up to 3.5 or even 4.5 percent. Those prisoners, the surveyors reported, were also taller and more aggressive, by and large, than the others.

What did it all mean? Many speculations were rushed into print. Were XYY boys doomed from birth to become criminals? Would that become a new defense at criminal trials? ("I couldn't help it; my chromosomes made me do it." Two defense lawyers — one in France, one in Australia — tried it, unsuccessfully.) Since then some of the speculators have modified their theories slightly, postulating that XYY boys are perhaps "inclined" to get into trouble, and that early intervention might deter them from that fate; the pontificators realized, belatedly, that there must be a good many XYY males in the United States who are *not* in prison and who have never been accused of any crime. Presently, in fact, based on population figures and the previously cited estimated incidence, there are some 103,000 to 309,000 American males, in all, who are XYY.

Obviously only a minuscule number of them are in prison. It must be assumed that the vast majority are living perfectly respectable lives. A theory that the XYY configuration might be correlated with such factors as socioeconomic class has, incidentally, been checked out and disproved. In fact, since this comment is intended to reassure parents who have discovered by some chance that they have XYY sons, possibly destined to grow up tall and aggressive, we might go further.

The present "average" height of the American male is five feet, eight inches, and was considerably less in the past. Yet, of all the United States Presidents, only five — the two Adamses, Madison (our shortest President, at five feet, four inches), Van Buren, and Benjamin Harrison — have been below that height; all but eight have in fact been above it. A certain amount of aggressiveness, we submit, is probably necessary for an individual to seek and win that office.

No one, to our knowledge, has studied the XYY incidence in the Congress, or among governors — or among directors and executives of large corporations. The results might be interesting.

And leading figures in the sports world — notably, in basketball and football — have frequently been tall, aggressive people, too.

sex-linked: See HEREDITY.

sex organs: These are the organs of reproduction, some internal and some external; the gonads (ovaries and testes) also have hormonal functions not directly related to reproduction (see ENDOCRINE GLANDS).

Female sex organs include the ovaries, which release eggs on a regular basis (see MENSTRUATION); the fallopian tubes, through which the eggs travel to the uterus; the uterus itself, which encloses the developing embryo if an egg is fertilized; the vagina or birth canal, the passageway through which sperm enter, a baby is born, and menstruation takes place; and, externally, the clitoris, labia (folds or "lips"), and lubricating glands. The external organs collectively constitute the vulva.

Male organs include the scrotum, the saclike tissue containing the testes or sperm-producing organs (sometimes called testicles); the epididymis, which collects sperm; the prostate gland, which manufactures semen, the fluid vehicle for sperm; the seminal vesicles, which store semen and release it when needed; the penis, containing the urethra through which sperm (as well as urine) are released; and, again, lubricating glands. Perfectly normal penises, incidentally, vary considerably in size and also, due to body build (e.g., whether or not surrounded by much fatty tissue), in *apparent* size — but there is very little difference in size among erect penises; unless your physician indicates that the size of your son's penis falls outside the normal range, it is not something about which either you or he should be concerned.

For problems, events, and conditions that affect or involve the female sex organs, see BARTHOLIN'S CYST; FISTULA; LABIAL ADHESIONS; MENSTRUATION; MONILIASIS; PAP TEST; PREGNANCY; VAGINAL DISCHARGE; VAGINITIS. For circumstances affecting the sex organs of boys, see CIRCUMCISION; HERNIA; HYDROCELE; HYPOSPADIAS; MEATITIS; MUMPS; PARAPHIMOSIS. Topics concerning both sexes are discussed under CONTRACEPTION; HERMAPHRODITISM; MASTURBATION; PUBERTY; VENEREAL DISEASES.

shigellosis: another name for bacillary dysentery; see DYSENTERY.

shingles: a viral infection causing a distinctive skin condition, also known as *herpes zoster;* it tends to afflict adolescents and adults much more frequently than younger children — it is in fact considered a rarity under the age of ten — and both the incidence *and* the severity of the illness increase with each decade of life.

There had long been strong evidence of a link between shingles and chickenpox; chickenpox epidemics have unquestionably been initiated by exposure of a youngster to someone with shingles. It is now certain that both conditions are caused by the very same virus, and that shingles is a "reactivation" of latent chickenpox. Symptoms of the two ailments, however, are quite different.

Shingles is an inflammation of nerve endings in the skin. Eruptions tend to follow nerve pathways on one side of the body; they consist of small blisters on a reddened area. In some cases, the eruption of the rash is preceded by fever. The rash is located on the chest in half the cases, but has been known to appear on the neck, face, or lower back. It is usually quite painful, and lasts for ten days to two weeks in a younger patient; pain is worse, and the duration of illness greater, with increased age.

As with chickenpox, antibiotics and similar drugs are ineffective. The physician can, however, prescribe analgesics, cortisone, and other medications.

Shingles is, as we've said, contagious; it can initiate chickenpox in someone who's never had it. Contagion is by direct contact with the eruption, with fluid from the blisters, or with clothing that has been in contact with the blisters; possible contagion persists until the blisters disappear.

It is believed rare, and perhaps impossible, to have shingles more than once.

shock: See ANAPHYLACTIC SHOCK; ELECTRICAL SHOCK; TRAUMATIC SHOCK. Insulin shock may occur accidentally in diabetes (see DIABETES MELLITUS) or refer to a form of therapy (see the following entry).

shock therapy: a form of treatment for some mental illnesses, involving the deliberate production of convulsions, either by injection of insulin or by means of an electric current. The former, which may have many hazardous side effects, is for all practical purposes no longer used. The second method, also called electroconvulsive shock therapy, is still considered useful in certain conditions, notably those involving extreme mania or depression (generally the patients are adults) — although use of some of the newer drugs (especially phenothiazines and antidepressants) has eliminated the need for this recourse in many cases. Shock therapy is not considered a standard form of treatment for children or adolescents, and it is employed only as a last resort and after extensive consultation.

shoes: There is no real need to put shoes on a child until the child is ready to walk outdoors (unless, of course, your floor is wont to shed splinters). Walking without shoes provides excellent foot-muscle development and exercise — and can be continued outdoors on grass or sand. Obviously, if the available grass or sand is likely to contain hookworm larvae, sharp seashells, or other harmful objects or entities, protection (which is the main reason for shoes in the first place) is needed.

When you buy your child shoes, make them inexpensive ones. We mean, by that, not rigid leather or plastic, but soft shoes with rubber soles; sneakers are fine. (Contrary to traditional thinking, your toddler's ankles do not need stiff supports — babies are, after all, born without shoes — and shoes that allow free movement while protecting the bottom of the foot from injury are best.) Buy the cheapest ones that fit; they are likely to be quickly outgrown. (*Don't* try to anticipate and buy shoes that are too large; they will make the child hobble while others are walking and running.)

Take the child with you when you buy shoes; nothing is as dependable a standard of measurement as the child's own feet. Try to ignore sales pitches. Once you have chosen a nice, flexible pair of sneakers or similar shoes, have the child put on both shoes and stand up; there should be half an inch of space beyond the big toe (if you can't feel the big toe, the shoe is too hard). If there is less space, a larger size is needed; if there's more — especially if the shoe flops up and down when the child walks (*have* the child walk) — a smaller size is needed.

If you don't spend a lot of money on children's shoes, you will probably buy shoes more often, which is better for your child's feet.

A word about corrective shoes. They shouldn't be prescribed by a salesperson. If such an individual insists that your child needs corrective shoes, express your appreciation for the concern and consult a physician; the salesperson may or may not be right — but only your doctor knows for sure.

shots: See IMMUNIZATION.

sibling: technically, another child of the same two parents; loosely, in a psychological and/or sociological context, another child who shares the same childhood environment (i.e., including stepchildren and adopted children).

sickle cell disease: a hereditary condition involving red blood cells of a peculiar sickle, or crescent, shape ("sickle cells"). It is associated with unusually high resistance to malaria, and is found chiefly among Blacks and other dark-skinned people living in, or descended from those living in, moist, tropical areas of Africa and the Far East.

If the recessive gene for this trait (see HEREDITY) is inherited from only one parent, there may be mild anemia, which exists in about eight percent of Afro-Americans (but up to one in four inhabitants of central Africa). When it is inherited from both parents, a serious anemia, called sicklemia, results, a condition afflicting perhaps one in five hundred Americans of African descent.

side effects: a broad term for results of drug administration that are not directly connected with the medication's intended therapeutic effect and are neither helpful nor beneficial. If aspirin is taken to relieve pain, for example, the fact that it also reduces fever (should fever be present) is an additional benefit, not a side effect; an allergic-reaction rash, or exacerbation of a peptic ulcer (both of which may result from use of aspirin) would be considered a side effect. Similarly so classed are intestinal upsets stemming from antibiotics, drowsiness caused by an antihistamine taken to relieve itching, etc. Potential side effects should always be considered by a physician in relation to the intended benefits for which a medication is prescribed.

sig.: See PRESCRIPTIONS.

sight: See VISION.

sigmoidoscopy: an examination of the sigmoid colon, the S-shaped part of the large intestine immediately above the rectum, with a special lighted tube made for this purpose; the physician can thus investigate the area visually.

sign: This word may seem synonymous, to you, with *symptom* — i.e., a clue to the diagnosis of an ailment. To a physician, it's not, and the phrase "signs and symptoms" is not as redundant as it may appear. A *sign* is medically defined as a symptom that can be objectively verified by the physician (or independently observed, in the absence of the patient's awareness of it). A thermometer reading that indicates fever, for example, is a *sign* (whereas "I feel hot" on the part of the child isn't), as is the detection of Koplik spots early in measles, or a visible swelling. For comparison, see SYMPTOM.

Sinequan: a trade name for doxepin; see ANTIDEPRESSANTS.

sinuses: a term that may refer to various parts of the body, but usually (in the absence of other qualification) refers to air-filled cavities in the head, connected with the nose-throat passage. There are four pairs of sinuses, three of which are present at birth. The *frontal sinuses,* above the eyebrows, don't develop until the age of two, three, four, or later. The others: the *ethmoid sinuses,* located behind the bridge of the nose; the *paranasal sinuses* (also called *antral* or *maxillary* sinuses), at the sides of the nose, behind the cheekbones; and the *sphenoid sinuses,* farther back toward the middle of the skull.

All sinuses can cause problems by becoming inflamed as a result of infection or allergic reaction, particularly the frontals and the paranasals; see SINUSITIS, following.

sinusitis: an inflammation of a sinus or sinuses resulting from infection or allergy that has caused swelling of the mucous membranes. Headache and fever are often present, especially if there is an accumulation of pus because of infection and blocked drainage; if the paranasal sinuses are involved, the pain may resemble that of a toothache.

If you suspect that your child has a sinus inflammation, give no medication beyond aspirin; especially avoid nose drops, sprays, cold pills, etc., without medical recommendation (for the reasons why, see COLD PILLS and DECONGESTANTS, NASAL). Do take the child to the doctor, who will determine the exact *cause* of the inflammation and will *then* prescribe or recommend appropriate medication: antibiotics or other drugs to combat infection, antihistamine in an allergic situation, decongestant spray or drops if such is required, and so on; if your doctor believes it's warranted, you may be referred to a specialist for further consultation or treatment. In some cases, drainage of the affected sinus or sinuses may be necessary.

If it's been determined that a youngster has some chronic problem — generally, allergy-related — affecting the sinuses, diving, which tends to aggravate the condition, should be avoided.

sinus medications, Sinutab: See DECONGESTANTS, NASAL.

sister: in Great Britain, the title by which a registered nurse is addressed.

Skelaxin: a trade name for metaxalone, a muscle relaxant; see SEDATIVES.

skin: the largest organ of the body. Yes, organ: the skin not only covers and protects the body but also helps to control the body's internal temperature, eliminates certain waste materials (through sweat and oil ducts), and plays a part in the utilization of vitamin D.

The color and condition of the skin can also be a helpful diagnostic barometer in a number of ailments not specifically affecting the skin itself. Yellowing of the skin, for example, may reflect problems in the liver or circulation; unusual dryness can signal certain endocrine difficulties affecting the body's chemical balances; certain eruptions are characteristic of specific infectious diseases.

About disturbances of the skin itself: the important thing is not to attempt to diagnose and treat any skin problems of unknown cause; very commonly, such attempts can make the situation worse — and make subsequent treatment by a physician harder, longer, and more complicated.

For discussion of specific skin conditions, see ACNE; ATHLETE'S FOOT; BEDSORES; BIRTHMARKS; BITES AND STINGS; BLACKHEADS; BLISTER; BLOOD BLISTER; BLOTCHES; BOIL; BRUISES; BURNS; CALLUS; CARBUNCLE; COLD SORE; CORNS; CUTS; DERMATITIS; DIAPER RASH; ECZEMA; FROSTBITE; HEAT RASH; HIVES; IMPETIGO; ITCHING; KERATOSIS; LICE, BODY; LIPOMA; MELANOMA; PARONYCHIA; PEELING SKIN; PEMPHIGUS; PITYRIASIS; POISON IVY; PSORIASIS; RASHES; RINGWORM; SCABIES; SCARS; SCRAPES AND SCRATCHES; SEBORRHEA; SHINGLES; SUNBURN; VITILIGO; WARTS; WHITEHEADS; XANTHOMA.

skin planing: See DERMABRASION.

skin, yellow: See CAROTENEMIA; JAUNDICE.

skull fracture: See HEAD INJURIES.

SLE: short for systemic lupus erythematosus; see LUPUS.

sleep: Many presumed authorities have spelled out, in books and articles, arbitrary sleep needs for children of various ages. These directives are, however, quite misleading; the fact is that children vary in their sleep needs just as adults do, and there are no hard-and-fast rules that can be applied to all youngsters of two, ten, or any other age. It's true that sleep is absolutely essential, at least as necessary as food, and perhaps more so; sleep is the only time the body can really relax. But how *much* sleep is needed varies with the individual.

An infant, of course, will simply sleep as much as he needs to; he'll go to sleep when he's sleepy and wake up when he's had enough sleep. Just to give you an idea of what "enough" may mean: a study in which 75 infants were observed continuously from the moment they were born until 72 hours later determined that the average amount of sleep per 24-hour period was 16½ hours — but that "average" emerged from an individual range varying from 10½ hours to 23 out of 24! Another study reported the sleep needs of two-and-a-half-year-olds; result: they were found to sleep anywhere from eight to more than fourteen hours at night (average, eleven), with total sleep time for a 24-hour period, including naps, averaging thirteen hours — but ranging all the way from eight to seventeen. The nighttime average is pretty consistent until kindergarten age; the need for daytime naps will gradually decrease (but again, it's a very individual matter, and one two-year-old may refuse to take daytime naps while another child of four may sleep every afternoon).

Getting babies to go to sleep when they need it is, as we've said, no problem. The difficulty for parents arises when the child's old enough to walk, talk, and become interested in the world around him. He still has his own sleep needs; the trouble is getting him to recognize them.

A preschool youngster will generally display sleepiness, which every parent learns to recognize: drooping eyelids, rubbing of eyes, and so on. The child may, however, be so interested in what's going on that a deliberate effort is made to stay awake. Sometimes the sensible solution is to let the child doze off in a corner of the family room, or to otherwise allow some connection with activity the child is reluctant to abandon (as by leaving the bedroom door open), rather than total exclusion from the scene.

As far as older children go, judge by the child's morning behavior. Does getting up in time for school pose undue difficulties? Can daily activities be carried on without fatigue or irritability? If the youngster seems to lack sufficient energy, and must be dragged out of bed in the morning, chances are more sleep is needed.

Also see INSOMNIA, if inability to sleep is a problem.

Sleep-Eze: an over-the-counter "sleeping aid"; see SEDATIVES.

sleeping pills: See SEDATIVES.

sleeping sickness: See ENCEPHALITIS; NARCOLEPSY. African sleeping sickness is a form of trypanosomiasis, discussed under PARASITES.

sleeplessness: See INSOMNIA.

sleepwalking: Don't be alarmed if it occurs; it's not uncommon in children. *Don't* scold or chastise a sleepwalking youngster. *Do* speak to him quietly and soothingly, take him back to bed, be very gentle, and stay with him until you're sure he's sleeping soundly. And *do* call your physician the next morning and discuss the question; follow whatever advice the doctor gives you.

"slow viruses": See MULTIPLE SCLEROSIS; SSPE.

"smack": a slang term for heroin; see NARCOTICS.

small-for-date: an adjective describing a baby born after 37 weeks of pregnancy, but weighing less than five pounds (2.3 kilograms) at birth. In many cases, the cause is not known, and the question is a subject of continuing research. There is, thus far, strong evidence that serious maternal malnutrition is one factor, and others are maternal cigarette smoking (causing a higher-than-normal carbon monoxide level in the mother's blood and possibly oxygen deprivation in the developing fetus) and overindulgence in alcohol. Whether other drugs may have this effect is not known.

A small-for-date baby may or may not need special neonatal hospital care; the physician will make that decision.

smallpox: a serious and highly contagious viral disease, also known medically as variola. It is an ancient scourge, known to have existed at least three thousand years ago; during the 1700s, it killed at least sixty million people in Europe alone, and those who survived were often horribly scarred.

Smallpox is now a medical curiosity in most nations of the world, including our own, and has in fact been declared officially eradicated from the Western Hemisphere by the World Health Organization (WHO). It is believed possible to use the word "eradication" when talking about smallpox because — unlike other diseases such as plague and yellow fever — smallpox may afflict only human beings. There was one report of the infection of two zoo apes during a 1949 Indonesia epidemic, and some authorities have speculated that a similar disease called monkeypox may be caused by a variant strain of the smallpox virus. But if there is no animal reservoir for the virus, *total* eradication is a real possibility and may become reality within the foreseeable future.

At this writing, there has not been a case of smallpox in the United States since 1949; the last Western Hemisphere case was reported from Brazil in 1971, and the hemisphere was declared smallpox free in 1973 (two years' surveillance following the last reported case is required before that official pronouncement is made). While over one hundred thousand cases (the figure was probably low) were reported to the WHO in 1973 and more than two hundred thousand in 1974, more than nine-tenths of them were clustered in India and the surrounding nations of Pakistan, Bangladesh, Nepal, and Afghanistan; the remainder were in Ethiopia (the rest of Africa has been free of the disease since 1970, and Indonesia attained official smallpox-free status in 1974). WHO immunization efforts concentrated on these areas, and 1975 saw a 90 percent decrease; 95 percent of the reported cases were in Bangladesh and the rest in India, Nepal, and Ethiopia. Early in 1976, WHO announced that the last case in Asia had been eradicated and the disease remained endemic only in Ethiopia.

Vaccination, once part of the preschool regimen for every American child, is no longer routine in the United States and is specifically not recommended unless there is high probability of exposure; under ordinary circumstances, the risk of adverse reaction to the vaccine — which is exceedingly small — is now considered higher than that of contracting the disease. Vaccination is, of course, essential for travel to an area where smallpox is still endemic. It is also still required for entry into many African, Asian, and Latin American countries, as well as for reentry into the United States if the traveler has been in a nation reporting smallpox within the prior two weeks. (Since the situation is changing, discuss your itinerary with your physician if there is a question concerning vaccination before a family trip.) The vaccination must be recorded on an official certificate stamped by the local health department; it is valid for three years.

smear: a sample of material swabbed or scraped from a mucous-membrane surface — e.g., the throat or the cervix — and spread on a glass slide for examination under a microscope, which may reveal the presence of abnormal cells or of infectious organisms.

The word is often used, too, in the term "blood smear" — a drop of blood placed on a slide and examined for cell type and morphology; it is part of the procedure called a complete blood count.

smell, sense of: At least partial loss of this sense is a familiar phenomenon in any situation involving inflammation of the nose; anyone who has had a cold knows the tasteless quality food assumes — really due to loss of the sense of smell, not of taste (which can detect only basics: sweetness, saltiness, sourness, and bitterness). But there are other, less obvious, things that can also cause such a loss, including a number of injuries, and afflictions involving the brain or nerves. If your child suffers a sudden loss of the sense of smell, and the reason isn't immediately apparent (as, a cold), you should consult your physician.

smoke inhalation: See GAS POISONING.

smoking: As everyone must know by now, the Surgeon General of the United States has established that smoking in general, and cigarette smoking in particular, is an extremely hazardous pursuit, and that there is a causal relationship between smoking and a variety of ills, including emphysema, heart disease, and cancer of the lungs (as well as other parts of the respiratory tract). It can also cause nicotine poisoning, a condition involving rapid pulse, dizziness, and nausea. If you smoke, you should make every effort to stop — and you shouldn't let your children take up the habit at all.

You should know, too, that smoking more than ten cigarettes a day while nursing has been associated with problems — and that smoking during pregnancy has been clearly implicated in the birth of babies abnormally low in weight.

snail fever: the popular name for schistosomiasis; see PARASITES.

snakebite: See the appropriate section under BITES AND STINGS.

sneezing: in older children, an involuntary reflex action resulting from any irritation of the nasal mucous membrane — by a cold, an allergen, or just something in the air. None of these things are necessarily true in an infant, though; infants sneeze a good deal simply to clear their noses, since they can't yet blow them as the rest of us can.

snoring: If a child's snoring is continual and chronic, it could be a symptom of enlarged adenoids; snoring that sets in suddenly, in a child who never snored before, is usually indicative of an infection in the upper part of the respiratory tract. In either case, it should be discussed with your doctor.

sodium bicarbonate: See ANTACIDS.

"soft spot": See FONTANEL.

Solacen: a trade name for tybamate, an anti-anxiety agent; see SEDATIVES.

Solar Cream, Solbar: See SUNSCREENS.

Soma: a trade name for carisoprodol, a muscle relaxant; see SEDATIVES.

soman: See PESTICIDES.

Sominex: an over-the-counter "sleep aid"; see SEDATIVES.

Somnafac: a trade name for the sleep-inducing drug methaqualone; see SEDATIVES.

Somnicaps: an over-the-counter "sleep aid"; see SEDATIVES.

Somnos: a trade name for chloral hydrate; see SEDATIVES.

Sonilyn: a trade name for sulfachlorpyridazine; see SULFA DRUGS.

sonography: See ULTRASONOGRAPHY.

Sopor: a trade name for the sleep-inducing drug methaqualone; see SEDATIVES.

sorbitol: See SWEETENERS.

sore throat: a general term covering any inflammation in the throat, or pharynx; the medical word for it is *pharyngitis.* The causes may range from a simple cold to infections of the larynx or tonsils to generalized infectious diseases. It may involve pain, coughing, and/or fever.

Any sore throat should be promptly reported to your doctor, along with other symptoms, such as cough (including the character of the cough), sneezing, headache, fever (take the child's temperature), or anything else, including the child's own description of how he feels and the color and appearance of the throat itself. The doctor should see the child as soon as possible (and will do so immediately if the symptoms are at all alarming); treatment may include cough medications, aspirin, and/or drugs to combat bacterial infection if it is present.

Acute pharyngitis, to a physician, is an infection of the throat itself, sometimes involving the tonsils and, in infants, the soft palate as well. It is quite painful; the child will find it hard to swallow, and an infant's cry may be disturbingly hoarse. The child may vomit and have fever — possibly as high as 104° F. (40° C.) — and the lymph nodes in the neck are often enlarged.

Consult the doctor promptly if you suspect this condition. The causative organism, viral or bacterial, must be identified, usually by throat culture. Once the doctor has made the diagnosis and prescribed medication if required, do what you can to make the child more comfortable; warm, nourishing fluids such as broths will help (the youngster won't want to swallow solid foods).

"*Strep throat*" is specifically an acute pharyngitis caused by streptococci, and is identical with scarlet fever except for the absence of a rash (the same group of bacteria are also responsible for a number of other infectious conditions). A strep throat can be accurately diagnosed only by an analysis of material taken from the throat; otherwise, the term is a misnomer.

If it is diagnosed, the doctor will treat it with antibiotics, usually penicillin or erythromycin, and you should keep the child at home for at least two days after treatment has started; any strep infection is highly contagious. Be sure, too, to see that the child receives the medication for *ten full days* — even if symptoms have disappeared.

See COUGHS for a discussion of medications to relieve them.

S.O.S.: See PRESCRIPTIONS.

Sparine: a trade name for promazine, a major tranquilizer; see SEDATIVES.

specialties, dental: Many dentists in general practice — all qualified dentists have either the D.D.S. or D.M.D. degree — also deal to some extent in the various specialties, depending upon their particular interests and abilities. Most dentists, in fact, perform simple extractions, take X rays, and treat some gum disorders.

Other dentists, however, have gone on through further training and experience to specialize in a certain area, problem, or type of service, and your own dentist may refer you or your child to one of them if it seems desirable. The specialties are as follows (the person who so specializes has a designation that ends in *-ist* — e.g., *periodontist* — except as otherwise specified):

Endodontics — disorders involving the nerves and other soft tissues within the teeth and related pathological conditions (also known as root-canal therapy)

Exodontics — extractions (an exodontist may also be an oral surgeon)

Oral surgery — more complex mouth surgery, including cysts, tumors, impacted teeth, and fractures of the jaw (the specialist is an oral surgeon)

Orthodontics — alignment and position of the teeth

Pedodontics — the treatment of children

Periodontics — problems involving the gums and other supporting structures

Prosthodontics — replacements such as bridges, crowns, and dentures

Radiodontics — diagnostic X ray

specialties, medical: Here, we list the areas of specialization currently officially recognized by the American Medical Association; physicians in these specialties may from time to time cooperate with your family doctor in caring for your child. (Often, now, your "regular" doctor may *be* a specialist, such as a family physician, a pediatrician in the case of your children, or an internist in the case of adult members of your family. These three are often referred to as "primary care" specialists.)

All of the people specializing in these areas have the degree of M.D. (Doctor of Medicine) or D.O. (Doctor of Osteopathy). They may offer—and it is desirable (from your point of view) that they do offer—substantiation of their expertise in their specialties in the form of certification by the appropriate bodies that testify to that expertise (see BOARDS). (Although the various specialty and subspecialty areas are supervised by M.D.s, D.O.s are permitted to take the qualifying examinations.)

The 22 specialties officially recognized as of this writing follow; their names correspond to those of the certifying boards. (We have not offered explanation where the listing is itself obvious. The term for the person pursuing a particular specialty ends in *-ist*—e.g., dermatologist or psychiatrist—unless otherwise specified.)

Allergy and Immunology—the entire area of the body's responses to—and problems caused by—challenge by foreign substances, including allergens, infectious organisms, and others

Anesthesiology—the administration of anesthesia and the maintenance of vital functions in emergency situations (surgical, traumatic, or other)

Colon and Rectal Surgery—(the specialist is of course a surgeon)

Dermatology—problems involving the skin, scalp, hair, and nails, both independently and in their relation to systemic illnesses

Family Practice—comprehensive primary care on a continuous basis—with attention to environmental and interpersonal as well as physiological factors—including all aspects of preventive medicine as well as coordination of other health services, including appropriate referrals to other specialists (the specialist is a family physician)

Internal Medicine—the diagnosis and (nonsurgical) treatment of systemic ills in adults (the specialist is an internist)

Since there are so many areas implicit in internal medicine that would lend themselves to full-time study, there have—understandably—developed a number of subspecialties (a certified subspecialist has previously been certified in the specialty). Nine of them, in fact, have been officially recognized. They are: Cardiovascular Disease, involving the heart and circulatory system; Endocrinology and Metabolism, basic biochemical phenomena; Gastroenterology, the gut; Hematology, the blood and blood-forming tissues; Infectious Disease; Medical Oncology, malignancies; Nephrology, the kidneys; Pulmonary Disease; and Rheumatology, connective-tissue and systemic disorders—including the various forms of arthritis—involving tissues in, around, or connected with the joints. Those specialists who have not subspecialized are sometimes said to practice *general* internal medicine.

Neurological Surgery—(the specialist is a neurosurgeon; also see Psychiatry and Neurology, this list)

Nuclear Medicine—the use of certain radioactive substances in diagnosis and therapy (the specialist is simply termed a specialist in nuclear medicine)

Obstetrics and Gynecology — pregnancy, childbirth, and all aspects of the female reproductive system and problems thereof (Physicians qualified in this area may choose, if they wish, to limit their practices; some — obstetricians — deal solely with pregnancy and childbirth, others on the contrary exclude that area and choose to treat only nonobstetrical patients.)

Ophthalmology — the eyes and all problems and disorders thereof

Orthopedic Surgery — the skeletal system and associated structures; a somewhat misleading specialty name, since the specialist — often referred to simply as an orthopedist — does not always perform surgery, but is as likely to employ various forms of physical therapy and/or other modes of treatment

Otolaryngology — the ears, nose, larynx, and upper respiratory tract in general (the individual is often referred to simply as an ENT — for ear, nose, and throat — specialist)

Pathology — the causes and development, including resulting functional and structural changes, of diseases and other abnormal conditions

Pediatrics — the growth and development, diseases and disorders, and general health of children (the specialist is a pediatrician, occasionally a pediatrist)

As is the case with internal medicine, a number of subspecialties are recognized, here six: Neonatal-Perinatal Medicine (see the definitions under NATAL); Pediatric Allergy; Pediatric Cardiology, heart malformation, malfunction, and disease; Pediatric Hematology-Oncology; Pediatric Nephrology; and Pediatric Urology. Here again, the pediatrician who is not a subspecialist is sometimes said to practice *general* pediatrics.

Physical Medicine and Rehabilitation — (the specialist is a physiatrist)

Plastic Surgery — (the specialist is a plastic surgeon)

Preventive Medicine — subdivided into four areas: Public Health, Aerospace Medicine, Occupational Medicine, and General Preventive Medicine (there are separate certifying examinations)

Psychiatry and Neurology — (the second area is the nervous system and disorders thereof)

These are two separate specialties (the Board includes representatives of both) but clearly overlap in part, with certain of the same basic knowledge required (parts of the examinations are in fact identical), so that a psychiatrist also has more than ordinary familiarity with the nervous system, and a neurologist has a degree of expertise in mental and emotional matters; some physicians are certified in both areas, but most choose one or the other. Each specialty also has a subspecialty and should your youngster require the services of either, you are likely to be referred to a pediatric (or child) psychiatrist or a pediatric (or child) neurologist.

Radiology — the diagnostic and therapeutic use of X rays and other forms of radiant energy

Surgery — treatment by operative procedure (as opposed to drugs, etc.), including the care of injuries; often, to distinguish it from certain other specialties, referred to as "general surgery." (The individual heading the emergency department of a hospital is usually a general surgeon. There is at this writing a movement afoot to designate "emergency medicine" as a separate specialty, dealing not only with accidental and other trauma but with initial treatment of all conditions of a sudden and critical nature.) The first certifying examinations in a new subspecialty, Pediatric Surgery, were given in 1975.

Thoracic Surgery — surgery involving structures within the chest

Urology — disorders of the urinary tract and of the genital organs in males

Also see, for others who may be involved to one degree or other in dealing with your child's physical or emotional problems, HEALTH PROFESSIONALS; INTERN; OPTICIAN; OPTOMETRIST; PHARMACIST; PSYCHOLOGIST; RESIDENT.

specimen: a sample — of urine, feces, blood, or sputum — taken from a patient for purposes of analysis. In some instances, a physician may ask you to bring such a sample with you when you come for an office visit. If the word "specimen" is used without further qualification, you may assume the doctor means a *urine* specimen (unless, of course, you have been discussing a specific question involving the stool); if the doctor wants a *stool* specimen, that will be specified (blood or sputum, of course, can easily be obtained at the doctor's office).

In either case, have the child urinate — or defecate, as the case may be — into a wide-mouthed jar or plastic container, and immediately put on an air-tight lid. Keep the urine refrigerated until you leave for the doctor's office.

An infant's stool sample can be on a soiled diaper; put the diaper in a plastic bag and close the bag securely. An older child's stool specimen may be easily obtained by filling the bowl with toilet paper, having the child defecate, and then removing a sample with a tongue depressor or a disposable utensil.

spectinomycin: See ANTIBIOTICS.

Spectrocin: a topical medication combining gramicidin and neomycin; see ANTIBIOTICS.

speculum: an instrument for enlarging the opening of a tract in order to examine the interior; the most familiar is the "duckbill" type, with two broad adjustable blades, used in examination of the vagina and cervix.

speech disabilities: What's a genuine disability, and what isn't, depends in part on a child's age — and sex. Girls, in general, learn to speak intelligibly earlier than boys do, just as they are toilet-trained earlier and develop earlier manual dexterity. We don't know why this is so; it just is. "In general," of course, means just that; there are plenty of exceptions to the rule.

At the age of two, most children can make themselves more or less understood by their own families; one in three, however, can't be comprehended readily by strangers. (If a child has *not* produced *any* intelligible words at all by the age of one year, you should arrange for a thorough examination. Don't assume there is retardation; the checkup may reveal a hearing problem — and it's important that it be discovered early.)

At three or four, stuttering or stammering is very common; generally, it means nothing more than that the child is in a hurry and can't keep up with his own thoughts. Don't make a fuss about it; in fact, if you ignore it, the child will outgrow it.

Additionally, a child coming from a home where a foreign language is spoken may have initial difficulties in pronouncing English sounds not found in the other language. A youngster from a Spanish-speaking home, for example, may have trouble with the short "i" sound in English, since the letter is pronounced "ee" in Spanish — and may for a time say "eet ees" for "it is." There is no "l" sound in Japanese. The French language has no "g" sound as in "George," or "ch" sound as in "chair." And so on. Generally these minor problems are quickly remedied by association with other youngsters. They should not, in our opinion, discourage you from having the child learn both languages; growing up bilingual cannot be other than an enriching experience.

By school age, most children have gradually developed good intelligibility, although there may be lingering difficulty with certain sounds (in general, consonant sounds are the last to be perfected). Nine out of ten seven-year-old girls and eight-year-old boys have achieved adult-level proficiency (remember we're talking about pronunciation, not vocabulary).

If a problem with speech persists beyond this age, it may require professional help — but don't leap to diagnostic conclusions. Among the causes of speech problems are hearing impairment, slight or severe (and some tonsil and adenoid problems can affect hearing); anatomical defects involving the teeth, tongue, or mouth structure (including temporary tooth gaps); disorders of the nervous system; respiratory problems; and emotional difficulties.

Don't get angry with a child who may have a speech problem, and don't overcriticize; do correct the youngster — patiently. If the problem persists — or if there is stuttering after the age of four or five — you should discuss it with your physician; the earlier it's dealt with, the better, whatever the cause.

speech therapist: See HEALTH PROFESSIONALS.

"speed": See AMPHETAMINES.

spermicides: See CONTRACEPTION.

sphenoid: See SINUSES.

sphincter: a ring of muscle that operates to open and close — or widen and narrow — a body passageway. Most passageways have them; there are, for example, a vaginal sphincter, an anal sphincter, a pyloric sphincter (between the stomach and the beginning of the small intestine) — and the lips might be called a kind of sphincter for the mouth.

sphygmomanometer: See BLOOD PRESSURE.

spider bite: See BITES AND STINGS.

spina bifida: a congenital defect involving incomplete formation or fusion of one or more vertebrae, the series of bones in the spine through which the spinal cord is threaded. Usually it occurs in the lower part of the back.

Often, the condition is so minor that it isn't noticed until — or unless — the child is X-rayed, perhaps years later, for some other reason. At this point, it's simply an interesting discovery for the doctor, and of no concern to you.

Only if there is an obvious deformity visible at birth, if fusion is so incomplete that the sheath of the spinal cord is unprotected, is there a real problem; in such a case, one or more specialists will be consulted as to the best mode of therapy.

Although spinal bifida is a familial condition, it is believed to be of multifactorial inheritance — i.e., resulting either from chance combination of a number of genes, or from interaction among several genes and unknown environmental factors. If you have had one child born with this defect, the statistical probability of your having a second with the same condition is quite low: no more than five percent, and possibly less.

spinal tap: the withdrawal of fluid from the spinal canal by insertion of a needle into the lower back, between the vertebrae; it's done if a physician judges it advisable as an aid in diagnosis. The fluid is analyzed for such characteristics as color, cell content, and so on (even as blood would be), and the findings may reveal to the doctor such things as the presence of infection or the seriousness of a head injury.

spirochete: See BACTERIA.

spitting up: See BURPING.

spleen: an organ in the upper left part of the abdomen, under the diaphragm. It functions in circulation and in the maintenance of normal blood volume: before birth, it manufactures blood cells; later, it mainly destroys old, worn-out blood cells but can also function as a blood-forming organ if necessary. Under certain circumstances, e.g., infection, it may become enlarged. The spleen may sometimes be removed, in case of injury or other circumstances in which it is judged advisable (the operation is called a *splenectomy*); there are no ill effects from the removal, and the body can adjust to the organ's absence.

splinters: How to handle them depends on how, and to what extent, they've penetrated the skin. Remember that you're not a physician; don't attempt any surgery, no matter how minor.

If the splinter's sticking out, remove it gently and carefully with tweezers, being sure to withdraw it along the same angle at which it entered. If you're not sure you've got it all out, take the child to the doctor. If you are certain it's out, simply cleanse the area with soap and water, and don't apply antiseptics or anything else; if it seems advisable to protect the site, put on an adhesive strip bandage.

If the splinter went in horizontally under the top layer of skin, so that it's entirely visible but not grabable, try soaking the foot (or whatever) in hot water — several times, in water as hot as the youngster can stand. This will often work the splinter to the surface, and you can then proceed as in the preceding paragraph. If the soaking doesn't do the trick, take the child to the doctor.

If the splinter is imbedded vertically, and not projecting above the surface of the skin, removal *must* be handled by a physician. And if it is very large, or very deeply imbedded, the injury is then a potentially serious puncture wound; the child should be taken to the doctor *immediately*.

Tiny splinters may be — and *should be* — left alone; with time and soaking, they will eventually work their way out.

splinting: See FRACTURES.

sponge: a word you may have heard used in connection with surgical operations. It is not, as you may have imagined, the sort of thing generally used in kitchen cleanups and car washing. Rather, it is simply something used to sponge away blood or other fluids, typically a piece of sterile gauze.

sports: Aside from directions you may receive from your physician regarding an individual child's participation in athletic activities generally or specifically, there is no harm in permitting a child of either sex to engage in any sport. That includes Little League baseball; athletic ability and potential are no different in prepubertal boys and girls — and girls of eight to twelve, in general, have reached a higher level of bone maturity than boys, thus are less subject to injury that may interfere with proper development. The only serious danger presented by competitive sports at this age is an emotional one, applicable to either sex: the possibility of parental overemphasis on winning (as opposed to the joy of playing the game) that places an excessive burden of responsibility on the child.

spotted fever: See TICK FEVER.

sprains: pulling or twisting injuries to connective tissues around a joint — ligaments, tendons, etc. — by overstraining or wrenching. The problem with sprains is that sometimes it's difficult for a lay person to tell the difference between this kind of injury and a broken bone. If you're in doubt about the nature of an injury to an ankle, knee, wrist, or elbow, assume a bone may be broken; see FRACTURES for what to do.

If an ankle or knee is involved, and you're reasonably sure there's no fracture, don't let the child try to walk. Have the youngster lie down with the affected leg elevated on pillows and, if the injury has just occurred, apply cold wet cloths for about an hour; if an hour or two has elapsed since the injury, make them *hot* wet cloths (or put the child in a hot bath) to reduce pain and swelling.

If it's a wrist or elbow, again apply cold if immediately following the injury, moist heat if time has elapsed — and put the arm in a sling.

If these measures effect no improvement after a few hours, and especially if the area has turned black and blue, there may be a minor fracture, and the child should be seen by a physician and X-rayed.

sprue: a fairly rare metabolic problem involving impaired absorption of fats; it occurs mostly, though not exclusively, in tropical areas. Typical symptoms include abdominal distension and cramps, diarrhea with a frothy stool, weakness, and weight loss; there may also be evidence of specific nutritional deficiency, since certain vitamins are fat-soluble.

Although symptoms are vaguely like those of cystic fibrosis or "celiac disease," sprue is not congenital, nor does it particularly afflict infants. Its cause is unknown. It is treated by various dietary measures, and usually also by supplementary water-soluble vitamins.

sputum: mucus and/or other matter spit out in illnesses involving the respiratory passages; analysis of it may reveal the presence of bacteria or other organisms causing the problem.

squinting: See NEARSIGHTEDNESS.

SSPE: short for subacute sclerosing panencephalitis, a progressive and invariably fatal disease of the central nervous system, also known as Dawson's encephalitis (it was first described by Dr. James Dawson of Vanderbilt University in 1933); it is commonly referred to simply by the initials. Its victims are children and young people, typically between the ages of five and twenty, 75 percent of them boys; there have been from thirty to fifty new U.S. cases reported annually in recent years, and it is believed that these figures represent fewer than half the actual number.

The illness strikes slowly and insidiously. Initial symptoms, appearing over a period of three to six months, include behavioral changes, irritability, restlessness, and forgetfulness; they are often first noted by teachers. As greater areas of the nervous system become involved, the muscles and sensory circuits are affected and the child stumbles and falls frequently, vision and speech deteriorate, convulsions occur, and finally, coma and death. There is no treatment.

Until the late 1960s, the cause of SSPE was a mystery. Now it is known that the villain is the measles virus; SSPE represents not an initial infection, but an apparent reactivation of viral activity in a child who has previously had measles, often before the age of two years. The average interval between the original infection and onset of SSPE is about six years. In the interim, the virus lies dormant or "smolders" both in the brain and in lymph tissues.

It is not known why or precisely how this phenomenon occurs so selectively (it is of course quite rare, and strikes only a tiny percentage of all children who have had measles — although the fact that it occurs at all is another good reason for vaccination). Nor has anyone explained SSPE's preference for boys — or its unusual prevalence in the Southeast, from which the majority of cases have been reported. Some have speculated that there is a "trigger" necessary, an environmental factor — perhaps an encounter with another pathogen — that "awakens" the virus; one study found an unusually high incidence, among a group of SSPE patients, of contact with dogs suffering from distemper.

Research on SSPE continues, within the context of a group of neurological conditions in which a "slow virus" etiology is known or suspected. The majority of them affect only older people or are practically unknown in this country, hence have not been included in this book; for one that is of great interest, see MULTIPLE SCLEROSIS.

stab wounds: See PUNCTURE WOUNDS.

staging: determination of the extent of involvement (areas and organs) in a disease process, especially in a disseminated malignant disease; see LYMPHOMA.

stammering: See SPEECH DISABILITIES.

stannous fluoride: See CAVITIES.

Staphcillin: a trade name for methicillin, a semisynthetic penicillin; see ANTIBIOTICS.

staph infections: various infectious conditions that may be caused by a number of different strains of staphylococci; some are trivial, others quite serious. You may have read that staph infections are always a threat in hospitals, and patients are carefully guarded against such infections, since the bacteria found in a hospital are likely to be especially virulent. But this particular type of organism is normally found just about everywhere, including in the air and on everyone's skin.

Sometimes staph infections involve only the skin; boils and impetigo are examples. But *internal* staph infections can be critical — if, for example, the bacteria enter the lungs, the nervous system, or the bloodstream via an unhealed wound. Whatever the area involved, treatment requires antibiotics; the organism should be tested in the laboratory to determine its sensitivity to various antibiotics.

starches: part of the carbohydrates; see NUTRITION and SWEETENERS.

stat.: See PRESCRIPTIONS.

steatorrhea: a descriptive term meaning the presence of fatty material in the stool; it may be a symptom of pancreatic disorder or of various conditions involving fat digestion.

Steclin: a trade name for tetracycline; see ANTIBIOTICS.

Stelazine: a trade name for trifluoperazine, a potent tranquilizer; see SEDATIVES.

stenosis: constriction or narrowing of a passageway; it may be negligible or quite serious, depending upon the passageway involved and the degree of constriction.

For examples, see PULMONARY STENOSIS; PYLORIC STENOSIS; STENOSIS OF THE ANUS; STENOSIS OF THE ESOPHAGUS; TEARDUCT STENOSIS.

stenosis of the anus: an uncommon congenital defect in which the anus, the rectal exit through which fecal matter is excreted, is abnormally narrow. It may or may not require treatment; if the child can have a reasonably normal bowel movement, there is generally no cause for concern (most babies, incidentally, strain in producing a perfectly normal stool, and such straining is not necessarily evidence of stenosis). If necessary, the condition can be corrected by various methods, and it is up to the physician to decide whether, and how.

stenosis of the esophagus: a narrowing of the food passageway between the throat and stomach; it may be a congenital defect, or it may be caused by injury — as, burns with subsequent formation of scar tissue resulting from swallowing a caustic poison. The condition is usually corrected by surgery.

Stental: a trade name for phenobarbital; see SEDATIVES.

sterilization: See CONTRACEPTION. For discussion of sterilizing feeding equipment, see BOTTLE FEEDING.

sternum: the anatomical term for the breastbone, the bone at the center of the chest below the collarbone, to which the ribs are attached.

steroids: technically, a large group of substances — mainly, though not exclusively, hormones — having similar chemical structure. Usually, however, when the term is used without further qualification, the reference is to specific adrenal hormones; see CORTICOSTEROIDS.

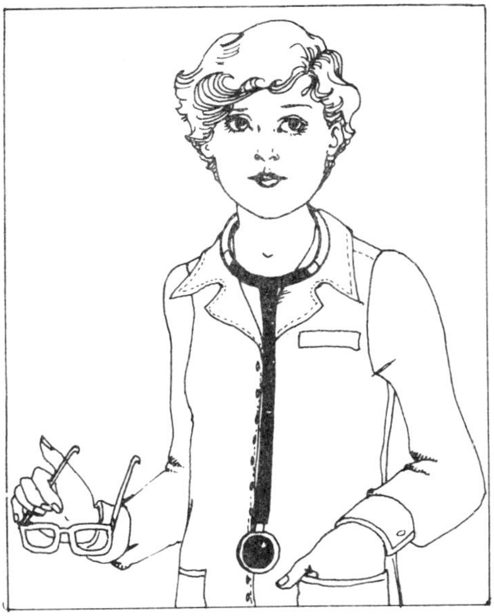

Physician Wearing a Stethoscope

stethoscope: that device doctors always have dangling from their necks; it's an instrument that conducts, and sometimes amplifies, sounds — of the heartbeat, the lungs, and so on — within the body, and serves the doctor as a diagnostic aid. When a woman is pregnant, her obstetrician can apply it to her abdomen and hear the heartbeat of her baby-to-be.

stiffness: This is a common, and predictable, result of unaccustomed muscular exertion, and nothing to worry about if there has been such exertion. A good hot bath before bedtime can sometimes prevent — or at least mitigate — the stiffness, which is usually a morning-after phenomenon.

If there's no apparent explanation for stiffness, *or* it doesn't depart after a day of rest, *or* there are other symptoms such as fever — the child should be seen by a physician.

Still's disease: See ARTHRITIS.

stings: See BITES AND STINGS.

stomach ache: See ABDOMINAL PAIN.

stomach virus: See INTESTINAL FLU.

stomatitis: an inflammation of the mouth, usually including the gums, and sometimes (there are various types) the lips, tongue, and throat as well; the causes vary and may include diet deficiencies, allergies, and certain kinds of poisoning, but generally the culprit is an infection, either bacterial or viral.

The mouth — and whatever specific areas are affected — is quite sore, and it is painful to eat and drink. There may or may not be fever; if there is, it can sometimes be high. The worst of the illness is usually over in four to six days, although complete healing takes about two weeks.

If you suspect stomatitis, see the doctor — who must diagnose the condition, and also determine the cause, in order to treat it properly. Pain relievers, local or systemic, are part of treatment; there may also be drugs given to combat infection (if it's bacterial).

Your doctor will tell you what else you should do. Despite the fact that it's hard for the child to swallow, it's important to see that enough fluids are taken to prevent dehydration. If the child's running a high fever and absolutely won't take any water, call the doctor promptly; special measures will have to be taken.

stool: the feces resulting from a single movement of the bowels. The appearance of a child's stool can be quite important in diagnosing a number of problems — its consistency, color, content (undigested food, blood, mucus, or whatever), and odor. If your child has a stool that seems unusual to you, save it for examination by the doctor; put it in a wide-mouthed jar or plastic container, or simply toss the dirty diaper into a plastic bag, and take it with you when you take the child to the doctor — as you should, if an unusual stool is coupled with other symptoms of illness.

Do remember, though, that it's normal for the character of an infant's stool to change when you change the baby's diet. And that color fed to a child is likely to turn up in the stool — red from beets, a greenish tinge from green vegetables, and so on. In general, if the youngster feels and acts perfectly well, there's nothing to be concerned about.

"STP": See PSYCHEDELICS.

strabismus: the medical term for a lack of focal parallelism in vision; it may take a number of forms, but the most familiar example is crossed eyes.

strangulation: If you've turned to this listing because there's been a forcible choking-off of breath in the child's windpipe, follow the instructions under HANGING, EMERGENCY PROCEDURE FOR. If something is stuck in the child's throat, see CHOKING.

The word also means a cutting-off of the blood supply to herniated tissue, and this too is a serious emergency; see HERNIA.

strawberry marks: See BIRTHMARKS.

Streptococcus: a genus of bacteria known to cause a number of infectious conditions ranging from nasty to critical. See ERYSIPELAS; IMPETIGO; RHEUMATIC FEVER; SCARLET FEVER; SORE THROAT.

streptomycin: See ANTIBIOTICS.

stridor: a narrowing of the trachea, or windpipe, usually characterized by loud, harsh breathing; the condition may be congenital or may happen later.

Congenital stridor, which is a temporary condition and needs no special treatment, results from a problem with the epiglottis, the elastic cartilage that closes off the windpipe during swallowing, but should snap back and permit free passage of air under other conditions. In some babies, for some reason, the cartilage is not as well developed and tends to flop (that's the only way to describe it), thus narrowing the passage somewhat. The condition isn't dangerous; the infant won't smother. The problem will gradually right itself by the time the child's about a year old.

Stridor can also occur as a result of some acquired obstruction — an infection of some sort, or the swallowing of a foreign body; such situations, of course, need prompt medical attention.

student nurse: See HEALTH PROFESSIONALS.

stuffy nose: See ALLERGY and COLDS for the most common causes of nasal stuffiness — and don't use nose drops or sprays unless your doctor specifically recommends them (the reasons for this warning are spelled out under DECONGESTANTS, NASAL).

A very small child may have a stuffy nose simply because he hasn't yet learned to blow it; if the environment is dry, mucus that's normally sneezed out dries and forms crusts that obstruct the youngster's nostrils — thus causing him to breathe harshly and with difficulty, or to resort to mouth breathing. It's a good idea to teach nose blowing as early as possible; the child who can learn it at the age of one year is extremely rare, but you should start trying to teach the technique by the age of two. (Many children, however, resist blowing their noses for many years, and there's not much you can do about it.)

stuttering: See SPEECH DISABILITIES.

stye: an infection at the root of an eyelash, appearing like a small pimple on the outer edge of the lid (it can be the upper or lower lid). If there's just one, and it's not gigantic, you needn't take the child to the doctor — and don't do anything yourself, except apply warm, wet compresses every three or four hours, if possible. Like a pimple, the stye will eventually come to a "head" (it will get yellow in the center) and go away.

If the stye is very big, though, or if there are more than one, do have the doctor look at the situation. And if the youngster gets styes frequently, discuss that with your physician, too.

For descriptions of other eyelid conditions, requiring different handling, see BLEPHARITIS; CHALAZION; CONJUNCTIVITIS; TEARDUCT STENOSIS; TRACHOMA.

subacute sclerosing panencephalitis: See SSPE.

subclinical: describing an infection insufficient to cause symptoms. The word may refer to the incubation period, or may denote an atypical instance of infection in which symptoms simply do not appear (or are so mild as to remain unrecognized).

subcutaneous: just under the skin, between the skin and the muscle beneath. The word may be used to describe a condition (as, "subcutaneous bleeding"), or the method of injecting something (some injections are given this way, others into muscle, still others directly into a blood vessel, depending upon the nature and purpose of the injection).

Sublimaze: a trade name for fentanyl, a morphinelike synthetic drug; see NARCOTICS.

Sucaryl: a trade name for a liquid solution of saccharin; see SWEETENERS.

succinimides: a class of antiseizure medications; see EPILEPSY.

sucrose: See SWEETENERS.

sudden infant death syndrome: a descriptive phrase for a condition of unknown cause in which an apparently healthy infant under the age of one year — typically, between the ages of two and five months — dies suddenly and unexpectedly, almost invariably while sleeping; it is also known, for the latter reason, as "crib death" (in Great Britain, where a crib is called a "cot," the phenomenon is termed "cot death").

Despite many years of research, the cause of crib death remains a mystery.

Aside from the foregoing, a number of facts are known:

• the phenomenon occurs all over the world, striking two or three of every thousand babies born and accounting for half of all infant deaths (the annual U.S. toll is eight to ten thousand);

• there is a seasonal pattern: the deaths are concentrated in the colder months;

• the infants do not suffocate, nor do they choke on food or other substances;

• a number of possible causes, including allergy and nutritional deficiency, have been ruled out;

• the deaths are eerily silent: the infants do not cry out or otherwise indicate pain or distress.

Needless to say, crib death does not result from any known failure, of commission or omission, on the part of the parents; the infant victims have all appeared happy, well-nourished and thriving, in many cases within hours — or even moments — of their sudden demise. Nor should parents who have experienced this tragic loss blame themselves for any lack of alertness; as we've mentioned, there is no cry or other warning.

A number of theories are presently being pursued in an effort to find the cause of — and thus, it is hoped, to prevent — crib death. Many feel the culprit may be an as yet unidentified infectious agent, one to which, for some reason, only young infants are susceptible. Some have speculated that crib death may represent an unusual response to one or more common, widespread organisms, such as common-cold viruses. Others are centering their investigations on the strange silence of crib death, postulating some event that simultaneously cuts off breath and prevents the infant from crying out. Still others believe that crib death will be traced to some congenital impairment of the heart or respiratory system.

Parents and other interested readers may wish to seek help and advice from, and/or lend support to, two nonprofit organizations concerned with aiding parents, informing the public, and furthering both publicly and privately supported research. They are: National Foundation for Sudden Infant Death, 1501 Broadway, New York NY 10036; and International Guild for Infant Survival, 6822 Brompton Road, Baltimore MD 21207.

suffocation: See, for first-aid procedures (depending upon the nature of the problem), CHOKING; GAS POISONING.

A child's deliberately holding his breath is *not* a cause for alarm, and he will *not* suffocate; see BREATH-HOLDING.

sugar in urine: a condition determined by urinalysis; it is usually — but not always — a signal of diabetes mellitus.

sugars: See SWEETENERS.

Sugracillin: a trade name for penicillin G; see ANTIBIOTICS.

sulfa drugs: a group of chemically related drugs, first developed in the 1930s, also known as sulfonamides. They are not bactericidal, but bacteriostatic; that is, they do not kill bacteria, but halt bacterial growth and multiplication. Sulfa drugs are effective against many things including a number of streptococcal infections and are especially useful in certain urinary and intestinal infections, although in many instances, they have been replaced by bactericidal antibiotics.

Among those currently in use are mafenide (Sulfamylon), salicylazosulfapyridine (Azulfidine), sulfacetamide, sulfachlorpyridazine (Sonilyn), sulfadiazine (Coco-Diazine), sulfadimethoxine (Madribon), sulfameter (Sulla), sulfamethizole (Thiosulfil), sulfamethoxazole (Gantanol), sulfamethoxypyridazine (Midicel), sulfisoxazole (Gantrisin), and a number of combinations of two or more such agents marketed under a variety of trade names; Azo Gantanol and Azo Gantrisin contain, in addition to the sulfa drug, a special urinary-tract analgesic to relieve pain and burning.

Allergic reactions to sulfa drugs are not uncommon, and some can be serious. If your youngster is taking any of them, *stop* the medication, and consult the doctor immediately, if any of the following develop: a rash, whether or not accompanied by itching and/or fever; other skin manifestations such as redness or scaling; nausea or vomiting; headache, dizziness, lethargy, or odd behavior.

Sulla: a trade name for sulfameter, a sulfa drug; see the immediately preceding entry.

"summer diarrhea": a dangerously misleading term that has been used by health authorities in some tourism-promoting nations to describe possibly serious endemic ailments that might well deter travelers, were their real nature known. The malady in question may indeed be a minor problem of intestinal adjustment to unfamiliar foods; it may, on the other hand, be something as major as dysentery, or even cholera. If you hear such a phrase in connection with a country you intend to visit, have a talk with your doctor about immunizations, or even a change of plans.

Sumycin: a trade name for tetracycline; see ANTIBIOTICS.

sunburn: It is, as we're sure you'll agree, best avoided. So we're going to talk about precautions and preventives first, before we discuss after-the-fact remedies. And do bear in mind that *anyone,* no matter how dark the skin, can under certain circumstances get a painful sunburn.

The noon sun — which includes a two-hour period on either side of noon itself — is by far the most dangerous; the higher the sun in the sky, the more intense its rays. A haze or overcast doesn't diminish this effect. And place as well as time is pertinent; any situation in which glare is reflected — snow, beach, water — increases the effect.

Infants should be exposed to direct sunlight for no more than five or ten minutes to start, and never during that dangerous noon period. A child with very light hair and eyes should be kept out of direct sunlight entirely until the age of a year or two; eye color is in fact a better clue to sunburn susceptibility than hair color — although redheads are quite susceptible whatever the color of their eyes.

After that age, you should still be extremely careful in exposing small children to the sun; those pale susceptibles shouldn't be exposed to high-noon sun at any time. Always take cover-ups along when you take a toddler to a beach — and again, whatever the child's coloring, try to avoid the noon period.

If a child — of any age — is taking medication of any kind, check with the doctor who prescribed it before you let the child out in the sun. Certain drugs — especially sulfa drugs and tetracyclines — have a tendency to increase photosensitivity.

Sunscreens are also helpful. See the entry following this one for a discussion of types, what's best to use — and, as important, what *not* to use.

What if this advice has come too late, and you've a sunburned youngster on your hands? How to cope depends upon the nature of the burn, plus the presence or absence of other symptoms. *Don't* apply any of those widely advertised sprays and other over-the-counter "remedies"; with few exceptions, they are multiple-ingredient products, and some of those ingredients are not only ineffective but may well aggravate matters.

Do remember that a sunburn is a burn — usually a first-degree or fairly mild one, but nevertheless a burn. First aid for a first-degree burn is coolness — cool compresses if one or two areas are involved, a cool bath or shower if it's an all-over sunburn; this will both draw out the heat and simultaneously numb the painful area. Then, after gently patting dry, you might apply (if the skin can be touched without pain) a simple emollient — meaning plain petroleum jelly, or a dry-skin lotion such as Alpha-Keri or Lubriderm — that will keep the skin soft and relieve tautness.

Sometimes even a first-degree sunburn is accompanied by chills or fever. Again, stick to simple measures. An older child or teenager can be given aspirin and, if the youngster feels up to it, warm, nourishing liquid such as broth. Sometimes about twenty minutes in a lukewarm bath can be helpful, too, in reducing fever. If these measures fail to effect any improvement, or if the feverish child is an infant or toddler, consult your physician before doing anything at all.

Any sunburn that goes beyond the first degree — i.e., if there is swelling, blistering, marked discoloration, broken skin, or any sort of eruption — in a child of any age calls for medical consultation; don't do anything without your doctor's advice.

Also see, for discussion of related problems, HEAT EXHAUSTION; HEAT RASH; HEAT STROKE.

sunscreens: Many products promise protection from the sun's ill effects, often along with a claim that the user will enjoy a "glowing" or otherwise attractive tan. Sometimes these promotional statements are true; frequently, they are not. It is vital to read the small print on the labels.

Unless there are other key phrases, "promotes tan" does not denote a product that offers protection. Nor should oil — baby oil or any other — ever be employed for this purpose; oil, remember, is used for frying. (The same applies to "butters" containing a variety of oils.)

If you have teenagers, they may be interested in the products, developed in recent years, that create an instant "chemical tan." Some tend in our opinion to produce somewhat inferior-looking tans — but esthetic considerations aside, they're perfectly safe. With just three precautions. They should never be applied to broken skin. They should not be used by anyone who has diabetes; they contain a chemical, dihydroxyacetone, that can affect the blood-sugar level. And it should be borne in mind that the tan they create is not a protection against sunburn, as is a naturally acquired tan; some protection must be employed until a natural tan has developed (some such products combine the chemical tanner with a protective agent).

There are two basic types of protective agents.

One is a sun block, a substance that is completely opaque, totally blocking light rays; this is the sort of protection you have perhaps seen on the noses of lifeguards. These *physical* sunscreens contain, typically, either zinc oxide or titanium dioxide.

The second type is a *chemical* sunscreen that works by filtering out certain rays of the sun's spectrum, those likely to cause burning; with continued use over a period of time, they will protect against burns while permitting the slow, gradual acquisition of some tan. The most effective such agent is para-aminobenzoic acid (often called PABA for short); also quite effective are padimate and glyceryl para-aminobenzoate. A group of chemicals called benzophenones — which include dioxybenzone, oxybenzone, and sulisobenzone — rate a little lower because they tend to be more readily removed by perspiration and swimming. (But actually, any sunscreen should be reapplied periodically and *always* after swimming.)

Products containing one or another of these six agents — others may appear from time to time, and now you know what to look for — include A-Fil, Block Out, Pabafilm, Pabanol, PreSun, Solar Cream (also contains titanium dioxide), Solbar, Sungard, and Uval.

sunstroke: See HEAT STROKE.

superior: anatomically, not "better," but above — in the direction of the head; the opposite of *inferior.*

suppositories: medications made to be inserted into the rectum or vagina rather than taken by mouth — either because the patient is unable to take medicine by mouth, or because the particular medication is meant to act in the rectal or vaginal area. *Never* give a child a suppository (or use one yourself, for that matter) unless it's on the specific advice of a physician.

Suppositories are designed to melt once they get inside, and room heat can affect them as well. If your doctor does prescribe a suppository, it should be stored in the refrigerator. Remove it from the refrigerator one hour before the scheduled insertion; it won't melt in that length of time, but will soften sufficiently so that it will be absorbed quickly once it gets inside the body. And do remember to remove the foil wrapping before you insert it!

If your child should swallow a suppository, call your doctor. Whether you should ignore it or do something about it depends upon the medication involved.

Sure-Sleep: an over-the-counter "sleep aid"; see SEDATIVES.

surgeon: See SPECIALTIES, MEDICAL.

Surgitube: See BANDAGES.

swallowing: Pain or difficulty in swallowing can be a symptom of many different things, ranging from various obstructions to sore throats to specific infectious diseases. If this occurs, talk to the child and see if anything else hurts, check for any other symptoms such as rashes, take the child's temperature, and call the doctor.

If your child has swallowed "the wrong way," or has swallowed a foreign object — whether or *not* it seems to be bothering him — turn to CHOKING.

swayback: an extreme arch, or curvature, of the spine; the medical term for it is *lordosis*. The immediate cause of the visible condition is an extreme forward curve of the lower part of the spine. It may be congenital or develop later, sometimes associated with substantial overweight, and sometimes connected with disease or malfunction of the hip joints. Treatment, if any, depends upon the judgment of your personal physician or an orthopedist.

Temporary "swayback" is perfectly normal when a child is first learning to walk; it takes time to achieve the muscular control necessary to hold the back erect, and that tends to develop after mastery of walking.

sweeteners: They fall into two categories: (1) naturally occurring substances — various sugars — and (2) synthetic substances, generally intended for substitution in the diets of those endeavoring to lose weight or who are advised for other reasons (e.g., diabetes mellitus) to limit their intake of carbohydrates. The latter reason is probably the only good one; a whole tablespoon of granulated sugar — perhaps three times as much as one would put into a cup of coffee — contains as many calories as a tomato, a tangerine, or less than one ounce of canned salmon. And there are unresolved questions concerning the safety of extensive use of the substitutes. But judge for yourself. Here are the facts about the two classes.

NATURAL SWEETENERS

Some form of carbohydrate occurs in all plant foods and is also present in milk, human and other. Carbohydrates are the energy sources in our diets (see NUTRITION); whatever form they come in, our bodies break them down into the only form that's usable, a sugar — more accurately (since "sugar" is what we usually think of as coming in a box or bag), a monosaccharide — called glucose.

There are a host of substances classified chemically as sugars or saccharides; you are likely to hear of only a few, those that play major parts in the human diet.

Monosaccharides are simple sugars that are used by the body without a great deal of chemical effort. One, as we've said, is glucose, which is also known as dextrose; it is the one form the body can use instantly, and you have doubtless encountered it in the form of corn syrup (which is essentially a concentrated solution of pure glucose, produced by combining cornstarch and water and breaking down the former by chemical processing). A second is fructose (a prime source, as you might suppose, is fruit), also called levulose, and the third is galactose; both fructose and galactose are converted to glucose in the body.

Disaccharides are substances in which two units of a simple sugar, or one each of two simple sugars, are chemically bonded; breaking that chemical bond requires an extra step in digestion, but not much extra time (unless there is a metabolic deficiency). Again, there are three that are really important. One is sucrose, which is table sugar, a combination of glucose and fructose; its breakdown requires an enzyme called sucrase. The second is maltose, a double glucose; the enzyme required here is maltase. The third is lactose, the form in which sugar occurs in milk, combining glucose and galactose; its use requires an enzyme called lactase, and people who have a lack of — or deficiency in — this enzyme may have difficulty digesting milk. (It should be noted that temporary deficiencies of these enzymes can occur, in some people, following intestinal ills — so that attempts to cope with double sugars, or disaccharides, at those times can cause additional discomfort.)

Polysaccharides are starches plus cellulose and pectin; the body can't digest the last two at all, unless they are previously broken down by cooking or other processing. Starch is stored by plants, prominently in their roots (e.g., potatoes) and seeds (e.g., corn). In our bodies, it's broken down to maltose and then to glucose and stored in the liver in a form called glycogen, to be drawn upon for energy when needed. (A vital substance called insulin plays a role at this stage; for what can go wrong when there is a lack of it, see DIABETES MELLITUS.)

Thus, a monosaccharide gets into the bloodstream very quickly — which is desirable if energy is needed quickly or if a diabetic is slipping into insulin shock; it is not desirable for a diabetic under other circumstances (and we trust the foregoing will explain why diabetics should restrict their intake of carbohydrates generally). The speed with which a carbohydrate is broken down and finds its way to the bloodstream depends in some part, too, upon the structure of the source: a liquid (e.g., orange juice) moves through the gastrointestinal tract much more quickly than a fibrous fruit such as an apple.

There are some natural substances we haven't mentioned. Honey, for one. We trust that despite a number of incredible tales that have appeared in print over the last few years, you realize that neither honey, honey combined with vinegar, nor honey combined with anything else can possibly cure chronic ills such as arthritis. Honey, like ordinary sugar, is simply a combination of glucose and fructose — except that the two are simply mixed rather than chemically connected; its only advantage — aside from its taste, which some people prefer — is that the enzyme needed to cope with table sugar isn't required for honey. Tablespoon for tablespoon, honey has more calories than ordinary table sugar (65 versus 40) and also more carbohydrates (17 grams versus 11 grams).

And what of other kinds of sugar — brown, "raw," and the rest? *Brown sugar* is less refined than white, has a different flavor because of trace minerals and a thin layer of syrup, has about 12 percent more calories and a tiny bit more carbohydrate measure for measure, and contains a little calcium (white sugar has none) and a smidgen of iron. ("Brownulated" sugar is the same thing in aggregate-crystal granules.) *Powdered sugar* is refined sugar that has been fine-ground into powdered form. *"Raw" sugar* is not really that, since real raw sugar is impure and not fit to eat; the "raw" sugar sold in some stores is sucrose with traces of cane fiber or beet pulp included to give it a different taste and texture, and chiefly benefits its manufacturers, since it is very expensive. *Colored crystalline sugar* is also sucrose in more expensive form.

SUGAR SUBSTITUTES

The whole subject of substitute sweeteners has been very much up in the air, and very hotly argued, for a number of years and remains so at this writing. We shall therefore be brief and must warn the reader that the status of the various agents may yet continue to change. There are, at this time, five that have been developed in liquid and/or crystalline form and/or incorporated in soft drinks and other processed foods.

Aspartame (Equa) was approved by the Food and Drug Administration in mid-1974 for sale in tablet and packet form and as a sugar-substitute sweetener in breakfast cereals, chewing gum, and instant-mix beverages, coffee and tea, toppings and puddings. Said to be 180 times as sweet tasting as sugar, aspartame contains the same number of calories as sugar (but obviously far less is required to attain the same degree of sweetness). It is made from two amino acids, aspartic acid and phenylalanine — the latter, extremely dangerous for children with PKU whose intake of this substance must be restricted (see PHENYLKETONURIA); if and when the product becomes generally available (wide marketing was postponed in mid-1975 pending results of safety studies on aspartic acid), labels will doubtless carry a warning to that effect.

Cyclamates (sodium cyclamate and calcium cyclamate), noncaloric sweeteners first marketed in the 1950s, were banned by the FDA, amid a great deal of controversy, in late 1969. About thirty times as sweet in taste, measure for measure, as sugar, cyclamates had over the years been incorporated in many products — notably, soft drinks — and had found great favor with consumers because of a lack of the somewhat bitter aftertaste that some had found with saccharin, the only other artificial sweetener that had been available for table use. During the middle and late 1960s, however, a number of studies had detected ill effects in experimental animals — including growth impairment and some birth defects — and there was some suggestion that the substances might be detrimental to certain people's blood pressure. Animal experiments had the greatest impact on both public and government; the ban resulted after bladder tumors in laboratory rodents fed massive quantities were confirmed in controlled studies. Evaluation of these substances continues, and in 1976 the FDA agreed to reconsider the ban following a report from the National Cancer Institute concluding that cyclamates probably do not cause malignancies in humans.

Mannitol, a sweetener about two-thirds as sweet as sugar (thus not practical for table use), is a naturally occurring substance; it's extracted from seaweed and other sources for use in a number of products — especially sugarless chewing gum. It also acts as a moisture-absorbing agent to prevent the gum from getting sticky; and although it is caloric, it is poorly absorbed by the human body and little utilized by bacteria in the mouth (which do use sugar and thus contribute to tooth decay).

Saccharin, a synthetic coal-tar derivative, has been available since the turn of the century as an artificial sweetener; it is about three hundred times as sweet as sugar, and is both incorporated in commercially produced foods and sold in the form of tablets and liquid (Sucaryl) for home use. The bitter taste we referred to earlier has been countered to some extent by the addition of small amounts of other substances. By 1972, however, studies had suggested that saccharin, like the cyclamates, may be carcinogenic; that year, it was removed from the FDA's GRAS (Generally Recognized As Safe) list and limits on the amount of saccharin included in packaged foods — as well as content-revealing labels — were mandated. Since that time, the National Academy of Sciences has been encouraging further research; saccharin may be (a) returned to the GRAS list, (b) restricted to use as a drug rather than a food additive, (c) banned, or (d) meet some other fate. The last might include specific recommendations as to safe use. In the meantime, the FDA suggests limiting per-day maximum consumption to fifteen milligrams per kilogram of body weight — which means, in a 125-lb (56.75-kg) person, some 851.25 mg, or the amount typically found in seven twelve-ounce bottles of a saccharin-sweetened soft drink. Saccharin crosses the placenta and should not be used by pregnant women.

Sorbitol, like mannitol, is a calorie-containing saccharide; it is obtained from a number of berries and other fruits, and is eventually converted to glucose, but has the peculiar property of being digested far more slowly than sugar. It is about two-thirds as sweet as sugar. It is thus useful for diabetics, but not designed to restrict calories. Like mannitol, it is of little use to mouth bacteria, and thus also plays a role in chewing gums designed to avoid cavities by eliminating sugar. There is little question about sorbitol's safety, although some investigators believe it may, in sufficient quantities, alter the absorption rates of some medications.

swelling: This is one of those symptoms that — like fever and pain — can signify a great many different things. Among them are abnormal cell growth, fluid accumulation, infection, allergic reactions, toxic effects of various substances, and severe injuries such as dislocations or fractures.

If swelling is connected with a specific accident or mishap, or you suspect a fracture, turn to that listing.

Any *unexplained* swelling means you should call the doctor *immediately;* you should do so especially fast if the swelling is in the abdomen — and *don't poke.*

swimmer's ear: a popular term for an infection in the outer ear acquired via swimming, medically termed *otitis externa;* see OTITIS.

swollen "glands": See LYMPH NODES.

Sydenham's chorea: See CHOREA.

sympathetic nerves: See NERVOUS SYSTEM.

symptom: a pain, or other departure from the norm, as experienced by a patient. It may or may not be evident to an observer; a limp would be, but a pain wouldn't. (For comparison, see SIGN.)

Symptomatic may mean two different things, depending upon how it's used. It may mean "indicative," as in, "A rash may be symptomatic of an allergy." Or, you may hear it in the phrase *symptomatic treatment,* which means treatment — as in many viral ills — that is given only to relieve symptoms, often the case when there is no specific treatment available.

Syncillin: a trade name for phenethicillin, a semisynthetic penicillin; see ANTIBIOTICS.

syncope: the medical term for a transitory loss of consciousness; most people call it fainting.

Vasovagal syncope is a not uncommon condition in children. It is characterized by fainting that is often brought on by a combination of physical and emotional stresses (as, anxiety plus heat plus hunger), and is marked by a drop in blood pressure and extreme slowing of the pulse (which may not be felt at *all* for a few seconds). Sometimes there is brief convulsion, and youngsters subject to this problem have often been misdiagnosed as epileptic and given medications and restrictions that are entirely inappropriate.

Very frequently, a youngster can control the condition, with a little practice. Fainting is caused — the precise mechanism is not fully understood — by a vascular-neural phenomenon. A child who feels such an attack coming on (and there is often an awareness) may be able to ward it off by a deliberate mental effort; "think angry" is, basically, the guide.

syndrome: a medical term with two somewhat different meanings.

It may refer to a group of symptoms and signs characteristic of a certain condition; such a group is often given the name of the physician or other researcher who first noted and described the condition — as, for example, Down's syndrome, also known as mongolism.

Or, a doctor might remark, "This is the usual mononucleosis (or hay fever, or chickenpox, or whatever) syndrome" — meaning that symptoms and signs displayed in the condition are typical ones, not peculiar to the individual patient.

synergism: a phenomenon in which the effects of two or more drugs taken simultaneously are greater than might be expected by simple addition — i.e., the whole is greater than the sum of its parts. Among substances known to have synergistic interactions and effects when combined are alcohol and almost any sedative or tranquilizer, which is why innocuous quantities of each, when taken together, have sometimes proved lethal.

synovitis: inflammation of the synovial membrane (also known as the *synovium*), the membrane lining a movable joint, which secretes lubricating fluid.

Syntetrin: a trade name for nolitetracycline, one of the tetracyclines; see ANTIBIOTICS.

syphilis: See VENEREAL DISEASES.

systemic: spread through, or affecting, the entire body; the opposite of *localized.* The word may apply to an ailment (as, "a systemic infection"), or to a medication which is given in such a way (as, by injection or by mouth) so as to spread through the body — as opposed to a medication that may be applied, for example, by swabbing it onto the skin (which is called *topical application*).

systemic lupus erythematosus: See LUPUS.

systolic: See BLOOD PRESSURE.

T

tachycardia: a pulse rate markedly above normal (the first part of the word comes from the Greek *tachos*, "speed"). Many things, including fever, excitement, and certain thyroid problems, can increase the pulse rate, and tachycardia does not necessarily suggest any cardiac dysfunction; sometimes, indeed, no cause whatever can be found. But a physician noting this phenomenon will generally wish to check further.

talking: See DEVELOPMENT; SPEECH DISABILITIES.

talus: the anatomical term for the ankle bone.

Talwin: a trade name for pentazocine, a potent analgesic; see NARCOTICS.

Tandearil: a trade name for oxyphenbutazone; see ANTI-INFLAMMATORIES.

tantrums: See TEMPER TANTRUMS.

tapeworms: See WORMS.

tarsus: the group of seven bones forming a connection between the talus and the metatarsals that form the arch of the foot; the instep.

Tay-Sachs disease: a rare, hereditary, progressive, and invariably fatal condition involving blindness and degeneration of the brain; it was first described in the 1880s by British ophthalmologist Warren Tay and American neurologist Bernard Sachs. Like a number of other hereditary conditions (see, for example, FABRY'S DISEASE; GAUCHER'S DISEASE; NIEMANN-PICK DISEASE), it is a metabolic problem classified as a lipid-storage disorder, caused by lack of a particular enzyme and resulting in accumulation — here, in the nervous system — of unmetabolized fatty substances; the missing enzyme in Tay-Sachs, identified in 1969, is one called hexosaminidase A. The condition usually first becomes evident, with obvious retardation and visual dysfunction, between the ages of four months and two years; there is no treatment.

Tay-Sachs disease is most common among Jewish persons of Eastern European (especially, Polish) extraction who have not intermarried with other groups; the condition is still extremely rare, though — about one in 3600 births in this group (one in thirty is believed to carry the gene — as compared with only one in four hundred among those not of this extraction). The trait is autosomally recessive (see HEREDITY for an explanation) — so that it cannot occur unless both parents are carrying the gene, and if that coincidence does occur, there is a 25 percent possibility for any of their children to have the disease (the mathematical chances remain the same for each child).

It is now possible to identify "carriers" of the genetic defect by special blood tests that can detect slight (but not total or disease-causing) deficiencies; the condition can be detected in an unborn child in the second trimester of pregnancy. And perhaps the illness itself will one day be curable by administration of the missing enzyme — although Tay-Sachs presents a special problem in this regard (see BLOOD-BRAIN BARRIER).

TB: See TUBERCULOSIS.

tearduct stenosis: the closure of a tearduct; the condition is congenital. Normally, tears drain from the eye into the nose through the tearduct — which is such a tiny pinhole it's amazing that stenosis doesn't happen more often. As it is, tearduct stenosis is fairly common. The baby's eye is obviously tearing, and tears run down the cheek; often the lids are stuck together upon awakening.

The condition isn't serious and is usually self-limited (the duct opens as the child grows). If you suspect your baby has this problem, do discuss it with your doctor.

For other problems affecting the eyelids, with quite different causes and symptoms, see BLEPHARITIS; CHALAZION; CONJUNCTIVITIS; STYE; TRACHOMA.

teeth: There are 32 permanent teeth; at least that's the number we all memorized when we were in elementary school. Actually, that's still true for seven out of ten people. For the other 30 percent, the figure is smaller. It's a matter of evolution plus heredity.

Gradually, the human species is doing away with the farthest-back molars — since they're no longer needed for such chores as grinding hunks of raw meat. At this point three out of ten people, approximately, will never develop all the "wisdom teeth" that round out the complement of 32, and will have 31, 30, or even fewer, when all their permanent teeth have erupted.

The first permanent teeth to arrive are the first molars, which come in just behind the temporary baby teeth (there are twenty of those, ten in each jaw); these four teeth, because they usually arrive between the ages of five and seven, are often called the "six-year molars."

After that, the baby teeth fall out and are replaced by their permanent counterparts. These are, in order: the eight incisors or cutting teeth (four upper, four lower); the eight bicuspids (with two cusps or points) or premolars; and the four cuspids or canines (the pointy ones). Then, four more molars, one behind each of the six-year molars. That makes 28, and the process may be completed by the age of twelve or thirteen, but perhaps not until fifteen or sixteen (the average rate, in other words, is three or four new teeth per year).

The very last group, the four third molars or "wisdom teeth," don't erupt — if they're going to erupt at all — until the late teens, or even the early twenties. Since they are vestigial, they sometimes tend to have unusually weak roots, or to come in crooked, or even to become impacted in the jaw; your dentist can, however, check for their presence and position by X ray and thereby anticipate potential problems.

Good care of the teeth should be instituted early. Brushing should begin at about the age of two — with a kiddie-sized toothbrush, of course. Don't do the brushing for the child;

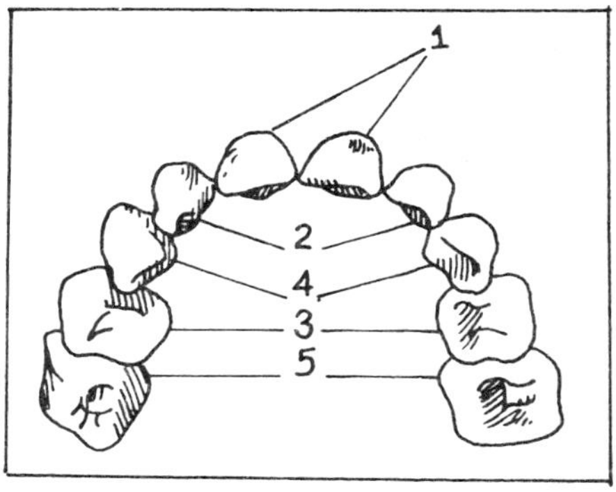

Baby or Deciduous ("Milk") Teeth
The numbers indicate the order in which a baby's teeth — the complete set of ten in one jaw is shown here — usually appear: (1) central incisors, often — unlike the case with subsequent teeth — lowers before uppers, at an age that varies considerably from one infant to another; (2) lateral incisors, typically between nine and fifteen months; (3) first molars, generally anywhere from twelve to seventeen months; (4) cuspids, in the spaces between the incisors and molars, between eighteen months and two years; (5) second ("two-year") molars, at the age of two or later.

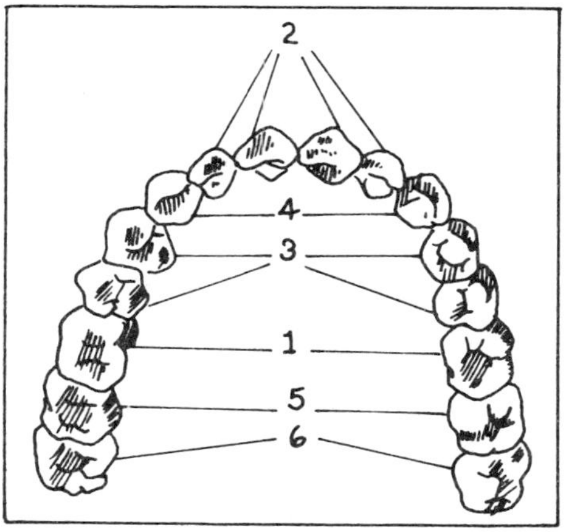

Permanent Teeth
The numbers (the sketch shows the full complement of sixteen teeth in one jaw of an adult) indicate the usual order of eruption: (1) first ("six-year") molars, five to seven years, behind the baby teeth; (2) incisors, the central ones typically first; (3) bicuspids; (4) cuspids or canines; (5) second ("twelve-year") molars, anywhere from age twelve to sixteen; (6) third molars or "wisdom teeth," in the late teens or early twenties — or perhaps never (see text).

you'll exert too much pressure on the gums. Instead, show him how to brush his own teeth — and see that it's done after each meal. And do use a stannous-fluoride toothpaste; such toothpastes are demonstrably helpful in reducing the incidence of decay (see the references at the end of this entry for more on that subject).

Care also includes *professional* care; we hope your children are not among the 50 percent of U.S. youngsters under fifteen who, according to the Children's Bureau of the U.S. Department of Health, Education, and Welfare, have never been seen by a dentist. Visits to the dentist should begin at the age of three, certainly no later than four; they should take place at least every six months, more often if the dentist judges it's necessary to cope with a special condition or problem.

Yes, all this should be done beginning with the baby teeth — even though, in the normal course of events, they'll later be lost and replaced by a permanent set. The reason that they must be kept in good condition, despite the fact that they're temporary, is so that they're not lost prematurely — which can cause drifting of the others. If that *does* happen, your dentist may want to insert a space maintainer so that the child's permanent bite won't be affected. If the *incisors* are lost prematurely, however, the space maintainer is generally not necessary.

Most tooth problems will be discovered by the dentist in routine examinations. There are, however, two that need brief comment here.

Broken teeth are quite common, and don't panic if your youngster breaks or cracks a tooth; it usually occurs with the upper incisors. If the tooth falls out of the mouth entirely, find it; it is possible that it can be successfully reimplanted. In any case, whether it's a loss, a break, or a crack, do get the child to the dentist as quickly as possible; the dentist will know what to do. Chips or cracks are usually corrected by means of fillings or crowns ("caps"), generally at some later date; again, your dentist will advise you as to when (this refers, of course, to *permanent* teeth).

Teeth-grinding, known to dentists as bruxism, doesn't usually signal some emotional disturbance, as you might suppose — at least not in children. What this habit — which typically evidences itself when the child is either preoccupied or asleep — generally means is that there is some problem with the child's bite; that is, the teeth don't come together properly. Sometimes, if a child's teeth have just recently arrived, it's merely a "discovery" phemonemon; the teeth are a new part of the youngster's body, and he's essentially playing with them. But don't assume the latter. If your child grinds his teeth, discuss the question with your dentist, who will know whether any corrective measures are needed.

For further discussion of teeth and their care, see CAVITIES; MALOCCLUSION; SPECIALTIES, DENTAL; TEETHING; TOOTHACHE. Also see GUM DISORDERS; you'll find additional cross-references there. And if your child's permanent front-of-the-mouth teeth have not yet arrived, be sure to see the special precaution, under ANTIBIOTICS, concerning tetracyclines.

teething: Your baby's first teeth may arrive at any age between three months and one year (or earlier, or later); the average is six to eight months. They will usually be the lower central incisors, the two teeth at the center front of the lower jaw.

The timing of the arrival of the rest of the baby teeth, also called milk teeth or deciduous teeth — twenty in all, ten upper and ten lower — varies considerably from child to child; bear that in mind in considering the ages we cite here (if you think your baby is *very* far off in tooth development, ask your pediatrician or family physician about it).

The next teeth to arrive are typically the upper central incisors, very soon after the lower ones. After that, the order and approximate ages are: the lateral incisors (one next to each of the central ones), usually the uppers before the lowers, somewhere between nine and fifteen months, generally ten to twelve months; the four first molars (there'll be a space between these and the lateral incisors), at twelve to seventeen months, on the average fourteen or fifteen; the pointy cuspids, in that space between the incisors and first molars, at eighteen to twenty months, or perhaps not until the age of two years; the second molars, one behind each of the first molars, at about two years (they're sometimes called "two-year molars") or some time thereafter.

Again — because parents tend to worry — we repeat: the time when teeth erupt varies a good deal. At the age of one year, a child may have anywhere from two to ten teeth. By and large, the timing of teething follows a hereditary pattern, and the ages at which you went through this process as infants may provide a rough guideline as to what to expect with your children. And incidentally, the later baby teeth arrive, the later they tend to be lost and replaced by permanent teeth (see the entry just before this one for data on the cutting of those).

Babies react in many different ways to teething. Some are fussy and irritable, and some of those may have other symptoms as well. Others aren't bothered at all.

One symptom that's not at all uncommon is a little diarrhea and slight appetite loss just before the eruption of each tooth; there may be a runny nose, as well. *Fever,* however, is *not* a normal accompaniment of teething, no matter what you may have heard or read, and if your baby does have fever, the doctor should be called.

Irritability simply means the process is making the baby uncomfortable, and there *are* things you can do to relieve the discomfort; there are *also* a couple of things you *shouldn't* do. *Don't* put any preparation, of any kind, on the baby's gums. *Don't* apply paregoric or any other opium derivative; they are narcotics and should never be used for this purpose. *Nor* should you use teething powders; such powders are rarely sold in the United States but are widely distributed in some parts of Europe. They generally contain mercury compounds, which can cause an extremely serious kind of poisoning affecting the function of the adrenal glands (see ACRODYNIA).

What's helpful and soothing is pressure on the baby's gums. If the child's old enough, let him gum a cold stalk of celery or a cold raw carrot. For a younger infant, biting on a pacifier can help, as can teething rings and biscuits (those biscuit crumbs, though, can be awfully hard to get out of rugs — and a stale bagel, if you live in an area where bagels are available, is an excellent substitute). Or simply rubbing the baby's gums with your finger can often make him feel better; the trouble with that is, he'll be upset when you stop. If the child's very fretful despite such measures, talk to your doctor about giving a little aspirin; the doctor will tell you whether you should and, if so, how much.

Once your baby has any teeth, be sure to see the special warning about nighttime bottles under BOTTLE FEEDING.

Tegopen: a trade name for cloxacillin, a semisynthetic penicillin; see ANTIBIOTICS.

Tegretol: a trade name for carbamazepine, an anticonvulsant; see EPILEPSY.

Teldrin: a trade name for chlorpheniramine maleate; see ANTIHISTAMINES.

temperature: There are a number of misconceptions about temperatures and the taking of them. We present here the basic facts you should have.

First of all, you should know what your youngster's *normal, well* temperature is. That temperature may or may not be the 98.6° F. (37° C.) commonly singled out as the crucial point, even on many thermometers. That figure represents only an average of normal human temperatures, which cover a range from a little over 97° to just under 100° F. (36° to 37.8° C.).

What makes temperature rise above this normal range? Infection, yes — although that's not completely consistent; a child can have a very high fever without being seriously ill, and on the other hand may be quite sick and have no discernible fever at all (or even a temperature that's lower than usual). And there are other things that can cause an increase in temperature: severe sunburn, some kinds of poisoning, a great deal of physical exertion (especially in warm weather), even the time of day; everyone's temperature is normally a little lower in the morning, a little higher in the evening — because of activity, not the time of day per se (it would be just the reverse if we slept all day and carried on our activities at night). So when you check your child's normal, not-sick temperature, do so both morning and evening — and in both instances, do so after the child has rested for half an hour.

When, aside from establishing the norm, should you take your child's temperature? There are three situations in which you should do so. First: if the doctor specifically tells you to. Second: if the child seems ill otherwise, and you are about to call the doctor; the child's temperature should be reported along with other symptoms. Third: if the child is recuperating from an illness involving fever, and the temperature should at this stage be dropping; if it goes up again, that might signal a secondary infection or some other complication, and the doctor should be called immediately.

There are two kinds of thermometers, and three places for taking temperature. One kind is an oral thermometer, made for use in the mouth, with a longish bulb; the other kind is a rectal thermometer, made with a somewhat rounded bulb, designed for insertion into the rectum. Aside from the bulb design, they are identical in the way they register temperature, have the same markings, and can in fact be used interchangeably if necessary (although it's not desirable, because the bulbs are designed for rapid registration of temperature in the particular place, and the bulb of the oral type is a bit sharp and fragile for the rectum of a wriggling infant). The third place is the armpit; either type can be used there.

Use a rectal thermometer only if the child is too young to hold a thermometer in the mouth; that includes all infants, of course. Use an oral thermometer if the child is old enough to understand your instructions and to cooperate in holding the thermometer in his mouth — usually after the age of three, four, or five. Take the child's temperature by armpit if for some reason neither of the other ways seems practicable, e.g., if an infant has diarrhea (some doctors also feel this is the best way for a child who's too young for the oral type but old enough to resist rectal insertion).

Either kind of thermometer should be shaken down before using it, to make sure it starts with a temperature reading below the child's normal one; this is done by holding the thermometer by the end opposite the bulb and using a brisk, snapping movement of the wrist. An oral thermometer should be slid under the tongue, and the

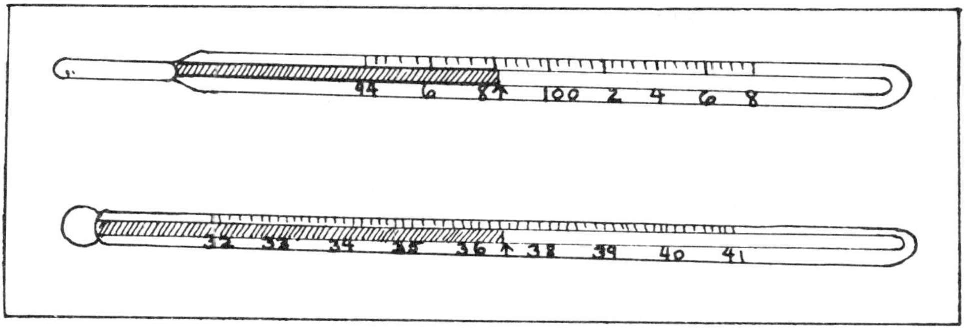

Thermometers
There are two types of thermometer, oral (top) and rectal; note the latter's more rounded bulb. See text for when and how to use each. The oral thermometer is marked in the familiar Fahrenheit scale, the rectal in the Celsius scale used in the metric system; you'll find conversion instructions in the text.

child cautioned to keep the mouth tightly closed. To insert a rectal thermometer, first dip the bulb into a little petroleum jelly; hold the baby across your lap on his stomach, gently insert the thermometer, and then hold it *and* the baby in place (so he won't squirm and hurt himself) by putting your hand firmly on the buttocks with the thermometer projecting between your fingers. To take the axillary (armpit) temperature, place the bulb of the thermometer (either kind) in the child's armpit, and hold the arm firmly against the side.

Temperature readings don't take as long as most people think. If a child has fever, it will register orally or rectally within thirty seconds — and a rectal thermometer needn't be left in any longer than that. One minute is sufficient for oral temperature-taking (it may change a tiny fraction of a degree after that, but a one-minute reading will be close enough if the child's mouth has been tightly shut). Only the armpit temperature needs a full three minutes to register accurately.

Sometimes the doctor may recommend measures to reduce an unusually high fever; such measures may include aspirin, sponging with tepid water or with a water-and-alcohol solution, etc. Don't take it upon yourself to do this, except in cases where it's a necessary emergency procedure; we've specifically mentioned it in certain entries where those situations are discussed (e.g., heat stroke, and certain types of poisoning). If such measures are necessary in other circumstances, your physician will advise you.

You may have, in traveling, encountered thermometers marked differently from those commonly in use in this country — or you may have been given such a thermometer as a new-parent present by the hospital where your baby was born. Quite a few U.S. hospitals have already switched to what is known as the metric system, which has been in use in the rest of the world (with the exception of Great Britain, which is changing over) for a long time. In the United States, we have been using the Fahrenheit temperature scale, on which the freezing point is 32°, the boiling point 212°. On the more widely used Celsius (sometimes called Centigrade) scale, the freezing point is 0°, the boiling point 100°. It is thus that a temperature of 98.6° F. is equal to 37° C.

To translate a Celsius temperature to Fahrenheit, multiply the Celsius temperature by 9, divide that result by 5, then add 32. To convert a Fahrenheit temperature to its Celsius equivalent, reverse the process; subtract 32, multiply by 5, and then divide by 9.

temper tantrums: They're not uncommon, and are usually quite purposeful. Typically the child will fling himself on the floor, kick his heels, scream, bang his head, and so on (although he will not hurt himself, and don't let him convince you that he will). He does this to get attention or to get something from you. If you become visibly upset, offer some reward for stopping the behavior, or give in to whatever the demand is, then he has achieved his aim — and he'll repeat the performance recurrently for a very logical reason: he knows it works. If you walk away and ignore him, he'll realize that the ploy is ineffective.

Temper tantrums in public introduce an additional factor: your embarrassment. It is admittedly unsettling to be the object of curious stares as you drag a screaming, kicking youngster along the street or down the aisle of a supermarket. Try not to show it. If the child knows that you'll capitulate to his demands in order to quiet him, the performance is bound to be repeated.

In rare instances, an apparent temper tantrum may be a symptom of something else. If our suggestions for coping with the problem don't work and, further, the tantrums are apparently unrelated either to a desire for attention or to frustration in achieving some special objective — then discuss the question with your doctor.

Also see BREATH-HOLDING, for discussion of another threatening technique.

temperomandibular: See JOINTS.

Tempra: a trade name for acetaminophen; see PAIN RELIEVERS.

tendons: fibers that connect muscles to bones and transmit the force exerted by the muscle. They're extremely strong; in a violent muscle pull, a bone may actually break before the tendon comes close to snapping.

Some tendons can be observed in action. One of the major ones is the cordlike structure in the bend of the elbow; it transmits the pull of the biceps muscle to achieve bending. The hamstrings at the back of the knee perform a similar service for the leg. And probably the most prominent of all is the Achilles tendon, the thick cord at the back of the ankle that connects the calf muscle to the heel bone; it functions chiefly in walking, so of course is undeveloped in infants.

tension relievers: See SEDATIVES.

Tenuate, Tepanil: trade names for the appetite-suppressant drug diethylpropion; see DIET PILLS.

TEPP: See PESTICIDES.

teratogenic: causing malformation in a developing fetus.

teratoma: a growth — not necessarily malignant — that includes types of tissues not normally found in the part of the body where the growth occurs; a dermoid cyst (see CYST) is an example, typically a benign one.

term: any limited period; medically, most often denoting the usual length of pregnancy, as in "carried to term."

Terramycin: a trade name for oxytetracycline, one of the tetracyclines; see ANTIBIOTICS.

Terrastatin: a product combining nystatin and a tetracycline; see ANTIBIOTICS.

testes (or testicles): See ENDOCRINE GLANDS; SEX ORGANS.

testosterone: a gonadal hormone; see ENDOCRINE GLANDS.

tetanus: an extremely serious, and potentially fatal, bacterial infection resulting from contamination of a wound with the tetanus bacillus, *Clostridium tetani;* the organism is found not exclusively on rusty nails, as many people suppose (although a rusty nail might indeed carry it), but in almost anything that isn't strictly clean, including manure, earth, and ordinary street dirt.

Tetanus infection may follow any wound at all, but since this particular bacterium thrives in the absence of oxygen, the deeper the wound (i.e., the less oxygen) the greater the danger, and a deep, narrow puncture wound — whether made by a knife, a nail, a needle, an animal's tooth — is the most dangerous of all. Once the organism gets into the system, it quickly reaches the spinal cord and releases a toxin that causes massive muscular spasm and rigidity; among the first muscles to be attacked are generally those controlling the jaw — hence tetanus's other name, lockjaw.

There is no first aid the lay person can give for the condition. Treatment must take place in a hospital and involves administration of serum antitoxin, antibiotics (generally penicillin), muscle relaxants, and, in extremely critical cases, placing the patient in a hyperbaric (super-high-oxygen) chamber to force oxygen through the entire body under pressure.

Any wound that involves even the possibility of tetanus infection means you should get the child to a physician, or a hospital, fast, whether or not there are any symptoms of infection. If the doctor judges that there is indeed a possibility of tetanus, and that the child is susceptible, antitoxin will be given immediately to prevent the problem. This used to be a risky procedure, since the antitoxin was always prepared from horse serum, to which a sizable number of people are allergic; now, however, there is a human-serum antitoxin available.

Nevertheless, you should not wait until such emergency treatment is necessary. There is also a vaccine for tetanus; vaccination should begin at the age of two or three months, with DPT shots, and thereafter be continued through life (see IMMUNIZATION for full details and the recommended vaccination schedule).

Don't confuse this with a similar-named noninfectious condition; see TETANY, following.

tetany: a condition like tetanus (see preceding) involving the muscles, but totally different in cause and treatment. Here, the immediate cause is calcium deficiency — not calcium that's deposited in bones, etc., but calcium (a very small percentage of the amount ingested) that circulates in the bloodstream. Normally, calcium in the blood is in a concentration of one part in ten thousand; if this concentration falls to half the normal figure, tetany

— characterized by violent muscular spasms and cramps, sometimes by convulsions — results.

The drop in circulating calcium is not generally due to a nutritional deficiency of calcium itself, but usually to one of two other problems — deficiency in vitamin D, which assists in the assimilation of ingested calcium (see NUTRITION), or parathyroid malfunction (see ENDOCRINE GLANDS).

Treatment will depend upon medical assessment of the problem and may involve administration of calcium and/or vitamin D and/or parathyroid hormone.

tetracycline, Tetracyn: See ANTIBIOTICS; the latter is a trade name for the former.

tetralogy of Fallot: a congenital defect — or rather, a combination of four specific defects — involving the heart and major blood vessels connected with the heart; it is not hereditary, but is a result of malformation (cause unknown) during pregnancy.

In this condition, the pulmonary artery, which carries blood to the lungs for oxygenation, is narrowed; there is an abnormal opening between the ventricles, or lower chambers, of the heart, so that venous blood mixes with arterial blood; the aorta or main artery is displaced; and part of the heart is enlarged. The result is a deficiency in oxygen supplied to the tissues and organs; since cyanosis is a symptom, the victims have been termed "blue babies."

Prior to 1945, such infants had little chance of survival. At that time, a new surgical technique was developed by Dr. Alfred Blalock and Dr. Helen Taussig, a surgeon and pediatrician respectively, at Johns Hopkins University. Now, "blue babies" can be saved by this operation, and these infants can look forward not to careers as professional athletes, but certainly to normal life expectancy.

Tetrastatin, Tetrex: See ANTIBIOTICS. The latter is a trade name for tetracycline; the former is a product combining a tetracycline with nystatin.

thalassemia: See ANEMIA.

therapist: Though sometimes used narrowly to denote someone dealing with emotional problems, the term is properly applied to any individual engaged in treating illness, either mental or physical; it comes from the Greek *therapeia,* "treatment."

thermography: a diagnostic technique utilizing the fact that differentials in skin temperature may reveal the presence of underlying disease; it has been found useful particularly in some circulatory disorders and in certain malignancies.

thermometers: See TEMPERATURE.

thiamine: one of the B vitamins; see NUTRITION.

thiopental: a barbiturate used primarily in anesthesia; see SEDATIVES.

thioridazine: a major tranquilizer; see SEDATIVES.

Thiosulfil: a trade name for sulfamethizole; see SULFA DRUGS.

thirst: Extreme, continuous thirst may be a symptom of a serious ailment, especially if it occurs in combination with excessive urination or with diarrhea; it may indicate extreme dehydration, which can occur in diabetes as well as other conditions involving glandular imbalance, and is a clear indication that a physical checkup is needed.

With children who have been very active in hot weather, the story is a little different. They have been perspiring a good deal — thus have lost liquid, and also salt. They need both — although they may be conscious only of the need for liquids. The salt need, however, is physiologically more important, and liquids alone could make the problem worse. They should be given salty snacks — pretzels, potato chips, and the like — followed by liquids.

thoracentesis: the withdrawal of fluid from the chest cavity by means of a puncturing device.

thoracic surgeon: See SPECIALTIES, MEDICAL.

thorax: the chest cavity, extending from the collarbone to the diaphragm (*not* to the waistline); it contains the ribs, heart, lungs, and, in infants, the thymus (see ENDOCRINE GLANDS).

Thorazine: a trade name for chlorpromazine, an antinauseant and major tranquilizer. See NAUSEA; SEDATIVES.

throat, sore: See SORE THROAT; TONSILLITIS.

thrombocytes: another name for platelets; see BLOOD CELLS.

thrombosis: a condition involving formation of a blood clot or clots in a blood vessel or within the heart; such a clot, which may of course seriously obstruct circulation or even the function of the heart itself, is called a *thrombus*.

"throwback": See the "Dominants and Recessives" discussion under HEREDITY.

thrush: a fungal infection of the mouth, medically termed *candidiasis*, tending to afflict babies within the first month of life; usually it is congenital, acquired while passing through the mother's vagina (a frequent site of such infection in adults, and teenage girls, as well). The first symptom may be reluctant feeding. In the mouth, the infection is visible as patchy white spots on the baby's lips, the inside of the cheeks, tongue, gums, and palate; there may also be fever and possibly gastrointestinal difficulties. The white patches look something like milk scum, but if an attempt is made to wipe them off, it can't be done easily, and the underlying membrane is inflamed and may bleed.

Thrush is not considered serious if it is caught early, and it can be treated with various drugs. If it isn't treated, however, it can spread to the gastrointestinal tract and through the respiratory tract to the lungs — and then becomes a serious matter indeed. If you suspect this condition in your baby, it's vital that you see your physician promptly.

As previously mentioned, the vaginas of older girls and women are susceptible to attack by the same organism, as is the skin in the diaper area of babies; see MONILIASIS.

thumb sucking: Many babies suck their thumbs, and there is little you can or should do about it. Although no damage is done by infant thumb sucking, the teeth can be pushed out of line if the habit continues after eruption of permanent front teeth (which may be as early as age five); pushing of the *baby* teeth won't have any permanent effect.

Thumb sucking often begins when a baby starts to teethe. What may happen then is that the habit continues until the age of three or so, when the child has begun to make friends with other youngsters; derisive comments of peers may discourage the habit.

If thumb sucking persists up to the age of four or five years, it does become a matter of concern since alignment of the permanent teeth is potentially threatened. By this age, dental visits should have begun. Sometimes the dentist can persuade the child to stop — and the dentist can also insert an appliance behind the upper front teeth that will make thumb sucking decidedly uncomfortable. If the problem persists, then it should be discussed with your physician as well.

thymosin, thymus: See ENDOCRINE GLANDS.

thyroglossal cyst: See CYST.

thyroid: See ENDOCRINE GLANDS.

tibia: the anatomical term for the shinbone, the larger of the two bones in the lower leg.

tic: a muscular twitch, especially of a facial, neck, or shoulder muscle. Usually such a twitch is due to emotional factors and is temporary and will gradually disappear by itself. But neither of these is always true. Sometimes a tic can result from nerve disease or injury. A tic that takes the form of blinking could be due to some vision difficulty. *Don't* call a child's attention to a tic; that may simply aggravate the problem. *Do* discuss it with your physician, who may refer you to an ophthalmologist or other specialist if necessary.

tick bites: See BITES AND STINGS.

tick fever: a rickettsial infection also known as Colorado tick fever, frequently as Rocky Mountain spotted fever, occasionally as "tick-borne typhus" (typhus is another rickettsial infection). The geographical names are very misleading. While tick fever was first identified in the Rockies, it is now considered endemic in a broad area that curves across the U.S. map from Idaho in the northwest through Colorado, Oklahoma, and Arkansas and all the way to the Atlantic coast, extending north to Cape Cod, south to Alabama and Georgia; it has, in fact, occurred in all states except Maine, Vermont, Alaska, and Hawaii — and the highest incidence in the past few years has been in the area from Maryland to the Gulf. Cases have been increasing steadily each year since 1968; there were 668 reported in 1973, 774 in 1974 (with 44 deaths), over 800 in 1975 — but reporting isn't mandated, and experts believe the actual numbers may be five times the reported figures.

As the preferred name of the disease suggests, it is transmitted by tick bite (both wood ticks and dog ticks), from a large wild-animal reservoir including birds and many wild rodents; like other rickettsial infections, it isn't communicable from person to person but is relayed only via its arthropod vector. Children have accounted for seven out of ten cases. The mortality rate in recent years has run about six percent, due chiefly to delayed or inaccurate diagnosis.

Tick fever can vary from mild to severe. Initial symptoms appear after an incubation period of two to twelve days, commonly four to eight. Fever, headache, and muscular aches are followed by the distinguishing feature, the characteristic rash — slightly raised pink spots that appear first on the wrists and ankles; the rash quickly spreads to the palms and soles, then to the rest of the body.

A mild case, aside from the rash, generally resembles flu, with a temperature that rarely rises above 102°

F. (38.9° C.); most cases of tick fever are of this mild type. In a more severe case, fever climbs to 104° F. (40° C.) or above, the rash may also appear on mucous membranes, and there are violent chills, intense pain, nausea, and sensitivity to light. Extremely serious cases (they are fortunately rare) involve the heart and central nervous system; one in five such cases can be fatal if it is not promptly treated.

Tick fever is, like other rickettsial diseases, treatable with antibiotics, in particular the tetracyclines; hospitalization may be required, depending upon the severity of illness. It must be added that the risk of fatal outcome soars significantly if treatment is delayed until the second week of illness. The Center for Disease Control has also taken pains to point out a serious hazard of misdiagnosis: penicillin, which is effective against many other infections, will accomplish nothing whatever against this one, and is tantamount to no treatment at all. If symptoms have set in, it is probably best to begin therapy rather than wait for results of blood tests (which can pinpoint the infection).

There are also two important aspects of the tick bite itself. It takes an hour or more for a tick to transmit the infectious organism; if it is quickly removed, there is small chance of infection. It should be removed very carefully, by covering it with butter or other grease to cut off its air — not by yanking or crushing, which leaves the tick's head buried in the skin and heightens the risk of infection.

If a tick *has* been clinging for an hour or two and is then removed, removal should still be done carefully; there is a test that can detect the infectious organism in the tick (its intact body and head are needed). Only about one tick in twenty is likely to be carrying the organism. The test is a fast one, and can eliminate the need for an unnecessary course of antibiotics — or, conversely, confirm the need for prompt treatment.

There is a vaccine that protects against tick fever, a series of three injections that is recommended if your family will be vacationing or camping in a tick-infested area (discuss the question with your own physician). Protection lasts for one year, at which time a booster is necessary.

t.i.d.: See PRESCRIPTIONS.

Tinactin: See ATHLETE'S FOOT.

Tindal: a trade name for acetophenazine, a major tranquilizer; see SEDATIVES.

Tine test: one of several skin tests for tuberculosis; see HEAF TEST for further comment.

tinnitus: ringing — or whistling, buzzing, clicking, or other odd sounds — in the ears; it can occur in infections involving the ears or eustachian tubes, as well as in adverse reactions to some medications. Whatever the cause, it demands prompt medical consultation.

tiredness: See FATIGUE.

titer: a measurement of the strength or level of a particular substance within a solution; used in a medical context, it often refers to antibody levels (to a specific infectious agent) in the blood, which may be measured either to assess the effectiveness of immunization, or to determine prior infection and development of immunity.

tobramycin: See ANTIBIOTICS.

tocopherol: the chemical name for vitamin E; see NUTRITION.

toe, broken: See FRACTURES.

toenail, ingrown: the growth of a toenail into the skin, causing great pain and tenderness; the toe involved is usually the big one. Ingrown toenail is caused by a combination of too-tight shoes and a nail cut too close at the corners (and conversely, can be prevented by cutting toenails straight across plus seeing that shoes are always properly fitted).

If your child has an ingrown toenail, consult your physician. Don't attempt to treat the problem at home, by using patent medicines or by any other means; ingrown toenail can lead to nasty infection (see PARONYCHIA).

Tofranil: a trade name for imipramine; see ANTIDEPRESSANTS.

toilet training: There are many social and cultural differences relating to toilet training throughout the world. In areas, for example, where a mother may have a baby annually and have to wash diapers herself, it becomes almost a necessity to have the older child out of diapers at the earliest possible moment; the mother may, therefore, place the infant on the toilet very frequently, simply to save the soiled or wet diapers. Surprisingly, the infants so raised seem to suffer no untoward psychological effects, and it is probably due to the fact that the mother is in no way torn about the "rightness" of her behavior.

If you are fortunate enough to have a diaper service or to use disposable diapers, the situation is quite different. It is then more trouble to undo the child's clothing twenty times a day and spend all that time in the bathroom than to change diapers at your convenience. If you never mention a word to your child about the toilet, training will eventually be accomplished, by emulating you and other children.

Never get into an argument with your child that you are bound to lose. Toilet training falls into this category. If the child gets the idea that you care dreadfully, bowel and bladder control can be used as a weapon against you, like a temper tantrum; stool, in particular, can be withheld as a means of getting attention. Don't let this happen.

If you have the patience to wait until the child is really ready, diapers can be discarded overnight — literally; no parent of a first child ever believes this, but it's true. Try not to be coercive; let pressure come (and it will) from peers.

When you are inclined to become annoyed with your toddler who may be quite verbal and may even understand some abstract concepts, but shows no interest in using the toilet, remember that it is quite a complicated procedure. Adults have done it so long that it has become reflex. But a small child must associate the feeling beforehand with the ensuing results — and then must be able to tighten the appropriate sphincter muscles until the appropriate place is reached (i.e., the bathroom) to urinate or defecate. Then, the sphincters must be relaxed in order to eliminate. It's pretty complicated! Before a child walks well, control of elimination can't be expected.

Boys usually are a bit slower at managing this complex process than girls, and often boys achieve bladder control — because they can stand up and see the results — before bowel control; with girls, who sit down to carry out both processes, it's usually the opposite. But: no normal child ever goes to kindergarten in diapers.

Unusually hard stools can sometimes cause a special withholding problem, possibly coupled with a physical complication; see ANAL FISSURE. And see BOWEL MOVEMENTS for some further pertinent points.

tomography: use of a diagnostic technique that results in a cross-sectional visualization of the body or an organ thereof. See COMPUTERIZED AXIAL TOMOGRAPHY; ULTRASONOGRAPHY.

tongue: The tongue functions in speaking and swallowing and is, of course, the organ of taste as well. Only four tastes, however, can be discerned, each by particular tastebuds, in specific locations on the tongue: sweetness and saltiness (at the tip), bitterness (at the back), and sourness (at the sides). Other so-called "tastes" are actually a result of smelling the aromas of foods — which is why we say food "tastes" flat when a cold or other condition interferes with the sense of smell.

The appearance of the tongue can sometimes be significant in diagnosis. "Strawberry tongue," white with red spots, for example, is typical of scarlet fever. A very bright red tongue may signal certain nutritional deficiencies. Small blistery sores, or whitish patches, may be symptoms of specific oral infections (see STOMATITIS and THRUSH).

Generally speaking, any unusual appearance of your youngster's tongue should be called to your physician's attention, whether or not there are any other symptoms of illness. Oddities of the tongue may not always be of medical significance; a common condition called "geographic tongue," for instance, in which the tongue resembles a relief map, is interesting, though of no importance whatever. But let your doctor do the judging.

Accidental biting of the tongue can occasionally occur in falls and in ordinary chewing; such an injury, whether cut or bruise, is generally nothing to worry about and normally doesn't require medical attention. If there's bleeding, it should stop, with a bit of pressure, within an hour (if it doesn't, do take the child to the doctor). The youngster can be given aspirin if the injury's very painful; sucking on a piece of ice (if the child's old enough) will have a helpful numbing effect on an aching bruise. A laceration on the tongue (or other mucous membrane) heals with a yellowish color; that's the normal shade, and not a sign of infection.

Congenital deformities of the tongue are quite rare, and there are only two you're ever likely to hear about. *Bifid tongue* is a condition similar to cleft palate or harelip in that the tongue is split in two parts at the front, rather than being properly joined; it's corrected by surgery. *Tongue-tie* results if the frenum, the vertical membrane that anchors the tongue underneath, is too short; it's a serious problem only if the baby is unable to suck and it's easily corrected, if necessary, by snipping the frenum.

tonsillitis: inflammation of the tonsils (see following), caused by bacterial or viral infection. About half the cases of tonsillitis are caused by streptococci, the same bacteria that cause scarlet fever and a number of other ailments; a prominent viral cause, especially in recurrent cases, may be the Epstein-

Barr virus. The most common victims are children between the ages of two and eight.

The infection's incubation period can vary; it's two to five days for strep, generally shorter — perhaps one to three days — for a viral infection. The main symptom is sore throat, particularly on swallowing and talking; in addition, there may be headache, stiff neck, and vomiting. The tonsils are visibly inflamed and enlarged, and there may be white spots on them; the lymph nodes, in the neck and elsewhere in the body, are commonly swollen. There is usually fever, which may range up to 106° F. (41° C.) and may be accompanied by convulsions.

If you suspect tonsillitis, it's important — as with any potential strep infection — to begin treatment quickly, before the bacteria migrate and start trouble in additional locations. Of course the child must be kept home; he'll voluntarily stay in bed, if he feels sick enough. The doctor will prescribe drugs to combat the infection and may also recommend regular doses of aspirin to bring down fever and relieve general discomfort.

Only a throat culture can accurately establish whether a given instance of tonsillitis is due to streptococcal (or other bacterial) or viral infection. If strep is involved, *ten days* of antibiotic therapy are necessary, even if symptoms have meanwhile vanished; an inadequately treated strep infection can result in subsequent rheumatic fever and/or nephritis.

Quinsy is a special and more acute type of tonsillitis involving abscess, usually on one side. There is often severe pain on that side of the neck, with more stiffness and even greater difficulty in swallowing than with the ordinary version. It of course requires immediate medical attention.

Severe tonsillitis with enlarged lymph nodes may suggest mononucleosis; that diagnosis can be confirmed by special tests.

tonsils: a pair of lymphoid structures at the back of the throat. Their basic function is protective, in that they release cells that meet and destroy invading bacteria; sometimes, however, the tonsils themselves are prey to infection (see the preceding entry).

tonus: See MUSCLES.

toothache: It usually means tooth decay — that is, a cavity. But not necessarily. It may also signify a problem in or around the root of a tooth, or somewhere in or near the jaw. Pain from a maxillary sinus infection, for example, can cause what seems to be a toothache in the upper jaw, a phenomenon physicians call *referred* pain; in that case, a particular tooth can't usually be pinpointed.

If toothache occurs, see your dentist as quickly as possible. In the meantime, do something to relieve the pain. Some things to relieve the pain: a wad of cotton saturated with oil of cloves (applicable only if you find a specific cavity in which to place the remedy), or aspirin, or hot or cold compresses (sometimes one works, sometimes the other).

topical: on the surface (of the skin or mucous membrane); the opposite of *systemic.* The word usually refers to an application of medication; an ointment, for example, is designed for topical application — as opposed to medications formulated for injection or oral administration.

TOPV: the abbreviation for trivalent

oral polio vaccine, formerly called Sabin vaccine.

torticollis: See NECK PROBLEMS.

Totacillin: a trade name for ampicillin, a semisynthetic penicillin; see ANTIBIOTICS.

tourniquets: See BLEEDING.

toxic: poisonous, and potentially lethal; the word may refer either to a substance introduced into the body via injection or ingestion, or to a substance that may be produced within the body. The diphtheria bacillus, for example, produces a toxin. *Toxin* refers to the actual substance that does damage to human cells; the diphtheria bacillus itself is not toxic — but snake venom is. A toxin generally causes more than just inflammation; it is actually destructive (often affecting vital areas such as nerve tissue or blood cells), and it usually moves quickly.

toxoid: a toxin treated to destroy its poisonous effects but still retain its ability to stimulate the production of antibodies; such a substance is typically used for immunization, as against diphtheria and tetanus.

toxoplasmosis: a parasitic infection by a ubiquitous protozoan — which may or may not cause symptoms of illness; it's estimated that one in three people has had this infection (that is, antibodies can be detected in that proportion of people). Toxoplasmosis can be acquired from excreta of birds and animals, and also from eating contaminated, undercooked meat. There is a good deal of interest in this infection among researchers, for it poses a very special and serious problem.

In victims other than newborn infants, symptoms generally appear — at least if the infection stems from eating undercooked meat — within a week or two, and may vary considerably. They are often flulike, with fever, headache, swollen lymph nodes and muscular aches. There may also be nausea, possibly a rash, and sometimes numbness in the hands and feet. The condition lasts about as long as flu does, although the aching may persist for a month. With such a vague and variable set of symptoms, toxoplasmosis is, understandably, often not diagnosed (although if it is suspected, there *are* tests that can confirm the diagnosis) — and even if it is, it's not considered serious, and there is no specific treatment for it.

The special and serious problem arises when the victim is a mother-to-be. She will not be any sicker than any other adult. And in the majority of cases, there will be no other ill effects. But in *some* cases toxoplasmosis during pregnancy can, like rubella, affect the unborn child, and congenital toxoplasmosis is an extremely critical matter: it may cause encephalitis, hydrocephalus or microcephaly, severe convulsions, permanent eye damage, and/or mental retardation. If it is diagnosed quickly enough, it can sometimes be arrested by the administration of sulfa drugs — but often irreversible damage will have already occurred.

You need be concerned about this question only if you are, or intend to become, pregnant, and have not had the illness (a blood test can tell); unlike rubella, toxoplasmosis cannot be communicated from one person to another. We suggest precautions in three areas.

First, avoid any possible contact with the wild carriers of the parasite, chiefly birds and rodents (it does not make them ill).

Second, be sure you do not eat raw or undercooked meat.

Third, be aware that the other major source is, specifically, cat feces, because it is mainly cats who seek out the aforementioned wild carriers. If you have a cat that is kept indoors at all times, fine. Otherwise, you should have someone else change the kitty litter; be sure your cat eats only commercial or other food provided by you and does not hunt outdoors; and avoid gardening during your pregnancy if there is any possibility of cat feces (your cat's or another's) in the soil, since the organisms can persist there for months.

So far as is known, toxoplasmosis can be contracted only once.

toys: There is mounting evidence that, despite the existence of certain regulations controlling the manufacture and distribution of playthings, present laws are inadequate to insure complete safety; it is necessary for parents to exercise care and judgment in selecting — and accepting gifts of — toys for their children.

Infants under the age of a year or so don't really need toys per se; a baby will be perfectly happy with a crib mobile or a "cradle gym" that he can reach out and touch and that moves.

For a crawler or toddler, it's important that the child's toys be nonswallowable (or such innocuous things as paper, that will be noninjurious if they *are* swallowed). Often, a child of this age will be delighted to play with ordinary household objects that aren't especially intriguing to *you,* but represent fascinating new experiences for *him:* wooden spoons, saucepans, empty boxes, hunks of tissue paper, and so on. Don't, though, give a tot anything to play with that is sharp, breakable, or mechanical (such as an eggbeater).

Some of the manufactured toys designed for various age groups are also quite good, well graded, dependably sturdy, and safely finished with nontoxic materials; among widely distributed lines are Childcraft, Creative Playthings, Playskool, and Tonka.

Any fuzzy animals your youngster plays with should be soft, have no metal parts (such as button eyes that can come out and be swallowed or aspirated), and should be machine washable.

Up to the age of at least four or five, in fact, anything small enough to swallow, or sharp enough to cut if handled carelessly, should be avoided. This includes plastic rattles with beads inside, as well as other things made of hard plastic — which can be bitten or broken and then display dangerously sharp edges.

Electrical toys of all types should of course wait until the child is old enough to understand fully how to operate them, and can be trusted to observe safety precautions — about six to eight years.

trachea: the windpipe that carries air from the throat to the bronchial tubes.

tracheotomy: an emergency surgical procedure in which an incision is made directly into the trachea or windpipe at the front of the throat, in order to permit air to reach the lungs; it is done if the passageway above that point has been blocked by injury, a foreign object, or obstructive inflammation and there is no other way to prevent fatal asphyxiation.

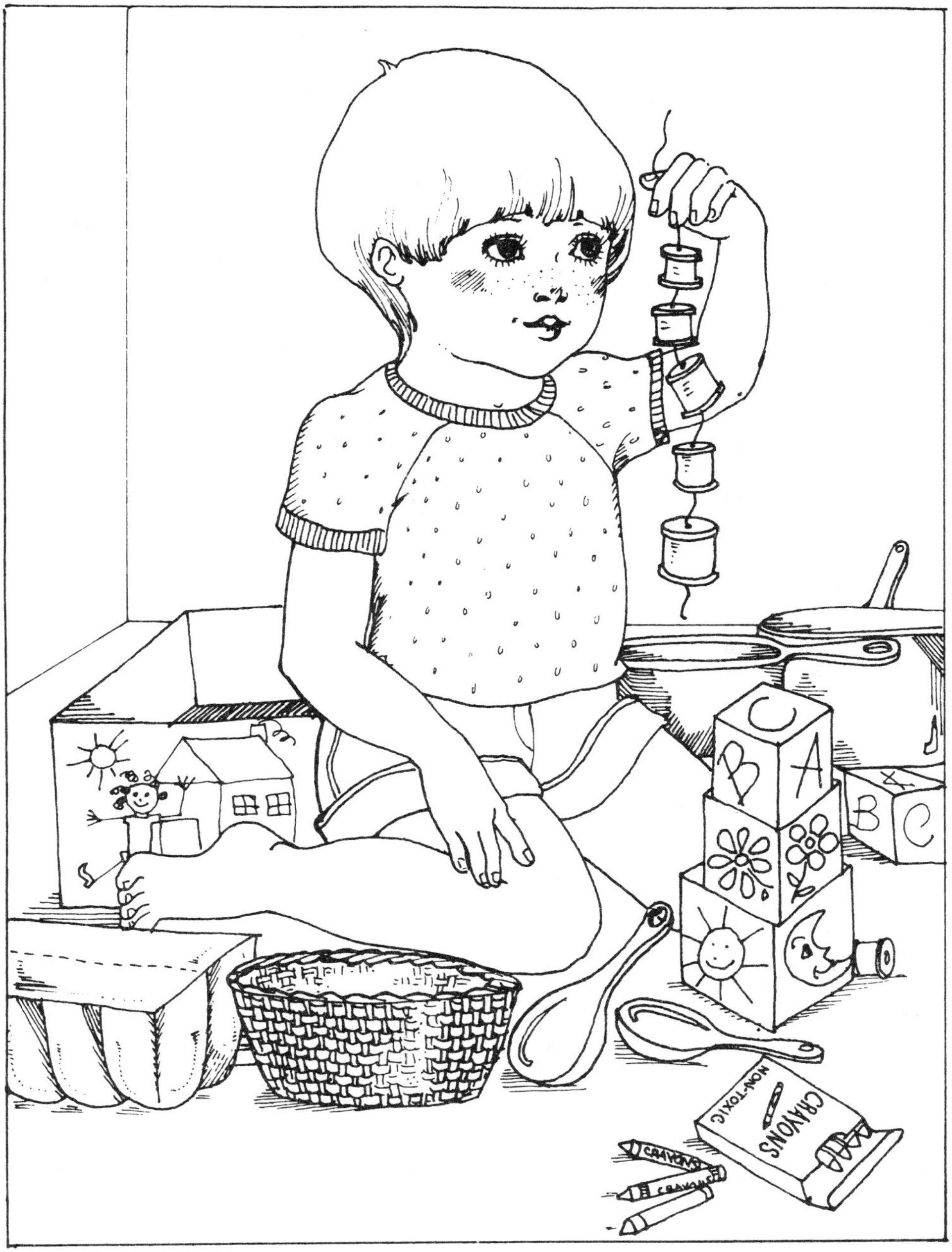

Toys for Toddlers
Household objects such as empty boxes, egg cartons, spoons, pots and pans, empty spools, and other nonswallowables and unbreakables make fine playthings for crawlers and toddlers. Exclude sharp-edged and mechanical items (such as eggbeaters), and make sure wooden objects are not splintery. Chunks of wood left over from craft projects can be smoothly sanded, painted, and decorated (use nontoxic materials, of course) to provide personalized sets ot blocks.

trachoma: an inflammation of both the conjunctiva (the mucous membranes around the eyes) and the cornea; it is a viral infection, related to conjunctivitis but far more serious and even more highly contagious. It is rare in the United States, except in a few isolated southern mountain areas, but is a major public health problem in certain other parts of the world, especially North Africa and the Near and Far East.

Trachoma can be successfully treated if it is diagnosed early enough; both sulfa drugs and topical applications of certain antibiotics — tetracyclines, in particular — are effective. If it goes untreated, it can cause severe scarring of the affected areas, with eventual blindness.

There is no immunization against trachoma. If your family travels to an area where it is endemic, stay far from anyone whose eyes are inflamed; the disease is contagious via both eye and nose secretions.

Trancopal: a trade name for chlormezanone, a tranquilizer; see SEDATIVES.

tranquilizers: See SEDATIVES.

transfusion: the introduction of a new supply of blood to replace blood loss from hemorrhage or disease. An *exchange transfusion* replaces a patient's blood, because of hemolysis or the accumulation of toxic elements, with healthy blood (a little at a time). A transfusion may, under emergency conditions, take place directly from person to person but is usually given from stored blood that has been preserved and prevented from clotting.

Matching of certain factors in the blood is essential; see BLOOD GROUPS and RH FACTOR.

transplants: one of the most intensive areas of medical research and investigation and, in recent years, probably the most widely publicized; transplanting of healthy parts or organs to replace diseased or damaged ones is an exciting medical frontier. At this writing, cornea, kidney, heart, larynx, liver, lung, and pancreas transplants have been attempted, with varying degrees of success. The kidney is the only one that can be obtained from a living person without serious damage to the donor; the others have involved removing the tissue or organ from a recently deceased donor (the transplant must be used within a short time, varying from minutes to hours).

The chief problem in transplanting tissue has been what is generally called — for lack of a more precise term — the "rejection mechanism." This reaction, still not completely understood, is apparently similar to the body's reactions to invading bacteria or other "foreign" proteins — i.e., the formation of antibodies that seek to fight off and destroy the invader; complicating the problem is the fact that drugs given to suppress such a reaction also suppress the body's resistance to ordinary infections. Research thus centers on seeking a way to persuade the body to accept the new organ yet maintain its hostility to bacteria, viruses, and the like.

This rejection mechanism does not occur if the transplanted tissue is genetically fully compatible with the recipient; thus a kidney transplant between identical twins is usually successful.

Tranxene: a trade name for clorazepate, one of the benzodiazepine tranquilizers; see SEDATIVES.

tranylcypromine: See ANTIDEPRESSANTS.

trapezius: See MUSCLES.

trauma: any injury from a source outside the body (not, as some think, a word limited to psychological phenomena), such as a cut, bruise, fracture, etc. A *psychic* trauma is, specifically, an event or experience that results in persisting emotional or mental ill effects.

traumatic shock: a threat to vital functions that can occur as a consequence of severe injury or hemorrhage; it must be anticipated, and considered a distinct possibility, in any gunshot or stab (or other major) wound, serious fracture, extensive burn, or automobile accident.

Shock (we'll just use the single word from here on) is a complex phenomenon; generally, it can be characterized as a severe impairment in circulation that grows progressively worse if untreated. Oxygen delivery is diminished by too low a supply to the body's cells to sustain metabolism; circulation is further slowed, and blood pressure drops to a dangerous level; the volume of blood being pumped by the heart is radically reduced. There follows a universal impairment of body processes, leading to general depression and, ultimately, complete failure of vital functions. The further the process has progressed, the more critical the threat.

SIGNS AND SYMPTOMS

Of course you can't determine blood pressure without special equipment. But there are ways in which you can judge the situation with reasonable accuracy, both general symptoms and clues as to the degree of danger.

In general, be alert for: rapid pulse; extreme weakness; paleness (rather than guessing at skin tones, check the conjunctiva, the mucous membranes around the eyes); "cold sweat," especially on the forehead, upper lip, and palms; a dull look to the eyes. There may be nausea, perhaps with vomiting, and the victim may express unusual thirst. Loss of consciousness is uncommon in shock, but it may occur.

Impending or mild shock is revealed chiefly by an increase in pulse rate, at least in older children and teenagers; a rise to 110 or 120 beats per minute is a definite danger signal. Pulse rates in small children are normally higher, as high as 130 in infants under the age of one year, and rectal temperature can provide better information (take it at frequent intervals); a slowly falling rectal temperature is often a key sign of impending shock.

There are also two tests you can perform.

(1) If the nature of the injury does not preclude it, and the child is old enough, have him rise quickly from a lying-down to a sitting-up position, and check the pulse rate in both positions; a definite increase after sitting up is an alarm signal. (This is known as the "tilt test.")

(2) If you have a watch or clock with a second hand, press the skin of the child's forehead with your finger, so it pales slightly; then see how long it takes for normal color to return. The time should be normal — one to one and a half seconds.

Second-stage ("moderate") shock is more critical. At this point, the pulse will be even faster (perhaps as high as 150), and noticeably weaker. A key sign — assuming the child is old enough to talk — is difficulty in speech; it will not be incoherent, but will definitely be slower than normal, and some words may be slurred.

Again, the two tests may be used. In the tilt test, not only does the pulse quicken, but there is dizziness or lightheadedness upon sitting up. And in the second test, the skin color takes longer than normal to return.

Severe shock involves a number of signs and symptoms, and there will be no doubt in your mind that there is a critical emergency. The pulse is even faster and weaker, breathing shallow and irregular. You won't be able to use the tilt test, because the child won't be able to sit up; if you press the skin on the forehead, it will simply remain paler than the surrounding area. The pupils are dilated, and if you shine a light into them they are very slow to contract or may not contract at all. Mental processes are also affected at this stage, and there is confusion and disorientation; any speech is likely to be either incoherent (perhaps just grunts and groans) or irrational.

WHAT TO DO

First, determine the victim's condition, using the foregoing clues.

If you are sure shock is not present or imminent, continue to be alert for signs, and take preventive measures. Act to conserve body heat by keeping the child comfortably warm; the ideal is a room temperature of 75° to 80° F. (24° to 27° C.). *Over*heating is *not* called for; a certain amount of lowered body temperature is helpful, since it decreases the need for oxygen. Also keep the victim lying down — with head lowered and feet raised, unless there is a head or chest injury and there is breathing difficulty. And stay with the youngster, remaining as calm as possible; your reassuring presence itself is helpful.

If the child is conscious and asks for something to drink, a little water is fine. If there is no chest or abdominal injury or possible skull fracture, juice, tea, or other clear fluid may also be helpful.

If you believe shock is present or imminent, you should lose no time in rushing the child to the nearest hospital emergency room, in the quickest possible manner — whether that means phoning for an ambulance or using whatever transportation you may have at hand. If you are waiting for an ambulance, take the foregoing protective measures while you wait; also do what you can to control extensive bleeding if it's present (see BLEEDING) and, if necessary, aid the child's breathing (see RESPIRATORY RESUSCITATION).

There is nothing else you can or should do. Professional treatment — involving transfusion, administration of plasma, and/or other procedures — is needed for shock.

If you are taking the child to the hospital yourself, don't stop to take time for anything. Simply transport him lying down, in the position mentioned earlier, if you can, and see that he's kept warm; if there is a second person available to accompany you, one of you should reassure the child, give resuscitation if needed, etc., while the other drives.

travel precautions: Depending upon where and how you're traveling, you'll find aspects of this subject discussed under ACCIDENTS, PREVENTION OF; FIRST-AID SUPPLIES; FOOD POISONING, PREVENTION OF; IMMUNIZATION; PARASITES. Poisonous creatures in and on the borders of the continental United States are described and illustrated under BITES AND STINGS; family travel elsewhere suggests a trip to the library to familiarize yourself with potentially hazardous flora and — especially — fauna.

Certain diseases are more prevalent in some parts of the world — or the United States — than in others. You might want to peruse the following entries to see if they apply to the area you plan to visit: CHOLERA; DENGUE; DYSENTERY; ENCEPHALITIS; HEPATITIS; HISTOPLASMOSIS; MALARIA; MENINGITIS; PARATYPHOID FEVER; PLAGUE; POLIO; Q FEVER; RELAPSING FEVER; SMALLPOX; TICK FEVER; TRACHOMA; TULAREMIA; TYPHOID FEVER; TYPHUS FEVER; YELLOW FEVER.

Here, some further thoughts, pertaining chiefly to foreign travel but applicable at least in part to domestic trips as well.

If anyone in the family has a chronic condition requiring continuing or emergency medication — such as drugs to combat severe allergic reactions, anticonvulsants, insulin, etc. — take along a supply sufficient to see you through, plus extras of anything prescribed for emergencies. Also take a *typed* prescription for each such medication indicating all applicable scientific names (both brand names and short generics may differ elsewhere), as well as exact dosage. Take an extra pair of glasses for anyone who wears them, and a typed prescription for those as well. If you are traveling by air, these things should be on your person or in carry-on luggage — not in checked baggage, which can be lost.

Take with you, too, any *non*prescription drugs which you might possibly need: remedies for headaches, skin problems, motion sickness, and the like. There is far less control in many other nations of over-the-counter patent medicines — and while many sold here leave a great deal to be desired, some available elsewhere are much worse. A number of countries, for just one instance, permit nonprescription sale of cold remedies containing chloramphenicol, an antibiotic with a high risk of severe, even fatal, effects; internal use of it here is strictly by prescription, and then only when deemed absolutely necessary. It's well to avoid buying nonprescription medications outside the United States and Canada.

You should have with you, in case of emergency, an up-to-date record for each member of the family noting immunizations (whether required or not), chronic medical problems (including allergies to medications), serious illnesses, and surgical procedures (with details and dates), as well as up-to-date data on your health insurance.

In case you must seek medical help in a land where you don't speak the language, it is handy to have a booklet listing English-speaking hospitals and physicians in close to a hundred countries; it's available without charge from the International Association for Medical Assistance to Travellers, 350 Fifth Avenue, New York NY 10001. And in case you can't locate an English-speaking physician and must nevertheless get professional medical help, there's another handy booklet, titled *A Foreign Language Guide to Health Care,* that provides French, German, Italian, and Spanish translations of a host of phrases that might be needed (ranging from "I have a pain here" and "Stop the bleeding!" to "I would not like the tooth extracted" and "Ouch!"); free on request from the Blue Cross Association (840 North Lake Shore Drive, Chicago IL 60611, and local offices across the country).

What about "traveler's diarrhea"? It does exist. It has been known under many aliases, among them "Delhi belly," the "Aztec two-step," "Montezuma's revenge," the "Turkey trots," the "Rome runs," the "Greek gallop," or simply "la turista." It's generally not serious, and typically doesn't last long — it's simply a reaction to unfamiliar foods — but it is common, and symptoms are decidedly unpleasant; many travelers like to have something along, just in case.

For a number of years, that something was a drug called Entero-Vioform — available only by prescription here, but often sold over the counter elsewhere. Experts have now concluded that reliance on this drug is a rather poor idea. For one thing, it isn't really helpful. For another, it has been known to cause highly toxic reactions, particularly of a neurological and muscular nature. The Center for Disease Control, which among others has warned against Entero-Vioform, suggests that the safest antidiarrheal is paregoric — used carefully, of course, according to directions.

There is, it should be mentioned, a difference between the relatively innocuous "turista" and much more serious ills that can be contracted in out-of-the-way places and may have similar initial symptoms. If symptoms appear rather quickly on arrival, after sampling the local fare, it's probably the common syndrome — and, if so, should be gone within days. If a person first experiences symptoms near the end of the stay or after returning home (or if there are additional symptoms, such as fever, or stools containing pus, mucus, or blood), something more serious is going on and you should seek medical help promptly.

We would also suggest that you (a) discuss an impending trip with your own physician, who may well have specific recommendations such as foods to avoid, medications to take along, and suggested immunizations and (b) take this book with you.

"trench mouth": See GUM DISORDERS.

triamcinolone: See CORTICOSTEROIDS.

Triavil: a trade name for a drug combining amitriptyline and perphenazine; see ANTIDEPRESSANTS.

triceps: See MUSCLES.

trichinosis: an illness caused by *Trichinella spiralis,* a tiny parasitic worm that infests animals, especially pigs. It can normally be prevented by making sure that your family never eats uncooked, or undercooked, pork or pork products. The meat need not be overcooked, however, since the organism is killed at a temperature substantially below the well-done stage; a reading of 180° to 185° F. (82° to 85° C.) on a meat thermometer is sufficient to dispose of any trichinella that may be present. Keeping the meat in a freezer at 0° F. (−18° C.) for 24 hours will also do the trick.

The parasite behaves in the human body the same way it behaves in the pig (which generally gets it by being fed uncooked garbage). It enters the body enclosed in cysts within the meat. Once the cysts reach the intestine, they dissolve, freeing the parasites — which proceed to multiply and send their offspring into the bloodstream; migration carries the organisms to striated muscle tissue, where they become encysted.

The result is muscular aches and pains, which may be preceded or accompanied by a variety of other symptoms, including fever, nausea, vomiting, diarrhea, dizziness, sore throat, and hives; there may also be myocarditis. There is treatment, which ideally takes place prior to muscle involvement, including corticosteroids and/ or a specific antitrichinella drug called thiabendazole — but therapy is lengthy, symptoms are extremely painful, and the whole thing is best avoided.

Although the feeding of raw garbage to pigs was outlawed in the United States in 1953, it has been estimated that perhaps one hundred thousand trichinella-infected swine are still marketed each year — which means that a lot of pigs are still being fed raw garbage (the chance of a grain-fed pig harboring the parasite is less than one in a thousand). If you hear of a program for irradiating slaughtered swine, support it; it can kill off trichinella — and there's no residual radioactivity, change in taste, or hazard to consumers. And we must also mention that travelers do not carry the protection of U.S. agricultural laws with them.

This final note, vis-à-vis avoiding the problem. The parasite does show a preference for pigs, but that doesn't mean it's limited to pigs. Assorted outbreaks of trichinosis in various parts of the world have been authoritatively traced to bear meat. The two most recent, as we write this, occurred in 1972 and 1974: the first was in Idaho and California and was traced to smoked (but uncooked) bear meat; the second, in Japan, involved a group of fourteen hunters who sampled raw slices. The latter incident made history of a sort: although trichinosis in humans has been recognized in this country for many years, it was Japan's first experience with it.

And don't feed your dog or cat possibly infected meat; all mammals are susceptible to trichinosis.

trichomoniasis: an annoying but not terribly serious inflammation of the vagina or urethra (it occurs in both men and women, although symptoms are often absent in males) caused by a parasitic organism present in the vagina and in the gastrointestinal tract of both sexes. Should you and/or your spouse be advised that you have been harboring such an infection, know that there are drugs that can banish it (which should of course be taken according to the prescribing physician's instructions). Know, too, that — as the treating physician may or may not have told you — you will feel extremely ill if you combine alcohol with such drugs.

Tridione: a trade name for trimethadione, an antiseizure drug; see EPILEPSY.

trifluoperazine, triflupromazine: two of the phenothiazine tranquilizers; the latter is also employed as an antiemetic. See NAUSEA; SEDATIVES.

Trigesic: See PAIN RELIEVERS.

Trilafon: a trade name for perphenazine, a phenothiazine tranquilizer that is also employed as an antivomiting agent. See NAUSEA; SEDATIVES.

trimethadione: an antiseizure drug; see EPILEPSY.

trisomy-21: See DOWN'S SYNDROME.

Trobicin: a trade name for spectinomycin; see ANTIBIOTICS.

trypanosomiasis: See PARASITES.

tuberculosis: a bacillary infection that may involve several kinds of body tissue but most commonly (in 90 percent of all cases) attacks the lungs. It is much rarer than it used to be, due to the development of modern techniques that make possible early diagnosis and effective treatment — and to public concern. At this writing, there are some 35,000 new cases in the United States each year — quite a lot, but not as compared with earlier figures. And over 90 percent are now totally curable, assuming treatment is obtained and the physician's advice followed. The problem is much more serious in some other nations; authoritative estimates put the probable world total at fifty million cases. It is well to remember that the bacteria are ubiquitous, and that no one is immune.

The illness is treated with special drugs that can rapidly render it noncontagious, and it is rarely fatal; nevertheless, you should see that your children are protected. One obvious measure is to keep them away from adults who have, or may have, the disease; symptoms in adults may include extremely low energy, weight loss, coughing (which may produce blood-stained sputum), and fever part of the day. If any member of the family has any of those symptoms, an immediate checkup is in order.

In children, the condition is less contagious and may be devoid of symptoms; it is even possible for a child to contract the illness and not display any symptoms until years later, when resistance drops for some reason. But there are skin tests that can detect the presence of the bacteria (the Heaf test, Mantoux test, and Tine test are three in common use), whether or not there is an active infection. Your child should routinely be given such a test at the age of six to twelve months, and as frequently thereafter as your own physician advises.

You may hear the term "active" especially in relation to tuberculosis among adults; the word has a specific meaning. An *active* case is a contagious one and can infect others; a *closed* or *arrested* one isn't contagious, although the person being treated is not yet completely well.

Should TB be diagnosed, it is important that medication be continued as long as the physician has instructed — even after arrest has taken place — in order to conquer the illness completely and to prevent a relapse. Various anti-TB drugs are used, and newer and more effective ones have generally taken the place of streptomycin. They include, prominently, isoniazid (Hyzyd, Niconyl, Nydrazid) and the antibiotic rifampin (Rifadin, Rimactane). Rifampin, incidentally, has a curious "side effect": it sometimes — but not always — turns all bodily excretions, including saliva, sweat, and tears, a bright red-orange.

There is no permanent method of immunization against tuberculosis. BCG vaccine, which gives temporary immunity, is used routinely for children in certain parts of the world, but is not used by, or even available to, private physicians in the United States; it is employed in this country only as a necessary public health measure.

Tuberculosis of the bone, which is uncommon, is usually evidenced by swelling, possibly stiffness and pain; it can be confirmed by X ray. Both it and the very rare tuberculosis of the skin are also treated with special anti-TB drugs.

One other pertinent point should be noted. Other primates — i.e., monkeys and apes — are also susceptible to tuberculosis and, it has been demonstrated, can transmit the disease just as people can.

Tuinal: a combination drug containing the barbiturates amobarbital and secobarbital; see SEDATIVES.

tularemia: a bacterial illness contracted from infected animals or their carcasses; its name was coined from its original discovery in Tulare County, California. It is also known as rabbit fever and, less commonly, deer-fly fever. Unlike most of the world's limited-area diseases, this one is *non*tropical; it's considered endemic in all of North America and Europe, and parts of northern Asia — including Japan — as well.

The bacteria are carried by a number of wild animals — not only rabbits and deer, but also squirrels, muskrats, opossums, foxes, skunks, and coyotes (hunters — and young finders of animals — take note: a slow animal is probably a sick one). Humans may get the infection in a number of ways: by handling the carcass of an infected animal (bacteria can enter through a small cut or abrasion and can actually penetrate unbroken skin as well); by being bitten by such an animal; by drinking contaminated water; through a bite by an insect or tick that has fed on the animal or its carcass; by eating undercooked meat from an infected animal. The bacteria are killed by a temperature of 130° F. (54.5° C.) — but *not* by refrigeration.

Tularemia's first symptom, if it has been contracted by contact or bite, is an ulcer that appears, in one to ten (usually about three) days, at the site of entry of the bacteria (if the infection is by ingestion, the incubation period is usually only one day). This is followed by swollen lymph nodes and additional symptoms that vary and may include fever, weakness, muscular aches, and vomiting. The illness lasts two or three weeks and is effectively treated with antibiotics, generally streptomycin or tetracyclines.

The disease is not contagious person-to-person, and having it once results in immunity. It is, however, best prevented by scrupulous care in dealing with wild animals and their carcasses — including strict instructions to your children never to go near such an animal or consider bringing one home as a pet.

tumor: any abnormal growth of a group of cells, usually similar in character to the surrounding tissue; it is also known medically as a neoplasm

— which simply means "new growth." A tumor may be either malignant or benign; most tumors are benign, and are considered harmful only when they exert pressure on other tissues or organs.

Tums: See ANTACIDS.

Turner's syndrome: like Klinefelter's syndrome (discussed under its own entry), an accident of embryonic development involving the sex chromosomes, but affecting girls, who are missing one X chromosome and are thus XO rather than the normal XX. Turner's is much rarer than Klinefelter's, occurring perhaps once in every five thousand female births; in Turner's, there are also a number of nonsexual physical abnormalities.

The girl with this syndrome is typically of short stature (and will always be so; growth hormone has no effect), with an unusually short neck and a low hairline in back. As in Klinefelter's, sexual maturity does not occur when it should, but that situation can be remedied by hormonal therapy. There may also be a variety of congenital problems involving the heart (especially coarctation of the aorta and pulmonary stenosis), kidneys, and/or eyes, which can often be treated successfully.

Another aspect of Turner's syndrome, of which parents of afflicted girls should be aware, is the possibility of hearing difficulties. It was previously believed that the syndrome frequently involved mental retardation. Now it is known that there is often congenital nerve deafness, possibly accompanied by learning disabilities; a recognition of that likelihood, with remedial measures and special schooling if necessary, can help such a child achieve her full intellectual potential.

Also see SEX CHROMOSOMES.

twins: There are two distinct kinds of twins, occurring in two different ways and with differing frequency.

Identical twins, medically termed *monozygotic* ("one-egged"), derive from a single egg fertilized by a single sperm. Such twins are always of the same sex and are genetically and visually identical or mirror images of each other; any differences stem from purely environmental factors, whether encountered before or after birth, with one exception: fingerprints, even in identical twins, are always unique — suggesting that these patterns are not hereditary, but are formed by chance during development in the uterus.

Fraternal (*dizygotic* or "two-egged") twins result when two eggs simply happen to be fertilized at the same time; they may or may not be of the same sex, and are no more closely related, genetically or in appearance, than any other siblings.

The incidence of twins varies. In the United States, twins occur once in about 80 births, and the rate seems to be substantially higher among older mothers than among very young ones (i.e., the chance of twins is higher for a mother-to-be of thirty-eight than for one of eighteen). In some other parts of the world, the statistics are quite different. Twins occur in the Scandinavian countries, for example, as often as once in 65 births, but only once in 110 births in Spain — and in the Orient, less than once in 170 births.

Three-quarters of all twins are fraternal. The incidence of identical twins is only once in 250 births, a figure that is consistent throughout the world and among all peoples. There is apparently a hereditary factor — or at least some familial influence — with fraternal twins, though not with identical twins.

Twins have no special medical problems by virtue of being twins — except that they are perhaps more likely than single babies to be below average in birth weight.

What's important is that you don't think of them, or treat them, as peas in a pod; twins should be encouraged, from the start, to develop their own identities and personalities. Insofar as you can afford it, it's preferable to dress twins differently, even if they are of the same sex; that way others are less likely to confuse them, and each child will be called by his or her own name — a distinction especially important to fraternal twins of the same sex, to whom mixups can be particularly irritating.

twitching: See TIC.

tybamate, Tybatran: an antianxiety medication or tranquilizer (the second word is a trade name); see SEDATIVES.

Tylenol: a trade name for acetaminophen; see PAIN RELIEVERS.

typhoid fever: an infection caused by a specific bacillus of the *Salmonella* genus; it is spread in a number of ways generally having to do with poor sanitation. Fortunately it is now rare in the United States, although it is still endemic in isolated areas here and is a definite threat in some other parts of the world.

Typhoid fever spreads via excretions from infected individuals and can be carried by contaminated milk, water, food, and so on, as well as by fish and shellfish from polluted water. It may be contracted by direct contact with someone who has the illness, too, and also from an asymptomatic carrier of the infection. Probably the best known individual carrier in medical history was "Typhoid Mary," a cook named Mary Mallon who spread the disease to hundreds in New York City in the early 1900s before the source of the epidemic was discovered.

It is not a pretty illness. The bacillus attacks the intestines chiefly. Symptoms, after an incubation period varying from one to three weeks, include severe abdominal pain, diarrhea (which may be bloody), high fever, intense headache, and a splotchy rash; all this goes on for several weeks if untreated. Typhoid can now be effectively treated with several of the antibiotics, but it's far better prevented and avoided.

By and large, pasteurization, controlled sewage disposal, and the like have helped to make typhoid the rarity it is. If your family is traveling to any area where there's a question about sanitation facilities and water purity, however, you should be vaccinated against the disease; such areas are numerous outside the United States, but include some swampy areas in the United States itself (discuss the destination with your physician). Vaccination is also advised in the event of flood or other natural disaster that threatens pollution of an otherwise safe community water supply. Vaccination gives protection for one to three years.

typhus fever: a term covering a group

of rickettsial infections, all carried by insects or other arthropods from animals to humans or from one human being to another. Typhus is not found in the United States, but it is endemic in eastern Europe, Africa, and the Near and Far East. There are three main types.

Epidemic typhus is carried by body lice and tends to thrive under dirty, crowded conditions; it was epidemic throughout Europe during World War I, and before the advent of antibiotics, up to 50 percent of its victims died. The disease is an extremely unpleasant one in any case. Symptoms, appearing after an incubation period of five to fifteen days, include high fever, chills, severe headache, vomiting, blood in the stool and urine; eventually a rash appears, consisting of dark red, flat spots, and there may be delirium.

Now, epidemic typhus can be cured in two to four days by the administration of antibiotics, especially certain of the tetracyclines. And insecticides can instantly halt an epidemic. There is also a vaccine — which your family should have if you are likely to be exposed to the disease in foreign travels (discuss your itinerary with your physician); immunity lasts for one year.

Endemic typhus, also known as *murine typhus,* is carried by fleas from rats; it is found along seacoasts in a number of temperate to tropical parts of the world. It is similar to epidemic typhus but is less severe and much less likely to be fatal. It is effectively treated in the same way as epidemic typhus and, again, there is a vaccine.

Scrub typhus is found primarily in Asia and the southwest Pacific area and is carried by mites from infected rats and mice. Its symptoms, appearing after an incubation period of a week or two, are very similar to those of a mild case of tick fever or Q fever, two other rickettsial diseases; there may also be a cough and other pneumonialike symptoms. Scrub typhus is considered much less serious than the other types, and there is no preventive vaccine. It is treated, like the others, with antibiotics, and the same antibiotics may also be given prophylactically after known exposure to the disease.

U

ulcer: a disintegration of skin or mucous membrane that leaves an open sore; there may or may not be pain, and the condition may or may not be associated with infection.

For some typical examples of ulcerative conditions, see BEDSORES; CANKER SORES; PEPTIC ULCER.

ulcerative colitis: See COLITIS.

ulna: the larger of the two bones in the forearm; its lower end is attached at the outer (little-finger) side of the wrist, and its upper end is the "funny bone" that suffers the not-so-funny pain when the elbow is sharply struck.

Ultran: a trade name for phenaglycodol, a tranquilizer; see SEDATIVES.

ultrasonography: a noninvasive diagnostic technique utilizing high-frequency sound waves that can be translated to a visual image. The principle on which it operates derives, essentially, from sonar or echolocation, and use of the technique in examining certain organs is often spoken of in such terms — e.g., echocardiography, echoencephalography. It is used for a variety of purposes, including visualization of fetal size, development, and position.

umbilical cord: See NAVEL IN NEWBORN BABY.

umbilical hernia: See HERNIA.

unconsciousness: a condition of complete unresponsiveness to stimuli — inability to hear, see, and move; it is like sleep, except that the victim can't be awakened. The term *coma* doesn't mean a different condition, just implies that the unconsciousness is longer lasting and carries a connotation of greater seriousness. *Fainting* is, on the other hand, much briefer, and is often due to postural hypotension (see BLOOD PRESSURE); treatment consists of lowering the person's head, loosening clothing, keeping the victim lying down until he feels better, and checking to see that no injuries were sustained in falling.

Aside from fainting, what to do about unconsciousness depends upon the cause, and also whether there are other apparent problems. If breathing is weak or failing, you should assist it without delay; see RESPIRATORY RESUSCITATION.

If breathing is all right or has been restored, see if you can find the *cause* of the unconsciousness. If you know that the person is a diabetic or an epileptic or has some other chronic problem, turn to that entry; if you are not sure, check for a necklace, bracelet, or identification card that might mention such a condition. If the pupils are unequal in size (pull up the eyelids and look), or you saw the head strike something, turn to HEAD INJURIES.

If you can't quickly determine any reason for the child's condition, loosen the clothing, cover lightly to maintain body warmth, and call the police or whatever number your community specifies for emergency ambulance service. Don't move or shake the child, and don't attempt to give *anything* — even water — by mouth.

underweight: In an infant or very small child, obvious underweight may mean that there is some factor interfering with normal growth or weight gain. In an older child or adolescent, it may — especially if there is a distinct and sudden weight loss — be a symptom of a number of different conditions, all requiring medical attention. In either case, it should be discussed with your physician.

undulant fever: See BRUCELLOSIS.

unilateral: involving only one side of the body, or only one of a pair of organs or limbs (such as eyes, kidneys, arms, legs, etc.); the opposite of *bilateral.*

Unipen: a trade name for nafcillin, a semisynthetic penicillin; see ANTIBIOTICS.

"ups" or "uppers": slang terms sometimes used by drug abusers to refer to stimulant drugs, especially the "pep pills"; see AMPHETAMINES.

urates: salts of uric acid that may, if there is an excess of the latter, be precipitated and deposited at various places in the body; see HYPERURICEMIA.

urea: a metabolic end-product that is one of the components of urine and can play a part in diaper rash. It is also produced in the chemistry laboratory and has proved useful in treating a few skin and other disorders (it is presently under investigation as a therapeutic agent in sickle-cell anemia). Determination of urea content in the blood is one useful measure of kidney function.

uremia: systemic poisoning resulting from accumulation of toxic wastes normally excreted by the kidneys; it is usually caused by serious and advanced kidney malfunction and can be fatal if it continues untreated. The symptoms, which generally come on gradually, include headache, nausea, vomiting, labored breathing, dizziness, dimmed vision, possibly jaundice, and a peculiar urinelike smell to the breath; subsequently there may be mental disorientation, convulsions, and coma. Any one of these symptoms, of course, should lead you to seek medical care immediately, and the condition shouldn't get to that final stage.

Treatment depends upon how far the condition has progressed and exactly what is causing the trouble with the kidney or kidneys (infection, poisoning of some kind, or degeneration); it may involve medications, removal of a kidney, and/or use of an artificial kidney either temporarily or permanently, or possibly a kidney transplant.

ureter: the tube through which waste materials excreted by the kidney travel to the bladder; each kidney has one.

urethra: the passage through which urine is excreted by the bladder.

URI: an abbreviation widely used by physicians, in both speech and writing; it stands for *u*pper *r*espiratory *in*-

fection — of which the common cold is an example, and is generally what the doctor has in mind when using the term.

uric acid: See HYPERURICEMIA.

urinalysis: the chemical and microscopic study of a specimen of urine, by a physician or technician, to determine such characteristics as acidity, specific gravity, and proportions of various waste materials and to check for the presence of such diagnostic clues as albumin, sugar, bacteria, or blood.

urination: Abnormalities with no ready explanation usually signal some problem. Sometimes weather or other circumstances can cause departures from a youngster's usual pattern; extreme cold, excitement, drinking a lot of liquids can all result in more frequent urination. About one in seven people excrete urine of a reddish hue after eating beets (it's hereditary, an inability to break down a particular pigment called betacyanin — and see ALCAPTONURIA for another hereditary oddity).

But generally speaking, you should call quickly to the physician's attention: excessive urination, in quantity or frequency; unusually scanty urination; pain or other discomfort experienced when urinating; any difference — even seemingly slight — in the color, consistency, or odor of the urine.

urologist: See SPECIALTIES, MEDICAL.

urticaria: See HIVES.

urushiol: See POISON IVY.

U.S.P.: the abbreviation for *United States Pharmacopoeia,* an official publication listing all drugs and medications approved by the Food and Drug Administration of the Department of Health, Education, and Welfare.

ut. dict.: See PRESCRIPTIONS.

uterus: See SEX ORGANS.

Uticillin: a trade name for penicillin V; see ANTIBIOTICS.

Uval: See SUNSCREENS.

uveitis: inflammation of the part of the eye containing the iris and blood vessels. Uveitis needs the immediate attention of an ophthalmologist, unlike inflammation involving only the mucous membrane and not the eye itself (see CONJUNCTIVITIS).

uvula: See PALATE.

V

vaccination: See IMMUNIZATION.

vagina: See SEX ORGANS. Vaginal itching, especially if it occurs at night, may be a symptom of pinworms; see WORMS. For other conditions, see the entries that follow.

vaginal discharge: The significance of a discharge from the vagina depends both on the girl's age and on the nature of the discharge itself.

Sometimes there is a bloody discharge, very like an adult menstrual flow, from the vagina of a newborn infant; although it looks alarming, it's no cause for concern — merely a result of the baby's getting a dose of maternal hormones — and will disappear within a few days.

Some one to three years before puberty and the onset of menstruation, some girls experience a vaginal discharge; if it's a clear fluid, there's nothing to worry about. If it's yellowy and/or odorous, though, take her to the doctor; it may mean there's an infection or a foreign body (such as a wad of toilet paper) in the vagina.

After menstruation starts, a vaginal discharge may mean any number of things (*leucorrhea* is the medical term describing any whitish discharge), some important, some not. If your daughter reports any discharge whatever between periods, the question should be discussed with the physician.

vaginal sprays: Having apparently exhausted their attempts to exploit people's insecurities concerning other body orifices, a number of manufacturers put on the market several years ago products purporting to "deodorize" or "freshen" this particular area. In fact, natural odors in and around the vagina are not unpleasant. Unpleasant aromas emanating therefrom are generally due to (a) deficiency of soap and water (like the armpit, the vulval area perspires a lot) or (b) some disorder that would benefit from medical attention. Further, the sprays have been responsible for many, many cases of severe irritation. We urge that you, if you are a woman, and your daughter resist the pleas of promoters and eschew the sprays. If there is persistent offensive odor from the vulvovaginal area despite the regular use of soap and water, the person to consult is your physician.

"vaginal thrush": See MONILIASIS.

vaginitis: an inflammation of the vagina, usually characterized by pain, redness, and a discharge; it is not uncommon in little girls. Generally it means there is an infection of the tract; if you suspect this condition, take the child to the doctor without delay; it may require treatment with sulfa drugs or antibiotics.

There are two frequent causes for such an infection.

One is simply scratching, with fingernails that are long enough to tear the mucous membrane and dirty enough to introduce bacteria into the area. Bear in mind that it is perfectly normal for little girls to masturbate (see MASTURBATION for a full discussion of that subject); you can avoid trouble by insistence on clean hands, and by trimming those troublemaking fingernails very short.

The other is incorrect wiping following bowel movements, and you should check to see how your daughter has been doing it. Girls should be taught to wipe toward the back, *away* from the vagina and the opening of the urethra (wrong-way wiping can cause trouble there, too); the reason is that there are normally bacteria in the intestinal tract and in the feces — which do no harm there but *can* create havoc if they're accidentally spread to the vagina or urinary tract.

In older girls who have passed the age of puberty (and in grown women, too), antibiotic therapy can sometimes trigger another type of vaginal inflammation; see MONILIASIS. And for still another, see TRICHOMONIASIS.

Valadol: a trade name for acetaminophen; see PAIN RELIEVERS.

Valium: a trade name for the tranquilizer diazepam; see SEDATIVES.

valley fever: a fungal infection of the lungs, medically known as *coccidioidomycosis;* it is also called San Joaquin Valley fever, and is endemic in that part of California but not limited to that specific area (it has sometimes been termed desert fever, and is now found throughout many parts of California, Arizona, and New Mexico).

Aside from its incubation period, generally one to three weeks, the illness itself is similar in all particulars to its counterpart in the central and eastern states; see HISTOPLASMOSIS.

Valmid: a trade name for the prescription hypnotic ethinamate; see SEDATIVES.

Vanobid: a trade name for candicidin; see ANTIBIOTICS.

Vanquish: See PAIN RELIEVERS.

vaporizer: a device designed to increase the moisture content of the air in a home or room. It is a worthwhile investment if someone in your family suffers from a chronic condition that makes breathing difficult or uncomfortable; increased humidity helps to loosen mucus and relieve nasal and bronchial congestion. There are two main types.

One is the hot-steam type or "croup kettle," which gives off hot steam when heated on the stove or electrically. This is the least expensive type, but there is a disadvantage in the possibility of accidental burns.

The other is the electric humidifier that breaks down cold water into minute particles, which are dispersed into the air — thus raising humidity without raising temperature, a distinct advantage.

For short-term or emergency humidity increase, in the absence of a special device, the most practical procedure is to take the child into the bathroom, close the door, and get the room steamed up by running hot water in the tub.

If you do have, or decide to get, a

humidifier, be sure to clean it regularly and thoroughly. The accumulation of molds — they can trigger allergic reactions as well as aggravate upper respiratory infections — has turned out to be a significant problem with neglected humidifiers (often creating the very problems they were intended, and purchased, to relieve!).

varicella: See CHICKENPOX.

variola: See SMALLPOX.

vascular: pertaining to the blood vessels.

vasectomy: See CONTRACEPTION.

vasoconstriction: narrowing of blood vessels. Such an event may or may not be helpful; it certainly is not if it has the effect of decreasing essential oxygen supplies to the body (vasoconstriction, generally peripheral, is one result of smoking). It may be helpful in conditions that involve vasodilation, such as migraine.

vasodilation: expansion (in diameter) of blood vessels. It may be an undesirable occurrence, or a sought-for therapeutic effect; see the immediately preceding entry.

vasopressin: a pituitary hormone; see DIABETES INSIPIDUS.

vasovagal syncope: See SYNCOPE.

V-Cillin: a trade name for penicillin V; see ANTIBIOTICS.

VDRL test: the standard blood test for syphilis; the letters stand for Venereal Disease Research Laboratory. See VENEREAL DISEASES for further comment.

vector: an organism, generally an insect or other arthropod, which carries bacteria or other infectious agents from one person (or animal) to another, but does not itself become ill. Ticks act as vectors in tick fever, for example, and lice perform the same vehicular service for organisms that cause epidemic typhus.

Vectrin: a trade name for minocycline, one of the tetracyclines; see ANTIBIOTICS.

Veetids: a trade name for penicillin V; see ANTIBIOTICS.

vegetarianism: If you are a vegetarian and wish to bring your children up similarly, that's your privilege; despite what you may have heard or read elsewhere, it's not necessarily going to hurt them — if you're careful. Your children do need protein; check the NUTRITION discussion for the reasons. It need not be *meat* protein. (Animal protein is animal protein, just as vitamin C is vitamin C whether it is extracted from rose hips or synthesized in a laboratory.) The advice that follows is derived from the considered opinions of major nutrition authorities.

"Vegetarian" may mean different things to different people. It may signify a totally vegetarian diet (sometimes called "vegan"). Or it may mean a diet that includes milk (and possibly eggs) but not any meats (i.e., animal flesh), often called lactovegetarian (or ovolactovegetarian).

Knowledgeable authorities in the field agree that a straight vegetarian (vegan) diet from birth is something less than desirable. For one thing, it means soybean milk rather than milk of animal origin; although that's sometimes necessary for infants who display an early intestinal sensitivity to animal milk and are being bottle-fed (allergy to human milk is extremely rare), it's not usually continued indefinitely, and other foods of animal origin (cheese, eggs, etc.) appear on the child's menu pretty early. Even after infancy, it is next to impossible — unless you are a highly trained nutritionist and a skilled mathematician as well — to assure a child proper nourishment, including all vitamins and minerals, on a vegan diet.

A lactovegetarian (or ovolactovegetarian) diet is something else; there is good evidence that many youngsters are thriving on such a diet. Since you are excluding a prime source of protein, however, some thoughtful planning is necessary to insure that your youngster's diet does include adequate amounts of this vital element from other sources. In other words, their daily menu should contain plenty of high-protein alternatives — eggs, nuts, milk and milk products (cheese, yogurt, ice cream, etc.), high-protein cereals, whole-grain breads, soybeans and other vegetable protein sources.

No extra vitamin or mineral supplements should be necessary on a lactovegetarian diet, if you balance things properly. On a vegan diet, supplements usually are necessary; such a diet is frequently deficient in cyanocobalamin (vitamin B_{12}), which comes only from foods of animal origin, and in major minerals such as calcium. And many essential amino acids derived from animal products may be missing as well, resulting in severe protein deficiency, or kwashiorkor (see DEFICIENCY DISEASES).

veins: See BLOOD VESSELS.

Velosef: a trade name for cephradine, one of the cephalosporins; see ANTIBIOTICS.

venereal diseases: There is no case for "not *my* child" complacency on the part of any parent as far as venereal disease is concerned. Probably well over eight million Americans are victims of these diseases each year. A quarter of them are under twenty; it has been estimated that another teenager is infected every two minutes. The problem is considerably broader than published figures indicate, since many cases undoubtedly go unreported (which is a great disservice both to individual contacts and to the community at large).

The fact is that, with the advent of "the pill" and other reasonably effective contraceptive measures, teenagers have become increasingly promiscuous — or at least willing to experiment — and careless; this is true, we hasten to add, at all socioeconomic levels. One thing must be made very, very clear to teenagers *and* their parents: contraceptive devices are designed to *prevent pregnancy only;* with the exception of the condom (which, if properly used, can prevent transmission of gonorrhea), they do *not* prevent *venereal disease.*

We would urge all parents of teenage sons or daughters, whatever you may believe their standards of behavior are, to discuss this subject with them. They should be fully alerted to the symptoms and dangers of venereal diseases. Most important, they should be told, if they suspect they may have contracted such an illness, to report that suspicion promptly, either to you or to a physician or VD clinic. Every one of these diseases is completely curable — *if it is caught and treated early.*

Any teenager who is infected with such an illness should also make it a point to alert recent sexual contacts; failing to do so is extremely cruel, and may doom those individuals — and others with whom *they* may have relations — to serious illness, permanent disability, or even death. And of course anyone who is the *recipient* of such a warning should have a medical checkup immediately.

Let us, at this point, dispel one serious misconception. A venereal disease need not be acquired by sexual intercourse in the classic "missionary position." The organisms are not fussy and do not demand a vaginal or penile entry route; *any* body orifice will do.

There are at least half a dozen diseases that are uniquely venereal in means of transmission. The minor ones tend to be the most obvious; that is, their symptoms appear so swiftly, and are so painful or visible, that medical consultation is invariably sought quickly.

One minor one that deserves mention here — since its symptoms, at least initially, are similar to those of many other ailments — is *bubo* or, as it is medically termed, *lymphogranuloma venereum.* It is a viral infection.

In this disease, there is usually a small sore in the genital area, but it normally heals quickly and, unless there is secondary infection, may go unnoticed. The chief symptom, however, is swollen lymph nodes, generally first in the groin, but subsequently in other parts of the body as well as infection spreads via the lymphatic circulation; the swellings are characteristically hard to the touch. There may also be stiffness and swelling in the genital area, fever, and other individually variable symptoms.

Fortunately, lymphogranuloma venereum is one of the few viral infections for which antibiotics are effective; certain tetracyclines are generally used.

Another that merits inclusion is *genital herpes,* which has increased to the point that it is now considered more widespread than syphilis. It is caused by a virus known as HSV-2, a variant of the *Herpes simplex* virus responsible for cold sores and the like, and it causes similar lesions in the genital area. While genital herpes does not result in the kind of ravage wrought by gonorrhea or syphilis, it can be painful, annoying, and difficult to treat; further, it is extremely contagious. But it is of concern chiefly for two other reasons.

One reason is a suspected connection between HSV-2 infection and cervical cancer. Some studies have suggested that women with herpes infection of the cervix are at significantly higher risk for eventual development of cervical cancer; the connection is not clear, and most researchers believe there are other factors involved and that the viral infection may in some way render the cells of the cervix more receptive to malignant changes. Yearly Pap smears are strongly recommended if there has been a diagnosis of HSV-2 infection; cervical cancer is now curable — if it is detected early.

A second reason for concern is that a mother with active vaginal or cervical herpes lesions at the time of delivery can transmit the virus to her child.

There is a 50 percent chance of such transmission, and at least 85 percent of infected infants die or are severely damaged, since the virus is capable of invading such internal organs as the liver, kidneys, and central nervous system. Infection can even occur before birth if several hours pass between rupture of the fetal membranes and delivery. If the mother has HSV-2 lesions in her genital tract, delivery by cesarean section prior to, or immediately after, membrane rupture is recommended.

Genital herpes is treated by scrupulous hygiene, avoidance of tightly fitting, nonabsorbent clothing, and sexual abstinence, until the lesions have disappeared, in order to prevent contagion. Once the infection has been contracted, it may recur unpredictably (just as cold sores do), without further contact with an infected individual. There is as yet no specific preventive or treatment. In 1976, however, there were encouraging reports of preliminary clinical trials of a new medication called inosiplex; they indicated that the drug, which is administered orally, may be useful both in speeding clearing of lesions and in prolonging intervals between recurrences.

The major public-health menaces among the venereal diseases are of course gonorrhea and syphilis; the former is by far the more widespread. Here are the facts about both.

GONORRHEA

Epidemic among young people for the past decade or more, gonorrhea is — if actual proportions reflect those of reported figures — perhaps thirty times more prevalent than syphilis (the Public Health Service estimates 2.7 million reported cases for 1974). It is caused by the bacterium *Neisseria gonorrhoeae.*

A major factor in the appalling incidence of gonorrhea is that there may not be any early symptoms — thus permitting infected persons to transmit the disease to others quite unknowingly. It has long been known that 60 to 80 percent of infected females are asymptomatic, and it was thought they served as *the* "hidden reservoir"; recent studies have shown, however, that at least 10 percent (some estimates run as high as 50 percent or more) of infected males may also be unaware that they are ill.

Even if they do appear — after an incubation period that may vary, but is usually three to five days — early symptoms in females may go unnoticed; generally the only one is a vaginal discharge, which may or may not be heavy enough to be obvious. Symptoms in males are usually quite apparent, with pain on urination and a visible discharge of pus.

Untreated, gonorrhea spreads through the body to other organs, eventually causing such complications as sterility, arthritis with irreversible crippling, heart disease, and blindness. (Infants can also be blinded while passing through the birth canal of a mother who has the disease; this tragedy can be prevented, however, by the administration of silver nitrate or other substances in the baby's eyes, and this precaution is now standard procedure in the United States and a number of other countries.)

Any suspicion of gonorrhea or of

exposure to possible infection — whether or not there are symptoms — means, of course, that a visit to a physician or to a VD detection center is in order. It used to be necessary to take a swab of material from the appropriate organ or orifice(s) and to culture it, which took a nerve-wracking matter of days. Since 1974, a while-you-wait blood test has been available; the diagnosis must still be confirmed by culture (there is a small percentage of false-positive results from the blood test), but a negative answer can be forthcoming immediately.

Treatment, upon confirmation of the diagnosis, is with pencillin G, ampicillin, or — if they are contraindicated — with spectinomycin or tetracycline. The infected individual can pass on the disease to others until follow-up cultures a week or two later confirm that the therapy has been successful and that no *N. gonorrhoeae* organisms remain. And we repeat, because it does bear repetition: anyone diagnosed as having gonorrhea should make sure all sexual contacts are alerted to the fact that they, too, may be harboring the disease.

Because the gonococcus is a first cousin to the bacterium that is responsible for meningococcal meningitis, and a vaccine has been found feasible for the latter, it is hoped that a similar preventive may be developed for gonorrhea in the not-too-distant future. Several formulations have been tested in the past and have not been successful, but one 1975 formulation seemed to hold promise of providing, if not total immunity, at least a degree of resistance.

SYPHILIS

Syphilis is caused by a spirochete, *Treponema pallidum,* and is a three-stage disease; it is curable in the first two stages. Although far less widespread than gonorrhea, syphilis is nonetheless also epidemic, and on the rise. The VD control division of the Center for Disease Control received a total of 84,000 case reports for 1974 — a figure believed by some authorities to represent only a quarter of the actual number — and final figures for 1975 (not available at this writing) were expected to be higher. A vaccine is theoretically possible, but it will probably be quite a few years before an effective one can be developed.

The first symptom, in either sex, is a chancre (pronounced "shanker") — an ulcerating sore — appearing at or near the site of entry of the infection, anywhere up to ninety days after exposure but usually about three weeks. In a male, the chancre generally appears on the penis, and is of course obvious. In a female, however, the chancre may be within the vagina, is usually not painful, and thus may not be noticed — posing the same threat mentioned in connection with gonorrhea.

There have been many odd rumors and old wives' tales about the transmittal of this disease, and it may be well to dispel them at this point. Syphilis is usually acquired in the usual way, by sexual intercourse; uncommonly, it can be contracted by simple kissing — in which case, the chancre appears in or near the mouth (as it does, of course, if the infection is acquired by oral-genital sexual activity).

Neither syphilis nor any other venereal disease has ever been shown to be acquired from toilet seats, swimming in polluted water, or the like. The only known sources of syphilis are (a) direct human contact and — rarely — (b) needles shared by drug addicts.

The disease can be halted at stage one by treatment with penicillin or certain other antibiotics. If it is not treated, the chancre will nevertheless heal within one to five weeks. The second-stage symptom, a rash that may be either general or localized, appears after another interval of about six weeks (the time is quite variable). Again, treatment at this stage will be successful.

If there is still no treatment, the rash disappears, but the disease itself simply remains latent for anywhere from two to fifty years — when it explodes into a variety of ugly conditions including heart and circulatory disorders, blindness, insanity, and death.

Diagnosed victims of syphilis — diagnosis is by blood test — whether at the first stage or the second, must bear in mind the sometimes lengthy incubation period; all sexual partners within a three-month period prior to the appearance of the first symptoms (or a six- to seven-month period prior to the rash stage) must be alerted and should have blood tests.

There are two types of blood tests used in establishing a diagnosis of syphilis. One, which is simple and inexpensive and is the standard technique in screening programs as well as the initial test in individual diagnosis, is the VDRL (it was developed by the Venereal Disease Research Laboratory of the Public Health Service); it tests for a particular substance in the blood (not antibody) based upon a reaction to an antigen (not bacteria). A negative reaction eliminates the possibility of syphilis. A positive reaction can, however, occasionally occur in certain other conditions, notably acute hepatitis and lupus (the false-positive VDRL is not uncommon in the latter). If there is such a reaction, the highly specific FTA (fluorescent treponemal antibody) test, in which serum is withdrawn and challenged with *T. pallidum,* is performed; it will reveal the presence of antibody to the bacterium.

Congenital syphilis, in which the disease is passed on to an unborn child, is now rare; in most of the United States, a blood test for syphilis is given routinely by obstetricians to all pregnant women. If the test is positive, the mother receives treatment *before* the birth of the baby.

ventral: toward the front, or belly side, of the body; the opposite of *dorsal.*

ventricle: See HEART.

Veracillin: a trade name for dicloxacillin, a semisynthetic penicillin; see ANTIBIOTICS.

vermifuges: substances to rid the body of worms. Never buy over-the-counter ones; see ACRODYNIA for the reasons why.

vernix: the white, cheesy film that covers all newborn babies; it's a lubricating substance that eases the baby's way through the vaginal passage. The mother may or may not see it, depending upon whether she is conscious during the birth as well as the hospital's procedure; some hospitals remove it immediately, while others don't.

verruca: See WARTS.

Versapen: a trade name for hetacillin, a semisynthetic penicillin; see ANTIBIOTICS.

vertebrae: the bones of the spinal column (the singular is *vertebra*), which enclose and protect the spinal cord. There are 24 of them: seven cervical vertebrae between the skull and the uppermost rib; twelve thoracic vertebrae, to which the ribs are connected; five lumbar vertebrae, between the thoracic vertebrae and the last two bones of the spine, the sacrum (which connects with the hipbones) and the coccyx (the "tailbone"). The nerve roots emerging from the spinal column do so between the vertebrae and are numbered to correspond (C1, T4, etc.).

vertigo: See DIZZINESS.

vesicle: See LESION.

Vesprin: a trade name for triflupromazine, an antinauseant and potent tranquilizer. See NAUSEA; SEDATIVES.

vestigial: describing a part or organ that has in the course of evolution lost whatever usefulness it may have once had, but is still present in the body; the appendix, the wisdom teeth, and the little toe are all considered vestigial.

Vibramycin: a trade name for doxycycline, one of the tetracylines; see ANTIBIOTICS.

Vincent's angina, or Vincent's disease: See GUM DISORDERS.

viral pneumonia: See PNEUMONIA.

viruses: the smallest and sturdiest kind of infection-causing organisms, often referred to as *filterable viruses* because they can pass through a filter capable of "catching" bacteria. Viruses grow and multiply only in living tissue, thus are difficult to study as compared with bacteria, which can be laboratory-grown in broths and other nutrients; such media as live animals, fertilized eggs, or tissue cultures must be used for virus research.

Many ailments, ranging from colds to flu to warts and including most of the contagious diseases of childhood, are caused by viruses (they are also among the prime suspects in some types of cancer). Most viruses shrug off attempts to banish them with antibiotics; there are a few exceptions, among them the viruses that cause psittacosis and trachoma.

There are, however, effective vaccines that can prevent a good many viral infections, notably those caused by a single virus or at most two or three distinct viruses. This group includes measles, rubella, mumps, polio, smallpox, yellow fever, and the various strains of flu.

You may, from time to time, see words or phrases incorporating the word "virus" or "viruses" that are a bit mystifying and do not seem very specific. They signify viruses, or groups of viruses, that have been specifically categorized on the basis of size, mode of transmission, or other factors. Among those terms:

Adenoviruses — the usual phrasing; it's short for "adenoidal-pharyngeal-conjunctival viruses," so called because they tend to persist in lymphoid tissue (tonsils, adenoids) even in the absence or cessation of symptoms. They thus tend to circulate pretty constantly among children. There are about thirty types (none with names, just numbers); together they probably account for a tenth of the respiratory ills in children, plus most sore throats and cases of conjunctivitis.

Arboviruses — another telescoped phrase; this one's short for "*ar*thropod-*bo*rne viruses," because of the fact that they are transmitted solely by arthropod vectors. There are about eighty of them known altogether (including those that affect only animals), but only a few connected with human ills are found in the Western Hemisphere; they include those that cause equine encephalitis, as well as those responsible for dengue and yellow fever.

Enteroviruses — a large group of viruses that, as you might suspect from the name, are generally domiciled in the alimentary tract — although that's not where they are likely to cause trouble. They circulate among people pretty continuously, although in temperate regions they are most active in summer and fall; having an illness caused by one of them bestows immunity (to that one only) — so small children are most susceptible to infection. The ills they cause, although some have specific names, are extremely variable in symptoms.

There are three subcategories of enteroviruses. Probably the best known members of the group are the three *polioviruses.* Also part of the clan are the *Coxsackie viruses,* the best known of which causes a poliolike late-summer illness (see COXSACKIE DISEASE); there are, however, some two dozen or more, which are known to cause herpangina as well as many early-fall illnesses that resemble influenza (the real "flu season" doesn't start until late fall/early winter). Third, there are some thirty *ECHO viruses;* the acronym is short for *e*nteric *c*ytopathogenic *h*uman *o*rphan viruses, the "orphan" part stemming from the belief, when they were first discovered in humans, that they didn't cause any diseases. They do. Most of the ills the ECHO viruses perpetrate are fairly minor febrile ones, some accompanied by rashes; they are, however, prominent causes of viral meningitis.

Epstein-Barr virus — a specific, herpeslike virus associated with — and considered almost definitely to be the cause of — a malignancy, prevalent primarily in Africa, called Burkitt's lymphoma; the virus is named for the two researchers who made that discovery. Epstein-Barr (EB) virus now is also considered the probable agent causing mononucleosis, as well as a good deal of recurrent tonsillitis. Why and how a single virus behaves in such radically different ways under different circumstances is not known.

Herpesviruses — a group of at least three (possibly more) ubiquitous agents, by and large causing ills that are more uncomfortable than critical. *H. simplex,* type 1 (HSV-1), is a major cause of cold sores and canker sores. Type 2 (HSV-2) is transmitted genitally, and can prove both annoying and difficult to treat; see VENEREAL DISEASES. (There is also some suspicion that it may be associated with precancerous cell changes in the cervix.) *H. zoster,* also known as the varicella-zoster virus, is the cause of both chickenpox and shingles.

Myxoviruses — the viruses that cause flu and flulike contagious diseases;

types A and B are the notorious ones, against which there are vaccines, but there is also a type C — a less prominent member of the family believed to cause occasional mild infections. The name of this group of viruses comes from the Greek *myxa,* "mucus"; they have a particular affinity for mucous membrances.

Parainfluenza viruses — a group of four viruses that can cause a variety of ills ranging from colds to — in infants — croup and bronchopneumonia; the severity of the conditions caused by these viruses is typically in inverse ratio to age.

Paramyxoviruses — a group including the measles virus, the mumps virus, possibly the rubella virus (it has not been definitely classified), and a number of others frequently associated with serious illness — including croup and bronchiolitis — in infants and very small children.

Poxviruses — a group of viruses that characteristically propagate in skin; they include the viruses that cause smallpox *(Poxvirus variolae)* and molluscum contagiosum, as well as a long list of similar ills that afflict other animal species.

Reoviruses — like some of the other category names, a condensation; this one stands for *r*espiratory *e*nteric *o*rphan viruses. They have been found in association with mild febrile illnesses, as well as occasional cases of diarrhea; it is not known, however, whether that's cause-and-effect or mere coincidence.

Respiratory syncytial viruses — like the parainfluenza viruses, a group — there are several strains — tending to afflict younger people far more severely than older ones. In older children and adults, these viruses typically cause colds; in infants and very small children, however, they are likely to set off serious lower respiratory conditions such as pneumonia.

Rhinoviruses — a group numbering well over a hundred, responsible for the vast majority of acute rhinitis cases in school-age children and adults — i.e., the common cold. The proportion is smaller in infants and preschoolers, simply because they are also susceptible to so many other infectious agents to which older folks have acquired immunity.

viscera: an umbrella word for all the internal organs.

vision: If a possible vision difficulty in your child is noted during a regular physical checkup, you will undoubtedly be referred to an ophthalmologist. Unless your pediatrician or family physician does complete vision testing (not just an eye chart), your youngster's vision should be checked by an ophthalmologist at age four to six, certainly no later than six; the doctor, if corrective eyeglasses or other measures are found necessary, will tell you when the child should be seen again (children's eyes grow, and can change, quite rapidly). If there is no abnormality discovered, you should have the child's eyes examined again at the age of ten or twelve — and again, follow the doctor's recommendation as to future checkups.

For comment on some specific vision problems, see ALBINO; AMBLYOPIA; ASTIGMATISM; BLINDNESS; CATARACT; COLOR BLINDNESS; CROSSED EYES; DEFICIENCY DISEASES; DOUBLE VISION; FARSIGHTEDNESS; NEARSIGHTEDNESS.

Vision in infants is discussed under DEVELOPMENT.

Visual acuity, or sharpness of vision, is tested by means of a chart bearing letters, words, figures, or pictures placed, typically, twenty feet from the subject (or employing mirrors or a projection device that accomplishes the distance effect optically). The rating, which is separate for each eye, is expressed in terms of a fraction; "20/20" means that what should be seen clearly at twenty feet *is* so seen at that distance. When the second figure is larger than twenty, it indicates less-than-normal acuity: a rating of 20/30, for example, means that what is seen clearly at twenty feet *should* be so seen at thirty. If the second figure is smaller than twenty, that's better-than-average acuity; a 20/15 value, for instance, denotes the ability to see at twenty feet what is usually seen only at fifteen feet. (The first figure is always 20, since that's the actual or projected distance from the subject to the chart.)

Vistaril: a trade name for the tranquilizer hydroxyzine; see SEDATIVES.

vitamins: See NUTRITION.

vitiligo: a condition involving spotty depigmentation of skin (but not hair or eyes, as in an albino); the condition seems to be more common among dark-skinned races and individuals — but possibly that's because it's more obvious under those circumstances. The cause of the affliction is unknown; for some reason, the pigment-forming cells in the skin lose their ability to produce melanin, the skin-coloring pigment, and the result is a complete absence of color. The condition is not dangerous, but it can be quite disfiguring.

Often, vitiligo disappears spontaneously; skin color comes back as mysteriously as it vanished. If it doesn't, treatment with a combination of certain drugs and ultraviolet light has been found effective in a small percentage of cases, generally those involving only a small area and of fairly short (less than five years') duration; cover-up makeup can, of course, also be used. If most of the skin is involved, and the condition has persisted for some time, the best course is often to deliberately extend the condition to the rest of the body; this can be done via special treatments.

If you suspect your child has this condition, discuss it with your family doctor or with a dermatologist.

Vivactil: a trade name for protriptyline; see ANTIDEPRESSANTS.

"voice box": See LARYNX.

voice changing: The change from the high-pitched voice of a small boy to the deeper voice of a male adult begins at the start of adolescence. The voice pitch depends upon the size of the vocal cords; the shorter the cords, the higher the tone. Women's vocal cords are shorter than men's, and children's are even shorter.

In the adolescent boy, there is a sudden increase in the size of the larynx (which includes the vocal cords, plus the cartilages to which they are attached). It may take place faster than the boy can master the muscles controlling the tension of the cords — thus, there is occasional faltering between high and low pitches. It may be embarrassing to the boy, but it's common and perfectly normal.

volvulus: See INTESTINAL OBSTRUCTION.

vomiting: the forcible ejection of the contents of the stomach; it usually signifies that the body wants to get rid of something. It may be an infectious agent, a poison, or something that causes an allergic reaction, and the vomiting is in that case helpful; or, it may signal a serious condition interfering with the normal downward progress of ingested food. What to do depends upon several factors, including the age of the child and other circumstances; see which of the following applies.

INFANTS

Repeated projectile vomiting in an infant under the age of two or three months — that is, repeated violent upheaval of the contents of an entire feeding — may signify something quite serious, an emergency situation; see PYLORIC STENOSIS.

Simple vomiting in an infant generally means little or nothing. Often, it's not true vomiting but a simple burp that has brought up some milk with the bubble of air (see BURPING). If the child looks all right otherwise, continue the feeding; the baby is probably still hungry. But if there are any other symptoms (fever, bloated belly, a sick appearance) call your physician (and stop the feeding). And if the performance is repeated, whether or not there are other symptoms, call the doctor.

OLDER CHILDREN

Vomiting after an accident or injury may or may not mean something serious. Turn the child on his side and get any vomit out of the mouth to prevent choking. Call the doctor. And don't give the child *anything whatever* by mouth.

Vomiting after taking medicine that the doctor has prescribed may mean there is some sensitivity to the medication. Try giving it mixed with milk, jam, or a soft drink (whatever the child likes and is permissible under the circumstances). If the youngster vomits again, call the doctor.

Unexplained vomiting means you should check for other symptoms of illness. Look at the vomited material; does it just contain food, or is there something peculiar, such as blood? Examine and question the child for other symptoms—pain (anywhere), fever, sore throat, paleness or flushing, a sick feeling, etc.

If there are *no* other symptoms, don't worry about it (but keep an eye out for the development of symptoms). If there are *any* other symptoms, call the doctor, and don't give the child anything at all by mouth (rinsing the mouth with a little room-temperature water to take away the bad taste is permissible).

Vomiting following flu or another similar respiratory infection may be the first symptom of a serious, potentially fatal, condition. Turn immediately to REYE'S SYNDROME, and get in touch with your doctor quickly if the description seems to fit.

Vomiting must sometimes be induced when a child has swallowed something poisonous, but even in case of poisoning, this is not always the safe or advised procedure; to find out if it is or it isn't for the particular substance swallowed, turn to POISONING, HOUSEHOLD SUBSTANCES AND MEDICATIONS.

Voranil: a trade name for the anorexiant clortermine; see DIET PILLS.

vulva: See SEX ORGANS.

W

Waldeyer's ring: a "collar" of lymphoid tissue; it includes the tonsils.

walking: See DEVELOPMENT for comment on when it usually begins; see LIMPING if the child has that problem.

warts: benign, circumscribed (limited) growths on the skin, medically called *verruca;* they are caused by viruses, but they're not contagious. Although warts may resemble moles more than skin lesions we normally associate with viral activity, the cause has been demonstrated without question. Further, some people seem to be more susceptible than others, and high levels of antibodies to the viruses have been detected in those whose warts disappear unusually quickly. Warts may be single or multiple, smooth or rough, large or small, and can occur anywhere on the body; they're considered neither serious nor dangerous.

Warts often disappear by themselves; in young children, they sometimes can be made to go away by the power of suggestion combined with the application of some potent-looking but innocuous substance (nobody, including physicians, knows why this works, but it does). They can also be removed in a simple doctor's-office procedure, but removal isn't usually recommended for a small child unless the wart is subject to frequent irritation. Warts should never be rubbed, scratched, or picked at, because that may lead to bleeding and to subsequent infection.

Plantar warts are a particular type that appear usually on the sole, occasionally on the palm or on the fingers; on the foot, they're often painful, just because they get constant pressure and can't grow outward. A lay person can sometimes confuse them with calluses (but your physician will know the difference). Because of the discomfort they often cause, plantar warts are usually removed — again, a simple doctor's-office procedure that does not require hospitalization; it may, however, involve a series of visits, over several weeks, including some at-home procedures.

Molluscum contagiosum is a condition involving multiple warts of a special description; they are raised, distinctly rounded, and umbilicated (that is, they have little depressions, like navels, at the center). They're usually in one area — most often the face, arms, or genitals — but may appear in scattered patches; "contagiosum" means that they often tend to spread on the same child, not that they're contagious to others.

Like ordinary warts, molluscum contagiosum is virus-caused, benign and not considered particularly serious, and may vanish spontaneously. If it doesn't, and the number and/or location of lesions poses a cosmetic problem, the warts, like others, can be removed; they also sometimes yield to certain topical medications.

Also see WHITEHEADS, with which warts can sometimes be confused.

wasp stings: See BITES AND STINGS.

"water on the brain": See HYDROCEPHALUS.

wax in ears: a substance produced by certain cells of the outer ear, and medically called *cerumen;* it's similar to sebum. Sometimes it accumulates and creates a plug, causing discomfort and/or diminished hearing; whether or not this happens depends upon the amount of wax produced and also the ear structure.

Don't ever try to remove ear wax yourself; your attempts could cause serious injury to the child's ears. Have the physician do it. The doctor may suggest (and we concur) that for a week or so prior to bringing the child to the office, you put a dropperful of hydrogen peroxide (3 percent solution, not the twenty-volume bleaching type), followed by a small amount of glycerine, in each ear once a day; that softens the wax and makes its removal easier for the doctor and more comfortable for the child.

weaning: When to wean your baby from breast or bottle to a cup should be discussed with your own physician. It may begin as early as the age of six months, but it's a very individual matter.

weight: Ideal weight for a child — or an adult, for that matter — depends upon a number of individual (and partly hereditary) factors, including height, bone structure, and muscular configuration; your own physician is the sole competent judge of whether or not a child's weight is right for that child.

Also see GROWTH RATES; OVERWEIGHT; UNDERWEIGHT.

wen: an obsolete word for a sebaceous cyst; see CYSTS.

wheezing: a symptom of some obstruction or constriction in the respiratory passages; the possibilities are numerous, and include infections such as sinusitis, allergic conditions such as asthma, and inhaled foreign objects or substances. If your child is wheezing, note any other symptoms that may be present and call the doctor.

whiteheads: True whiteheads occur at puberty or later; they are plugs in oil ducts — and are essentially incipient blackheads that have not yet been discolored by oxidation. Sometimes they are confused with small warts, and vice versa. See your physician; don't try to remove them yourself.

"Whiteheads" in an infant, tiny, shiny, and usually on the face, are something else; they are the result of still-closed sweat glands and are common during the first few months of life, especially if the weather (or the house) is quite warm. Nothing need be done about them; they'll eventually go away by themselves.

white spots: See VITILIGO.

whooping cough: a contagious disease of childhood, caused by the bacillus *Bordetella pertussis;* the medical term for it is pertussis. It is considered quite serious in infants, far less so in older children.

During its incubation period of five days to three weeks (the average is fewer than ten days), pertussis behaves like a persistent cold. Then the characteristic "whooping" cough begins (rarely, a child can have the infection without the cough) — a loud, spasmodic cough with difficulty in catching the breath. The typical whooping sound is made when the child inhales between coughs. There may also be vomiting following the coughing spells. There is generally little or no fever unless complications occur.

The infection persists for a month or two, and is quite contagious while the cough lasts. Antibiotics have little effect against whooping cough (it's in that sense unlike most bacterial infections), but may be given to guard against secondary infection and to decrease the severity of the illness somewhat, especially in an infant; there is also a special gamma globulin that is often helpful in small children. Other measures may also be taken to guard an infant against possible complications, which can include pneumonia and encephalitis. A baby or very young child may also require additional relief via steam inhalations, administration of oxygen, or special medications.

In addition to these medical measures, which are of course up to the physician, the child must be fed a good, balanced, but easy-to-digest diet, best given in very small amounts many times a day rather than via the usual number of full meals. Strained meats and vegetables, broths, juices, puddings, gelatin, and the like are good, and it's wise to feed the child fifteen or twenty minutes after a coughing spell has subsided.

If whooping cough is diagnosed in one child, other susceptible children in the family should be given gamma globulin. Once an individual has the infection, there is a long — though not lifelong — immunity.

Because whooping cough can be so serious in infants and very small children, periodic vaccinations beginning at two or three months and continuing to about five years are recommended (see IMMUNIZATION for the suggested schedule). After that, because older children tend to have severe reactions to the vaccine and also because the illness is milder in older children, pertussis injections are generally discontinued.

Wigraine: See MIGRAINE, for which this combination-of-ingredients medication is used.

Wilms' tumor: a malignant tumor of the kidney; it is the third most prevalent solid tumor in children and is found *only* in children. It is believed to be congenital, arising (for unknown reasons) from embryonic tissue, and typically becomes evident before the age of six; its appearance after the age of eight, while not unknown, is extremely rare.

Generally Wilms' tumor — it's named for Dr. Max Wilms, a turn-of-the-century German surgeon — is first brought to medical attention by a parent who has noticed a lump or swelling toward one side of the child's abdomen, or has felt such a swelling while bathing the child. There may or may not be other symptoms preceding or accompanying that discovery, such as malaise, fever, loss of appetite, abdominal pain, or blood in the urine; usually, there aren't.

The tumor is typically encapsulated within the kidney, so there is a very good possibility of complete surgical removal. Metastasis can take place, though, via individual cells that break away and travel to other parts of the body in the bloodstream — and that process can be initiated by physical pressure. So if you suspect your child may have this kind of tumor, *don't poke* — and do seek prompt diagnosis, which is confirmed by careful examination, blood counts, urinalysis, X rays, and IVP.

Treatment in addition to surgery may or may not be necessary, depending upon the size of the tumor and whether or not metastasis is suspected. Sometimes drugs may be given before the operation to shrink the tumor; they will generally be given after surgery if the physician feels there may still be some roving malignant cells. Usually there is a postoperative course of irradiation treatments, unless the child is less than a year old *and* there's no doubt whatever that every last bit of cancerous tissue has been removed.

The prognosis in Wilms' tumor is quite good. While phrases such as "five-year survival rate" and "ten-year survival rate" are typically used in discussing most other malignancies, here the word "cure" is actually employed — and is now being applied to two-thirds of the cases. A major factor is that 95 percent of all metastases or recurrences appear, if they are going to appear at all, within a two-year period — so that if a child is perfectly healthy two years after surgery, it is highly probable that the child has, in fact, been cured.

For general discussion of malignancies in children, and cross-references to other major forms, see CANCER.

Wilpo: a trade name for phentermine; see DIET PILLS.

"witch's milk": See BREAST DEVELOPMENT.

workup: You may hear a physician use this term. It refers to a series of tests which, combined with the patient's medical history and physical examination, are designed to clarify the diagnosis of the particular disease or condition in question. A workup may or may not require hospitalization.

worms: These parasites that can afflict both animals and humans are ubiquitous, and are part of a large group of organisms of various sizes that use other, larger organisms in stages of their life cycles, usually to the detriment of the latter. Generally part of the life cycle is spent in the outer environment, part in the host.

Some such organisms can't be seen, even in the adult stage, with the naked eye, but can nevertheless cause trouble (see PARASITES and TRICHINOSIS). The parasites discussed in this entry, however, are closer to what we think of when we use the word "worm"; they're considerably less obtrusive than an earthworm, but they are nonetheless large enough to be seen (although their eggs are strictly microscopic).

It's true that the spreading of worms among children can be prevented to an extent by good personal hygiene (such as hand washing after bowel movements) and public-health measures such as control of water pollution, adequate sewage disposal, and laws regulating the handling of foods. Despite these precautions, children do sometimes acquire worms one way or another, and it's nothing that you need be ashamed of; the discovery that your youngster has worms is not necessarily any reflection on you, your home, or your family, and you should not let embarrassment deter you from seeking proper treatment, if you suspect such a condition.

Do go to your physician for diagnosis and treatment, and *don't* use over-the-counter vermifuges (antiworm preparations); some of the latter are very dangerous (see ACRODYNIA).

There are four major types of worms found in the United States. In rough order of prevalence, they are pinworms, roundworms, hookworms, and tapeworms; the last three afflict, and can be spread by, dogs and cats as well as humans.

PINWORMS

These worms, also sometimes called threadworms, are quite common in temperate climes, and a child can pick up the microscopic eggs almost anywhere. It is estimated that pinworms infest or have infested some 75 percent of all New York City children in the three-to-five-year age group; the figures for other cities are probably similar.

Once on the hands, the eggs find their way to the intestinal tract very easily: little children put their hands in their mouths. The eggs hatch in the lower intestine, grow into white threadlike worms about ⅛ inch to ½ inch (0.3 to 1.2 centimeters) in length, and are fruitful and multiply.

The females then crawl out through the rectum, usually at night, to lay their eggs around the anus, and itching in this area is usually the first (and may be the only) symptom. Sometimes they get lost and can't find their way back; they may then wander, in a girl, to the vagina (which causes itching there, too), or even onto pajamas, underwear, or bedclothes, where the worms may sometimes first be discovered even before the child has complained of any discomfort.

If the child scratches, there is risk of secondary infection (as we've said in a number of other places in this book: keep children's nails trimmed very short); even fingering the itchy area, then putting the fingers in the mouth, of course perpetuates the worms' cycle. The only other symptom, if there is one, may be a mild "upset stomach."

Pinworms can be banished by prescription medications given by mouth. If pinworms are diagnosed in a child, all members of the family should be examined and, if necessary, treated, since the eggs may have found their way readily to others.

ROUNDWORMS

The second most common kind of worms, known medically as *ascaris,* are a good deal larger than pinworms; the female can be as long as fifteen inches (38 centimeters), the smaller male about six or seven inches (15.2 to 17.8 cm). Roundworm eggs are found in soil; the eggs find their way to the human intestinal tract via unclean food grown in contaminated soil, or like the eggs of pinworms, by way of little hands put into little mouths.

Roundworms normally make their home in the small intestine. The eggs hatch, progress through a barely visible larval stage, then grow into adults, which are wont to curl up in a ball and brace themselves against the intestinal wall like a coiled spring. The females lay some two hundred thousand eggs a day, which are excreted in the feces, which then find their way back, through careless sewage disposal, to soil, and the cycle continues.

If there are only a few roundworms in the intestine, and no other untoward events, there may be no specific symptoms (although of course the eggs can be found by stool analysis). There can be complications, however. A great many roundworms inhabiting a stretch of intestine can cause a tumorlike mass that obstructs the tract. And like pinworms, roundworms may wander beyond their usual haunts. The larvae can slip into the bloodstream and be carried to the respiratory tract and lungs, where they can cause pneumonia. The adult worms can migrate upward to plug the bile duct or esophagus.

Various medications, given orally, can get rid of the infestation.

HOOKWORMS

Like roundworm eggs, the eggs of hookworms are found in soil contaminated by sewage — but in this case, a particular type of soil: warm, sandy, and moist; hookworms are found predominantly in the Southeast. Once in the soil, the eggs hatch in about a day. The minute larvae can enter the human body either via contaminated food or water or directly through the skin, even if the skin is unbroken (often the victim has been barefoot); in the latter case, itching and inflammation at the site of entry may be the first sign of the invasion.

Like other worms, hookworms head for the intestine. If the larvae have entered through the skin, their method of accomplishing this adds an extra dimension to the troubles suffered by their human host. They ride the bloodstream as far as the lungs, where they cause a pneumonialike inflammation that's accompanied by coughing; then, when they're coughed up into the throat, a number of them manage to be swallowed — and they're on their way to their destination.

Once in the small intestine, they swiftly become adults, varying in size from ¼ inch to ½ inch. True to their name, they have hooklike appendages which enable them to hang onto the intestinal wall — which they do, living by sucking blood. They also excrete a toxic substance that has the nasty faculty of causing capillaries to burst and interferes with normal coagulation of blood.

In any quantity at all, hookworms produce a definite anemia. Commonly, symptoms include fatigue, weakness, dullness and dryness of hair and skin, and a feeling of hunger; this kind of anemia is never fatal, but it can be completely debilitating. Similar symptoms, of course, may be caused by other conditions; hookworm infestation can be diagnosed, however, by analysis of the stool — which reveals the eggs (each female worm may produce up to fifteen thousand eggs a day).

Treatment, depending upon the stage at which the infestation is discovered, may include medications to combat lung inflammation or anemia, as well as drugs to banish the worms themselves.

TAPEWORMS

These are long, flat worms like tape measures, and when we say long, we mean long: they can be fifteen feet (four and one-half meters) or more in length. There are actually about forty different species of tapeworm, but only five or six are really common, and they all behave in about the same way.

Tapeworms are acquired by ingestion — of the flesh of animals or fish that have been infested (often by feeding on contaminated material), or of feces-contaminated food or water. The worms settle in the intestine; like hookworms, they are equipped with attachment devices and are bloodsuckers.

Symptoms vary with the number of worms and the child's general health, but they typically include weight loss, anemia, and weakness; there may also be diarrhea (or sometimes constipation) and/or a large appetite (or sometimes a loss of appetite). Such symptoms are suggestive of a number of other ailments, but as with other worms, the condition can be quickly diagnosed by stool analysis, which reveals eggs and/or segments of the worms (bits and pieces tend to break off, which unfortunately doesn't faze the tapeworms).

As with other worms, there are a number of effective medications the physician can prescribe.

wounds: Turn to the specific type of wound to see what measures should be taken, as BULLET WOUNDS; CUTS; FRACTURES; SCRAPES AND SCRATCHES; etc.

wrist, broken: See FRACTURES.

wry neck: See NECK PROBLEMS.

Wygesic: an analgesic combining propoxyphene (see NARCOTICS) and acetaminophen (see PAIN RELIEVERS).

X

xanthoma: a symptom of a hereditary condition involving fatty deposits, primarily and particularly in the skin; it doesn't appear, usually, until well after infancy. Like some other hereditary conditions, its nature depends upon whether it is inherited from both parents or only from one.

If it is inherited from only one parent, there are yellow spots or patches in the skin, especially on the eyelids. These are fatty tumors, but they're benign. They can be easily removed via minor surgery; they may recur, but the condition still isn't considered serious.

If the gene is inherited from both parents — a situation even rarer than the simple skin condition — the deposits in the skin are not mere patches but nodules, and there may also be similar fatty deposits in internal organs; such a condition is, of course, a good deal more serious. How serious it is, and what's to be done, depends upon the organ(s) affected and the number and location of the tumors.

Should xanthomas be diagnosed in a child, it is extremely important that blood tests be done; see LIPIDS.

xeroderma: unusual dryness of the skin, especially upon exposure to sunlight; it is believed probably due to hereditary factors.

xerophthalmia: an eye condition caused by deficiency of vitamin A; see DEFICIENCY DISEASES.

X rays: radiation beamed at specific areas in order to treat (as, in malignant growths) or to diagnose (the rays can be focused on a photographic plate and thus register certain internal conformations). It is true, as you may have read, that radiation in large doses can be harmful. Be assured that your physician and your dentist are at least equally aware of this fact; they will advise and use X ray only when necessary for treatment or for maintenance of your child's health.

Y

yaws: a tropical infectious skin disease involving multiple ulcerations; it sometimes resembles ringworm. It is caused by a spirochete that is a first cousin to the one that causes syphilis; yaws, however, is not a venereal disease.

"yeast" infection: See MONILIASIS.

"yellow babies": See RH FACTOR.

yellow fever: a viral infection transmitted by the bite of a specific mosquito; it's endemic in some parts of Central and South America as well as parts of central Africa, but has been successfully eliminated from many areas simply by destroying the mosquito vector and its breeding places. Travelers should know that it also affects other primates — i.e., apes and monkeys — in areas where it is prevalent.

The disease is an extremely unpleasant one, including (after a three- to six-day incubation period following the bite) high fever, headache and back pain, and internal bleeding; it can be fatal.

If your family is traveling to an area where yellow fever is endemic you should be vaccinated, and such vaccination is in fact required by the World Health Organization for travel to certain areas. The vaccine is — unlike some others — 100 percent effective, and protection lasts ten years; it is available in the United States only through vaccination centers designated by the Public Health Service, and not through private physicians. Your own doctor can tell you, however, where to obtain the vaccination.

yellow in eyes or skin: See JAUNDICE.

"yellow jackets": a slang term, sometimes used by drug abusers, for the barbiturate pentobarbital; see SEDATIVES.

yellow jacket stings: See BITES AND STINGS.

yellow spots: See XANTHOMA.

Yersinia: a genus of bacteria, the most prominent of which *(Y. pestis)* causes plague.

Z

Zactane, Zactirin: trade names that signify, respectively, the analgesic ethoheptazine and a combination of that drug and aspirin; see NARCOTICS.

Zarontin: a trade name for ethosuximide, an antiseizure drug; see EPILEPSY.

ZIG: the abbreviation for *z*oster-*im*mune *g*lobulin; see CHICKENPOX.

zoonoses: animal diseases that can be — and are — transmitted to man; that is, the animal has the disease, and doesn't simply act as a vector. The plural form, the one you're most likely to see, is used here; the singular is not zoonose, but *zoonosis,* and is pronounced "zoh-on-oh'-siss" (the plural is "zoh-on-oh'-sees").

Probably the best-known zoonosis is rabies. A number of ailments common to man can also afflict other primates (apes and monkeys). Other zoonoses include brucellosis, equine encephalitis, psittacosis, ringworm, trichinosis, and tularemia.

zygote: a fertilized egg. For explanation of some other words stemming from this one, see HOMOZYGOUS; TWINS.

Appendix A.

How to Choose and Use a Doctor

You should, let us say at the outset, have a physician who takes care of your children on a regular basis — someone they see periodically for checkups, who is available in case of illness or injury, whom you can call to ask advice and who can answer questions concerning your youngsters' physical and emotional health. The kind of physician you choose will depend in part upon the age(s) of your children, in part upon where you live.

Chances are, if you live in a small community with few physicians, there will be few narrow specialists. Your children's doctor is likely to be *your* doctor as well, a specialist in family practice — one who attends all members of the family both young and old, including prenatal care.

In a larger community, there is more stratification. Although an increasing number of family physicians are practicing in larger cities, the physician attending adults in your family will probably be an internist and, although many teenagers choose to remain with the doctor who cared for them when they were younger, some may feel that they want a "grown-up doctor"— so that your internist may be your older children's physician as well. The physician responsible for your baby's and younger children's health will almost always be a pediatrician.

RECOMMENDATIONS

Whatever the *kind* of physician you are seeking, there are a number of good routes to follow — and one rather poor one. *Don't* pick an M.D. from the yellow pages. Two reasons. One is that the people listed there are not always duly licensed physicians. Yes, that statement is really true. In early 1973, it was found that in New York State, from 7.0 to 13.8 percent of those listed (there were variations from one metropolitan area to another) were not, in fact, licensed to practice medicine; the telephone company has since submitted listings to the state's medical society for verification. A subsequent survey in Washington DC revealed a similar situation. But even if every "M.D." listing in your local telephone directory is, in fact, an individual duly licensed to practice medicine in your state, you may make an awful lot of calls before you find a physician in the category you're seeking; see SPECIALTIES, MEDICAL for a sampling of the people your calls might turn up.

(It should be noted that physicians are listed by specialty in a few areas, and such listing is under consideration in some others. Do not suppose such a listing guarantees anything. Such names may, again, not be cross-checked even for licensing. And if they are, the "specialty" practice claimed may be no more than wishful thinking. A 1975 survey followed up over eleven thousand physicians listed as specialists in the phone directories of eight California counties; just 56.9 percent had actually passed a specialty examination. Some of the remainder may have in fact been highly qualified, skilled, and about to take their exams. Others clearly were not: one general practitioner, styling himself a "plastic surgeon," was successfully sued after maiming a patient, escaped by declaring bankruptcy, and at this writing was reported back in business employing the same *modus operandi* — and, incidentally, still listing himself as a specialist with the county medical society.)

How *should* you go about looking for a physician to care for your children? The situation is a little different, as far as recommendations are concerned, depending upon whether you're moving, or staying in the same community; in the latter instance, you may be looking for a doctor because you have, or are expecting, a new baby, or because the physician who has been caring for your children is moving away or retiring, or just because you want to change.

If you are moving, a good source of recommendations is the physician you are now seeing, who may well know — or know of — competent colleagues in other areas; by all means, ask. A physician who is retiring or moving away will be similarly happy to recommend a replacement. And an obstetrician caring for an expectant mother is generally able to suggest the names of several pediatricians.

One reason that a physician you know is a good source of recommendations is that the physician knows *you.* As we shall point out in more detail a little later, a degree of rapport between doctor and patient (and/or parent) is a very important part of the picture. For the same reason, if your present physician cannot offer any names — or if you have decided to change doctors, thus precluding any such discussion — others who know you can be helpful: friends and relatives, business or professional associates, new neighbors if you have moved to a new community. (Naturally, it is well to exercise a little discretion. A physician will presumably be a reasonably good judge of a colleague's competence. A friend or neighbor may or may not be. If your friend's or neighbor's children seem sickly, markedly under- or overweight, have never had any vaccinations, or otherwise appear to be continuously in something less than good health, a recommendation from their parents is perhaps not awfully valuable.)

Assuming that for some reason none of the foregoing sources are available to you, where do you turn if not to the telephone directory?

There are a couple of good possibilities.

One is the county medical society. In most places that office will have a list of practicing physicians and will happily provide the names of two, three or more of the kind you seek. There is one disadvantage. Physicians who have been in practice for some time and are kept busy around the clock by their regular patients often remove their names from county lists. Thus, the names you receive will likely be those of young, less experienced physicians, who may not yet be Board-certified — or, sometimes, those of older, behind-the-times physicians. At the same time, there's another side to that very coin: medicine has changed quite a bit over the past couple of decades, and a *young* doctor listed with the medical society, one who has recently emerged from medical school, internship, and residency, may well be more familiar with up-to-date techniques and thinking than another who has been in practice for twenty years and has been Boarded for ten, but who has not made any further self-education efforts. (At this writing, incidentally, there is talk of required recertification in all the specialties; the American Board of Family Practice already mandates it, and family physicians must be recertified every six years.)

Another good source may be the young interns and residents at the nearest good hospital. (By "good" we mean preferably affiliated with a medical school in some way, operated on a nonprofit basis by private citizens or local government, and certainly accredited by the Joint Commission on Accreditation of Hospitals.) These are the very young white-coated people who usually regularly staff emergency rooms and walk-in clinics. Don't bother them if they're busy. But if you can wander in and corner them when they're not, they will be able to give you the names of those physicians who are guiding them during their postgraduate training. While there are some physicians who are full-time faculty members at medical schools, there are many more — generally designated as "attending" (or some degree thereof) — who are in private practice and donate a portion of their time to teaching. They are almost invariably Board-certified, they have had experience in patient care as well as continuing contact with the academic and research areas, and they are pretty good bets.

Whatever source or sources you turn to, try to get at least two or three names. That will save you time, in case the first one doesn't work out.

MAKING A CHOICE

Your first step is to pick a name from your list and phone for an appointment. (*Don't* put it off until your child falls ill; at that point, you will not want to take the time to shop around.) Be frank about the reason for your call, and make an appointment to talk with the doctor. You may be told that a minimal fee will be charged for the visit, and that's perfectly legitimate (although some physicians do not charge for such a visit, they are fully entitled to do so).

It's smart to arrive a little early for that initial appointment; that way, you'll have an opportunity to look around, get a feel of the atmosphere, observe other patients and parents, see how people are treated by the nurse or receptionist — in short, to get an idea whether or not you feel comfortable. If your child is over the age of three years, it's a good idea to bring the child — who is, after all, the prospective patient — with you.

Some questions to ask yourself: Do other parents seem relaxed? Are they treated cordially? Do the children in the waiting room seem happy, or terrified? Does the place — allowing for the havoc wrought by youngsters tossing toys and magazines about — meet your particular standards of cleanliness and order?

Once you are in the physician's office, don't hesitate to ask any and all questions concerning both the doctor's qualifications and habits of practice. You have every right to — and, in fact, an obligation to your children to do so. Is the doctor licensed to practice? The license is usually displayed; if you don't see it — and have no background information, such as a faculty position, to reassure you — *ask.* How about Board certification, whether in Pediatrics, Family Practice, or Internal Medicine? Again, such a certificate is usually displayed — but if you don't see one, *ask.* You may be told that the doctor is "Board-eligible." (The specialty board exams cannot be taken immediately after completing a residency; a certain amount of actual practice experience is required.) Does that mean that the examinations will be taken very soon? *Ask.*

How about the physician's hospital connection(s) — i.e., where will your child be placed by this doctor if hospitalization is necessary? Again, you may have background information on this point — but if you haven't, *ask.* Is the hospital affiliated with a nearby medical school? That's good. If not, is it a hospital that has a working relationship with a not too distant medical school? Not bad. That means there are officially approved residency programs and that someone other than the proprietors is judging the place. Is it run privately, strictly for profit? Not good; chancy, anyway. Interns and residents in such a hospital — these are the physicians with prime responsibility for around-the-clock care of hospitalized patients — are often there because they were not accepted by the more desirable programs at teaching hospitals.

(This may be as good a place as any to explain a few terms many people have found confusing concerning various types of hospitals. *Municipal hospitals, county hospitals,* etc., are hospitals supported by public funds; they may be, and many are, teaching hospitals as well, by affiliation with a medical school. *Voluntary hospitals* are nonprofit institutions, also frequently associated with medical schools. *Proprietary hospitals* are privately owned and operated by a single physician or, more often, by a group of physicians; such hospitals do not accept patients of other physicians.)

How about the physician's availability? Is there a "call hour" — many pediatricians and family physicians have such an hour, often first thing in the morning — when you can phone to ask nonurgent questions? More important: how about the situations that do involve urgency? Is the physician's phone answered 24 hours a day? By whom? Who returns the calls, if a physician is not doing the answering? How about house calls: does this doctor make them? If not personally, is there someone on call who does? (Although there is a lot of joking about this topic, most physicians do in fact make house calls — if and when it's necessary and desirable to do so. Many times, it is neither. A generation ago, a critically ill child might have been as well off, or even better off, in his own bed, since the hospital had little more to offer.

Now, a physician who believes a child is critically ill may well prefer to treat the child in the hospital, where sophisticated diagnostic techniques, emergency equipment, and the newest medications are at hand.)

Especially if you are a new parent, you want to feel that the physician is not only qualified to look after your child, but will evidence some patience and understanding in dealing with you, no matter how minor your concerns may seem. If you are fortunate enough to be sitting in the doctor's office when a call comes in, pay attention.

How does the doctor react to the call? Is a call refused when the nurse or assistant urges the doctor to take it? If it is accepted, how is it answered? Does the doctor seem truly concerned about the person at the other end of the line? Would you like to *be* the person at the other end of the line?

If your child is with you, you will want to be sure that there is an affinity there, as well. *You* should feel comfortable with the physician — *and so should your child.* How do they react to each other? Does the child seem frightened or repelled — or relaxed and interested? Does the physician talk "over the child's head" as if the latter were not there? Or do you sense an interest in really establishing a relationship with the child? If the child asks questions — about equipment or anything else — are they curtly dismissed, or pleasantly and honestly answered?

Whether the interview lasts five minutes or forty-five minutes, do you feel that you are welcome — or that each visit is part of an assembly-line operation, to be terminated as quickly as possible?

And do ask about money. Doctors do charge fees, and you are entitled to know what they are. It is not at all out of line to ask the costs of various services — an office visit to have a cut finger stitched, a complete checkup, immunizations, house calls, etc. Typically, the fees of physicians practicing in the same specialty in the same community will be roughly similar — although a doctor who is a diplomate of the appropriate board and spends part of the time instructing future physicians at a medical school may, deservedly, feel entitled to charge slightly more than someone who has a license to practice, period.

If, at the end of the interview, you feel that the physician is not for you, or you're not sure, it's perfectly all right to indicate that three different doctors were highly recommended to you and that you would like to talk with the others before you make your decision. And do so, repeating the process each time. If you can't find someone whose personality delights you, you're probably wise — other things being equal — to choose on the basis of professional qualifications.

THE FIRST VISIT

Once you have come to a decision, you should schedule a visit to the office of the physician you've selected, for a complete physical and history. It should include a full head-to-toe examination of the child, including vision and hearing. And it is now the doctor's turn to ask questions, because certain information is vital if your child is to be cared for properly. (Most of this applies, incidentally, to initial contact of an adult with a new doctor.) If they are not asked, that should give you pause.

Here are the main things the physician *should* want to know: Where and when was the child born, and who was the attending physician? What serious ills has the child had, and when? How about surgical procedures, fractures, other major injuries? What immunizations has the child had, and when? Has there been evidence of any allergies or other idiosyncratic reactions, and if so, what? Is there any family history of diabetes or heart disease? Or other hereditary conditions? Are the child's grandparents living? If not, when did they die, at what age, and of what illness? Is the child generally happy? If not, what seems to be the problem? Do you feel the child has any physical — or other — problem? Does the child? Obviously, depending upon the child's age, some of these questions should be directed to the child.

THE ONGOING RELATIONSHIP

Assuming all this goes well, you will now have a regular doctor. Since you have gone to all sorts of trouble to select that physician carefully, you will want to use his or her expertise to your child's best advantage. Here are a few pointers to that end.

Follow the physician's advice. While that may seem so obvious that it doesn't bear mentioning, agonized discussions of the possible reasons for something called "patient noncompliance" take up almost as much space in medical journals as learned discourses on newly discovered drugs and diseases. They add up to, "We tell them what to do, so how come they don't do it?" For your child's sake, be sure to: return for a follow-up visit, or report by phone, if the doctor asks you to; give the child a medication just as the doctor has directed, for *as long as* directed (many antibiotics banish symptoms long before they have chased away the infection); see that your child has periodic checkups and immunizations on the schedule recommended by your doctor (which may differ, for good reason, from the general ones presented in this book).

Be fully familiar with your child's normal, usual appearance and behavior, so that you'll be aware of any *departure* from that norm (*your* child's norm, not that of the child down the block or an "average" we've recorded in this book). Any unusual condition or symptom should mean a prompt call to the doctor. (See the separate discussion of phone calls a bit later.)

Never give your child any medication without your doctor's advice, unless you've previously been given general instructions that apply to the particular situation. If your physician has indicated that any time Johnny has a headache, he may be given a certain dosage of aspirin at particular intervals, what is meant is just that; it does *not* mean that you may arbitrarily increase the dosage or shorten the intervals, *nor* does it mean that you may apply the same remedy if Johnny has an *ear*ache.

If a medication has been prescribed or recommended, and your child (a) fails to respond or (b) develops new symptoms after receiving the medication, that also means the doctor should be called promptly. Failure to respond may mean there hasn't been sufficient time, or that the condition may require more or different medication — but let the doctor be the judge. New symptoms may be related to the illness, or may mean allergy or other reaction to the medication — but again, let your physician make the judgment.

If you should happen to take your child to another physician to whom you have not specifically been referred by your child's regular doctor, ask that physician to write the regular doctor and give a report of whatever is diagnosed, prescribed, etc. Should your pediatrician or family physician refer you to another specialist, such a report will doubtless be requested. But if, for example, you take your teenage daughter to your gynecologist for an examination, or the entire family visits your ophthalmologist for eye tests and examination — simply ask that a report be sent to the primary-care physician. (You should also do this, by the way, for yourself.) It's important, because your child's basic, primary-care physician should have a *complete* record to which you, or anyone, can turn in an emergency.

When you are reporting a problem to the doctor, mention *any*thing out of the ordinary, whether or not you think it has any relevance. Let us say, for example, that you are wondering what to do about your daughter's stomachache and fever. There are many, many causes for that particular set of symptoms. It may be quite helpful if you mention any recent event in your daughter's life that has not been part of her usual routine, whether or not it seems truly exotic. If she has been on an African safari, it will probably occur to you to bring that up. But you should also mention such events, if they apply, as a camping trip, an overnight stay at a new friend's home, a change of lunch menu at her school, a meal at a previously unvisited restaurant. (Obviously — we hope — depending upon your child's age, you may have to do a bit of detective work. You probably know where your five-year-old has been, but it's unlikely that you know everything your fifteen-year-old has eaten within the past twenty-four hours.) Other things that may be important, varying with the child's age: a new pet; possibly a new toy; a sick child in the neighborhood; a new child in a class at school; anything else — let your imagination wander — that might have introduced some new (and possibly harmful) factor into your child's life.

Encourage older children to talk to the pediatrician or family physician, if they seem reluctant to talk to you, about physical or emotional problems. Most pediatricians and family physicians are receptive, sympathetic, and trustworthy; that last means — to reassure teenagers who may be reading this book — that their motive is to help the patient, not to report them (to their parents or to anyone else). A knowledgeable physician will give reliable, up-to-date advice on such subjects as drugs, can counsel a young person on relative risks of sexual activities, and in most states can provide contraceptive prescriptions and treat venereal disease without parental consultation (those same teenagers are advised, however, that if the bills are sent to their parents, and they are queried, it's up to them).

TELEPHONE CALLS

Sooner or later, just about every parent is faced with the question: Should you call the doctor, or not? Typically, the problem arises at four o'clock in the morning, when you are reasonably sure your physician is fast asleep. Let us offer, at the outset, some reassurance that is also a guideline: most pediatricians and family physicians would rather be phoned, at any hour of the day or night, for something that turns out later to be trivial, than not be called about a condition that is found to be serious.

To specifics.

Here are some things that do *not* merit a wee-hours phone call and should wait until you can call the doctor's office in the morning:

• an ordinary cold (assuming you're sure that's what it is and it is not the first cold in a young infant);

• one episode of vomiting;

• one loose stool;

• apparent constipation with no other symptoms;

• a rash, with no other symptoms, that does not appear to be causing discomfort;

• behavior problems;

• future immunizations;

• anything else that obviously has no bearing on your child's well-being at that moment.

Here are some things that *do* mean a call to your physician is in order:

• serious, or possibly serious, injury;

• abdominal pain, especially if it's accompanied by loss of appetite (appendicitis is not uncommon in children over the age of two years, and it can be life threatening if it's not promptly diagnosed and treated);

• loss of consciousness, convulsion, or difficulty in breathing;

• a marked change for the worse in a child who is already ill (a sudden rise in fever, for example, or the appearance of a new and unexpected symptom);

• any abnormal discharge from any body opening;

• persistent diarrhea, vomiting, or both;

• persistent earache;

• fever of 103° F. (39.4° C.) orally or 104° F. (40° C.) rectally — or, in an infant who has never been ill before, 100.5° F. (38° C.);

• two or more unexplained symptoms, whatever they may be.

(We should add that if emergency care is clearly needed immediately — if the child has suffered an extensive burn, for example — you should *not* take the time to phone your doctor, because treatment cannot be given either at your home or in the doctor's office. You should take the child — or call for an ambulance to take the child — to the nearest hospital emergency room. If you are waiting for an ambulance to arrive, call your doctor while you wait. If you are taking the child to the hospital yourself, phone your physician from there.)

Despite the foregoing guidelines, there are going to be some situations that do not fit neatly into either list. If you are in doubt, *make the call.*

Finally, a few tips on getting full value from phone calls to your physician, whatever the problem or the hour. While some of these pointers may seem pretty obvious, they are often just the things that are overlooked in stressful situations.

First, before you place the call, think what the doctor will want to know, as well as what *you* want to know. If there is an abdominal pain, for example, *where* in the abdomen? Is it continuous, or intermittent? Is it sharp, or dull? How is the child reacting to it? Does it hurt more in one position than in another? Are there other symptoms? If you believe your child has fever, take the temperature, so you can report it exactly. If there's a rash, exactly what does it look like? When did it start? *Where* on the child's body did it start? What parts of the child's body does it cover now?

Next — still before you pick up the phone — get pencil and paper. Leave space to write instructions the doctor may give you. Write down the child's temperature, plus the name and phone number of your pharmacy (or one that is open at the hour at which you're calling, if yours isn't), in case the doctor wants to order some medication. Also get out, and have near the phone (so you can read the label), any medication you think might be relevant — e.g., something previously prescribed for the child (if you think the condition might be the same), or prescribed for another child in the family (if you think the one you're phoning about might have caught something from a sibling).

You may or may not reach your doctor immediately. Depending upon the hour and other circumstances, you may find yourself talking to a nurse or assistant, to an answering service that promises to relay your message, to a recording device that invites you to leave a message (don't be intimidated; those machines are very reliable), or to an announcement referring you to another physician (which means yours is out of town or otherwise totally unavailable; a substitute has always been selected with care, and you should write down the name and number and use it). If you must leave a message, whether with a human being or a machine, make it both succinct and informative (and if it's a machine, mention the *time* of your call) — and don't forget to mention both your full name *and* your child's name. And if you are waiting for a physician to return your call, *stay off the phone.*

When you do have the doctor on the phone, get to the point as quickly as possible, and answer the doctor's questions as accurately as you can. If the child is old enough to talk, and physically able to do so, after you have described the situation briefly and reported such details as temperature, *put the child on the phone;* it is often quite important for the doctor to know exactly how the child feels, and the child's own description is better than one that comes secondhand (the doctor may also be able to elicit additional information by putting questions you would not think of). Then, get back on the phone and *write down* the doctor's instructions; be especially careful to write down *numbers* accurately (repeat them back as you do so), since they're easily forgotten under stress.

Appendix B.

Root Clues to Medical Terms

Although we have defined hundreds of terms in this book, you are bound to encounter some, sooner or later, that you won't find discussed, if only because new ones are constantly being coined. With some knowledge of the coinage sources, it's often fairly easy to deduce the meaning of a lengthy and seemingly unfathomable expression by breaking it down into its component parts.

The list that follows includes most of the parts from which medical words have been compounded in the past and are likely to be in future. Virtually all are from Greek or Latin; we haven't specified which, or traced each one back, but the etymologies can be found in any unabridged dictionary.

Hyphens indicate the typical placement within a word. Thus, *auto-* means typically employed as a prefix, *-ase* as a suffix or ending; hyphens at both ends (as, *-ceph-*) signify a component that may occur at either end of a word, or that is as likely to be somewhere in the middle.

a- lack or absence of; equivalent to the English "un-" or "in-" prefix, or the suffix "-less"; e.g., ASEPTIC

ab- from, away from; e.g., ABRASION (the rest of that word is from the Latin for "scraped")

actin- pertaining to rays, of light or of energy; e.g., ACTINIC KERATOSIS, one caused by exposure to the sun

aden- gland or, more commonly, glandlike; e.g., ADENITIS, ADENOIDS

alb- white or whitish; e.g., ALBINO

-algia pain; e.g., CEPHALALGIA

an- same as *a-*, used before vowels; e.g., ANOREXIA

andr- male; e.g., ANDROGEN

ante- before; e.g., ANTENATAL

anti- against; e.g., ANTIVENIN

arter- referring to the arteries as distinct from veins

arthr- the joints; e.g., ARTHRITIS

-ase an enzyme, the first part of the word denoting the substance upon which the enzyme acts; e.g., LACTASE

aud- hearing; e.g., AUDIOLOGIST

aur- the ears, but now almost entirely replaced by *oto-* (the latter is from Greek, the former from Latin), since it can be so easily confused with other terms (e.g., aura)

auto- the self, the final vowel often dropped when placed before another vowel; e.g., AUTISM

bi- two; e.g., BILATERAL; often used, as well, to reflect details of anatomical or chemical structure, as in BICEPS, BICARBONATE, BICUSPID

-bio- life; e.g., ANTIBIOTIC, biology

bronch- the branches of the windpipe, i.e., the bronchial tubes; e.g., BRONCHITIS

-card- the heart; e.g., ELECTROCARDIOGRAM

-centesis puncturing (of a cavity or structure in order to withdraw fluid); e.g., AMNIOCENTESIS

-ceph- the head; e.g., ENCEPHALITIS

chir- the hands; e.g., CHIROPRACTOR

chole- the gall bladder; e.g., CHOLECYSTECTOMY

chondro- cartilage; e.g., CHONDRODYSTROPHY

circum- around; e.g., CIRCUMCISION

contra- against, opposite; e.g., CONTRACEPTIVE, CONTRALATERAL

cryo- extreme cold; now used almost exclusively in coined words relating to research and therapeutic techniques, as CRYOTHERAPY

-cyst- bladder, or fluid- or semisolid-containing sac; e.g., CYSTITIS

-cyte, cyto- cell; e.g., ERYTHROCYTE; CYTOTOXIN

dent- teeth; e.g., DENTIST

-derm- the skin; e.g., DERMATOLOGIST

dis- away from, separated from; e.g., DISEASE, DISLOCATION

-dont- same as **dent-,** used later in a word; e.g., PERIODONTIST.

-dys- difficult, something amiss; e.g., DYSMENORRHEA, DYSENTERY

ecto- outside; e.g., ECTOPIC PREGNANCY

-ectomy surgical removal, the first part of the word denoting the part removed; e.g., TONSILLECTOMY

-emia the blood; e.g., ANEMIA

en- in; e.g., ENDEMIC (the rest of the word is from the Greek for "people," hence "in the people" or native)

endo- within, inner; e.g., ENDOCARDITIS

-enter- the intestines; e.g., PARENTERAL

eryth- red; e.g., ERYTHEMA

ex- from, out of; e.g., EXODONTIST

gast- stomach, belly; e.g., GASTRITIS, GASTROCNEMIUS (the second part of the latter word is from the Greek for "leg," hence the muscle is literally "the belly of the leg")

-gen- producing, causing, in broad sense; e.g., GENES, ALLERGENIC

-gram, -graph inscription or visual depiction, the first part of the word denoting the thing depicted, the agent producing the inscription, or both; e.g., ELECTROENCEPHALOGRAM

haem-, hem- same as **-emia**, used at beginning of word; e.g., HEMATOLOGIST

hepat- the liver; e.g., HEPATITIS

hetero- other, different; e.g., HETEROZYGOUS

hom- same; e.g., HOMOSEXUAL

hydr- water; e.g., DEHYDRATION

hyper- to a high degree, greater than normal; e.g., HYPERTENSION

hypo- lower or less than normal; e.g., HYPOTHYROIDISM

idio- peculiar to the individual; e.g., IDIOPATHIC

intra- within; e.g., INTRAVENOUS

iri- the iris of the eye; e.g., IRITIS

-itis inflammation, the first part of the word denoting the location; e.g., EPIPHYSITIS

lact- milk or related thereto; e.g., LACTIC ACID

leuc-, leuk- white; e.g., LEUCORRHEA, LEUKEMIA

-lys-,-lyt- loosening, dissolving, breaking up or destroying; e.g., HEMOLYTIC ANEMIA

mal- wrong, bad; e.g., MALNUTRITION

(malaria, incidentally, was so named because it was once believed to stem from "bad air")

medi- middle; e.g., OTITIS MEDIA (the word "medicine" is from a different Latin root)

meta- beyond, after; e.g., METACARPALS, METASTASIS

mono- one; e.g., MONONUCLEOSIS (the coining refers to particular cell structures found in blood tests)

-myo- muscle; e.g., DERMATOMYOSITIS.

neo- new; e.g., NEONATAL

-nephr- relating to the kidney(s); e.g., NEPHRITIS

neur- the nervous system; e.g., NEURITIS ("neurosis" isn't a literally correct coinage, but essentially a bestowing of respectability on a popular euphemism, i.e., "nervous condition")

-oid -like, the first part of the word denoting what is presumably resembled; e.g., DERMOID CYST

-ology study of (it stems from the Greek for "treatise," which in turn derived from the word for "word"); e.g., CARDIOLOGY and many others you can form yourself from this list

-oma swelling or mass, often—though not always—a neoplasm; e.g., SARCOMA, LIPOMA, HEMATOMA

oophor- the ovaries; e.g., OOPHOROMA

-opia vision; e.g., HYPEROPIA

orch- the testes; e.g., ORCHITIS

ortho- straightening and, by extension, correction of deviation—whether physical or figurative—from the optimal or norm; e.g., ORTHODONTIST, ORTHOPEDIST (if you conclude, from this listing, that the latter originally pertained strictly to children—you're right)

-osis condition (yes, an extremely broad term), the first part of the word giving further information as to the location or nature of it; e.g., HYPNOSIS, PSYCHOSIS

oste- pertaining to bone; e.g., OSTEOCHONDROSIS

ot-, oto- the ears; e.g., OTOLOGIST

-otomy involving surgery; e.g., TRACHEOTOMY

par-, para- beside, apart from; e.g., PARANASAL SINUSES, PARASITES

-path-, -pathy suffering, by extension disease; e.g., PATHOLOGIST

-ped- children; e.g., PEDIATRICIAN

peri- around; e.g., PERICARDITIS

-plasm, -plast- growth or shaping; e.g., NEOPLASM, RHINOPLASTY

-pod- foot; e.g., PODIATRIST

post- behind, after; e.g., POSTNASAL, POSTPRANDIAL

pro- before; e.g., PROPHYLAXIS (the second part of the word comes from the Greek for "guard")

pseud- deceptive; e.g., PSEUDOHERMAPHRODITISM

psych- the mind; e.g., PSYCHIATRIST (the second part of the word comes from the Greek for "physician")

-pyr- heat or fire; e.g., HYPERPYREXIA

rheum- stream, a derivation that no longer makes any sense but that stems from the ancient theory of assorted liquids coursing about the body and causing various ills (see HUMOR); e.g., RHEUMATOID

-rhin- the nose; e.g., RHINITIS

-rrhea flow(ing); e.g., DIARRHEA

-scler- hard; e.g., SCLERODERMA

-scope, -scopy view, viewing; e.g., BRONCHOSCOPY

seps-, sept- contaminated; e.g., SEP-

TIC ("septum" derives from a different root)

-som- the body (i.e., physically, tangibly); e.g., PSYCHOSOMATIC

stom- the mouth, by extension any remotely similar opening anywhere, whether natural or contrived; e.g., STOMATITIS

-stomy an opening created surgically, the first part of the word denoting the site; e.g., COLOSTOMY

sub- under; e.g., SUBCUTANEOUS

super-, supra- above, toward the head (a Latin counterpart of the Greek *hyper*)

ur-, -uria, uric-, uro- relating to urine or components thereof; e.g., HYPERURICEMIA, PROTEINURIA, UROLOGIST

vener- related to loving or making love (derived originally from the Roman goddess Venus); e.g., VENEREAL DISEASES

xero- dry; e.g., XERODERMA

zo- pertaining to animal (as opposed to plant) life; e.g., ZOONOSES

Appendix C.

Other Recommended Reading

What follows is a highly selective list of publications (along with some sources for additional ones). All are familiar to one or both of us, and are listed here because we think they are of value; there are doubtless dozens of others that are equally interesting and/or informative, and no aspersions are implied by, or should be inferred from, their omission.

Books of commercial publishers are available at, or may be ordered through, bookstores and book departments. Federal publications may be bought at Government Printing Office bookstores in Atlanta GA, Birmingham AL, Boston MA, Canton OH, Chicago IL, Dallas TX, Detroit MI, Kansas City MO, Los Angeles CA, New York NY, Philadelphia PA, San Francisco CA — or, ordered by mail (check or money order must be enclosed) from Superintendent of Documents, U.S. Government Printing Office, Washington DC 20402. (In a number of instances, we have omitted prices on federal publications, because they are constantly revised and updated; if you want to order these, or later publications on the same topic, write and inquire regarding prices.)

CHILD CARE, GROWTH, DEVELOPMENT

The First Five Years, by Virginia E. Pomeranz, M.D., with Dodi Schultz. Doubleday, 1973; Dell (paperback), 1976. Our subtitle is "A Relaxed Approach to Child Care," and that's what it's all about. Covers all the infancy and preschool basics — from bathing and feeding to behavior problems and coping with what we call "sticky sex questions," as well as many less crucial matters that can nevertheless loom large for first-time parents. Some reviewers have been kind enough to call it witty as well as practical; we never argue with reviewers.

A Child's Mind, by Muriel Beadle. Doubleday, 1970. Subtitled "How Children Learn During the Critical Years from Birth to Age Five," this book is not a how-to guide but a highly informative and very readable review of what is known of this fascinating field, and the studies from which the facts emerged. Ms. Beadle is a thorough researcher and a lucid writer.

What Every Child Would Like His Parents to Know to Help Him with the Emotional Problems of His Everyday Life, by Lee Salk. McKay, 1972; Warner (paperback), 1973. While we have some disagreements with the author (e.g., his rather rigid stance on working mothers, and such pejorative phrases as, among others, "a physical examination or some other unpleasant medical procedure"), Dr. Salk, a child psychologist, does offer some sound advice on dilemmas ranging from coping with grandparents to communicating the facts of death and divorce.

How to Help Your Child Get the Most Out of School, by Stella Chess, M.D., with Jane Whitbread. Doubleday, 1974. The authors — Dr. Chess is a distinguished child psychiatrist, Ms. Whitbread a leading writer and editor in the area of parent-child relations — approach their subject with sense and sympathy (for both parent and child). Down-to-earth, detailed pointers on every problem a parent is likely to meet, from preschool education (and evaluating day-care centers) to dealing with sometimes incompetent guidance counselors at the senior high school level.

The Pocket Guide to Babysitting, by the Office of Child Development, Department of Health, Education, and Welfare. U.S. Government Printing Office, 1974; 70¢ (see note at beginning of this appendix). An attractive, well written, and highly informative 48-page booklet slim enough to slip into a jeans pocket but bulging with good guidelines on everything from basic safety and bottle feeding to coping with injuries, illness, temper tantrums, and nonstop crying. And the first publication we've seen that realizes boys can be baby-sitters, too.

PHYSIOLOGY

The Human Body, by Isaac Asimov. Houghton Mifflin, 1963; New American Library (paperback), 1964. ***The Human Brain,*** by Isaac Asimov. Houghton Mifflin, 1964; New American Library (paperback), 1965. These companion volumes by the brilliant and prolific Dr. Asimov — who has the uncanny ability to understand *and* clearly explain practically anything on or off earth, from Shakespeare to the secrets of outer space — remain unexcelled in the realm of lay-language explanations of human structure and inner workings. The works are enhanced by his linguistic precision and brief but intriguing etymological digressions, as well as by Anthony Ravielli's well executed anatomical illustrations.

Behold Man, by Lennart Nilsson in collaboration with Jan Lindberg; text by David H. Ingvar, Stig Nordfeldt, and Rune Pettersson; translated from the Swedish by Ilona Munck. Little, Brown, 1974. Not for everyone (in either price or content), but this colorful tour of the human interior by the photographer of baby-in-the-womb fame (some of those are included) will intrigue and awe those who can find beauty in the structure of a bile duct or in contemplation of the incredible landscape of the scalp seen through a microscope. We can.

FOOD AND NUTRITION

How to Buy Food, by the U.S. Department of Agriculture Marketing Service. U.S. Government Printing Office, 1973; $4.45 (see note at the beginning of this appendix). A neatly packaged set of fourteen "How to Buy . . ." booklets ranging in size from 8 to 28 pages, each dealing with a particular category (poultry, eggs, potatoes, dairy products, fresh fruits, etc.). Explaining, as appropriate, types and categories, official grading of qualities, packaging and labeling, storing for safety and retention of nutritive value; many cooking and menu suggestions, as well. Clear photographic illustrations.

Nutritive Value of Foods, by the U.S. D.A. Consumer and Food Economics Research Division. U.S. Government Printing Office, 1971; 30¢ (see note at the beginning of this appendix). A booklet of charts covering just about anything you'd think of feeding to your children, revealing for each: calories; protein, carbohydrate, and fat content (fatty acids are also broken down into saturated and unsaturated); amounts of calcium, iron, vitamin A, vitamin C, and three major B vitamins.

Metabolics, by Lawrence E. Lamb, M.D. Harper & Row, 1974. An in-depth exploration, by the cardiologist who devised and carried out the medical criteria and examinations for the selection of the Gemini and Apollo crews, of just what happens to the food you eat — down there at the molecular breakdown and buildup level. A complex tale requiring careful reading, but the reward is new understanding of the whys and wherefores of good nutrition guidelines (and the fallacies of some of the farther-out diet ideas).

A Consumer's Dictionary of Food Additives, by Ruth Winter. Crown (paperback), 1972. ***Eater's Digest,*** by Michael F. Jacobson. Doubleday, 1972; Anchor (paperback), 1972. The two books cover the same territory (the second is subtitled "The Consumer's Factbook of Food Additives"), and both are done quite competently; Dr. Jacobson is a researcher in microbiology, Ms. Winter a respected and knowledgeable writer on health topics. Differences are largely in size and approach: Dr. Jacobson's book contains, as might be expected, a good deal of background and research data; Ms. Winter, whose book is larger, uses terser language and packs more facts, as well as more substances, into her listing.

Home Canning of Fruits and Vegetables (45¢) and ***Home Canning of Meat and Poultry*** (30¢), by the U.S. Department of Agriculture. Booklets detailing safe and effective procedures that will insure your avoiding the risk of botulism. (See ordering note at the beginning of this appendix.)

SAFETY

Lead Poisoning in Children, by Jane S. Lin-Fu, M.D., F.A.A.P. U.S. Government Printing Office, 1967. Free on request from Office of Information, Health Services and Mental Health Administration, Parklawn Building, Rockville MD 20852. Booklet discusses causes and consequences, plus ways for the individual and the community to combat the scourge.

Coast Guard Official Recreational Boating Guide. U.S. Government Printing Office, 1971; 60¢ (see note at the beginning of this appendix). A fat 94-page booklet covering everything anyone would need to know about safe boating activities, including legal requirements, recommended safety equipment, tested emergency procedures, and much more.

EARS AND HEARING

Noise Pollution, by the U.S. Environmental Protection Agency. U.S. Government Printing Office, 1972; 35¢ (see note at the beginning of this appendix). A booklet detailing the physical and psychological dangers of elevated noise and suggesting solutions, including action by individual citizens.

Facts About Hearing and Hearing Aids, by the National Bureau of Standards. U.S. Government Printing Office, 1971; 60¢ (see note at the beginning of this appendix). A 32-page booklet explaining the causes, effects, and detection of hearing loss, with specific guidelines for choosing and using a hearing aid (emphasis is on the latter). Extremely useful for the parent whose child must wear such an aid.

Other Sources of Information

American Speech and Hearing Association, 9030 Old Georgetown Road, Washington DC 20014

National Association of Hearing and Speech Agencies, 919 Eighteenth Street NW, Washington DC 20006 (data on centers and clinics)

Deafness Research Foundation, 366 Madison Avenue, New York NY 10017

DRUGS

Licit and Illicit Drugs, by Edward M. Brecher and the editors of *Consumer Reports.* Little, Brown, 1972. An exhaustive report on the history and present picture of nonmedical use of mind-affecting drugs in the United States, including — as the title page emphasizes — not only narcotics, hallucinogens, and the like, but also caffeine, nicotine, and alcohol. A masterful job of medical journalism by an extremely able writer, and an authoritative source book for those seeking a picture both broad in scope and concise in detail.

Is the Grass Greener?, by Dorothy V. Whipple, M.D. Robert B. Luce, 1971. A point-of-view book — not, as the title would suggest, restricted to marijuana, but covering all the illicitly used drugs, plus alcohol — in question-and-answer form. Dr. Whipple, a practicing pediatrician (and university professor) who has over several decades established a unique rapport with young people, concludes her straight-talking presentation of the facts with thoughtful proposals for the future.

Marihuana: A Signal of Misunderstanding, report of the National Commission on Marihuana and Drug Abuse. U.S. Government Printing Office, 1972; $1.00 (see note at the beginning of this appendix). The full text of the report to the President examines physiological, psychological, and sociological aspects and implications of marijuana use (the federal government spells it with an "h" instead of a "j") and offers specific recommendations for changes in federal and state laws.

SEX ET CETERA

The Wonderful Story of How You Were Born, by Sidonie Matsner Gruenberg. Doubleday, 1971 (new edition). Designed to be read by children of nine or ten, the late Ms. Gruenberg's book is also an excellent guide for shy parents who are at a loss for words and ideas in explaining the subject to a younger child.

The Sex Book, by Martin Goldstein, M.D., and Erwin J. Haeberle, M.D., with photographs by Will McBride.

Herder & Herder, 1971. Designed for somewhat older children, this book speaks frankly, in words and pictures, about all aspects of sexuality. Although it has been hailed by many as an innovative success, we must add that it may not be your particular cup of tea; it should be scanned before buying, rather than ordered sight unseen, to be sure its approach meets with *your* approval for *your* children.

Microbes and Morals, by Theodor Rosebury. Viking, 1971; Ballantine (paperback), 1973. Subtitled "The Strange Story of Venereal Disease," this scholarly but smooth-reading book by an eminent bacteriologist relates a saga that is strange indeed. Dr. Rosebury (who was a principal advisor for the TV production "VD Blues") traces the tortuous paths of gonorrhea and syphilis through human history from ancient times to the present — dropping many a prominent name en route — to reveal the curious societal factors that have ironically prevented the conquest of VD.

Other Sources of Information

Sex Information and Education Council of the U.S., 1855 Broadway, New York NY 10023

Planned Parenthood Federation of America, 810 Seventh Avenue, New York NY 10019, and local chapters (data on contraception, infertility problems, abortion, other aspects of family planning)

HEREDITY AND GENETICS

Heredity in Humans, by Amram Scheinfeld. Lippincott, 1972. If you are intrigued by our discussion of the subject, you'll find it covered just about completely (but in clear, nontechnical language) by this able writer who has specialized in the various aspects of hereditary mechanisms. Some of the information therein is slightly out of date, having been superseded by new knowledge — but that is a minor quibble and doesn't detract from the book's value.

Other Sources of Information

The National Foundation–March of Dimes, Box 2000, White Plains NY 10602 (data on birth defects, hereditary and other)

National Genetics Foundation, 250 West 57th Street, New York NY 10019 (data on genetic counseling facilities)

SPECIFIC PROBLEMS

Arthritis, by Sheldon Paul Blau, M.D., and Dodi Schultz. Doubleday, 1974. Covering all the major arthritic disorders, their causes (so far as known) and treatments. Dr. Blau is Chief of the Arthritis Clinic and Director of the Division of Rheumatic Diseases at Nassau County (New York) Medical Center, and Associate Professor of Clinical Medicine at the State University of New York.

How to Live with Diabetes, by Henry Dolger, M.D., and Bernard Seeman. Pyramid (paperback), 1970 (revised edition). Dr. Dolger is a prominent diabetologist, his co-author a skilled medical writer; this book provides much valuable guidance for the parents of a diabetic child — both in physical management of the illness and in emotional ramifications for the child who has diabetes mellitus.

The Headache Book, by Arnold P. Friedman, M.D., and Shervert H. Frazier, Jr., M.D., with Dodi Schultz. Dodd, Mead, 1973. Dr. Friedman is a world-famous neurologist and authority on this subject, Dr. Frazier, Professor of Psychiatry at Harvard. (If you are in The Netherlands, you can buy it under the title *Het Hoofdpijn-boek;* isn't that interesting?)

Rh: The Intimate History of a Disease and Its Conquest, by David R. Zimmerman. Macmillan, 1973. The absorbing story of the ailment that frustrated generations of parents and physicians, the major mother-fetus incompatability, told by a talented science writer.

Other Sources of Information

The U.S. Government Printing Office publishes small booklets or folders on a variety of ills, on a continuous basis. They are revised as new research information becomes available. Among recent offerings are *Mongolism: Hope Through Research; Epilepsy: Hope Through Research; Muscular Dystrophy: Hope Through Research; The Child with Cerebral Palsy; CF: Facts About Cystic Fibrosis; Food Allergy; Phenylketonuria; Hypertension: High Blood Pressure.* Write (see the address at the beginning of this appendix) for information regarding topics in which you have a special interest.

Allergy Foundation of America, 801 Second Avenue, New York NY 10017

National Cystic Fibrosis Research Foundation, 202 East 44th Street, New York NY 10017

National Kidney Foundation, 315 Park Avenue South, New York NY 10010

American Diabetes Association, 18 East 48th Street, New York NY 10017

Muscular Dystrophy Association of America, 1790 Broadway, New York NY 10019

National Association for Retarded Children, 2709 Avenue E East, Arlington TX 76010

National Hemophilia Foundation, 25 West 39th Street, New York NY 10018

Epilepsy Foundation of America, 1828 L Street NW, Washington DC 20036

United Cerebral Palsy, 66 East 34th Street, New York NY 10016

The Arthritis Foundation, 475 Riverside Drive, New York NY 10027

American Foundation for the Blind, 15 West 16th Street, New York NY 10011

MISCELLANY

Life on Man, by Theodor Rosebury. Viking, 1969; Berkley (paperback), 1970. In this book, Dr. Rosebury does for human ecology what he did for humans-versus-bacteria in his aforementioned study of VD. "On" means, literally, cozily subsisting upon the skin — of both sexes, of course. (Dr. Rosebury would probably have titled his book differently had it been written later; he is no sexist, simply an extraordinarily intelligent and informed person who is — happily for the rest of us — continually fascinated by phenomena that everyone else seems to overlook.)

Source Book of Medical History, by Logan Clendening. Dover, 1960 (reprint of a 1942 publication; paperback).

The renowned Dr. Clendening, who was Professor of the History of Medicine at the University of Kansas, died in 1945; his research and writings span the breadth of his chosen field. If you're interested in the background of historical events we've necessarily referred to only briefly in this book, this is a marvelous extension of that interest — not an at-one-gulp reading, but an endless source of information into which one might dip from time to time, including original sources.

Metrics: Measurement for Tomorrow, by Helmer A. Ronningen. Collier (paperback), 1972. We have consistently provided kilogram equivalents for pounds, centimeters for inches, and degrees-Celsius counterparts for degrees-Fahrenheit, in this book. It's all part of what's bound to occur: practically every other nation in the world uses the metric system (chances are, your child is learning it in school, along with our pounds-and-inches arrangement). This book is a well-organized, handy guide. You're going to need one.

Advertising of Proprietary Medicines, paperback reprints of hearings on over-the-counter drugs before the subcommittee on monopoly of the select Senate committee on small business. U.S. Government Printing Office, 1971, 1973. A set of real eye-openers. If you were astonished by the small precautions we have included in this book, you will be dumbfounded by the revelations offered by these transcripts. (You may also share our annoyance that no significant consumer protection resulted; do not expect to view television commercials with anything approaching peace of mind, after perusing these volumes.) Order from the Government Printing Office (see the note at the beginning of this appendix). Part 1 (analgesics), $1.75; Part 2 (sedatives, etc.), $2.25; Part 3 (cough and cold remedies, etc.), $2.35.

Other Sources of Information (Continuing)

There are some extremely helpful continuing advisories available, at little or no cost, from our government in Washington. We have mentioned a number of government publications, representing only a small proportion of those that our tax monies pay for. It seems smart, to us, to take advantage of them. The four that follow are especially valuable. For ordering, see the note on the first page of this appendix.

Price List of Government Consumer Publications. Free. Revised from time to time.

Selected List of Publications. Also free, a list that arrives monthly, noting newly issued publications and their prices, which may be ordered via a convenient form from a designated fulfillment center. A lot of the federal publications mentioned here were obtained that way.

FDA Consumer. A magazine published monthly; subscription price, at this writing, $8.55. The official publication of the agency that monitors all sorts of things, ranging from medications to safety in other areas, that can seriously affect the health of your children. Each issue includes a listing (not really totally up-to-date, since legal actions take time) of products singled out for prosecution.

Consumer News, a twice-each-month publication of the Office of Consumer Affairs, part of the U.S. Department of Health, Education and Welfare; the subscription price, at this writing, $4.00 a year. The mailing is a newsletter announcing various relevant events/decisions/advisories — not all, but many, relating to your family's health.

Appendix D.

Poison Control Centers

The numbers listed here are those available from the National Clearinghouse for Poison Control Centers of the Department of Health, Education, and Welfare at the time this book went to press. Since telephone numbers may change, it is wise to call the indicated number and confirm its currency before entering it on the last page of Appendix E. Also, if you do not find your town (or the town where the nearest hospital is) listed here, you might call the nearest hospital, the local health department, or your physician to see if an additional Poison Control Center has been established in your area since this list was published.

Alabama

Anniston:
237–5421, ext. 307

Auburn: Day: 826–4037
Night: 887–6778, 887–3235

Birmingham: 933–4050

Dothan: 794–3131, ext. 521

Florence:
764–8321, ext. 206, 207

Gadsden:
492–1240, ext. 205

Huntsville: 539–9411

Mobile: 473–3325

Opelika: 745–4611

Alaska

Anchorage: 277–6671

Fairbanks: 456–6655, ext. 15

Juneau: 586–2611

Ketchikan: 225–5171, ext. 31

Sitka–Mt. Edgecumbe: 966–2411

Arizona

Douglas: 364–8473

Flagstaff: 744–5233, ext. 255

Ganado: 755–3411

Kingman: 757–2101, ext. 247

Nogales: 287–2771, ext. 94

Phoenix: 252–6611, ext. 111
267–5011
252–5911
277–6611, ext. 2481
258–7373, ext. 291

Prescott: 445–2700, ext. 25, 58

Tucson: 624–2721, ext. 220
882–6300
622–5833, ext. 724
327–5461, ext. 428

Winslow: 289–4691

Yuma: 344–2000, ext. 221

Arkansas

El Dorado: 863–2266, ext. 221

Fort Smith: 782–3071, ext. 210
441–4381

Harrison: 365–6141, ext. 124

Helena: 338–6411, ext. 271

Little Rock: 664–5000, ext. 415
Osceola: 563–2611, ext. 53
Pine Bluff: 535–6800, ext. 225

California

Fresno: 233–0911, ext. 2431
Los Angeles: 664–2121
Oakland: 652–8171
654–5600
Orange: 997–2722
Sacramento: 453–3692
453–3797
San Diego: 294–6000
San Francisco: 553–1574
558–3881
San Jose: 393–0262, ext. 318, 319

Colorado

Denver: 893–7771

Connecticut

Bridgeport: 334–3566
334–1081
Danbury: 744–2300
Hartford: 566–3456
Middletown: 347–9471
New Britain: 224–5672
New Haven: 772–3900
436–1960
Norwalk: 838–3611
Waterbury: 756–8351

Delaware

Wilmington: 655–3389

District of Columbia

Washington: 835–4080, –4081

Florida

Apalachicola: 653–3311
Bartow: 533–1111, ext. 237
Bradenton: 746–5111, ext. 466
Daytona Beach: 255–0161, ext. 256
Fort Lauderdale: 525–5411, ext. 513
Fort Myers: 334–5286
Fort Walton Beach:
242–1111, ext. 106
Gainesville: 372–4321
392–3261
Jacksonville: 389–7751, ext. 315
Key West: 294–5531
Lakeland: 683–0411
Leesburg: 787–7222, ext.221
Melbourne: 727–7000, ext. 704
Miami: 325–7429
Miami Beach: 674–2121
674–2200
Naples: 649–3131, ext. 221
Ocala: 732–1111, ext. 15
Orlando: 841–8411, ext. 656
Panama City: 769–1511
Pensacola: 434–4011, ext. 4811
Plant City: 752–1188
Pompano Beach: 941–8300, ext. 710
Punta Gorda: 639–3131, ext. 129
Rockledge: 636–2211, ext. 506
St. Petersburg: 894–1161, ext. 242
Sarasota: 955–1111, ext. 1241
Tallahassee: 599–5100
Tampa: 253–0711
Titusville: 269–1100, ext. 474
West Palm Beach:
655–5511, ext. 341
Winter Haven: 293–1121, ext. 222

Georgia

Albany: 883–1800, ext. 158
Athens: 549–9977, ext. 357
Atlanta: 659–1212, ext. 893
Augusta: 724–7171, ext. 2176
Columbus: 324–4711, ext. 431

Macon: 742–1122, ext. 3144
Rome: 232–1541, ext. 223
Savannah: 355–3200, ext. 455
Thomasville: 226–4121, ext. 169
Valdosta: 242–3450, ext. 717
Waycross: 283–3030, ext. 240

Hawaii

Honolulu: 537–1831

Idaho

Boise: 376–1211, ext. 707
Idaho Falls: 522–3620, ext. 208
Pocatello: 232–2733, ext. 244

Illinois

Alton: 462–8851
Aurora: 896–3911
Belleville: 233–7750, ext. 250
Belvidere: 547–5441, ext. 367
Berwyn: 797–3159
Bloomington: 828–5241, ext. 395
662–3311, ext. 356
Cairo: 734–2400, ext. 42
Canton: 647–5240, ext. 240
Carbondale: 549–0721, ext. 341
Carthage: 357–3131, ext. 84, 85
Centralia: 532–6731, ext. 716
Champaign: 337–2533
Chanute AFB: 495–3133
Chester: 826–4581
Chicago: 942–5969
649–4161
633–6542, –6543, –6544
567–2017
791–2810
542–2030
774–8000, ext. 401
770–2419
978–2000
996–6885, –6886
947–6231
Danville: 443–5221
442–6300, ext. 647, 674, 736
Decatur: 877–8121, ext. 676
429–2966, ext. 731, 732, 733, 742
Des Plaines: 297–1800, ext. 1000
East St. Louis:
874–7076, ext. 216, 232
274–1900, ext. 204, 268
Effingham: 342–2121, ext. 211, 212
Elgin: 695–3200, ext. 348
742–9800, ext. 681
Elmhurst: 833–1400, ext. 550
Evanston: 492–6460
492–2440
Evergreen Park: 445–6000, ext. 221
Fairbury: 692–2346, ext. 248
Freeport: 235–4131, ext. 228
Galesburg:
343–8131, ext. 336, 356, 386
343–3161, ext. 255, 256
Granite City: 876–2020, ext. 421
Harvey: 333–2300, ext. 5295
Highland: 654–2171, ext. 297, 298
Highland Park: 432–8000
Hinsdale: 887–2600
Hoopeston: 283–5531
Jacksonville: 245–9541
Joliet: 725–7133, ext. 679, 680
729–7563
729–7565
Kankakee: 933–1671, ext. 606
939–4111, ext. 735
Kewanee: 853–3361, ext. 219
Lake Forest:
234–5600, ext. 684, 685, 683
La Salle: 223–0607, ext. 14
Lincoln: 732–2161, ext. 346
Macomb: 833–4101, ext. 433
Mattoon: 234–8881, ext. 29
Maywood: 531–3000

McHenry: 385–2200, ext. 602
Melrose Park:
681–3000, ext. 226, 239
Mendota: 539–7461, ext. 225
Moline: 762–3651, ext. 233
Monmouth: 734–3141, ext. 224
Mt. Carmel: 263–3112, ext. 211
Mt. Vernon: 242–4600, ext. 521
Naperville: 355–0450, ext. 326
Normal: 829–7685, ext. 274
Oak Lawn: 425–8000, ext. 382
Oak Park: 383–6200
Olney: 395–2131, ext. 226, 228
Ottawa: 433–3100, ext. 227
Park Ridge: 696–5151
Pekin: 347–1151, ext. 241
Peoria: 672–5500
691–4702, ext. 791
672–2109, –2110, –2111
672–4950
Peru: 223–3300, ext. 253
Pittsfield: 285–2113, ext. 238
Princeton: 875–2811, ext. 311
Quincy: 223–5811, ext. 255
223–1200, ext. 260
Rockford: 968–6861, ext. 441
226–2041
968–6898, ext. 534
Rock Island: 793–1000, ext. 2106
St. Charles: 584–3300, ext. 229
Scott AFB: 256–7595
Springfield: 528–2041, ext. 460
544–6464, ext. 210
Spring Valley:
663–2611, ext. 464, 466
Streator: 673–2311, ext. 221
Urbana: 337–3311
337–2131
Waukegan: 688–4181
688–6181
Winfield: 653–6900, ext. 556
Woodstock: 338–2500, ext. 215, 232
Zion: 872–4561, ext. 239, 240

Indiana

Anderson: 649–2511, ext. 251
Angola: 665–2141, ext. 42
665–2166
Crown Point: 738–2100
East Chicago: 392–1700
392–7203
Elkhart: 294–2621
Evansville: 426–3405
477–6261
426–8000
Fort Wayne: 484–6636, ext. 7800
423–2614
Frankfort: 654–4451
Gary: 886–4710
Goshen: 533–2141, ext. 462
Hammond: 932–2300
Huntington: 356–3000
Indianapolis: 639–6671
924–8355
Kokomo: 453–0702, ext. 444
Lafayette:
742–0221, ext. 428, 421
La Grange: 463–2144
La Porte: 362–7541, ext. 212
Lebanon: 482–2700, ext.44
Madison: 265–5211, ext. 14
Marion: 662–4694
Mishawaka: 259–2431
Muncie: 747–3241
Portland: 726–7131, ext. 159
Richmond: 692–7010, ext. 622
Shelbyville: 392–3211, ext. 52
South Bend:
234–2151, ext. 253, 264
284–7458

Terre Haute:
232–0361, ext. 397, 398

Vincennes: 885–3348

Iowa

Des Moines: 283–6212

Dubuque: 588–8210

Fort Dodge: 573–3101

Iowa City: 356–1616

Kansas

Atchison: 367–2131

Dodge City: 227–8133

Emporia: 342–7120, ext. 330

Fort Riley: 239–2323

Fort Scott: Day: 223–2200
Night: 223–0476

Great Bend: Day: 793–3523
Night: 792–2511

Hays: 628–8251

Kansas City: 831–6633
287–8881

Lawrence: 843–3680

Parsons: 421–4880

Salina: 827–5591, ext. 112

Topeka: 234–9961, ext. 150

Wichita: 685–2151, ext. 7515

Kentucky

Ashland: 325–7755, ext. 444

Berea: 986–3061

Fort Thomas: 292–3215

Lexington: 278–3411, ext. 152
233–5320

Louisville: 589–8222

Murray: 753–7588

Owensboro: 683–3511, ext. 275
(night, ext. 232)

Paducah: 444–6361, ext. 284
(night, ext. 541)

Whitesburg: 633–2160

Louisiana

Bogalusa: 735–1322

Lake Charles: 478–1310, ext. 210

Monroe: Day: 325–6454
Night: 325–2611

New Orleans:
524–3617, –3618, –3619

Shreveport: 222–0709

Maine

Portland: 871–0111

Maryland

Baltimore: 955–5000
528–7701

Bethesda: 530–3880

Cumberland: 722–6677

Easton: 822–5555

Hagerstown: 797–2400

Massachusetts

Boston: 232–2120

Fall River: 674–5789

New Bedford: 997–1515

Springfield: 788–7321
787–3200

Webster: 943–2600

Worcester: 756–1551

Michigan

Adrian: 263–2412

Ann Arbor: 764–5102

Battle Creek: 963–5521

Bay City: 895–8511

Berrien Center: 471–7761

Coldwater: 278–2359

Detroit: 494–5711
864–5400, ext. 417

Eloise: Day: 722–3748, –3749
Night: 274–3000, –6232

Flint: 766–0111

Grand Rapids: 774–7854
774–1774
247–7123
774–6794

Hancock: 482–1122

Holland: 396–4661

Jackson:
783–2771, ext. 221, 222, 298

Kalamazoo: 383–7333
383–6401

Lansing: 372–5112

Marquette: 228–9440

Midland: 631–7700

Monroe: 241–6509

Petoskey: 347–7373

Pontiac: 858–3000, ext. 256

Port Huron: 987–5555

Saginaw: 755–1111

Traverse City: 947–6140

Minnesota

Bemidji: 751–5430

Brainerd: 829–2861, ext. 211

Crookston:
281–4682, ext. 202

Duluth: 727–6636
727–4551, ext. 359

Edina: 920–4400

Fergus Falls: 736–5475

Fridley: 786–2200

Mankato: 387–4031

Marshall: 532–9661

Minneapolis: 332–0282
347–3141
588–0616
874–4233
296–5276

Morris: 589–1313

Rochester: 285–5123

St. Cloud: 251–2700, ext. 221

St. Paul: 224–9121
227–6521
228–3132
291–3348
298–8201
222–4260
291–3139

Virginia: 741–3340

Willmar: 235–4543

Worthington: 372–2941

Mississippi

Brandon: 825–2811, ext. 287, 288

Columbia: 736–6303, ext. 217

Greenwood: 453–9751, ext. 633

Hattiesburg: 544–7000, ext. 565

Jackson: 968–1704
982–0121, ext. 345
354–6650

Keesler AFB: 377–2516
377–6555, –6556

Laurel:
649–4000, ext. 207, 218, 220, 248

Meridian: 483–6211, ext. 54, 71

Pascagoula: 762–6121, ext. 654

University: 234–1522

Vicksburg: 636–2131, ext. 250, 276

Missouri

Cape Girardeau: 334–4461, ext. 49

Columbia: 882–8091

Hannibal: 221–0414, ext. 213

Joplin: 781–2727, ext. 276

Kansas City: 471–0626, ext. 383
421–8060, ext. 257, 235

Kirksville: 665–4611, ext. 240

Poplar Bluff: 785–7721, ext. 33

Rolla: 364–3100, ext. 31

St. Joseph: 232–8461, ext. 277

St. Louis: 865–4000, ext. 468
367–6880, ext. 220

Springfield: 836–3193
881–8811, ext. 248, 241

West Plains: 256–3141, ext. 8

Montana

Bozeman: 586–5431

Great Falls: 761–1200

Helena: 442–2480, ext. 137

Nebraska

Lincoln: 483–3244

Omaha: 553–5400

Nevada

Las Vegas: 385–1277

Reno: Day: 785–4129
Night: 785–4140

New Hampshire

Hanover: 643–4000

New Jersey

Atlantic City: 344–4081

Belleville: 751–1000

Boonton: 334–5000

Bridgeton: 451–6600

Camden: 795–5554

Denville: 627–3000

East Orange: 672–8400

Elizabeth: 527–5059

Englewood: 568–3400

Flemington: 782–2121

Livingston: 992–5161

Long Branch: 222–2210

Montclair: 746–6000

Morristown: 538–0900

Mount Holly: 267–7877

Neptune: 988–1818

Newark:
926–7240, –7241, –7242, –7243

New Brunswick: 828–3000
545–8000

Newton: 383–2121

Orange: 678–1100

Passaic: 473–1000

Perth Amboy: 442–3700

Phillipsburg: 859–1500

Point Pleasant: 892–1100

Princeton: 921–7700

Saddle Brook: 843–6700

Somers Point: 927–3501

Somerville: 725–4000

Summit: 522–2232

Teaneck: 837–3070

Trenton: 396–1077

Union: 687–1900

Wayne: 684–6900

New Mexico

Alamogordo: 437–3770

Albuquerque: 843–2551

Carlsbad: 887–3521

Clovis: 763–4493

Las Cruces: 522–8641

Roswell: 622–8170

New York

Albany: 445–3131

Binghamton: 772–1100, ext.431
729–6521

Buffalo: 878–7000

Dunkirk: 366–1111, ext.414, 415

East Meadow:
542–2323, –2324, –2325

Elmira: 737–4194
733–6541, ext.213, 271, 289, 535

Endicott: 754–7171, ext.66

Glens Falls: 792–3151

Ithaca: 274–4011
274–4383
274–4411

Jamestown: 487–0141

Johnson City: 773–6611
Kingston: 331–3131, ext.250
New York City: 340–4495
Niagara Falls: 278–4511
Nyack: 358–6200, ext.451, 452
Oswego: 343–1920
Rochester: 275–5151
Syracuse: 476–3166
473–5831
Watertown: 788–8700

North Carolina
Asheville: 255–4660
Charlotte: 372–5100
Durham: 684–8111
Greensboro: 379–4109
Hendersonville: 693–6522
Hickory: 328–2191
Jacksonville: 353–1234, ext.211
Wilmington: 763–9021, ext.311

North Dakota
Bismarck: 223–4700
Dickinson: 225–6771, ext.329, 259
Fargo: 237–8115
Grand Forks: 775–4241
Jamestown: 252–1050
Minot: 838–0341, ext.253
Williston: 572–7661

Ohio
Akron: 379–8562
Canton: 452–9911, ext. 203
Cincinnati: 872–5111
Cleveland: 231–4455
Columbus: 228–1323
Dayton: 461–4790
878–6623
Lorain: 282–2220
Mansfield: 522–3411, ext.545
Springfield: 325–0531, ext. 371
Toledo: 382–7971
Youngstown: 746–2222
Zanesville: 454–4000

Oklahoma
Ada: 332–2323, ext. 200
Ardmore: 223–5400
Lawton: 355–8620
McAlester: 426–1800, ext. 240
Oklahoma City: 271–5454
Ponca City:
765–3321, ext.584
Tulsa:
584–1351, ext.598

Oregon
Portland: 225–8500

Pennsylvania
Allentown: 433–2311
821–3252
Altoona: 944–1681
Bethlehem: 691–4141
Bloomsburg: 784–7121
Bradford: 368–4143
Bryn Mawr: 527–0600
Carlisle: 249–1212
Chambersburg: 264–5171, ext. 431
Chester:
494–0721, ext.232
Clearfield: 765–5341
Coaldale: 645–2131
Coudersport: 274–9300
Danville: 275–6116
Doylestown: 345–2281
Drexel Hill: 259–3800
DuBois: 371–2200
Easton: 258–6221
East Stroudsburg: 421–3194

Erie: 864–4031
459–4000
455–6711, ext.521
455–3961

Gettysburg: 334–2121

Greensburg: 837–0100

Hanover: 637–3711

Harrisburg:
782–3639
782–4141, ext.4132

Hershey: 534–6111

Indiana: 463–0261

Jeannette: 527–3551
527–1511

Jersey Shore: 398–0100

Johnstown: 535–7541
536–6671
536–5353

Kittanning: 542–5011

Lancaster: 299–4546
299–5511

Lansdale: 368–2100

Latrobe: 539–9711

Lebanon: 272–7611

Lehighton: 377–1300

Lewistown: 248–5411

Muncy: 546–8282

Nanticoke: 735–5000

Oil City: 644–1211

Paoli: 647–2200

Philadelphia: 823–8460

Philipsburg: 342–3320

Pittsburgh: 681–6669

Pittston: 654–3341

Pottstown: 327–1000

Pottsville: 622–3400

Reading:
376–4881
378–6218

Sayre: 888–6666

Scranton: 346–3801
961–4205
343–5566

Sellersville: 257–3611

Sewickley: 741–6600

Sharon: 981–1700, ext. 281

Somerset: 443–2626

State College: 238–4351

Titusville: 827–1851

Tunkhannock: 836–2161

Uniontown: 437–4531

Washington: 225–7000

Wellsboro: 724–1631

Wilkes-Barre: 823–1121, ext. 222

Williamsport: 322–7861

York: 843–8623

Rhode Island

Kingston: 792–2762
792–2775

Pawtucket: 724–1230

Providence: 277–4000
521–5055

South Carolina

Charleston: 792–4201

Columbia: 765–7359

South Dakota

Aberdeen: 225–5110

Sioux Falls: 336–3894

Tennessee

Chattanooga: 755–6100

Columbia: 388–2320, ext.49

Cookeville: 528–2541

Jackson: 424–0424

Johnson City: 926–1131

Knoxville: 971–3261

Memphis: 522–3000

Nashville: 322–3391

Texas

Abilene: 677–3551, ext.266,267
Amarillo:
376–4431, ext.501, 502, 503, 504
Austin: 478–4490
Beaumont: 833–7409
Corpus Christi:
884–4511, ext.556, 557
El Paso: 544–1200
Fort Worth: 336–5521, ext.17
336–6611
Galveston: 765–1420
765–1561
Grand Prairie: 641–1313
Harlingen: 423–1224, ext.23
Laredo: 722–2431, ext.29
Lubbock: 792–1011, ext.315
Midland: 684–8257
Odessa: 337–7311, ext. 250
Plainview: 296–9601
San Angelo: 653–6741
San Antonio: 223–1481
Tyler: 597–0351, ext.255
Waco: 753–1412
756–6111
Wharton: Day: 532–2440
Night: 532–1440
Wichita Falls: 322–6771

Utah

Salt Lake City: 581–3711

Virginia

Alexandria: 370–9000, ext.555
Arlington: 558–6161
Blacksburg: 951–1111
Charlottesville: 296–9888
Danville: 799–2100, ext.3869
Falls Church: 698–3111
698–3600
Hampton: 722–1131
Harrisonburg: 434–4421, ext. 225
Lexington: 463–9141
Lynchburg: 846–6511, ext.203
Nassawadox: 442–8000
Norfolk: 489–5111
Petersburg: 732–7220, ext.327, 328
Portsmouth: 397–6541, ext.418
Richmond: 770–5123
Roanoke: 981–7336
Staunton: 885–0361, ext.209, 247
Waynesboro:
942–8355, ext.440, 500
Williamsburg: 229–1120, ext.65

Washington

Aberdeen: 533–0450, ext.277
Bellingham: 676–8400
Longview: 636–5252
Madigan: 967–6972
Olympia: 491–0222
Richland: 943–1283
Seattle: 634–5252
Spokane: 747–1077
Tacoma: 272–1281, ext.59
Vancouver: 256–2064
Yakima: 248–4400

West Virginia

Beckley: 252–6431, ext.213
Belle: 949–4314, ext.261
Charleston: 348–4211
Clarksburg: 623–3177, ext.251
Huntington: 696–6160
696–2224
696–2573
Martinsburg:
267–8981, ext.201,216
Morgantown: 293–5341

Parkersburg: 424–2212
424–4251, ext.251

Pt. Pleasant:
675–4340, ext.252

Ronceverte:
647–4411, –4412, –4413

Weirton: 748–3232, ext.208

Welch: 436–3161, ext. 264

Weston: 269–3000, ext.201, 228

Wheeling: 243–3281

Wisconsin

Eau Claire: 835–1511

Green Bay: 432–8621

Kenosha: 656–2201

Madison: 262–3702

Milwaukee: 344–7100

Wyoming

Casper: 577–7201

Cheyenne: 634–3341, ext.220

Appendix E.

Vital Statistics and Emergency Phone List

The information on the following pages, to be filled in by you, is in all cases helpful, in many essential; in some, it could save your child's life. Be sure it is completely filled in, and that it is kept up to date. Take it with you when you take your child to the doctor, both to supply needed medical-history data and to record such facts as may emerge from the visit itself.

Be sure, too, that baby-sitters and others caring for your children know where to find this information, and also tell such a person where to find any medications that might be required in case of emergency. Of course you should always leave a telephone number where you can be reached if you are out for the evening. And leave money with a babysitter in case a taxi must be taken to get emergency medical aid, or if medication must be ordered, etc.

Child's Full Name ______________________________

Date and Place of Birth ______________________________

Attending Obstetrician at Birth ______________________________

Physical Checkups (Enter in Pencil)

Date of Most Recent: ______________ Next Scheduled: ______________

Height at Last Checkup: ______________ Weight at Last Checkup: ______________

Diseases and Serious Illnesses (don't include colds; do include flu, childhood diseases, infections of major organs, etc.):

Illness	Month, Year	Illness	Month, Year

Surgical Operations:

Name or Nature of Operation	Month, Year

Fractures, Other Major Injuries:

Nature and Location	Month, Year

Allergies (list medications, accidents such as stings or bites, conditions such as asthma):

Nature of Allergy	Special Precaution, Procedure or Medication

Immunization Record (those already appearing are necessary and basic; fill in dates in pencil):

DPT ______________________ (Booster Due ______________)

DT ______________________ (Booster Due ______________)

Tetanus ______________________ (Booster Due ______________)

Rubella ______________________ }

Measles ______________________ } or MMR ______________

Mumps ______________________ }

Polio ______________________ (Booster Due ______________)

TB Test ______________________ (Next Due ______________)

Other: ______________________

Other Special Conditions or Problems, with Precautions or Special Instructions:

Child's Full Name ______________________________

Date and Place of Birth ______________________________

Attending Obstetrician at Birth ______________________________

Physical Checkups (Enter in Pencil)

Date of Most Recent: ______________ Next Scheduled: ______________

Height at Last Checkup: ______________ Weight at Last Checkup: ______________

Diseases and Serious Illnesses (don't include colds; do include flu, childhood diseases, infections of major organs, etc.):

Illness	Month, Year	Illness	Month, Year

Surgical Operations:

Name or Nature of Operation	Month, Year

Fractures, Other Major Injuries:

Nature and Location	Month, Year

Allergies (list medications, accidents such as stings or bites, conditions such as asthma):

Nature of Allergy	Special Precaution, Procedure or Medication

Immunization Record (those already appearing are necessary and basic; fill in dates in pencil):

DPT ______________________ (Booster Due ______________)

DT______________________ (Booster Due ______________)

Tetanus ______________________ (Booster Due ______________)

Rubella______________________

Measles______________________ } or MMR ______________

Mumps ______________________

Polio ______________________ (Booster Due ______________)

TB Test ______________________ (Next Due ______________)

Other: ______________________

Other Special Conditions or Problems, with Precautions or Special Instructions:

Child's Full Name ______________________________

Date and Place of Birth ______________________________

Attending Obstetrician at Birth ______________________________

Physical Checkups (Enter in Pencil)

Date of Most Recent: ______________ Next Scheduled: ______________

Height at Last Checkup: ______________ Weight at Last Checkup: ______________

Diseases and Serious Illnesses (don't include colds; do include flu, childhood diseases, infections of major organs, etc.):

Illness	Month, Year	Illness	Month, Year

Surgical Operations:

Name or Nature of Operation	Month, Year

Fractures, Other Major Injuries:

Nature and Location	Month, Year

Allergies (list medications, accidents such as stings or bites, conditions such as asthma):

Nature of Allergy	Special Precaution, Procedure or Medication

Immunization Record (those already appearing are necessary and basic; fill in dates in pencil):

DPT ______________ (Booster Due ______________)

DT ______________ (Booster Due ______________)

Tetanus ______________ (Booster Due ______________)

Rubella ______________ }
Measles ______________ } or MMR ______________
Mumps ______________ }

Polio ______________ (Booster Due ______________)

TB Test ______________ (Next Due ______________)

Other: ______________

Other Special Conditions or Problems, with Precautions or Special Instructions:

Child's Full Name ______________________________

Date and Place of Birth ______________________________

Attending Obstetrician at Birth ______________________________

Physical Checkups (Enter in Pencil)

Date of Most Recent: ____________ Next Scheduled: ____________

Height at Last Checkup: ____________ Weight at Last Checkup: ____________

Diseases and Serious Illnesses (don't include colds; do include flu, childhood diseases, infections of major organs, etc.):

Illness	Month, Year	Illness	Month, Year

Surgical Operations:

Name or Nature of Operation	Month, Year

Fractures, Other Major Injuries:

Nature and Location	Month, Year

Allergies (list medications, accidents such as stings or bites, conditions such as asthma):

Nature of Allergy	Special Precaution, Procedure or Medication

Immunization Record (those already appearing are necessary and basic; fill in dates in pencil):

DPT ______________ (Booster Due ______________)
DT ______________ (Booster Due ______________)
Tetanus ______________ (Booster Due ______________)
Rubella ______________
Measles ______________ } or MMR ______________
Mumps ______________
Polio ______________ (Booster Due ______________)
TB Test ______________ (Next Due ______________)
Other: ______________

Other Special Conditions or Problems, with Precautions or Special Instructions:

Child's Full Name ______________________________

Date and Place of Birth ______________________________

Attending Obstetrician at Birth ______________________________

Physical Checkups (Enter in Pencil)

Date of Most Recent: ______________ Next Scheduled: ______________

Height at Last Checkup: ______________ Weight at Last Checkup: ______________

Diseases and Serious Illnesses (don't include colds; do include flu, childhood diseases, infections of major organs, etc.):

Illness	Month, Year	Illness	Month, Year

Surgical Operations:

Name or Nature of Operation	Month, Year

Fractures, Other Major Injuries:

Nature and Location	Month, Year

Allergies (list medications, accidents such as stings or bites, conditions such as asthma):

Nature of Allergy	Special Precaution, Procedure or Medication

Immunization Record (those already appearing are necessary and basic; fill in dates in pencil):

DPT ________________ (Booster Due ________)
DT________________ (Booster Due ________)
Tetanus ________________ (Booster Due ________)
Rubella________________
Measles________________ } or MMR ________
Mumps ________________
Polio ________________ (Booster Due ________)
TB Test ________________ (Next Due ________)
Other: ________________

Other Special Conditions or Problems, with Precautions or Special Instructions:

Child's Full Name ______________________________

Date and Place of Birth ______________________________

Attending Obstetrician at Birth ______________________________

Physical Checkups (Enter in Pencil)

Date of Most Recent: ______________ Next Scheduled: ______________

Height at Last Checkup: ______________ Weight at Last Checkup: ______________

Diseases and Serious Illnesses (don't include colds; do include flu, childhood diseases, infections of major organs, etc.):

Illness	Month, Year	Illness	Month, Year

Surgical Operations:

Name or Nature of Operation	Month, Year

Fractures, Other Major Injuries:

Nature and Location	Month, Year

Allergies (list medications, accidents such as stings or bites, conditions such as asthma):

Nature of Allergy	Special Precaution, Procedure or Medication

Immunization Record (those already appearing are necessary and basic; fill in dates in pencil):

DPT ______________ (Booster Due ______________)
DT ______________ (Booster Due ______________)
Tetanus ______________ (Booster Due ______________)
Rubella ______________
Measles ______________ } or MMR ______________
Mumps ______________
Polio ______________ (Booster Due ______________)
TB Test ______________ (Next Due ______________)
Other: ______________

Other Special Conditions or Problems, with Precautions or Special Instructions:

Emergency Phone Numbers

Ambulance, Community Emergency Number ______________________

Private Ambulance Service ______________________

Dentist ______________________

Address ______________________ Phone ____________

Central Number, Dental Emergency Service ______________________

Doctor (pediatrician or family physician) ______________________

Address ______________________ Phone ____________

Alternate Doctor and Number ______________________

Central Number, Medical Emergency Service ______________________

Drugstore ______________________ Phone ____________

24-hour Drugstore ______________________

Electric Company Emergency Number ______________________

Father's Phone Number at Work ______________________

Fire Department or Designated Emergency Number ______________________

Gas Company Emergency Number ______________________

Hospital (nearest) ______________________

Insurance, Hospital and Medical

Company	Type	Policy No.	Agent and Phone

Mother's Phone Number at Work ______________________

Neighbors (nearest available)

Name	Address	Phone

Poison Control Center Number(s) ______________________

Relative(s) to Notify in Case of Emergency

Name	Address	Phone (include area code)

Taxi, Number(s) to Call ______________________